RATIONAL MANUAL THERAPIES

RATIONAL MANUAL THERAPIES

EDITORS

JOHN V. BASMAJIAN

O. Ont., M.D., F.R.C.P.(C), F.A.C.A., F.A.C.R.M.(Australia), F.A.B.M.R., F.S.B.M.
Professor Emeritus of Medicine and Anatomy
McMaster University
Former Director of Rehabilitation Programs
Chedoke-McMaster Hospitals and Chedoke Rehabilitation Centre
Hamilton, Ontario, Canada

RICH NYBERG

P.T., M.M.Sc.
Atlanta Back Clinic-OPT-TC
Tucker, Georgia
Associate, Division of Physical Therapy
Emory University
Atlanta, Georgia
Instructor
Institute of Graduate Physical Therapy, Inc.
St. Augustine, Florida

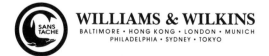

WILLIAMS & WILKINS
BALTIMORE · HONG KONG · LONDON · MUNICH
PHILADELPHIA · SYDNEY · TOKYO

Editor: John P. Butler
Managing Editor: Linda Napora
Copy Editor: Mary Kidd
Designer: Dan Pfisterer
Illustration Planner: Lorraine Wrzosek
Production Coordinator: Charles E. Zeller

Copyright © 1993
Williams & Wilkins
428 East Preston Street
Baltimore, Maryland 21202, USA

Accurate indications, adverse reactions, and dosage schedules for drugs are provided in this book, but it is possible that they may change. The reader is urged to review the package information data of the manufacturers of the medications mentioned.

Printed in the United States of America

Library of Congress Cataloging in Publication Data

Rational manual therapies
  editors, John V. Basmajian, Rich Nyberg.
      p.— cm.
    Includes index.
    ISBN 0-683-00420-4
    1. Manipulation (Therapeutics) I. Basmajian, John V., 1921-——. II. Nyberg, Richard E.
    [DNLM: 1. Manipulation, Orthopedic. 2. Physical Therapy—methods. 3. Spinal Injuries—therapy. WB 535 R236]
RM724.R38 1993
615.8'2—dc20
DNLM/DLC
for Library of Congress
                                                                        91-47927
                                                                          CIP

                                              93 94 95 96 97
                                  1 2 3 4 5 6 7 8 9 10

To the multitude of patients who have been

the Rosetta stone in solving the puzzles of back problems.

J. V. B. and R. N.

To Jim—My friend, brother, and teacher—thanks for

the lessons and inspiration; and

to Pam, Caila, Travis, and the rest of my family—I love you.

RICH

Preface

Rational Manual Therapies has been written for those interested in the art and science of manipulation, spinal motion, and soft tissue mobilization. All who practice or wish to learn about the principles and art of the "healing touch"—including manual therapists, back pain specialists, physical therapists, osteopathic physicians, chiropractors, and trainers will find this a comprehensive resource.

A multidisciplinary team of authors has provided solid rationale and, wherever available, modern scientific evidence on manipulation and mobilization; anatomy and assessment of low back; techniques, exercise, and training; ergonomic considerations and more.

We have attempted to be objective, even critical, of unsupported clinical success stories. The manual therapy vehicle is already desperately overloaded and we were determined to eliminate most of the "junk" while retaining material of value to all health professionals and their patients. Some of our work has its roots in Basmajian's *Manipulation, Traction and Massage, Third Edition*, but the bulk of *Rational Manual Therapies* is completely new.

Readers must judge our rate of success here. We hope you will come away better informed and better prepared but no less cautious of clinical success stories that are not validated. Manual therapy is a lively topic of wide interest and controversy. We will have served an enormous population of sufferers if we have been able to clarify the *pros* and *cons* of these approaches.

We offer special thanks to our authors. In addition, the constant striving for excellence of John Butler, our Williams & Wilkins editor, has done much to improve the product. Many others, too, have influenced our decisions, but in oblique ways that only they will spot. To all our warmest thanks.

J.V.B.
R.N.

Contributors

JOHN G. ARENA, Ph.D.
Director, Pain Evaluation and Intervention Program
Veterans Administration Medical Center
Associate Professor, Department of Psychiatry
Medical College of Georgia
Augusta, Georgia

JOHN V. BASMAJIAN, O.Ont., M.D.,
 F.R.C.P.(C), F.A.C.A., F.A.C.R.M.
 (AUSTRALIA), F.A.B.M.R., F.S.B.M.
Professor Emeritus of Medicine and Anatomy
McMaster University
Former Director of Rehabilitation Medicine Programs
Chedoke-McMaster Hospitals and
 Chedoke Rehabilitation Centre
Hamilton, Ontario, Canada

ROBERT CANTU, M.M.Sc., P.T.
Orthopedic Rehabilitation Center
Atlanta, Georgia

ALAN GRODIN, P.T.
Orthopedic Rehabilitation Center
Atlanta, Georgia

JAMES D. HARRIS, D.O., F.A.O.C.R.M.,
 Board Certified, P.M. & R.
Chairman, Department of Rehabilitative Medicine,
 Osteopathic Rehabilitation Medicine, Inc.
Tulsa, Oklahoma

GREGORY S. JOHNSON, P.T.
Director of Institute of Physical Art
Mill Valley, California

WILLIAM L. JOHNSTON, D.O., F.A.A.O.
Professor Emeritus
Department of Family Medicine
College of Osteopathic Medicine
Michigan State University
East Lansing, Michigan

RANDALL S. KUSUNOSE, P.T., O.C.S.
Encinatas Physical Therapy and Sports
 Rehabilitation, Inc.
Encinatas, California

PAMELA MAY, P.T.
Atlanta Back Clinic
Tucker, Georgia

MARY McCLURE, M.M.Sc., P.T.
Atlanta Back Clinic
Tucker, Georgia

FRED L. MITCHELL, JR., D.O., F.A.A.O.
Professor Emeritus
Department of Biomechanics
College of Osteopathic Medicine
Michigan State University
East Lansing, Michigan

RICH NYBERG, M.M.Sc., P.T.
Atlanta Back Clinic-OPT-TC
Tucker, Georgia
Associate, Division of Physical Therapy
Emory University
Atlanta, Georgia
Instructor, Institute of Graduate
 Physical Therapy, Inc
St. Augustine, Florida

DANIEL ORTIZ, M.P.H., C.P.S.
Georgia Tech Research Institute
Georgia Institute of Technology
Atlanta, Georgia

WRAY PARDY, M.M.Sc., P.T.
Atlanta Back Clinic
Tucker, Georgia

VICKI L. SALIBA, P.T.
Institute of Physical Art
Mill Valley, California

RICHARD A. SHERMAN, Ph.D., Major,
  U.S. Army
Chief, Biometrics and Research Design Service
Department of Clinical Investigation
  Fitzsimons Army Medical Center
Aurora, Colorado

RUSSELL SMITH, M.M.Sc., P.T.
Private Practice, Physical Therapy
Dover, Delaware

ANDREW J. TATOM III, B.S., P.T.
Director, Associated Physical Therapists P.C.
President, Injury Control Technologies
Lynchburg, Virginia

ROBERT C. WARD, D.O., F.A.A.O.
Professor, Department of Biomechanics
College of Osteopathic Medicine
Michigan State University
East Lansing, Michigan

CHERYL F. WARDLAW, M.M.Sc., P.T.
Physical Therapy Department
Emory University Hospital
Atlanta, Georgia

LOIS B. WOLF, M.M.Sc., P.T.
Division of Physical Therapy
Atlanta Back Clinic
Tucker, Georgia

Contents

1

Introduction:
A Plea for Research and Validation

JOHN V. BASMAJIAN

Among the everyday therapeutic tools that have been most widely accepted and simultaneously condemned are the topics of this book: manipulation (including mobilization, stretching, and traction) and massage in its variety of forms. They have no exclusive claim on this bizarre "love-hate" category, but lacking the drama of surgery and life-saving pharmaceuticals, and often prescribed as a last resort, these tools just get ignored by the scoffers. When confronted with good results, the skeptics fall back on a demand for double-blind controlled studies for validation of efficacy; ironically, this caution flies out the window when they are advised by their surgeons to undergo some complex operation or to take some dangerous drug.

Prejudice and human behavior aside, the need for research and validation indeed is great for any treatments that bear a cost of money, time, and human hopes. This book is based on the premise that the successful techniques described provide legitimate therapeutic services; of these, some may be based on interventions that have direct pathomechanical and pathophysiologic bases, and others may have indirect (even "placebo") effects that a significant number of the patients find worthwhile.

Investigations of therapeutic efficacy of pharmaceuticals are difficult enough even though governments, drug companies, physi-

cians, and scientists have a vested interest and where double-blinding is quite practicable. But where there are physical procedures, especially procedures where there is direct contact between patient and therapist, these add a new dimension of difficulty. This increases exponentially as the difficulty of scientifically describing the underlying disease or disorder increases. Because many of the indications for manipulation and massage are often couched in exotic language usually unknown to the medical scientist, the problem of research becomes almost—but not completely—impossible. In fact, the frequent use of glib, fallacious, or irrelevant pathomechanics to address the medical problem may pose a threat that is greater to progress in research than an absence of truly scientific pathologic explanations.

PLACEBO EFFECTS

Placebos are defined in the old sense as anything given to please the patient—for the word placebo means "I please"—with a strong suggestion that the inert substance given has a powerful therapeutic effect. The therapist or physician, in the old definition, knew that the treatment was inert but gave the patient a strong suggestion that it was an effective treatment, possibly even a powerful treatment. When the patient recovered from the symptom rapidly, or apparently as a result of the treatment, then it was said that a "placebo response" had occurred. In this type of definition great emphasis was placed on the therapist's knowing that the treatment was nonspecific and more clearly that it was by use of an inert substance or procedure. Little attention was paid to any possible psychoneurophysiologic influences that might actually have brought about an effect in the body of the patient. A more useful modern definition of the placebo response would be:

> a response in a conscious patient to the treatment of a symptom or sign (or possibly a disease and/or condition) where the administrator of the treatment has no scientific basis in demonstrated fact that the treatment has a specific effect on the target, sign, symptom, disease, or condition.

From this, the definition of a placebo can be derived as the substance or procedure received by the patient for the purpose of treatment which will bring about a placebo response, whether it is planned as deliberate deception, suggestion, or in good faith without scientific proof of efficacy in advance. It can be seen from this last definition that ideas about placebos are changing. Because the purpose of this chapter is not to obtain a placebo effect, let us now examine whatever scientific basis we have for the power of the placebo in any type of treatment and, as much as possible, treatments carried out in the rehabilitation setting. Placebos and the use of placebos, with strong faith on the part of the practitioner in their efficacy are as old as medicine itself. As suggested before, it is not necessary for our conception of placebos to include planned deception.

"No More, Gentlemen!"

In 1799, as George Washington, father of his country, lay dying, some of the greatest physicians in America were gathered around his bedside. After great debate at the highest level of medical ethics and science, the physicians

decided to bleed their patient. When he did not recover any strength, once more they bled him—and still once more. It was the considered opinion that he needed high colonic irrigation, so he had one or two of those as well on that same day. Finally the patient himself, mustering what strength remained, asked his concerned physicians to forbear. "No more, gentlemen," he said. And soon after, in spite of—or, perhaps, because of—the best efforts of his doctors, he died. Fresh debate ensued over whether the doctors had been remiss in their duties in not trying out further attempts to "save the President's life."

Similar stories abound in the history of medicine. And yet, ironically, the high regard for the physician in the Middle Ages and Renaissance was far beyond the regard now given doctors in modern times. Even though much of what physicians did for many centuries now is known to be absolutely contrary to physiology and scientific management, nevertheless they were credited with many cures and substantial improvements due to their activities.

How can this be? Much of what they did was inert or harmful by scientific standards, and yet it worked! Perhaps it worked better than much of what medicine does today except for the very specific target-oriented therapies such as antibiotics for specific bacteria, vaccination against specific viral and bacterial infections, replacement therapy for hormonal deficiencies, and various other specific replacement therapies. We may include some of surgery as well, while quite clearly reserving judgment on about half of the surgery done in North America, and I mean not just the "improper" surgery, as it might be called, but also the advocated and well-regarded surgery which is done for many conditions in the partial treatment of disease conditions.

Quite correctly, our defense for many of the treatment procedures used today is that it is the best state of the art. This, of course, is also the argument for much of what goes on in television, advertising, politics, and so on. But it is the best state of the art that we must keep on improving.

The Powerful and Mysterious Placebo

While rehabilitation (including the subjects of this book) does not stand alone in its use of and unknowing dependence on the art of placebo, perhaps half of what is done in therapy departments is either useless or harmful—but we don't know which half. Intensive research to determine the specific effects of everything we do is essential. While we may advocate and admire the nonspecific effects of placebo treatments, science and plain honesty demand that we learn as much about specific effects as possible while also learning to harness and drive the powerful tool of the placebo response.

Placebo Effect of Machines and Manual Therapies

Lest physical and manual therapists congratulate themselves on the fact that they do not use drugs but rather use techniques and machines, consider the placebo effect of machines. Schwitzgebel and Traugott[1] reported experiments with normal subjects who were attached by arm electrodes to electronic machines. It was implied that their performance on special tasks would be improved when the current was on and would decrease when it was off. As you will have guessed, there was no current ever turned on, and again you have guessed correctly that the hypothesis was borne out. When the subjects thought the current was on, their performance increased markedly. And no doubt, in a manual therapy setting, the surroundings, the equipment, and the assured way in which the therapists handle the equipment have a very strong influence on the patient.

There is no question that approaches other than chemotherapy have strong placebo influences. In 1976, Henry Byerly[2] pointed out that placebos seemed to work like magic incantations in that both require an object of concentration, and virtually anything can function as an object. Further, the improvement need not be simply of a subjective nature. Byerly cites a rheumatoid arthritis study in which placebos achieved the same level of effectiveness as aspirin in objective improvement in the swelling of the joints. It is conceivable that physical agents other than ingested chemicals might have the same influence as a placebo response, as difficult as it may be for some to accept.

In a research study on the treatment of back problems,[3] the electronic gear of the recording devices (inserted electrodes, EMG equipment, various electronic devices, and a computer) raised the placebo response for sugar pills in almost 200 patients with back problems from the usual 30% (or so) to about 50%.

The Therapist's Role

The therapist—whether a physical therapist, manual therapist, or physician—is vital. It is the human being, surrounded by the mystique of a profession, who has the strongest influence. If that therapist is knowledgeable about the procedures employed, is confident, and, above all, comes in close contact with the patient, success of almost any treatment occurs in 30% to 50% of patients. If the therapist touches and manipulates the patient, this greatly enhances the effectiveness, regardless of whether the current fad is carried out correctly or incorrectly. Hence, many patients will recover from disabilities of the musculoskeletal system by having an "improper" manipulation or traction rather than the "proper" manipulation advocated by some charismatic healer. It does not seem to matter whether transcutaneous electrical nerve stimulation or acupuncture are done absolutely "correctly"—a large number of patients will achieve substantial success or cure. The important element seems to be a close contact between the patient and the therapist. This is at least as important as the specific effect of the treatment.

LOW BACK PAIN AND EMG ACTIVITIES LEVELS

Low back pain in its many manifestations represents a process which particularly requires research both for its pathomechanics and for the modes of efficacy of techniques used in manual therapies. Holt[4] found that 54% of 2000 people questioned had low back pain. Fisk[5] showed that 80% of all Americans suffer from low back pain at one time or another.

Various classifications of low back pain, including viscerogenic, vascular, neurogenic, psychogenic, and spondylogenic have been described. Yet for patients with chronic back problems, approximately 39% show radiographic evidence of disc degeneration, primarily at the fourth and fifth lumbar discs.[6] Surgical management of patients with proved lumbar disc disease indicates that expected improvement will occur in 70%, while 90% of similar patients treated conservatively will show improvement.[5] Data from long-term studies reveal that only 10% of patients treated surgically demonstrate a full return to their previous lifestyles without developing a problem secondary to their original injury.[7] Moreover, results of the various nonsurgical treatments, including rest, traction, physical therapy (heat and massage), trigger point stimulation, medication, occupational changes, and joint mobilization[8] indicate that such procedures are at least as beneficial as surgery and, in many cases, are more effective.[9]

Information about mobility and muscle activity in the back can improve our understanding of biomechanical principles underlying posture and provide valuable data that will aid in developing more appropriate treatment plans. The mobility of the spine and actions of the erector spinae, composed of the transversospinalis (multifidus and rotatores), and the sacrospinalis (longissimus and iliocostalis) muscle groups, are described in some detail in Chapter 4. Careful studies have demonstrated a profound reduction of low back EMG activity during painful muscle spasms.[3,4,10]

RESEARCH ON MANIPULATION FOR LOW–BACK PAIN

Research on the effectiveness of manipulation began in earnest during the past two decades.

A randomized trial of a single manipulation compared with "placebo" by Glover et al.[11] was inconclusive though it tended to favor manipulation. Doran and Newell[12] found less support, concluding that manipulation, "physiotherapy," corsets, and analgesia were all about the same in a randomized study of 456 patients. Other, more recent, randomized studies with small groups[4,13–17] have yielded mixed conclusions.

Perhaps the latest available report is the most scientific and the most negative; in it, Godfrey et al.[16] describe a single-blind, randomized controlled clinical trial of rotational manipulation for low back pain of recent onset in 81 adults. The control treatments which the authors believed to be placebos (they probably were) were minimal massage and low-level electrostimulation. Both "treated" and "control" patients improved rapidly in the 2- to 3-week observation period. At retest, there was no statistically significant difference between the improvement scores of the two groups.

No absolutely impeccable study has yet been reported on the efficacy of any treatment for low back pain, let alone on manipulation. This important area of medical science is a morass into which the naive investigator stumbles at his own peril. Yet science must be recruited to establish the pathomechanics and pathochemistry as well as the rationale of various specific and nonspecific treatments. Meanwhile, patients rely on their own perceptions of the dollar-value of treatments received or available. As individuals, they are guided by personal results and word-of-mouth advertising of the effectiveness of this or that treatment. Dogmatism—both pro and con—is a paramount characteristic among almost all who deal with potential manipulation therapy; against that background scientific analysis remains our best hope to lead us out of the morass. Thus issues raised in Chapter 3 are of vital importance.

Generally, 70% of all low-back pain patients will improve in 2 months regardless of the treatment intervention, but many patients develop pain behaviors that have grave psychosocial, economic, and personal impact. Physical interventions including traction, mobilization, heat, massage, and ultrasound will provide minimal effective remediation for this group. Most therapeutic applications are characterized by the same theme—the patient plays a passive role as the modality or technique is applied *to* him. My colleagues and I believe that to assist in reducing a patient's perception of low back pain intensity the patient must play an active role and therefore do activities *for* himself. Toward this end we spent several years obtaining normative data on low back mobility using surface electrodes to monitor EMG activity of lumbar erector spinae during dynamic and static trunk movements, as reported in Chapter 4. We verified the findings of previous investigators regarding electromyographic activity during movement. Specifically, using surface electrodes we did not see EMG activity during quiet standing, but the erector spinae muscles were active during forward trunk flexion, became silent at full trunk flexion, and were activated at 60° of trunk flexion during a flex to fully extended movement.

We then expanded our studies to chronic low back pain patient populations[10,18] where we consistently observed that the patterns of EMG recorded from lumbar paraspinal muscles were different from those of normal individuals, particularly with respect to flexion and extension as well as trunk rotatory movements. Specifically, most chronic back pain patients are unable to eliminate paraspinal EMG activity during quiet standing and forward trunk flexion. In addition, the typical pattern of increased activity from paraspinal muscles opposite to the side to which the patient rotates does not prevail. We believe that these differences might eventually be used as part of (e.g., electromyographic feedback) training strategies to change movement patterns and through appropriate postural corrections, to alleviate pain perception. (See Chapter 8).

Because our clinical studies and most preceding electromyographic studies have used surface electrodes, the specificity of paraspinal muscles contributing to trunk movements remains unclear. A need exists to verify our findings from surface electromyography with percutaneous, indwelling fine wire electrodes because skin electrodes placed over the paraspinal musculature may result in recordings that are nonspecific. Verifying quantitative measures of paraspinal muscle activity previously recorded with surface electrodes would lend more credence to a biofeedback training technique designed to ameliorate low back pain.

REFERENCES

1. Schwitzgebel RK, Traugott M. Initial note on the placebo effect of machines. Behav Sci 1968; 13:267.
2. Byerly H. Explaining and exploiting placebo effects. Perspect Biol Med 1976; 19:423.
3. Basmajian JV. Effects of cyclobenzaprine HCl on skeletal muscle spasm in the lumbar region and back: two double-blind controlled clinical studies. Arch Phys Med Rehabil 1978; 59–58.
4. Holt L. Cervical, dorsal and lumbar spinal syndromes: a field investigation of a nonselected material of 1,200 workers in different occupations with special reference to disc degeneration and so-called muscular rheumatism. Acta Orthop Scand, suppl 17, 1954.
5. Fisk JR. The clinical history as a diagnostic level prognostic tool in low back pain. Second Annual Conference on Physical Impairment and Disability, "Back Pain." Atlanta: Emory University School of Medicine, Nov. 17, 1977.
6. Friberg S, Hirsch C. Anatomical and clinical studies on lumbar disc degeneration. Acta Orthop Scand 1950; 19:222.
7. Gottlieb H, Strite L. Comprehensive rehabilitation of patients having chronic low back pain. Arch Phys Med Rehabil, 1977; 58:101.
8. Finneson BE. Low back pain. Philadelphia, J.B. Lippincott Co., 1973.
9. White AWM. Low back pain in men receiving workmen's compensation. Can Med Assoc J, 1966; 95:50.
10. Wolf SL, Basmajian JV. Assessment of paraspinal electromyographic activity in normal subjects and in chronic low back pain patients using muscle biofeedback device. In: Asmussen E, Jorgensen K, eds. Biomechanics VI-B, Baltimore: University Park Press, 1979.
11. Glover JR, Morris PP, Khosla T. Back pain: a randomized clinical trial of rotational manipulation of the trunk. Br J Ind Med 1974; 31:59.
12. Doran DML, Newell DJ. Manipulation in treatment

of low back pain: a multicentre study. Br Med J 1975; 2:16.

13. Evans DP, Burke MS, Lloyd KN, et al. Lumbar spinal manipulation on trial, part I—clinical assessment. Rheum Rehabil 1978; 17:46.

14. Farrell JP, Twomey LT. Acute low back pain: comparison of two conservative approaches. Med J Aust 1982; 1:160.

15. Sims-Williams H, Jayson MIV, Young SMS, et al. Controlled trial of mobilization and manipulation for patients with low back pain in general practice. Br Med J, 1978; 2:1338.

16. Godfrey CM, Morgan PP, Schatzker J. A randomized trial of manipulation for low-back pain in a medical setting. Spine 1984; 9:301.

17. Hoehler FK, Tobis JS, Burger AA. Spinal manipulation, JAMA, 1981; 245:1835.

18. Wolf SL, Basmajian JV, Russe CTC, et al. Normative data on low back mobility and activity levels. Am J Phys Med, 1979; 58:217.

2

History and Development of Manipulation and Mobilization

JAMES D. HARRIS

Manipulation is defined in *Dorland's Medical Dictionary*[1] as "Skillful or dexterous treatment by the hand. In physical therapy, the forceful passive movement of a joint within or beyond its active limit of motion." Manipulation is currently an area of great interest for many different groups of medical professionals. The enthusiasm for manual treatment is on the increase in the 1980s and '90s, exemplified by such new organizations as the American Association for Orthopedic Medicine. Numerous seminars, books, and videotapes are being used by health care professionals to teach the art of manipulative medicine.[2]

CLASSICAL PERIOD

Historically, the "hands on" approach to medical care is not new. Although the laying on of hands is well documented in the Old Testament and other historical documents, so-called modern medicine had its birth with the development of the Hippocratic School of Medicine, a logical starting place for this discussion.

Born in Asia Minor in 460 BC, Hippocrates became a physician and teacher of great skill and is recognized as the Father of Medicine. The Hippocratic Oath taken by many physicians before entering practice is a tribute to the Father of Medicine, who focused attention on the patient. In his *Aphorisms*, he re-minded his students not to meddle with or to hinder nature's attempt toward recovery. The idea of focusing full attention on the patient rather than just on the scientific theory of disease or on elaborate laboratory and radiographic testing has considerable merit.

There were many different schools and philosophies of medicine which affected the course of today's medical care. Even though Hippocrates dominated his time in medicine, there were others who believed that he was too philosophical and who advocated a more practical approach. Their approach was more specifically disease-oriented; they believed that disease was an "outside intruder" that caused the condition which existed within man. However, the Hippocratic School emphasized the study of health in man as an individual and steered attention away from the outside intruders or disease that afflicted man. The theoretical battle in medicine of "inside" versus "outside" persists today. With the renewed interest in manipulative medicine, the philosophies behind the use of manipulation must be explored.

Hippocrates did not agree with the treatment of lumbar kyphosis of his time. He advocated the use of steam heat, followed by traction from both the head and the foot while the patient lay in a prone position. Pressure was to be sharply applied on the kyphosis while the traction was maintained. The direction of force was dictated by the condition that occurred in the patient. This manner of readjustment proved to be beneficial for selected patients. He also advocated different types of treatment rather than just a single-force thrust; prolonged pressure by sitting on the patient, shaking movements, and a foot being applied to the prominence. A padded board with a long lever arm to apply local pressure across the patient's back (Fig. 2.1) was another device. He related that a thrust without traction could be satisfactory. Hippocrates did not limit manual treatment of patients to the low back area. His most famous successor, Galen (AD 131–202), preached the use of manual medicine in the treatment of the extremities, as well as for problems in the cervical vertebrae.

In the Middle Ages, the Arabian physician, Abu'Ali ibn Sina (980–1037), accumulated and wrote a summary of medicine that survived as the authoritative textbook until the 17th century. It included the manual medicine approach to the treatment of backs advocated by Hippocrates. The famous antiquarian Chinese physician, Chang Chung-King, referred to as the Chinese Hippocrates,

also advocated treating the patient with manual medicine.[3]

Other notables in medicine such as Thomas Sydenham (1624–1689), an Englishman, and Samuel Hahnemann (1755–1843), a German doctor who founded homeopathy, also deviated from the cnidian principle of disease-oriented medicine. Hahnemann developed a medical treatment that often advocated the use of extremely small doses of drugs. This was a counter-movement to the megadoses of medicinal agents that were being used by his contemporaries. Herman Boerhaave (1668–1738), son of a Dutch country pastor, was described as being "poor in money, but pure in spirit." He chose the Hippocratic philosophy of medicine as his guide and encouraged patient observation rather than disease-oriented medicine.[4]

The use of spinal traction, as well as medieval Turkish manipulation during traction, were recorded in the leading textbooks of the Renaissance (Fig. 2.2). Ambroise Paré wrote about "vertebral dislocations" thus:

> When the vertebrae are dislocated outwards, forming a prominence, the patient should be tied down prone to a board with ropes under

Figure 2.1. Ancient method of treating kyphosis (see text).

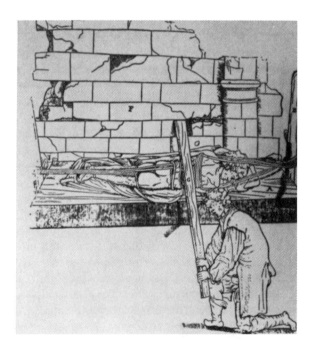

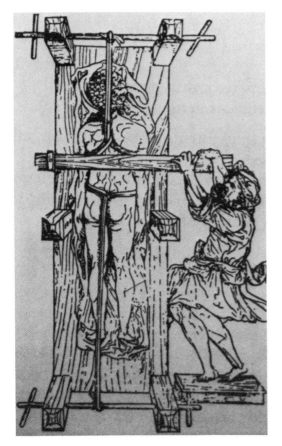

Figure 2.2. Combined suspension and pressure on the lumbar spine by means of a board (The scamnum Hippocratis).

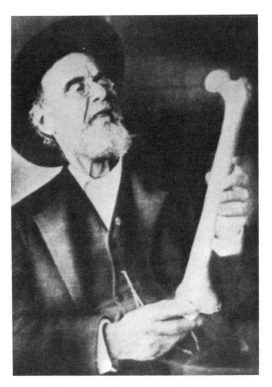

Figure 2.3. Dr. A. T. Still, originator of osteopathy.

the armpits, the waist, and the thighs. He is then pulled and stretched as much as possible from above and from below, but not violently. If traction is not applied, cure is not to be expected. The operator then places his hand on the kyphosis and presses the prominent vertebra in.

John Shultes (1595–1645) advocated Paré's method of treatment. But from the 17th and 18th centuries until the latter part of the 19th century, the treatment by manual means lost favor in the medical profession.

Andrew Taylor Still (1828–1917) (Fig. 2.3) the founder of osteopathic medicine, was a rough-hewn frontier doctor from the midwestern United States. He was an eccentric and nonconformist, but he pursued his beliefs with intensity and devoted himself to the phi-

losophy of medicine and the study of man as a total unit. He did not believe that disease was strictly an outside agent, afflicting evils on the body, but instead considered that disease was a normal body response to an abnormal body situation. During Still's lifetime and to the present, the basic philosophical principle of osteopathic medicine and the term osteopathy has been a focal point of medical controversy and debate.[5–7]

BONE-SETTERS

The contribution of the bone-setters cannot be ignored. In central Europe, the art of bone-setting was handed down from one generation to another. Gypsies of central Europe were known for their bone-setters. The Indians of Mexico employed various manipulative techniques, such as "the shepherd's hug" or the "farmer's push." There also were such techniques as "stamping or trampling," which are practiced in some countries even today. A mystique existed about who had the "great power to heal" or the "right to manipulate." For instance, it was believed that a "stamper" has to be born foot first. Other folklore in many European and Asian countries maintain superstitious beliefs, e.g., that a stamper has to be a virgin or of a certain numerical order of birth (e.g., seventh son).

Related to the above, "Lomi-Lomi" is an ancient Hawaiian version of massage, over eight centuries old. Its main feature is that the masseur walks on the patient's back, and while he walks, he kneads the flesh and regulates his weight by holding on a bar above the massage table.

In a similar technique in East Africa, women who led camels would lie in a prone position while their cohorts stood on their backs, trampling and kneading with their toes. In European countries such as Norway, Sweden, and Finland, there has been for many years a folklore manual-type of medicine, which appeared to be successful. The technique of "weighing salt" is well documented in Swedish folklore medicine, and time has justified these methods of treatment.

Bone-setters have existed for hundreds of years with their techniques often handed down through families. The first of these bone-setters about whom details exist was a woman called Sarah Mapp, who practiced her skills in Great Britain in the 1700s. She was a very well-known character of her time. She was described by the *London Magazine* (Aug. 2, 1736) as being "enormously fat and ugly," and her nicknames were "Crazy Sally" or Crosseyed Sally."[8]

Whorton Hood gave the first formal description of the bone-setting craft in the 19th century, as taught to him by Richard Hutton and based on anatomy. In his writings, he insisted that legitimate practitioners failed to meet the desires of the sick. Bone-setting was a major topic at the annual meeting of the British Medical Society in 1882.[8]

Sir Herbert Barker (1869–1950) (Fig. 2.4) of Great Britain enjoyed the support of many individuals, including at least one surgeon who had been president of the British Medical

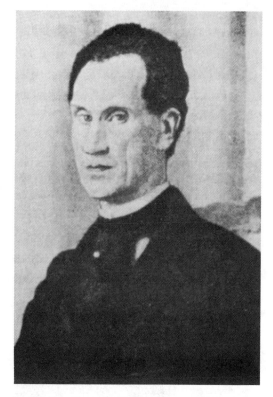

Figure 2.4. The most famous of all bone-setters, Sir Herbert Barker.

Association. Barker lacked a formal medical education, but practiced in London until 1927. He had learned his skills from his cousin, a bone-setter named John Atkinson, who in turn was taught by Robert Hutton, a nephew of Richard Hutton. The Huttons came from a farming family in England that had practiced bone-setting for over 200 years. Although Herbert Barker was refused an honorary medical degree, King George V honored him with a knighthood. In 1925, Dr. George M. Laughlin arranged for the Andrew Taylor Still College of Osteopathy and Surgery to give him an honorary D.O. degree, which Sir Herbert referred to as his "American Knighthood." In his autobiography,[9] he wrote:

Strong as the love of service to suffering is among many doctors as a whole, there existed some things much stronger and less worthy in prejudice and jealousy which have from time immemorial darkened the pages of surgical history and smirched its record of noble endeavors. . . . I am certainly not prepared to be condemned by men who are culpably ignorant of what it is their business to know, and which they are too arrogant, or too prejudiced to learn. . . . It is still true that the faculty has neglected the study of methods and are today incapable of relieving sufferers who resort to them. Yet they persist still in their refusal to accept the help of those who can instruct them in this beneficial branch of the healing art. . . .

"I cannot afford the time and strength demanded for demonstrations for the benefit of individuals. When I desire to bring the method before the faculty as a whole, secure them a place in the curricula of the medical schools . . . obtain for the entire body of students a thorough and practical training in the work. . . . I contend unreservedly that the method of the manipulative art . . . are quite unknown to the general practitioner, and even to the specialist in surgery . . . they have no real or effective knowledge even in its rudimentary principles. . . .

The Lancet in 1925 recognized Barker in an editorial thus: "The medical history of the future will have to record that our profession has greatly neglected this important subject. . . . The fact that must be faced, that the bone-setters had been curing multitudes of cases by movement . . . and that by our faulty methods we are largely responsible for their very existence."

CHIROPRACTIC

The history of the chiropractic profession is traced back to Daniel David Palmer (1845–1913) (Fig. 2.5), who practiced his own magnetism business for 10 years until 1895. D.D. Palmer wrote his first textbook, *The Chiropractic Adjuster*, in 1910, in which he advocated the art of replacing subluxed vertebrae to cure disease. He claimed to be the first to replace displaced vertebrae by using the spinous process and transverse process as levers, which he thought was a revolutionary theory in the healing art. In Palmer's own account, he related that in his readings of the Hippocratic method of treating backs and from his visits to France, he revived this method of treatment. It is reported that his first patient was cured of deafness in September, 1895, by his adjusting a large subluxation of the cervical vertebrae. His son, B.J. Palmer, described this historical event as, "The bump was adjusted, and within ten minutes he had his hearing and has had it ever since."

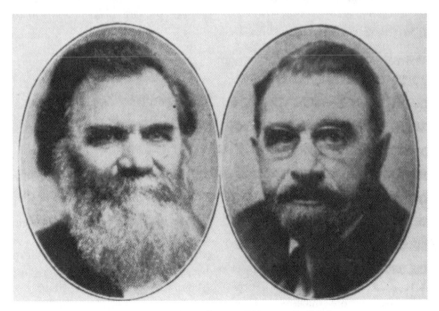

Figure 2.5. David D. Palmer and his son, B. J. Palmer.

D.D. Palmer opened the first chiropractic school in Oklahoma City in 1897. He advocated not only manipulating the spinal column, but also the extremities. His followers were known as "mixers" or as adhering to the "the Carver method of chiropractic." In later years this included physical therapy, dietetics, megavitamins, and other nonprescription medications.

B.J. Palmer, the son of D.D. Palmer, started his own school in Davenport, Iowa in 1907. It has been reported that he was a student in the Osteopathic College in Kirksville in 1900, but did not finish his course of study, but Dr. Charles Still has reported that Palmer obtained his knowledge from a Mr. Stother, an osteopathic student from Kirksville. B.J. Palmer advocated manipulation of the spine only, and his supporters were called "straights" who followed "the Palmer Method of Chiropractic." In time, the straights lost out to the mixers.

B.J. Palmer was very enterprising; in 1924 he developed the "neurocalometer" which would register variations of skin temperatures along the vertebral column. It was used to identify more accurately where the nerves were compressed. This, according to B.J. Palmer, indicated the level of the vertebra in which dislocation had caused the trouble. This instrument was not for sale, but was rented to his graduates and formed an integral part of the teaching of the International Chiropractic Association. The chiropractic doctrine states that chiropractic treatment achieves two ends, "one, to remove the cause which has facilitated the onset of disease and let it gain a foothold in the body; two, to permit a normal flow of life energy from the brain to the tissues, thus preventing the disease from spreading further."[8]

In the *British Medical Journal*, chiropractic was described as "a branch of Osteopathy, first, designed to maintain Osteopathic dogma in its most primitive form, and second, maintaining its commercial character."[9] Dr. Morris Fishbein in 1925 staunchly opposed both chiropractic and osteopathic concepts, and his

summation was, "Chiropractic is the malignant tumor on the body of osteopathy." In the next half century the training for the chiropractic profession has progressed from a two-week course to a much more extensive syllabus that includes anatomy, physiology, biochemistry, pathology, bacteriology, public health, and hygiene, as well as diagnosis and treatment.

The mixers have defined chiropractic as "the science of healing human ailments by manipulation and adjustment of the spine and other structures of the human body, and the use of such other mechanical, physio-therapeutic, dietetic, and sanitary measures, except drugs and major surgery, as are indicated to care for the human body." Their theory or philosophy underlying spinal adjustment is summed up in five principles: (a) that a vertebra may become subluxed; (b) that this subluxation tends to impinge on the structures (nerves, blood vessels, and lymphatics) passing through the intervertebral foramen; (c) that as a result of such impingement, the function of the corresponding segment of the spinal cord and its connecting spinal and autonomic nerve is interfered with and that the conduction of the nerve impulse is impaired; (d) that, as a result thereof, the nervous tone in certain parts of the organism is abnormally altered, and such parts become functionally or organically diseased, or predisposed to disease; and (e) that the adjustment of the subluxed vertebra removes the impingement from the structures passing through the intervertebral foramen, thereby restoring to diseased parts their normal nervous stimuli and rehabilitating them functionally and organically.

Via newspapers, television, and radio advertisements, the chiropractic profession impresses on the public that subluxation of the spine produces certain diseases and that the adjustment of these vertebral segments can cure the disease. They claim that chiropractic recognizes the true and primary cause of the disease, but even today some chiropractors discourage vaccination of their family members and choose to treat them by adjustment.

NAPRAPATHY

Naprapathy is an offshoot of chiropractic that started approximately in 1908. Its original school was in Chicago, and it adhered to the principle that ligamentous contracture draws the vertebrae too closely together and causes disease by obstructing nerves and blood vessels. The major premise is that by stretching out these ligaments normal neural and blood flow can be established through a manual thrust type of treatment.

ORTHOPEDIC MEDICINE

James Cyriax, M.D. (Fig. 2.6) devoted his professional life to orthopedic medicine, the treatment by manipulation, massage, and injection. He pursued his beliefs with intensity and had written extensively. He defines manipulation as "a method of treatment that consists of different sorts of passive movement performed by the hands in a definite manner for a prescribed purpose." His main purpose for manipulation is the correction of internal derangement. He lectured extensively on his "parallelogram of force" in reference to the intervertebral disc and advocated extension-

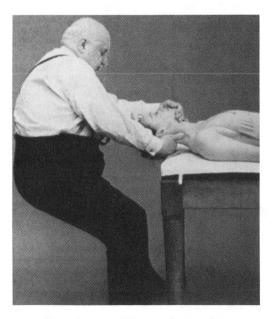

Figure 2.6. Dr. Cyriax treating a patient.

type exercises and distractive-type forces to "suck back up" the nucleus pulposus, and certain passive movements to maneuver the displaced fragments of the disc. His choice of maneuver is based on three uncontestable criteria: (*a*) the most likely one to succeed, (*b*) the least painful, and (*c*) the most informative. He worked on the premise with a basis of a trial and end-feel, and effect.[10]

Cyriax repeatedly classified osteopathic physicians as lay manipulators and has requested that osteopaths drop the notion of practicing an alternate system of medicine and to forget anatomical tone in curing visceral disease. "They would have to withdraw from the osteopathic lesion as an important factor in the development of disease, and agree that fixation of the spinal joint has a local effect only."[10] He also insisted that chiropractors who had taken over the panacea effect of manipulation should seek medical guidance and supervision. Cyriax strongly advocates manipulation by physical therapists, as they are taught by doctors and work with doctors, and have a mutual regard established. In his writings he relates that he has taught thousands of people to manipulate through his long stay at St. Thomas' Hospital, and also through his teaching books, videotapes, and guest lectureships. Although the British Chartered Society of Physiotherapists decry the term manipulation and have substituted the word *mobilization*, Cyriax feels that manipulation is a much more preferred term.[8]

Cyriax believes that a book written by a Dr. Riadore on *Irritation of the Spinal Nerve* in 1842, probably provided the inspiration for the first osteopath:

> If an organ is deficiently supplied with nervous energy or blood, its function is decreased, and sooner or later its structure becomes endangered. . . .
>
> When we reflect that every organ and muscle in the body is connected and dependent more or less upon the spinal nerves for the perfect performance of their individual functions, we cannot otherwise prepare to hear of a lengthened catalogue of maladies that are either en-

gendered, continued, or the consequence of spinal irritation.

Riadore also gave the first account for root pain emanating from "contact" at the intervertebral foramen. He recognized disc degeneration.

Manipulation became unethical in 1858 with the passage of the Medical Act in Great Britain. Until then, doctors had sent their patients to bone-setters for manipulation. Dr. James Paget delivered a lecture in 1868 entitled, "Cases That Bone-Setters Cure," in which he pointed out how neglectful doctors were of manipulation, thereby leaving patients with no alternative but to consult laymen. In 1871, the first English book on manipulation appeared, written by a Dr. Hood, about the work of Hutton, the well-known bone-setter.[8]

CYRIAX ON OSTEOPATHY AND ORTHOPEDIC MEDICINE

Cyriax in his writings tried—unsuccessfully—to discredit Dr. Still for his deep religious background, using such terms as "hallucinations" and such statements as "when he was shown that spinal dislocation would cause paraplegia long before it had this effect, he changed his hypothesis to pressure on a nerve."

According to Dr. Cyriax, "*The Lancet* in 1871 collected articles and lectures in book form the same year (surely a gold mine for the first osteopaths); also, Howard March and R. Dacre Fox, both in 1882 and Hugh Owens Thomas and Sir Robert Jones." However, Cyriax described Edgar F. Cyriax as a prolific author of articles, and claimed that he was the first to describe the displacement of the intervertebral disc as a cause of clinical symptoms.[10] He quotes David LeVay:

Current medical families such as the Cyriax's arose to occupy themselves in successive generations chiefly with the advancement of mechanotherapeutics. For the first time, these techniques were probably related to a sound knowledge of anatomy and pathology. The

bone-setters, their clothes stolen, could only impugn the accuracy with which their very personal tradition had been translated into medical jargon.

In conclusion, Cyriax relates that—

For hundreds, even thousands of years, manipulative treatment for low back pain has been common practice—by very different methods and with entirely different theoretical aims: Hippocrates straightened a kyphosis; Galen replaced outward dislocated vertebrae; and Ambroise Paré wrote about subluxation of the spine. Patients have been trampled upon by women chosen on sexual grounds (virgins, mothers of seven children, etc.); birth by presentation of the foot has been regarded as a given magical power to the stamper. Sufferers have been given blows on the back with different tools from hammers to brooms and steel yards and have been lifted back to back and shaken. Bone-setters have replaced small bones out of place; osteopaths have treated the 'mysterious osteopathic lesion'; chiropractors have replaced subluxed vertebrae; orthopedic surgeons have manipulated 'subluxation of the sacroiliac joint'; and neurologists have 'stretched the sciatic nerve.' Curiously enough, all concepts and methods have met with some degree of success. Clearly, the mechanism has been a fragment of disc which has become dislocated and was put back into position, or when a protrusion of the disc was 'sucked back' (or perhaps when a jammed or blocked joint was 'unlocked,' or perhaps when a nerve root was shifted off the apex of a prolapsed disc).

In the publication, *Illustrated Manual of Orthopedic Medicine*,[11] Cyriax suggests that orthopedic medicine may have been born in 1929 but only now is it coming of age (Fig. 2.7).

This was the challenge facing me in 1929. I then found, starting as an orthopedic house surgeon, that patients were divided into two categories—those whose defects showed up on the x-ray, and those who x-rays were normal. At that time it was the custom to pass the latter on for physical therapy, consisting of various kinds of heat therapy, general diffuse massage, and exercise. It was a question of divided responsibility. No diagnosis was made or at-

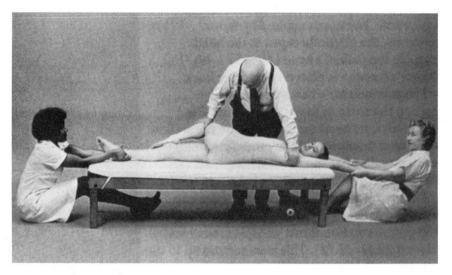

Figure 2.7. Spinal manipulation by Dr. Cyriax and associates.

tempted in either the orthopedic or physical therapy departments, and the treatments were not given because they were indicated or even specified, but simply because they were available . . . . Whenever a patient is sent for physical therapy, it must be with the diagnostic certainty, not only that physical therapy is the appropriate recourse, but also that the physiotherapist knows the work, that is, how to treat the right tissue in the right way. In such an informed context, the relationship between physician and physiotherapist becomes complementary; he can inject were she cannot; she can take much time-consuming work off his hands by massage or manipulation. Between the two of them, nearly all patients can be dealt with on the spot; generally the last thing needed is to call in a specialist, least of all a specialist outside the field of soft tissue lesions.

A. T. STILL

The roots of manipulative therapy in the United States began with A. T. Still[12] and his philosophy of health care, stressing the wellness and wholeness of an individual. Still's life and political views from early manhood kept him in the center of controversy; he lived in Missouri, a border state, the son of a Methodist minister, and both he and his father were ardent abolitionists. In 1853, the elder Still

was appointed a missionary to the Shawnee Indians and with his family moved to Kansas, where Andrew joined his father in the fight against slavery. In 1857 he was chosen by the people of Douglas County, Kansas, to represent them in the Kansas legislature. There, he quickly aroused the anger of the proslavery groups.

Dr. Still, a staunch supporter of Lincoln, enlisted in the Ninth Kansas Cavalry and saw active duty in the war, rising to the rank of Major. The thoughts of slavery and equal opportunity were ingrained in his background and when he founded the American School of Osteopathy, he declared the institution open to Negroes. Always controversial, he fought for women's suffrage as well.

Dr. Still's medical education was typical of the time—much of it by preceptorship, some from formal training. Before the Civil War, he had attended the College of Physicians and Surgeons of Kansas City, but before completing his course he left to enlist. He acquired other related experiences and had literally grown up in the medical field where he helped take care of the Shawnee Indians. In his autobiography[13] he wrote:

. . . one day when about 10 years of age I suffered from a headache. I made a swing of my father's plow lines between two trees, but my head hurt too much to make the swing comfortable; so I let the rope down to about 8 to 10 inches off the ground, threw the end of a blanket on it and lay down on the ground and used the ropes for a swinging pillow. Thus, I lay stretched on my back with my neck across the ropes. Soon, I became easy and went to sleep. I got up in a little while with the headache gone. As I knew nothing of anatomy at the time, I took no thought of how the rope would stop a headache and the sick stomach which accompanied it. After the discovery, I roped my neck whenever I felt those spells coming on. I followed the treatment for 20 years before the wedge of reason had reached my brain and I could see that I had suspended the action of the great occipital nerves and given harmony to the flow of the arterial blood to and through the veins, and ease was the effect.

Still held to the statement of Alexander Pope, "the proper study of mankind is man"; to provide himself with material for dissection, he exhumed bodies from the graves of Indians. As he later recorded, "a thousand experiments were made with bones until I became quite familiar with the bone structure." It was a personal tragedy, however, that convinced Dr. Still that the status of medicine was inadequate. In the spring of 1864 there was a severe epidemic of meningitis in which thousands of people died, including three of Still's children. This tragic event served to drive him relentlessly on to the study of man and led him to develop the philosophy that occupied his mind for the remainder of his life.

In 1874, Dr. Still was ready to present his concepts to the medical world, first to the doctors at Baker University in Baldwin, Kansas. Although he and his brothers and father had donated land to the University, Still was rejected by the University. In spite of his reputation as a good medical doctor and his service in the Civil War, and also his good record as a state legislator, the doors of the University were closed to him.

Dr. Still returned to Missouri determined to continue developing his ideas and incorporating them into his medical practice. He be-

lieved that the structure of the body was reciprocal and related to its function. He believed that the body's musculoskeletal system, bones, ligaments, muscle, and fascia, form a structure that when disordered may affect a change in the function of other parts of the body. This effect could be created through the irritation and abnormal response of the nerve and blood supply to other organs of the body; the body of man is subject to mechanical disorder.[5]

Dr. Still's fame grew, and people from all over the United States came to Kirksville, Missouri for treatment by the "lightening bone-setter." The first formal class in the teaching of osteopathic medicine met in Kirksville in November of 1892, under a charter taken out in May of that year. A second charter was issued October 30, 1894, to the American School of Osteopathy. The object of the school was to improve the existing system of surgery, obstetrics, and treatment of disease generally, and place the same on a more rational scientific basis and to impart information to the medical profession and to grant and confer such honors and degrees to the students that completed courses of instructions.[5]

The centennial celebration of osteopathic medicine in 1974 brought out the concept that osteopathic medicine was holistic in nature and was based on five major premises: (a) *unity of the body*—each system both in function and dysfunction depends upon others and influences other systems; (b) *healing power of nature*—there are substances within the body that, when they are in proper balance, preserve health and protect against disease; (c) *somatic component of disease*—the musculoskeletal system is truly the 'machinery of life,' and its reciprocal communication to other systems of the body is an important anatomical physiological principle of medical care; (d) *structure-function concept*—structure and function cannot be separated in human physiology, but there is interdependence; and (e) *manipulative therapy*—its application to restore and maintain normal structural functional relationship of the musculoskeletal system is important

(Fig. 2.8), not only to the function of the musculoskeletal system itself, but important also to the neural-hormonal communication with other body systems.

Manipulative therapy was recognized as a potentially useful therapeutic medium for both the maintenance of normal function and the correction of dysfunction. It was pointed out clearly that manipulative therapy and osteopathic medicine must be viewed in totality of their philosophy, not as things set apart. Manipulative therapy, like drugs, surgery, physical therapy, and diet are tools with which the basic fundamentals of osteopathic medicine can be expressed. Manipulation is a therapeutic means, no more and no less, and the American Academy of Osteopathy has set up a program for certification in manipulative skills. Special recognition is given to those who have more or less specialized in structural problems of the musculoskeletal system and special skills in manipulative therapy.[5,13]

In 1975 and 1977, the National Institute of Neurological and Communicative Disease and Stroke of the National Institute of Health funded workshops on the research status of spinal manipulative therapy. At the first workshop, 58 scientists and clinicians of national and international status from the United States and eight foreign countries, including doctors of medicine, osteopathy, and chiropractic, and specialists in 11 basic sciences, usually Ph.D.'s, met. The workshop was held in 1977 at the Kellogg Center of Continuing Medical Education at Michigan State University sponsored by the College of Osteopathic Medicine, Michigan State University to consider mechanical disorders of the musculoskeletal system (particularly the spinal area) which might cause pain and/or alter physiology, both local and at remote points.[14]

Since the pioneer paper by Korr,[15] many more workers around the world have added their experiments and observations to recent discoveries. The description of what amounts to an intraneural circulation opens the door to much neural biologic investigation, not the least of which is relevant to the neural biologic basis for manipulative therapy.

MANIPULATION BY M.D.'S

John McM. Mennell, M.D. has long been a proponent of manipulative therapy in the allopathic medical profession.[3,16] He writes:

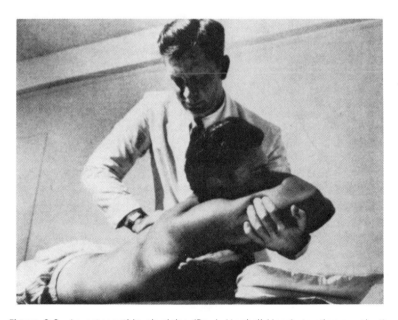

Figure 2.8. An osteopathic physician (Dr. J. Marshall Hoag), treating a patient's back by "mobilizing" the upper thoracic vertebrae.

It has always seemed to me that the main reason why the medical profession has been reluctant to accept manipulative treatment of joint pain is because the proponents of manipulative treatment have never clearly emphasized that manipulative maneuvers and treatments are designed solely to restore something which is normal anatomically and physiologically to a joint—something which is unconcerned with voluntary joint movement, but is solely concerned with mechanical joint play, and which is essentially present only in life and absent in death. The prerequisite for successful treatment in any field of medicine is accurate diagnosis. The condition of joint dysfunction is the only pathologic condition that will respond to the treatment of manipulation. So, before manipulative therapy is ever used, the normal range of joint-play movements must be learned as carefully as the range of voluntary movement as now taught and learned in routine anatomy classes. That joint play movements are small, often not more than 1/8 of an inch in extent in any plane, does not mean that they are unimportant.

He further states that

. . . manipulating joints is an art and, as with so many arts, not everyone can expect to be able to learn to use it. Perhaps there are two main reasons why joint manipulation has not found the wide acceptance that it merits in the practice of medicine; first, the user has not learned the proper techniques; and second, the user is simply inept at the art. It is so much easier to blame a modality of treatment for failure than it is to blame someone who perhaps never should be using the modality in the first place. . . . Any pathological joint condition, whether simple joint dysfunction, or some serious joint disease, affects to some extent all the anatomical structures that play a part in the functioning of the joint. All the affected structures need attention in treatment if a return to normalcy is to be expected.

Dr. Mennell further points out, ". . . so, joint manipulation is one modality of treatment that may or may not have a place in the treatment of a painful joint. If it is not used when it is indicated, treatment will fail to alleviate the patient's symptoms; if it is used when it should not be, treatment will also fail

to relieve the patient's symptoms and, indeed, many even make them worse."[3,16]

Outside the osteopathic profession, manipulative therapy is applied to joint injury, postural imbalance, and neuromuscular rehabilitation. The physiologic basic of manipulation in osteopathic medicine includes reestablishing normal function of joint relationships, relieving tension and contracture, stimulating improved circulation and tissue drainage, and restoring functional capacity and is well documented. Much interest recently has been directed toward "myofascial trigger zones," and entire texts have been devoted to this topic. It is believed that those who practice manipulative therapy in medicine must have detailed knowledge of functional anatomy including the planes of joint motion, neuroanatomy, neurophysiology, and neurology, along with biochemistry and pharmacology. The purpose of manipulation is not just restoring fragmented disc parts or a herniated nucleus pulpsus, but it is to restore or improve structure and function inter-relationships, to normalize function by normalizing structure, to improve circulation including arterial, venous, and lymphatic in localized areas, and to decrease noxious afferent impulses that are being fed into the central nervous system. It also may improve the effectiveness of the body's immune mechanism, develop a helpful psychological attitude and emotional response, and to use the techniques and phenomena of "biofeedback." The time has come for manipulative therapy to achieve its proper place in the total medical care system.

The tool of manipulation is being more liberally used in the allopathic institutions. Different terms have been attributed to manipulative treatment, such as adjustments, mobilization, release techniques, and manual medicine. Physicians have the obligation to evaluate the musculoskeletal complaints, diagnose, and set up a treatment program. The question of manipulative treatment has been deliberated over the centuries. If manipulative treatment is indicated, then the physician has the option to treat the patient himself or to delegate this treatment to others. In the United States today, the physical therapist has shown a strong interest in mobilization.[17]

The federal government also has an enormous responsibility in reference to whether manipulative treatment will be paid for. The economics of health care delivery have escalated astronomically. If the physicians are given the responsibility for health care, then, they also must have the authority to render the most effective and efficient treatment. Manipulative treatment takes time and energy, as well as learned skill. If there is negative reimbursement for this type of treatment, then it will stagnate and be delegated to lesser-trained individuals, or not be done at all.

REFERENCES

1. Dorland's medical dictionary. 26th ed. Philadelphia: Saunders, 1981.
2. Hoag JM. Osteopathic medicine. New York: McGraw Hill, 1969.
3. Mennell J. Back pain: diagnosis and treatment using manipulative technique. Boston: Little, Brown & Co., 1960.
4. Stoddard A. Manual of osteopathic practice. London: Hutchinson, 1969.
5. Adler P, Northrup G. 100 Years of osteopathic medicine (1874–1974). Squibb & Sons Inc., Medical Community, Inc., 1976.
6. Northrup GW. Osteopathic medicine & American reformation. Chicago: American Osteopathic Association, 1966.
7. Young WR, assoc. ed. Osteopaths. Life, Sept. 29, 1960; 108–118.
8. Schiotz E, Cyriax J. Manipulation past and present. London: Heinemann, 1975.
9. Barker H. Leaves from my life. London: Hutchinson, 1928.
10. Cyriax J. The textbook of orthopedic medicine, Vol. II. Treatment by Manipulation, Massage and Injection. 10th ed. London: Bailliere Tindall, 1980.
11. Cyriax J. Illustrated manual of orthopedic medicine. London: Butterworth's, 1983.
12. Gevitz N. The D.O.'S: osteopathic medicine in America. Baltimore: Johns Hopkins University Press, 1982.
13. Continuing Medical Education 1990 Calendar. College of Osteopathic Medicine, Michigan State University, 1990.
13a. Still AT. Autobiography, Kirksville, 1908.
14. Kellogg JH. The art of massage: its physiological effects and therapeutic applications. 12th ed. Battle Creek, 1919.
15. Korr IM. Axonal delivery of neuroplasmic components to muscle cells. Science 1967; 155:342.
16. Mennell J. Joint pain: diagnosis and treatment using manipulative technique. Boston: Little, Brown & Co., 1964.
17. Nyberg R. In: Basmajian, JV (ed.), Manipulation, traction and massage. 3rd ed., Baltimore: Williams & Wilkins, 1985.

3

Manipulation:
Definition, Types, Application

RICH NYBERG

The basis for understanding the role of spinal manipulation in helping manage back pain is dependent on fundamental knowledge of spinal manipulation terminology, use, explanation, and research. The following objectives are presented to clarify the purpose for each area.

1. To define the various types of manipulation utilized for spinal orthopedic problems.
2. To provide explanation and rationale for the mechanisms of manipulative therapy.
3. To identify the criteria for successful application of spinal manipulation.

Practitioners of manipulation, past and present, report undeniable evidence of the clinical results of manipulative therapy despite the criticism of many who claim there is no scientific basis for the use of manipulation. Determining whether manipulation is an effective tool for helping patients with back pain requires an understanding of terminology used by practitioners of manipulation and the establishment of controlled, properly designed studies. The defining of manipulation is critical to the development of manipulative therapy. The scientific community must identify with a a testable, reliable, clear language to investigate the clinical observations of manipulative physicians and therapists. Without identifying terminology that is common to all involved in manipulative care, the ability to effectively communicate is impaired and research efforts to establish validity are hindered.[1] Moreover, physicians and researchers who may not receive the theory, terminology and practical skills of manipulation in the course of an academic program are inclined to have difficulty accepting the therapeutic value of manipulation.[2] The first assignment, therefore, is to identify and clarify the nomenclature associated with manipulative therapy.

DEFINITIONS

Manipulation is generally defined as any manual operation or maneuver.[3] More specifically, manipulation is a skilled therapeutic use of a passive movement designed to restore motion. Manipulation justifiably falls into the basic classification of passive movement, which means motion not under voluntary control, but occurring in response to an external or outside force.[4] Passive motion therapy is utilized to maintain or restore range of motion. As the biomechanical nature of back pain became understood and the recognition of abnormal motion behavior identified through advances in x-ray technology, acceptance of motion therapy for the treatment of back conditions increased. Restoration of range of motion, however, is one of many parameters which determine normal motion behavior. Therefore manipulative practitioners must be aware that motion control, direction, quality, power, and velocity are also essential in the management of a back condition. As a result, therapeutic rehabilitation programs are a requisite component of any manipulative therapy treatment for back pain.[5]

The underlying foundation of the rationale for manipulation use is in the detection of motion impairment. Clinical practitioners of manipulation must be able to determine abnormal motion. Although stereoscopic radiography has helped to identify the existence of abnormal spinal motion, few clinical motion tests have been substantiated with regard to reliability and validity. One of the first dilemmas in justifying manipulative therapy is consequently the confirmation of the problem.

A biomechanical problem in spinal motion can interfere with range of motion and/or motion control. The ability of a manipulative therapist is dependent upon an accurate assessment of motion quantitatively and qualitatively. Quantitatively, abnormal motion can be regarded to be either hypomobile—meaning decreased movement—or hypermobile—meaning increased movement. Qualitatively, abnormal motion is defined to mean either resistance or ease to motion. The skill of a manipulator is related to the accurate assessment of motion behavior. Clearly, the type of manipulation therapy chosen for a motion restriction and/or resistance disorder is different than for a motion instability where normal tissue restraints are inadequate.

TYPES OF MANIPULATION

The word manipulation takes on different meanings among health practitioners and lay people. The ambiguity and lack of clear definition of manipulation results in communication problems which ultimately lead to misconceptions. To some, manipulation is the use of a vigorous high-speed manual maneuver which repositions displaced bones into place and results in a pop or crack. To others, manipulation may mean a gentle, refined motion which increases joint motion or soft tissue extensibility. The language of manipula-

tion must be specifically delineated and defined. The following section identifies the various and most common forms of manipulation used. The purpose is to define each manipulation type so that the language of manipulation can be understood and communication among health practitioners enhanced.

An overview of manipulation types is presented in Table 3.1. The first differentiation to make is between general (regional) or specific (localized) manipulation.

General vs Specific Spinal Manipulation

A general spinal manipulation involves a load applied to more than one joint and usually more than one spinal segment. The manipulative pressure is transmitted to a number of joints/segments which have been determined to be hypomobile. Therefore the indication for regional manipulation is in improving motion in an area of the spine which is generally stiff. The problem that complicates general manipulation is the possibility of increasing motion in an unstable joint not detected during the evaluation.

Table 3.1
Types of Manipulation

General (regional)	Specific (localized)
Indirect	Direct
Noncontact	Contact
Soft tissue	Joint
Mobilization (nonthrust)	Manipulation (thrust)
Types of motion application:	Types:
Graded oscillation	Under anesthesia
Progressive loading	General
Sustained loading	Specific
Types of mobilization:	
Joint mobilization	
Soft tissue therapy	
Soft tissue mobilization	
Myofascial release	
Neuromuscular therapy	
PNF	
Muscle energy	
Positional release therapies	
Strain/counterstrain	
Functional or active	
Assistive motion therapy	

Specific spinal manipulation is meant to influence only one segment or spinal joint. Its intent is to localize forces to one segment or one spinal joint and minimize force transmission through uninvolved spinal segments. Proponents of specific spinal manipulation employ locking procedures to protect uninvolved spinal segments, thereby concentrating the force to the restricted segment. Theoretically, this is safer and perhaps more effective than the general technique. Opponents, however, claim that localization of force to the involved vertebral level through locking procedures is not possible. They argue that manipulative forces to the spine are always regional, thus dismissing the specificity theory. The other issue regarding the specificity of spinal manipulation relates to the accurate determination of the restricted spinal segment and delineation of the motion direction restriction. For example, the inability of L3–4 to side bend to the left may be due to a restriction in superior motion of the right inferior process of L3, a restriction in inferior motion of the left inferior process of L3, or to restrictions on both sides. The application of specific spinal manipulation to an incorrectly identified spinal joint/segment or in the wrong direction may not help the condition and possibly could worsen the situation. Figure 3.1 demonstrates the normal arthrokinematic behavior of L3 and L4 during left side bending.

Direct vs Indirect Manipulation

Direct manipulation involves a force applied into the direction of motion restriction or barrier.[6] Direct action manipulation engages the restricted barrier to normal motion and applies a force to move through the restrictive barrier to restore normal active and passive range of motion. In the case of C3–4 where the left inferior process of C3 does not slide superiorly, a direct manipulation would move the left inferior process of C3 superior to the position of resistance and then apply additional force to restore superior glide. Direct manipulation methods are logical and effec-

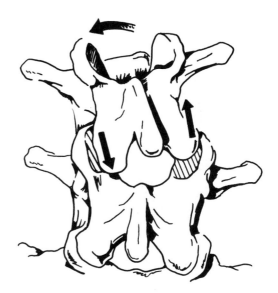

Figure 3.1 Normal arthrokinematic of L3 and L4 during left side bending.

tive, but sometimes painful, especially during acute conditions when localized muscle guarding interferes. Figure 3.2 illustrates the force applied in a direct manipulation to restore superior glide of the left inferior process of C3 on C4.

Indirect manipulation involves movement in the opposite direction of the motion restriction.[7,8] Utilization of indirect manipulation to restore superior movement of the left inferior process of L4 on L5 would involve moving the left inferior process of L4 inferior. In other words, the left inferior process of L4 would be moved away from the motion barrier. More simply, if a motion segment is restricted in left rotation, an indirect manipulation approach would mobilize in right rotation. Figure 3.3 demonstrates an indirect manipulation force to restore superior movement of the right inferior process of L4 on L5.

At first the idea of indirect manipulation may appear strange. To understand the concept of indirect manipulation, consider how a stuck, skewed drawer in a chest is successfully pulled out of the chest. Often the movement that eventually frees the drawer after repeated attempts to pull the drawer out is an inward

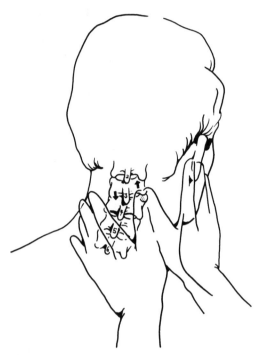

Figure 3.2 Direct manipulation to restore superior glide of the right inferior process of C3 on C4.

push. In other words, the drawer is pushed in first, before pulling it out—an indirect procedure. A restricted spinal joint often unlocks in the same manner.

Indirect manipulation is usually safer than the direct approach and has less tendency to produce an adverse reaction. During acute stages of a condition where muscle activity and pain interfere with direct action manipulation, indirect method may be effective. The principles of painless and opposite motion in spinal manipulation have been advocated as a safe, effective means for restoring range of motion and reducing pain.[7,8,9] A general rule of thumb when in doubt about using a direct or indirect method is to choose the indirect approach. Remember, however, after unlocking a fixed joint with indirect manipulation movement, the range of motion in the restricted direction may still need to be restored through direct manipulation. As a result, combined methods of indirect and direct manipulation are often necessary.

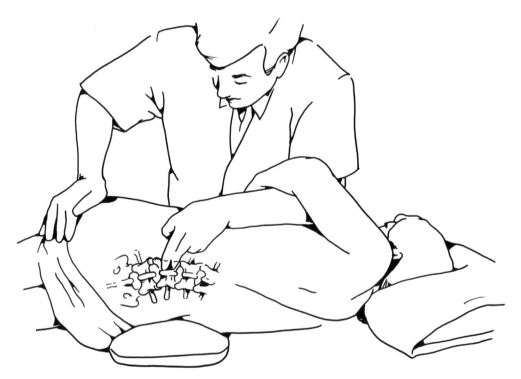

Figure 3.3 Indirect manipulation involving inferior glide of the left superior process of L5 on L4 to restore superior glide.

Contact vs Noncontact Manipulation

Manipulation can also be classified as being contact or noncontact. The *contact manipulation approach* requires hand or finger placement on the involved area and/or spinal segment. Vertebral contacts are frequently made on the spinous process, laminas, facet joints, and sometimes transverse processes. In the thoracic and lumbar spines the accessible contact points are the spinous and transverse processes. With respect to soft tissue manipulation, specific contact can sometimes be made directly to tender and/or trigger points to effect change in soft tissue tonicity. When specific contacts to involved tissue areas are too sensitive, contact to uninvolved tissue regions are used to transfer force to the hypersensitive areas. This strategy employs a noncontact technique. Contact is recommended for enhancing specificity of action, assisting in localized force transmission, enhancing control, and for monitoring tissue response. In some cases, however, the involved area may be too sensitive to contact and contact away from the lesion is necessary. In other situations, additional leverage is required to affect a soft tissue or joint release and contact needs to be away from the involved area. Figure 3.4 illustrates the use of direct contact on the involved spinal segment for the purpose of restoring extension motion at that vertebral level.

Noncontact manipulation involves hand or finger placement away from the spinal segment or area in lesion. The major indications for the use of noncontact manipulation is when contact is painful or when additional leverage is needed to achieve a soft tissue or joint release. Frequently additional or different manipulative force is achieved in the spine when the extremities are contacted and used for leverage. Opponents of noncontact manipulation insist that noncontact methods are unsafe, nonspecific and more difficult to monitor with respect to tissue response. Figure 3.5 shows noncontact manipulation of the lumbosacral spine by utilizing both lower extremities for leverage and force generation.

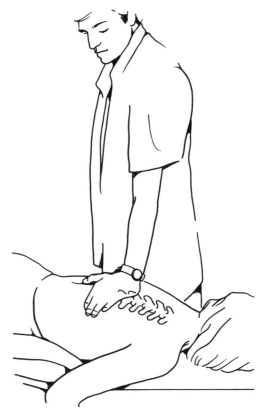

Figure 3.4 Contact manipulation at T6/7 to restore extension range of motion.

Soft Tissue vs Joint

Manipulation is also categorized as being soft tissue or joint, based upon the primary objective and effect.

Soft tissue therapy does not involve high velocity motion and therefore is identified as soft tissue mobilization or myofascial release. Soft tissue therapy is aimed towards enhancing proper tonus (activity state) and/or extensibility in soft tissues. Manual therapy of soft tissue may have mechanical, physiologic, and/or neuroreflexive effects. Restoration of soft tissue extensibility and/or the inhibition of hyperactive musculature helps promote motion function which in turn leads to a reduction in pain. Soft tissue therapy can be used during acute, sub-acute, and chronic musculoskeletal conditions. In multifactorial problems soft tissue mobilization can be used as a preparatory procedure to decrease muscle

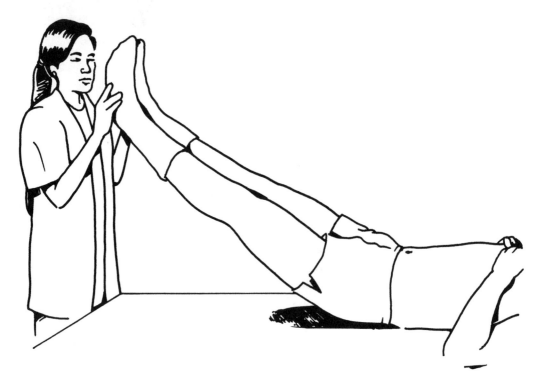

Figure 3.5 Noncontact manipulation to improve lumbo-sacral flexion range of motion.

guarding so that joint manipulation is effective in improving vertebral mobility. In many situations, the force necessary during joint manipulation can be substantially reduced if adequate soft tissue therapy is employed first.

Joint manipulation may or may not involve the use of high-velocity movement. Joint manipulation using a high-velocity, low amplitude movement is also sometimes referred to as *thrust manipulation*. More recently, in osteopathic manual medicine, the term *mobilization with impulse* has been utilized as well. Joint manipulation without thrust or impulse is referred to as joint mobilization.

Joint mobilization involves slower motion activity than manipulation with thrust. The principal objective of joint manipulation (thrust) or joint mobilization (without thrust) is to restore range of motion to a joint with altered motion function. Specifically, joint manipulation may unlock a joint in which motion is blocked or improve range in a restricted joint. Joint manipulation may also im-

prove joint position as well as distribute mechanical stress to a joint more evenly. A repositioning and/or redistribution of stress to a joint often results in a reduction in pain in addition to improving joint motion function.

Joint manipulation can be useful during all stages of joint conditions—acute, subacute, or chronic. The stage of the joint condition, however, determines the type of manipulation employed. As a general rule, joint mobilization is usually more helpful for acute or subacute problems, whereas joint manipulation is usually more effective with chronic conditions, provided that the motion restriction is not too severe. In the case of a considerable joint limitation, soft tissue and joint mobilization should precede joint manipulation. During the immediate period of joint injury where inflammation and swelling exist, joint mobilization and manipulation are generally contraindicated.

In mobilization (nonthrust) three types of motion application can be used: graded oscillation, progressive loading, or sustained loading.

Graded Oscillations

Graded oscillation is a form of cyclic loading whereby alternate pressure, on and off, are delivered at different parts of the available range.[10] Oscillatory motion application is graded on a 1 to 4 scale based on the amplitude of the motion and part of the range reached (Fig. 3.6).

Grade 1 oscillations are small in amplitude and delivered at the initial available restricted active range.

Grade 2 oscillations are large amplitude motions delivered from initial to middle ranges of available active movement. Although restoration of full range of motion is possible when using grade 1 and grade 2 oscillations, the principal effect is theorized to be neurophysiologic. The cyclical loading nature of graded oscillation movement is performed at a certain, set speed according to patient comfort. The rhythmical, vibratory activity produced most probably activates sensory mechanoreceptors, helping to reduce pain and improve propioceptive function.

Grade 3 oscillations are large in amplitude and delivered from mid to end range of the restrictive passive motion barrier.

Grade 4 oscillations are small amplitude motions delivered into the end range of the restrictive passive motion barrier. The primary effect of grade 3 or grade 4 oscillations is speculated to be mechanical; however, neurophysiologic responses are also possible. The cyclic nature of end range oscillations is analogous to the "try, try again" philosophy which ultimately leads to a progressive increase in movement. Caution must be exercised when using end range graded oscillations on an acute joint condition. Sometimes an irritable joint structure is agitated by cyclic loading, especially grade 3 or 4 oscillations.

Progressive Loading

Progressive loading mobilization involves a successive series of short amplitude, spring type pressures.[11] The pressure is imparted at progressive increments of the range and is defined on a 1 to 4 scale as is graded oscillation. The pressures used with progressive load mobilization are transmitted at different ranges; however, the amplitude of each pressure is the same (Fig. 3.7). Progressive loading is utilized for mechanical and/or soft tissue restrictions, and therefore the pressure depth reached is determined by the established objective as well as the tolerance of the patient. For example, if a reflex muscle contraction developed during a grade 2 progressive load, then the therapist is advised to limit the progressive load to a grade 1 or choose an alternate mobilization type. Any motion gain resulting from grade 1, 2, or 3 progressive load mobilization is likely to be the result of neurophysiologic change, whereas a grade 4 may actually lengthen restrictive tissue. Note that grade 1, 2, and 3 progressive loading occur within the available active range of motion. Grade 4 goes beyond the restrictive physiologic barrier and into the passive motion barrier.

Progressive loading requires skill in consistent reproduction of short amplitude, spring pressures at different range increments. Although the amount of spring may vary according to the condition, the amplitude is always small. Unfavorable patient reactions should always first be assessed from the standpoint of improper application. Adhesive joint restrictions sometimes require a spring-like pressure to unlock. Easily agitated motion segments or irritable tissue, on the other hand, may not tolerate the spring nature of progressive loading mobilization.

Sustained Loading

Sustained loading is continuous, uninterrupted pressure or force which may remain the same intensity, gradually increase, or decrease depending on the patient reaction. If motion is being restored during a sustained loading pressure, the therapist maintains the same loading force. If proper motion is not being facilitated, the therapist slowly and gradually increases or decreases the load ap-

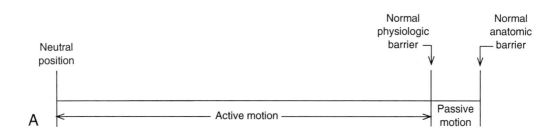

NORMAL RANGE OF MOTION

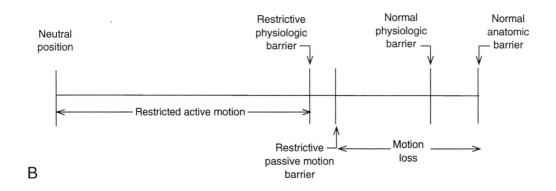

MOTION RESTRICTION

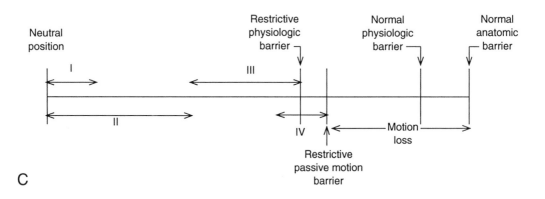

GRADED OSCILLATION RANGES
AND AMPLITUDES

Figure 3.6 A. Normal active and passive range of motion within physiologic and anatomic barriers, **B.** Abnormal active and passive range of motion with restrictive physiologic and passive motion barriers, **C.** Arrows depict the amplitude of each graded oscillation and the position in the available range.

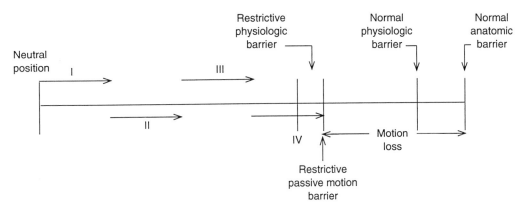

Figure 3.7 Progressive loading ranges and amplitudes. Note grade 1, 2, and 3 progressive loading occur within the available active range of motion.

Grade 4 goes beyond the restrictive physiologic barrier and into the passive motion barrier.

plied until the desired motion develops. Maintaining a sustained, uninterrupted load enhances sensory perception to tissue response. In acute, easily provoked conditions, immediate tissue feedback is desired, and therefore sustained loading is recommended. In addition, the viscoelastic properties of adaptively shortened soft tissues can be influenced by the use of sustained loading, particularly if the concept of low load, long duration load application is utilized. Sustained loading mobilization, however, may not be sufficient to mobilize a joint that possesses an intra-articular restraint to motion such as an adhesion or cartilagenous interlocking problem.

JOINT MOBILIZATION

Various types of mobilization have developed within manual therapy and medicine. The importance of defining each type is essential to communication among and between clinical disciplines. Research efforts to substantiate the effect of mobilization on specific conditions requires clear understanding of the definition and language utilized in mobilization. The following section defines and delineates the role of each mobilization type. Further detail is provided in subsequent chapters.

Joint mobilization is a nonthrust manipulation. In osteopathy, joint manipulation performed without impulse is referred to as mobilization or articulatory procedure.[8] Joint

mobilization pressures may vary from gentle to vigorous, but are imparted slowly as opposed to thrust or high-velocity manipulation. Since the pressure utilized is slow, controlled, begins gently, and gradually increases, the patient can report about the effect during the time of application. The instantaneous feedback mechanism provides a sense of security for the patient and helps to increase the safety feature of mobilization.

Joint mobilization is performed within the available active and passive physiologic range of the restricted joint. The intent of joint mobilization is to regain normal active range of motion as well as restore passive joint play action. Repositioning of a joint may also come about by joint mobilization, thus improving alignment and stress distribution. Motion recovery, joint realignment, and uniform stress distribution improve joint function which often leads to a reduction in pain. The improvement in joint function increases a joint's adaptive potential to mechanical stress, whether normal or abnormal, and reduces the possibility of re-injury.

SOFT TISSUE THERAPIES

Soft tissue therapies involve manual contacts, pressures, or movements, primarily to myofascial tissues. The purpose of soft tissue directed therapy is to normalize activity status, restore extensibility, and reduce pain. The scientific and theoretical basis for the effects of soft tissue therapy are presented later in the book. Soft tissue work is classified into 2 categories, *soft tissue mobilization and myofascial release*. *Soft tissue mobilization* is simply defined as the manual manipulation of soft tissues administered for the purpose of producing effects on the nervous, muscular, lymph, and circulatory systems.[12] The various types of soft tissue mobilizations include: classical massage, connective tissue massage, Rolfing, acupressure, and soft tissue stretching. The soft tissue characteristics influenced by soft tissue mobilization are tone (the tension status) and extensibility (the ability to realign or elongate).

Different types of hand contacts and movements are used, depending on the objective. As a general principle, with the exception of Rolfing and acupressure, soft tissue mobilization uses low intensity manual pressure and should not cause pain. For decreasing soft tissue tone, slowly applied sustained pressure is recommended. For improving soft tis-

sue extensibility the following maneuvers are suggested: effleurage, kneading, petrissage, friction, and stretching. If applied properly all soft tissue techniques should result in local and general relaxation, thus reducing tone.

The type of soft tissue condition not only determines the type of maneuver used, but the direction of mobilization, as well as the amount of pressure. For example, a painful muscle exhibiting increased tone and restriction in lateral expansion to the right may require indirect, transverse pressures. Therefore, slowly applied mobilizations perpendicular to the muscle fiber alignment in a contralateral direction are necessary to avoid pain, decrease tone, and increase extensibility. On the other hand, a nonpainful, adaptively shortened muscle may respond to mobilization parallel or perpendicular to the fiber alignment as well as to stretch elongation procedures. Fig. 3.8 illustrates medial to lateral perpendicular kneading of the right erector spinae musculature.

Connective tissue massage is a subcategory

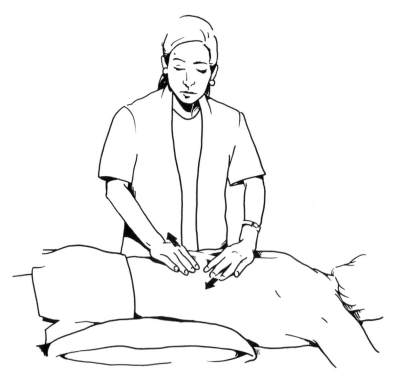

Figure 3.8 Medial to lateral perpendicular kneading of the left erector spinae musculature.

of soft tissue therapy developed by the German physical therapist, Elisabeth Dicke. Connective tissue massage (CTM) is a specific manipulation applied to the connective tissue close to the body surface. CTM involves light, short or long superficial strokes to the skin and underlying subcutaneous tissue. Physical effects in the form of mobilizing connective tissue and reflex effects such as circulatory changes are possible both locally and generally.[13] The basic short paraspinal stroke is demonstrated in Fig. 3.9.

Rolfing is a form of soft tissue treatment which used deep manual pressure and stretching. Ida Rolf felt that "order" in structure allows defined and appropriate function. The greater the order in the structure, the lower its entropy and higher its energy content.[14] Structural integration of the body's fascia through deep tissue mobilization is used to reduce abnormal stress from postural deviation and restore vertical alignment. Rolfing is believed to be able to normalize the directional pulls of the fibers within connective tissue and improve muscle tone, extensibility, and contractility. Rolfing pressures along the spine of the scapula are utilized to realign the shoulder girdles (Fig. 3.10).

Acupressure is a method of point massage to acupuncture points for the purpose of analgesia. Fingertip pressure is used over a finite acupuncture point of highly discernible tenderness. The pressure can be applied in a circular, a transverse, or in a deep, constant pressure. The magnitude of pressure should be sufficient to elicit extreme tenderness or pain, although the sensitivity of the point usually decreases during the treatment. The duration of pressure is typically 30–90 seconds when a number of points are treated; however, one point can be treated as much as 3–4 minutes.[15]

One possible explanation for the mechanism of pain relief by acupressure is the modulation of endorphin levels. Thus, acupressure affects our awareness of pain. Acupressure may also affect the electrical current through cutaneous nerves altering the point's resistance to external stimuli. Pressure application

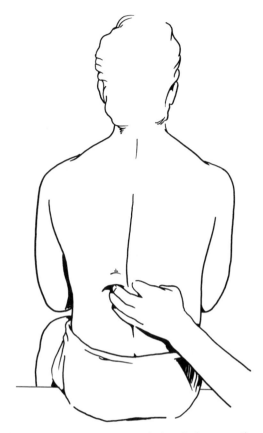

Figure 3.9 Basic short paraspinal stroke in connective tissue massage.

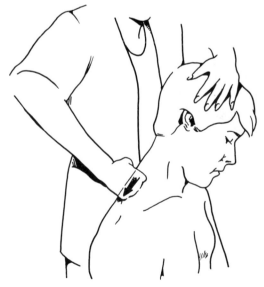

Figure 3.10 Rolfing pressure along the spine of the scapula to realign shoulder girdle.

to myofascial trigger points may restore local circulation by removing a fluid obstruction and facilitating venous flow. In addition, nociceptor activity may be reduced by the activation of sensory mechanoreceptors in the involved myofascial area. Fig. 3.11 demonstrates acupressure applied to the acupuncture point, K3, for the purpose of decreasing neck and shoulder pain.

Soft tissue stretching is the lengthening of

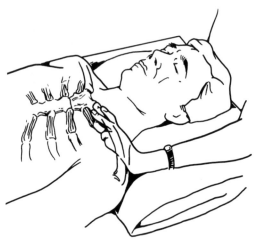

Figure 3.11 Acupressure point inferior to sternoclavicular joint.

soft tissues, primarily muscles, for the purpose of restoring muscle balance among muscle groups as well as joint range of motion. Universal to all soft tissue stretching procedures is the concept that muscles must be in a state of optimal relaxation before effective stretching can occur. Low intensity isometric contraction in a painfree position prior to the stretch facilitates the stretch by postcontraction relaxation and enhances the safety of the procedure. After the isometric contraction and subsequent relaxation either the patient or therapist stretches within pain tolerance to the point of resistance.[16] At the resistance point the sequence is repeated. Passive stretching may also be utilized. Low load, prolonged duration stretch times are recommended for the best results. The lengthening of the soft tissues obtained is thought to be due to the realignment of fibers within the connective tissues exterior and interior to the muscle as well as the actual elongation of muscle fibers. Fig. 3.12 illustrates passive stretching to the left hip adductors and medial hamstring musculature as well as to the related connective tissue.

Myofascial release is a form of soft tissue therapy which is based upon neuroreflexive

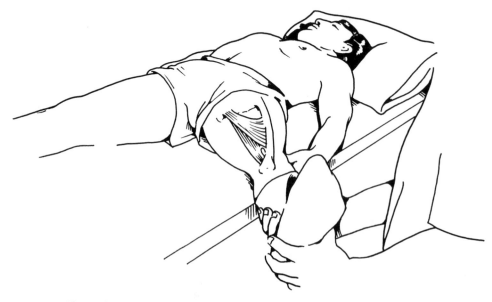

Figure 3.12 Passive stretching to left hip adductors and medial hamstrings.

responses that reduce tissue tension. The appropriate application of manual contact requires the determination of the best point (location) of entry into the musculoskeletal system, selection of the most suitable types of stress to induce the inhibitory effect, and the sensitivity in palpation to react properly to tissue response. The net result is a relaxation of tissue tension and subsequent decrease in myofascial tightness. The reduction in activity which occurs to the agonist through myofascial release indirectly helps the antagonist(s), since the reciprocal inhibition influence is lessened. Positional and functional symmetry is improved as a result of balancing myofascial tensions in the involved area.

Myofascial release is a safe, effective method to normalize myofascial activity, regain tissue extensibility, and reduce pain. Since the patient's own inherent tissue forces are being tapped for the corrective changes, myofascial release is usually tolerated well. The effect can be local or regional, and frequently it is distal to the area of contact. In cases where considerable tissue irritability is present myofascial release can be used in nonirritable areas to affect the involved area. Myofascial release is not always painless. However, in many situations, the initial discomfort subsides as the contact is maintained over time, provided the therapist is responding appropriately to the induced, inherent tissue motion changes. Typically a patient having a good response to myofascial release offers a favorable comment during the procedure. Hand position and force direction for a thoracolumbar myofascial release is demonstrated in Fig. 3.13.

Neuromuscular Therapies

Two types of neuromuscular therapies for spinal motion-related problems exist, propioceptive neuromuscular facilitation (PNF) and muscle energy.

PNF was developed by Herman Kabat M.D. and Margarett Knott P.T. during the late 1940s and early 1950s primarily as an alternative treatment approach for patients with neurologic conditions. The application of PNF principles to patients with orthopedic problems evolved in physical therapy as knowledge of the nature of musculoskeletal dysfunctions increased.

The origin of *muscle energy* is credited to Fred Mitchell, Sr. who described the technique in 1958.[17] The basic, underlying principle of muscle energy as first practiced by Dr. Mitchell was that muscular activity could be utilized to restore physiologic joint motion. For the purpose of introduction to neuromus-

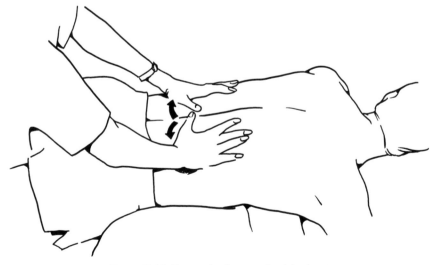

Figure 3.13 Thoracolumbar myofascial release.

cular therapy, operational definitions and basic concepts for each type are presented. Further in-depth descriptions and principles of PNF and muscle energy are provided in succeeding chapters.

Proprioceptive Neuromuscular Facilitation (PNF)

PNF is a method of promoting or hastening the response of the neuromuscular mechanism through stimulation of proprioceptors.[18] Specific motor recruitment is enhanced or facilitated by specific demands which activate proprioceptors within tissues in the body. The application of a manual stimulus is used to elicit efficient neuromuscular responses. The primary objectives of PNF are to develop trunk or proximal stability and control as well as to coordinate mobility patterns. PNF therefore can be used to help stabilize vertebral motion segment instabilities and to improve spinal movement control.

The manual contacts used in PNF should use pressure in an exact way to obtain the desired neuromuscular response. Painful stimuli are avoided so as to prevent a withdrawal reaction. The pressure used serves as sensory feedback to help the patient understand the motion direction desired. The specific procedure utilized in PNF is determined by the objective. To obtain greater force in muscle contraction, a stretch stimulus or maximal resistance is used.

If the purpose of PNF is to sequence muscle activity properly during a motor function, timing is emphasized. With respect to spinal dysfunction, timing is often required to develop trunk stabilization. Delayed muscular responses of the trunk must be improved before distal motion deficiencies are reestablished. With spinal joint injury, proprioceptive activity may be disturbed. Traction and approximation of joint surfaces during PNF may restore joint receptor activity, enhancing both joint position and motion awareness.

PNF is also used to bring about relaxation of antagonist muscle groups. The contraction of a muscle or muscle groups to facilitate one pattern of movement will demand a relaxation of muscles used in the antagonistic pattern. The PNF techniques of repeated contractions, slow reversal hold, and rhythmic stabilization during patterned motion activity will stimulate the agonist and relax the antagonist according to the laws of reciprocal innervation proposed by Sherrington.[19] Fig. 3.14 illustrates a pelvic PNF which is used to normalize lumbar and pelvic neuromuscular activity.

Thus, PNF is used for a variety of spinal dysfunctions. If properly executed it can reduce pain from motion impairment, restore muscle balance, facilitate proper motor control/recruitment, and enhance spinal stability.

Muscle Energy

Muscle energy is a form of manipulative treatment using active muscle contraction at varying intensities from a precisely controlled position in a specific direction against a distinctly executed counterforce. Muscle energy techniques are used to mobilize joint restrictions, strengthen weak musculature, stretch tight myofascia, reduce muscle tonus, and improve local circulation.[20] Precise positioning is achieved when the initial restrictive barrier is engaged during passive motion. Four types of muscle contractions can be used, isometric (same length), isokinetic (same speed), isotonic (same force), or isodynamic (same force, variable speed and length).[21]

The most common contraction force used in muscle energy application to the spine is isometric. To treat an area of myofascial and/or joint restriction, isometric contractions of the muscle(s) opposing the restricted movement are used. For example, Fig. 3.15 demonstrates a direct muscle energy technique to improve right rotation of T7/8 by using an isometric contraction of the left erector spinae.

The localization of muscle force during contraction is very important in obtaining the desired result. The amount of force and counterforce is established on the basis of the size and strength of the involved muscle(s), the

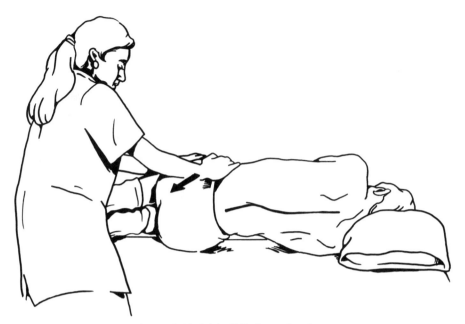

Figure 3.14 Pelvic PNF diagonal pattern.

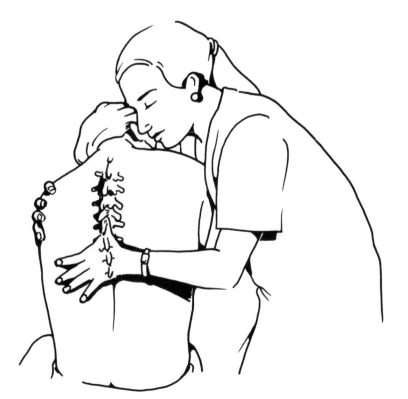

Figure 3.15 Direct muscle energy to improve right rotation of T7/8.

type of motion impairment, and the stage of the condition. In general, a small amount of force is used, 1 lb. (about .5 kilogram) or less, especially when beginning. Too much force may result in activation of too many muscles about a joint and cause joint compression instead of restoring therapeutic movement.

By restoring joint movement and improving neuromuscular activity in an area of motion dysfunction, motor performance is enhanced. Motion patterns become efficient, and work expenditure for motion activity is lessened with successful application of muscle energy. In both PNF and muscle energy the patient is actively involved as a participant in the corrective process. Involvement of the patient during the treatment allows and encourages the patient to assume responsibility for self-care.

Positional Release Therapies

Fundamental to the concept of Positional Release Therapies is the presence of neuromuscular motion disorder. Its advocates contend that improper neuromuscular mechanisms are responsible for establishing and/or maintaining joint motion abnormality. The concept of motion dysfunction created or perpetuated by abnormal neuromuscular reflex changes is in departure from the mechanical-structural problem identified by practitioners of high-velocity manipulation. Although modifications of Positional Release Therapy have evolved, two basic types exist, Strain/Counterstrain and Functional Technique or active assistive motion therapy.

Strain/Counterstrain, as developed by Lawrence Jones, D.O., is the passive placement of the body in a position of greatest comfort to reduce pain. According to strain/counterstrain theory pain relief is achieved by the reduction and arrest of continuing inappropriate proprioceptive activity which maintains the motion dysfunction.[22] The position of spontaneous release resulting in pain reduction is typically away from the motion restriction or in the direction of motion ease and comfort.

The underlying basis for Strain and Counterstrain is that every neuromuscular disorder has a palpable point of tenderness as well as a position which can be obtained for comfort. The position of injury is one of strain which places some muscle(s) in a shortened state and (an)other muscle(s) in a lengthened state. According to Korr's muscle spindle theory for neuromuscular disorder the gamma motor neuron activity to the intrafusal fibers of the shortened muscle(s) is turned up instead of decreased. The resultant tension in the intrafusal mechanism of the shortened muscle(s) causes excitation of the CNS, stimulation of alpha motor neurons, and the maintenance of extrafusal fiber contraction.

The counterstrain position is a position of comfort which further shortens the already shortened musculature. The movement into and out of the position of release is done passively and slowly so as to allow the CNS to continually monitor muscle spindle responses. The position of release is held 90 seconds to allow the gamma motor neuron activity to decrease and the spindle to reset to normal activity status. The tissues are returned to neutral position very slowly so as to prevent re-activation of the facilitated neuroreflexive pathways. The corresponding point of tenderness is often less sensitive to palpation pressure after an effective release. A counterstrain procedure for a hyperactive, tender left piriformis muscle is shown in Fig. 3.16.

Strain and counterstrain is a gentle, nontraumatic type of manipulation which is especially effective when irregular neuromuscular activities have maintained and perpetuated abnormal mechanical stress to tissue. Shortened muscles have developed as a result of hypertonicity. A return to normal length is achieved through positional release of abnormal neuroreflexive activities. The essential effect is a re-ordering of CNS activity and resultant normalization of neuromuscular behavior.

Functional Technique (or active assistive motion therapy) is based upon the patient's self correction abilities. Fundamental to the func-

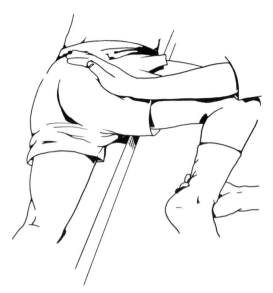

Figure 3.16 Counterstrain for a hyperactive, tender right piriformis muscle.

tional or active assistive approach is that a motion response is the result of the demand placed upon the body. For the spine the demand or stimulus evokes a movement response from each motion segment. A normal movement response elicits full, painfree, efficient, and controlled motion activity. In the functional approach identified by Hoover, normal movement behavior in response to a demand was characterized by an ease of motion. Protest to motion demand is called *bind*.[23,24] Features of bind in motion segment(s) of the spine include restriction, increased work effort, disturbance in direction or tracking difficulty, uncoordinated movement activity, and sometimes pain.

The underlying theory for functional approach is based upon altered neural activity. Altered neural activity can cause or be the result of abnormal motion behavior. Attention to spinal motion segment dysfunction in the form of some type of nonintrusive stimulus (typically physical) encourages motion activity. Therapeutic responses result in motion ease of performance. Therapeutic motion activity supplies the central nervous system (CNS) with normal input regarding motion patterns and sequences. The return of proper

afferent motion signals to the CNS presumably enables a reorganization of efferent activity with a subsequent improvement in movement in the area of dysfunction.[25]

A key element in successful use of functional methods involves utilization of the least intrusive stimulus to evoke a motion response. The therapist may need only to establish contact on the lesioned spinal segment to facilitate motion activity. If contact alone is not sufficient, a motion demand in any one of several planes can be used to bring about a movement reaction.[26] Typically, the first motion elicited is in the opposite direction of the restriction or bind.

The second criterion for effective application is dependent upon the therapist's ability to perceive and sense the resultant motion activity produced by the patient. The motion response to the stimulus selected is therefore generated by the patient's neuromuscular-skeletal system.[27] The therapist "listens" to the motion response through palpation, but does not create motion for the patient. If the motion is determined to be therapeutic the activity is allowed to continue or can be assisted or amplified. Thus, the motion is actively determined by the patient, but can be assisted by the therapist. Nontherapeutic motion patterns elicited by the patient can be discouraged by the therapist. Resistance to unwanted movement or guidance towards desired movement is used to restore functional ease in motion performance. The participation of each spinal segment, especially segments previously exhibiting movement dysfunction, is critical. Fig. 3.17 illustrates the application of Functional Technique in restoring lumbo-sacral flexion, right side bending, and right rotation.

In some functional types of therapy the motion brought about eventually ceases. The position obtained allows a balancing of neuromuscular activities to take place. The patients are encouraged to relax through their own respiratory activities until an optimal release in tissue tension is felt in the area of dysfunction.

The goal in functional manipulation is to

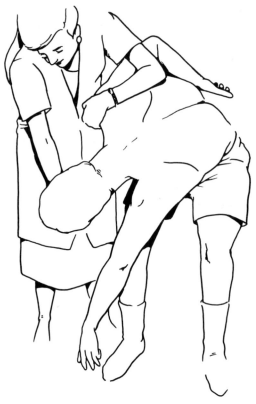

Figure 3.17 Functional technique improving lumbo-sacral flexion, right side bending and right rotation.

restore motion ease in functional performance by re-ordering neural activity to and from the CNS. Individuals with reflexogenic, protective muscle guarding, and joint motion dysfunction respond to Functional Technique quite well. Chronic, rigid joint fixations are less receptive to the functional approach.

Thrust Manipulation

Thrust manipulation is the use of high velocity, low amplitude motion delivered at the end of the restricted physiologic limit of a joint's range of motion. The purpose of thrust manipulation is to restore accessory or involuntary joint mobility. Thrust manipulation may create a distraction (separation) of a translation (gliding) of joint surfaces which may help to restore full, painless motion activity to a joint in dysfunction.

The use of thrust or impulse in manipu-

lation requires skill in force application, especially in regard to amplitude. The thrust action should never be forced or be imparted in the direction of pain. Appropriate patient selection is critical in successful outcome, perhaps more so than the actual application of the maneuver. Not all patients are structurally, biomechanically, or psychologically candidates for thrust manipulation. In addition, the stage and duration of the condition needs consideration. An acutely inflamed joint fixation or a 20-year-old joint restriction of significant magnitude will most likely react adversely to a sudden thrust manipulation. Preparation of reactively involved surrounding joint tissues is often a necessary, preliminary step. Thrust manipulation can snap an adhesion binding the joint, alter vertebral position, normalize joint motion by stretching periarticular tissue (ligament, capsule and deep, short musculature), and reduce pain by normalizing mechanoreceptor activity.

Three types of thrust manipulations are used:

1. Under Anesthesia. Thrust manipulation can be performed under anesthesia, but it is controversial. Under general anesthesia with loss of all sensation and nerve function the patient has no reflex mechanism to protect a joint structure. Resistance to passive movement is due solely to the restriction with the joint itself, since involuntary and voluntary muscle guarding is eliminated. Extreme caution must be exercised to prevent overstretching and injury.

An indication for manipulation under anesthesia is prolonged, intractable pain with motion impairment unresponsive to intensive spinal manipulation without anesthesia in a patient who has failed to respond to physical therapy of any kind, medication, injection, and bedrest. In other words, manipulation under anesthesia is usually one of the last steps in treatment for patients with motion restriction and intolerable pain.

For cervical motion disorders manipulation under anesthesia is contraindicated until sternocleidomastoid reflexes have returned. Partial analgesia permits protective reflexes yet provides muscle relaxation. To prevent the possibility of manipulating beyond normal motion capabilities of the cervical spine, non-thrust mobilization is recommended.

Some degree of inflammation usually develops after manipulation under anesthesia. Anti-inflammatory medication is recommended to reduce post manipulative pain and inflammation. Motion activity through exercise as well as manipulation are suggested after the anesthetic procedure to maintain the range of motion achieved.[28]

2. General Thrust Manipulation. This involves a high-velocity, low-amplitude stretch to more than one joint and possibly more than one segment. Multijoint or segmental manipulation of the spine is sometimes helpful in the thoracic region when three or four segments in a row become fixed. With the notable exception of Cyriax, most manipulative therapists and physicians advise against general manipulation in the cervical and lumbar areas because of the possibility of an existing joint hypermobility.

3. Specific Thrust Manipulation. This involves three criteria:

(a) The first is the use of spinal locking procedures designed to minimize force on uninvolved spinal segments and maximize force on the involved segment. To accomplish spinal locking, the mechanical behavior of the spinal motion segment must be understood. To achieve locking the facet joints must be apposed on both sides by backward bending or on one side by rotation. Approximation of the articular processes theoretically opposes further motion at the uninvolved segments. Facet apposition is one method used by "specificity manipulators" to protect normal or hypermobile motion segments and localize the thrust to the involved spinal level. Another mechanism by which spinal locking is attained is through ligamentous, myofascial tension.[29] Ligamentous, myofascial tension locking is accomplished by forward bending of the spine above and/or below the segmental dysfunction.

Spinal locking should never lock the segment to be manipulated. Poor localization of forces due to overlocking may lead to the use of ex-cessive manipulative force. When precise localization of force is achieved through spinal locking, manipulative force is minimized. In fact, in some situations a joint release is obtained at the level of dysfunction during the locking procedure. The thrust is therefore no longer necessary. An L2/3 left rotation thrust manipulation is shown in Fig. 3.18.

(b) The second criterion involves the use of a high-velocity movement. Consider the fact that the faster a performer is able to pull the tablecloth, the less likely is the table setting affected. Similarly, the quicker the manipulative thrust the less chance of affecting adjacent spinal levels. A skilled manipulative therapist has quick-acting hands capable of high speed, low force activity.

(c) The third criterion for specific thrust manipulation deals with the amplitude of the overpressure. All thrust techniques require overpressure at the end of the restricted joint range. Therefore, motion slack must be removed at all uninvolved spinal levels and within the segment to be manipulated before the thrust. A prerequisite for effective safe thrust manipulation is the exact identification of the spinal position needed to take up the tissue slack. Positioning to take up the slack in adjacent tissues and to reach the motion barrier requires deliberate, slow movement activity in multiple dimensions.

In specific thrust manipulation the overpressure is of very short amplitude and of very low force. The safety features of thrust manipulation therefore include: high velocity, short amplitude, low force, and precise localization. The intent of specific thrust manipulation is to restore motion to one joint or segment without adversely affecting adjacent segments. The theroretical intention is admirable, but whether spinal specificity in manipulation actually occurs is unknown.

APPLICATION OF SPINAL MANIPULATION

The criteria for successful application of spinal manipulation are presented in Table 3.2. The following section discusses each factor in relation to the actual application of spinal manipulation.

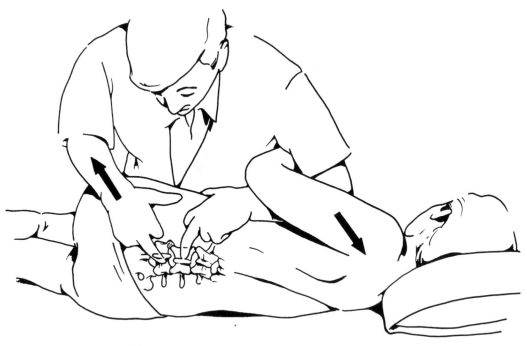

Figure 3.18 An L2/3 left rotation thrust manipulation.

Table 3.2
Criteria For Manipulation and Technique

Criteria
  Appropriate choice
  Rationale
  Appropriate sequencing
  Appropriate adjustments
  Appropriate time length
  Evaluation of effect
Technique criteria
  Patient position
  Therapist position
  Hand placement
  Specificity
  Recruitment of tissue
  Motion direction
  Control
  Amount of force
  Sensitivity to tissue response

Appropriate Choice

The choice is largely governed by the stage of the condition, the type of dysfunction, and the attitude of the patient. Generally speaking, the more acute the condition the less manipulation should be done. If performed immediately after an acute episode manipulation is intended to facilitate repair and offer pain relief. The types of manipulation most likely to help during the acute stage include nonthrust grade 1 or 2 oscillations, myofascial release and functional technique.

Direct, invasive manipulation is not absolutely contraindicated at the time of acute injury, especially if a mechanical restriction is present. Special care must be taken to prevent muscle reactivity when applying direct manipulation during an acute condition. A tendency of some manually trained physicians and therapists is to do too much with respect to manipulation during the acute stage of a spinal condition. In many instances of acute spinal pain, the best approach initially is to encourage rest from function. The pain from acute spinal conditions will often resolve in a week's time with bedrest. Once the pain subsides a biomechanical assessment of spinal motion performance is suggested to determine the type of motion therapy needed.

Subacute, settled, or chronic conditions may respond to a nonthrust progressive or sustained loading mobilization to increase joint range of motion. An adhesive joint condition with a rather abrupt end feel to passive motion testing may be receptive to a thrust manipulation which breaks the adhesion. Thrust manipulation, however, can cause an adverse, postinflammatory reaction with a resultant increase in muscle activity if performed on a chronic considerably restricted point.

Vertebral motion limitation due principally from soft tissue restriction may respond to soft tissue mobilization or neuromuscular therapies such as PNF and muscle energy. The decision to use soft tissue or neuromuscular treatment is based on the clinical assessment of soft tissue involvement. The presence of abnormal muscle tone, localized muscle bands, trigger or tender points, and hypo- or hyper-extensibility may indicate the use of soft tissue therapy. Mechanical instabilities, muscle weakness, or imbalance as well as motion control problems often require neuromuscular therapy and therapeutic exercise instruction.

Treatment selection is also determined by the mental state or psychologic set of the patient. The first requirement in any effective therapeutic relationship is establishing trust. In manual therapy, trust is conveyed through the type of hand contact made and the way movement is facilitated by manipulation. Patient confidence in the manual approach to treatment of motion disorder is essential from day one; otherwise, muscular tension interferes. Patient relaxation, although difficult to achieve, is essential for effective manipulative therapy.

An inclination of manipulative practitioners is to take for granted the psychologic impact of manual contact on patients, solely because of the regular use of their hands-on approach. Constant awareness of and sensitivity to the reasons for tactile defensive behavior is important in developing trust. For example, a frightened, anxious, somewhat timid individual is not likely to respond well to an aggressive manipulation approach.[6] In fact, a thrust manipulation may correctively release a joint fixation in a worried patient, but lead to an increase in pain because of the resultant fear, anxiety, and subsequent muscle tension. Patients with musculoskeletal problems and past/present history of physical abuse also have difficulty in relaxing during manual therapy. Frequently, many treatment sessions involving very gentle manipulation are necessary before the physically mistreated person accepts the manual contact as therapeutic. As a general rule, patient initial acceptance of manipulation is higher when hand contact and motion therapy is gentle.

Rationale

Little evidence exists to validate one type of manipulative therapy as being more effective than others for a specific dysfunction,[1,30,31,32] especially with respect to long term results. Therefore, establishing rationale for the use of a particular manipulation type is important. Identifying the reason for using a manipulation therapy clarifies the intent or objective. The plan of action for use of manipulation should be logical and based upon mechanical, neurophysiologic, and psychologic effects. For example, in a condition which involves a significant degree of soft tissue irritability and muscle spasm, motion may be painfully impaired. The use of soft tissue mobilization or myofascial release may be beneficial in reducing tissue excitability and improving motion function. Without scientific support of manipulative therapy, the clinician must establish clear, rational, analytical judgments to determine the usefulness of a particular manipulation for a specific dysfunction.

Sequencing

A treatment plan often entails a series of manipulative procedures. How one sequences the treatment may affect the outcome. A facilitated, hyperexcitable, stiff motion segment with associated muscle spasm and soft tissue restriction may require the ordering of a number of different strategies. The first objective may involve using a soft tissue therapy to inhibit the hyper-responsive muscle activity.

Myofascial release can, therefore, be chosen as the first strategy to lessen muscle tension. Soft tissue mobilization to improve extensibility may follow to decrease the soft tissue tightness about the motion segment. The spinal joint restriction is then treated by joint mobilization to increase vertebral range of motion. As a final step, PNF may be employed to normalize neuromuscular functional performance in the involved area. Sequencing in this manner might reduce the potential for an adverse response such as increased tissue irritability, muscle spasm, or further motion restriction.

A mechanical instability, on the other hand, often necessitates a different sequencing of manipulative therapies. If a vertebral positional fault exists, the first strategy may involve a nonthrust manipulation to reposition. However, since the spinal segment is hypermobile, neuromuscular approach must be instituted to stabilize the segment. Muscle energy and/or PNF activities are usually helpful in improving motor control at unstable motion segments. Although special care is taken not to stretch a hypermobile spinal segment, other areas of spinal restriction must be treated to prevent localization of stress to the unstable level. Therefore, additional therapy to restricted motion segments above or below the instability might include the use of soft tissue and/or joint mobilization.

Adjustment

The ability to adjust the manipulative technique during a treatment or during a series of sessions is dependent upon experience and expertise. The determination of whether a procedure is effective is based upon patient feedback, tissue response, and knowledge of condition. A reduction in soft tissue tension along with a feeling of less resistance to movement indicates a positive response to manipulation, especially if the patient provides unsolicited positive feedback with respect to pain relief. Conversely, an increase in soft tissue tension accompanied by greater resistance to movement clearly signals an unfavorable re-

action. Ongoing palpatory assessment is essential during manipulative therapy to monitor tissue response and make necessary adjustments. Some novice practitioners make the mistake of criticizing the manipulative technique as being ineffective when in fact their application of the technique is at fault. Every manipulative approach is to be analyzed at the time of application for proper positioning, hand placement, tissue recruitment, force direction, force control, and force amount. Altering one or more of the criteria for manipulation will often result in a successful effort to normalize motion performance. Always consider evaluating your application of a manipulative procedure before changing strategies.

Knowledge of various types of manipulation is important in becoming flexible in approach. Skill and proficiency in many manipulative methods are necessary in order to change strategies when the condition warrants. Some clinicians are extremely talented in certain types of manipulative therapies, but have shortcomings in other procedures. The best manipulators of joint fixations may not be able to help a patient with a mechanical instability in the absence of skill in the neuromuscular approach or therapeutic exercise. No substitution exists for the hours required to become an experienced, skilled, and multifaceted therapist. A truly talented clinician is open and well-versed in all manipulative approaches.

Time and Evaluation

The length of time necessary to achieve a desired result with manipulation is variable. Clearly, if the sole intent of manipulation is to relieve pain, the clinician relies on the testimony of the patient before, during, and after application of the manipulation. The choice, adjustments, and application of the manipulation can therefore be determined by the patient's pain report. Sole dependence on pain status for determining manipulation modus operandi is not suggested for chronic pain patients since the focus on pain is not conducive to positive therapeutic change.

To evaluate the mechanical effects of manipulation the clinician observes and palpates for motion change. An increase in range of motion accompanied by a decrease in resistance to motion represents improved function at a previously hypomobile segment. Changes in range of motion are verified by observing active spinal motions and palpating passive segmental mobility during or after the manipulation. Continuous, ongoing evaluation at the time of manipulation determines the length of time necessary to obtain the desired result. Little experimental evidence exists for identifying the specific amount of time required for an effective manipulative result. Therefore, the therapist must depend on observational and palpatory skills. From a personal standpoint, if a positive response in the form of tissue or motion change is not forthcoming within 3–5 minutes, an alternate strategy is used.

TECHNIQUE CRITERIA

Patient Position

Correct body position of the patient is essential in promoting relaxation as well as ensuring safety and success in the maneuver. Patient comfort brought about by proper positioning either eliminates or reduces muscle activity. A decrease in muscle activity enhances the effectiveness of manipulation, since less resistance is encountered. A nonthrust mobilization to a mid-cervical facet joint that does not glide inferiorly may be perfectly correct in all aspects of technique application, but not tolerated because of the prone position of the patient. Patient relaxation through proper positioning is therefore a prerequisite for use of manipulation. The more relaxed a patient becomes the greater the success in manipulation.

Therapist Position

The therapist's position for manipulation must be comfortable. Balance is necessary to minimize work expenditure in maintaining position. Reducing muscular effort in performing manipulation permits the operator to sense tissue response. Unnecessary physical exertion by the clinician interferes with sensory-motor discrimination and often results in a poor delivery of manipulation. Therapist balance and relaxation can often be achieved by using an adjustable height table. Lowering the table enables the shorter clinician to have control, while raising the table eliminates the bending necessary for the tall clinician.

Hand Placement

Therapeutic hand contact is painless, soft, and yet secure. The art of touch for manipulative therapy determines patient confidence in the clinician. Hand placement onto a painful, readily agitated area should be comfortable. The hand conforms to the area contacted and essentially becomes part of the patient, allowing for sensory reception in both directions. Tension in the hand, wrist, and forearm is easily transmitted to the patient and therefore must be eliminated. The hand serves as a conduit for force delivered centrally from the body, but does not generate force itself. Distal pressure from the fingers, hand, wrist, or forearm distorts one's sensory discrimination and interferes with the ability to alter the procedure as needed.

Accurate placement of the hand for manipulation is achieved by knowledge of surface landmark anatomy and enhanced through visualization of deeper tissue structures. The skilled manual practitioner has "x-ray vision" as well as heightened sensory abilities. Precise contact often determines whether manipulation is tolerated and effective. Special care and understanding is required for the tactile defensive patient. The manual physician or therapist must recognize the possible factors for patient protective behaviors and responses from touch such as may occur with persons who have been physically abused. Despite the therapeutic intent, physical contact applied to a sexually abused patient is frequently not accepted until trust and confidence are established. Acceptance of the manual therapy approach therefore may require many treatment sessions.

Specificity

The specificity of manipulation refers to the exactness of the procedure within the context of the therapeutic goal. If the objective is to restore range of motion to 4 segments of the thoracic spine a one-level directed manipulation may serve no purpose. The specific intent is to mobilize a thoracic region. Conversely, a one-level or joint fixation neighbored by a segmental hypermobility necessitates manipulation specificity so that the hypermobile level does not become unstable.

To facilitate the manipulation action at a specific place, spinal locking procedures are suggested. As indicated previously the uninvolved section of the spine can be locked by joint apposition or soft tissue tension. A tight locking of spinal levels above and below the involved segment will help localize the manipulation. Care is taken during the locking set-up not to elicit a muscle response. However, positioning to lock spinal segments may excite an easily facilitated, protective muscle response, which in turn resists the manipulation.

Some clinicians recommend positioning for the purpose of protecting neighboring segments only to the point of ensuring relaxation of soft tissues and avoiding muscle reactivity. Obviously, untying a knot in a line holding a boat to a dock is more difficult when the line is taut rather than loose. If the same knot were used to tie up a horse, additional tension caused by frightening the horse might further interfere with the attempt to untie. Patient relaxation is therefore a prerequisite to positioning for specificity.

Recruitment of Tissue

The recruitment of tissue during manipulation is accomplished by the development of force. The rate at which force is developed is determined by the goal of manipulation, but it is a function of tissue reactivity. If the goal is to tear an intra-articular adhesion or to facilitate a strong muscle contraction, a quick stretch may help. In the presence of pain with associated reflex muscle contraction a slow, smooth, controlled development of force is required. Forces applied at low, even rates allow the patient to feel comfortable about the procedure. Given a sense of control, the patient is able to relax.

The skill in tissue recruitment during manipulation is largely related to what is called *taking up the slack*. In taking up the slack for the purpose of improving joint mobility the soft tissues in the immediate area are prepared. A slow, steady recruitment of soft tissue gives the therapist constant feedback and brings about a relaxation response. The inhibitory effect obtained by proper tissue recruitment is requisite for successful manipulation.

In addition, the deliberate recruitment of soft tissues enables the clinician to detect the restrictive passive motion barrier accurately and to localize forces. The manner in which a motion barrier is engaged determines how the restriction behaves. A forceful confrontation may result in a guarded tissue behavior whereby the restriction defends itself from outside movement influences. A gentle encounter of the motion barrier which fosters two-way communication is the preferred type of interaction and is promoted by proper tissue recruitment.

Motion Direction

The motion direction for manipulation is chosen on the basis of the type of movement-related problem and the tissue response. As mentioned previously, manipulation can either be direct or indirect, depending on the irritability and duration of the condition. In cases of motion restriction, restoration of movement in the plane(s) of the limitation is the objective. With mechanical instability, motion control is a problem which often leads to inconsistent direction of movement. Instabilities benefit from manual treatment which helps improve the control and direction of movement.

A clinician encountering pain, muscle contraction, or increased resistance to the manipulation should consider a change in force direction. Slight alterations in the direction of manipulation may permit a joint to position properly or move more freely. Forcing a movement through resistance increases the chance of causing additional tissue irritation and frequently results in more restriction.

Traditionally in manipulation the motion direction is either parallel or perpendicular to the joint surfaces. A force directed in the plane of the joint attempts to slide while forces at right angles separate the two surfaces. In reality, a joint disengagement frequently requires force(s) at angles between 0° and 90°. On occasions, a 90° joint compression force may actually produce the unlocking. The difficulty in predicting which specific direction of motion will be permitted in the restricted area necessitates an open minded approach to establish the pathway to motion freedom.

Control

The successful application of any manipulation requires control during the execution of the procedure. The patient must feel secure in order to relax or perform effectively. The area of contact should be sufficient to offer the patient security and knowledge that the procedure is safe. For patients fearful of movement or extremely sensitive to pressure development, the area of contact should be diffuse. For patients requiring specific proprioceptive feedback, contact should be precise and definite. Unlocalized contact for patients in need of exact proprioceptive input will lead to inappropriate responses, such as the use of undesired muscular contraction(s) in PNF.

With the exception of high-velocity manipulation, manipulative movements should be slow, deliberate, and evenly regulated. Irregular movements lacking control are likely to bring about protective responses by excitation of the patient's central nervous system. Smooth, methodical, conforming movements allow for greater sensitivity to tissue response

for the therapist and greater acceptance of movement by the patient.

Amount of Force

The amount of force varies according to many factors: Age, sex, stage of the condition, general health status, type of movement disorder, degree of the dysfunction, personality type of the patient, and manipulative style of the therapist. For example, a fearful, 60-year-old female with an osteoporetic spine and an acute intercostal muscle spasm requires a very gentle manipulative approach. On the other hand, a 20-year-old athlete who compresses a facet joint from an extension injury may respond favorably to a high velocity manipulation. Although it is desirable to have multiple manipulative strategies to employ, a clinician often becomes more proficient in certain types. The amount of force therefore varies with experience. Perhaps the issue is not the amount of force utilized, but whether the patient accepts the pressure. If the force is appropriate, regardless of the amount, movement is facilitated. If the force is inappropriate, regardless of the amount, movement is inhibited.

Adverse reactions to spinal manipulation are more likely when greater force is used, particularly if tissue resistance is not identified. For some, the philosophy is to use as much force as required, but as little as necessary. Others contend that the skill of a therapist is inversely proportional to the amount of force utilized. The higher the skill level the less force is needed. As a general statement, most agree that a safe, effective, physiologic tissue change occurs when slow, even, gentle forces are applied. A therapist involved in manipulative care should be always aware of the first rule of medicine which says *to do no harm*.

Sensitivity to Tissue Response

The key to successful use of manipulative therapy is the clinician's recognition and reaction to tissue response(s) from the manipulation. All biologic tissue possesses an inherent responsiveness to pressure or motion stimuli. If the objective is to achieve a release of tissue tension, then a reduction in tissue tone and muscle tightness should be felt during the maneuver. An increase in tissue tension or the development of a reflex muscle contraction signifies incorrect selection of a manipulation type or improper application. Tissue receptivity to manipulation is therefore an ongoing evaluative process.

The manual therapist determines the duration of a manipulation endeavor by the response of the tissues engaged. Restoration of motion activity, a reduction of soft tissue tension, a release of heat, an improvement in motion control, or an increase in strength are some indicators used to determine when a manipulative procedure has been successful. Relief of pain at the time of a manipulation is always a welcomed response and is also used as a monitoring mechanism.

The skill of a practitioner of manipulation is closely connected to the ability to detect ongoing responses of the body to the imparted stimulus. Failure to recognize and respond to unfavorable tissue reactions often interferes with achieving the desired therapeutic goal. Moreover, an increase in symptoms may result. Conversely, the development of a heightened sensitivity to tissue behavior leads to a greater ability to respond to the needs of the patient.

CONCLUSION

The various forms of manipulation have been identified and defined. The descriptions given for each manipulation are intended to delineate the different types used in manual therapy practice. The indications for use are presented along with suggestions regarding specific problems. Support and rationale is provided for each manipulation type. The principles for successful application of spinal manipulation are also addressed. In addition, the criteria for technique are outlined and described. In summary, this chapter attempts to provide clarification to manipulative therapy by defining terms, identifying rationale for use, and indicating criteria for application.

REFERENCES

1. Hadler NM, Curtis P, Guillings DB, et al. A benefit of spinal manipulation for acute low-back pain: a stratified controlled trial. Spine 1987;12:703–706.
2. Parker GB, Tupling H, Pryor DS. A controlled trial of cervical manipulation for migraine. Aust N Z U Med 1978;8:589–593.
3. Stedman's medical dictionary, 21st Edition. Baltimore: Williams & Wilkins, 1970.
4. Dorland's illustrated medical dictionary, 25th Edition, Philadelphia: W. B. Saunders, 1974.
5. Farfan HF. The scientific basis of manipulative procedures. Clin Rheum Dis 1980;6:159–177.
6. Kappler RE. Direction action techniques. J Am Osteopath Assoc 1981;81:239.
7. Mitchell FL, Moran PS, Pruzzo NA. An evaluation and treatment manual of osteopathic muscle energy technique, Valley Park MO: Mitchell, Moran and Pruzzo Associates, 1979.
8. Greenman PE. Principles of manual medicine. Baltimore: Williams and Wilkins, 1989.
9. Maigne P. The concept of painlessness and opposite motion in spinal manipulation. Am J Phys Med 1965;44:55–69.
10. Maitland GD. Vertebral manipulation, 3rd ed. London: Butterworths, 1973.
11. Paris SV. Introduction to spinal evaluation and manipulation, S-1 course notes, Institute Press, St. Augustine, FL: 1990.
12 Beard G, Wood EC. Massage—principles and techniques. Philadelphia: W. B. Saunders Co., 1964.
13. Ebner M. Connective tissue massage, theory and therapeutic application. Edinburgh: Churchill Livingstone, 1975.
14. Rolf I. Rolfing. Santa Monica, CA: Dennis Landman Publishers, 1977.
15. Rumsey J. Guidelines for acupuncture massage—neck pain. Sports Medicine Section Bulletin of the APTA 1977;4:8–9.
16. Evjenth O, Hamberg J. Muscle stretching in manual therapy. A clinical manual. Vol. II. Sweden: ALFTA Rehab, 1984.
17. Mitchell FL Sr. Structural pelvic function. AAO Yearbook 1958:71–89.
18. Knott M, Voss D. Proprioceptive neuromuscular facilitation, 2nd ed. New York: Harper and Row, 1968.
19. Sherrington C. The integrative action of the nervous system. New Haven: Yale University Press, 1961.
20. Goodridge JP. Muscle energy technique: definition, explanation, methods of procedure. J Am Osteopath Assoc 1981;18:249–254.
21. Kroemer KH. An isoinertial technique to assess individual lifting capability. Hum Factors 1983; 25:493–506.
22. Jones LH. Strain and counterstrain. Colorado Springs, CO: The American Academy of Osteopathy, 1981.

23. Bowles CH. A functional orientation for technic. Yearbook of the Academy of Applied Osteopathy, 1955:177–191.
24. Hoover HW. Functional technique. Yearbook of the Academy of Applied Osteopathy, 1958:47–51.
25. Bowles CH. A functional orientation for technic—Part II. Yearbook of the Academy of Applied Osteopathy, 156:107–114.
26. Bowles CH. Functional technique: a modern perspective. J Am Osteopath Assoc 1981;80:326–331.
27. Bowles CH. A functional orientation for technic—Part III. Yearbook of the Academy of Applied Osteopathy, 1956:53–58.
28. Grieve GP. Modern manual therapy of the vertebral column. New York: Churchill Livingstone, 1986:777–786.
29. Stoddard A. Manual of osteopathic technique, 8th ed., London: Hutchinson & Co, 1974.
30. Jayson MIV, Sims-Williams H, Young S. et al. Mobilization and manipulation for low back pain. Spine, 1981;409–415.
31. Sloop PR, Smith DS, Goldenberg E, et al. Manipulation for chronic neck pain: a double-blind controlled study. Spine 1982;7:532–535.
32. Riches EW. End results of manipulation of the back. Lancet May 3, 1930;957–960.
33. Light KE, Nuzik S, Personius W, et al. Low load prolonged stretch vs high-load brief stretch in treating knee contractions. Phys Ther 1984;64:330.

4

Functional Anatomy of the Spine and Associated Structures[1]

JOHN V. BASMAJIAN

Biomechanics, Body Postures, and Dynamics Associated with Pain and Discomfort

BIOMECHANICS

This branch of mechanics is the science that deals with the motion or non-motion of living matter from molecules to whole organisms including the human body. It is divided, as is the science of mechanics, into *Statics* and *Dynamics*.

Statics deal with conditions in which objects are at rest or in equilibrium, i.e., they may be moving in a straight line at constant speed under the action of balancing forces.

Dynamics, however, come into play when objects are under the action of unbalanced forces that result in movement. In turn dynamics is divided into branches: *kinematics* and *kinetics*.

Kinematics embraces geometric descriptions of motion in terms of displacement, velocity, and acceleration against time without regard to the forces that cause the motion.

Kinetics, however, is specifically concerned with the forces responsible for causing the motion, changing it, or stopping it.

Although the human body has hard and soft parts that as physical structures respond to kinetic forces in different ways, bioengineers, orthopedic specialists, manipulation practitioners, and other kinesiologists ranging from physical therapists and athletic trainers to rolfers and Alexander technique specialists generally accept the bones as being the rigid bodies on which both internal and external forces act to impel all or parts of the body. Of course muscles either move the bones or hold them steady at the joints.

Postures

The definition of posture can be altered for the sake of argument according to how broad or how narrow one wishes to make it. In the narrowest sense, posture may be considered to be the upright, well-balanced stance of the human subject in a "normal" position. In this sense, the EMG of posture would deal with the maintenance of the erect subject's position against the force of gravity. The present account will, of necessity, emphasize this aspect of posture, but a broader, more generous, and more palatable definition would not exclude the multiplicity of normal (and abnormal) standing, sitting, and reclining positions that human beings assume in their constant battle against the force of gravity. In the final analysis, the intrinsic mechanisms of the body that

[1]The illustrations for this chapter are reproduced with permission from Primary Anatomy, 8th edition, by J. V. Basmajian, 1982; © J. V. Basmajian.

counteract gravity make up the essence of the study of posture. One of these, the muscular mechanism, shall be our chief concern.

CENTER OF GRAVITY (CG) AND LINE OF GRAVITY (LG)

Generally CG is accepted for the erect adult to be a central point at the level of the second sacral vertebra, i.e., 5 cm or less behind a line joining the hip joints. A vertical line through it (as traditionally viewed from the side) passes midway between the following bilateral structures: (a) the mastoid processes; (b) a point just in front of the shoulder joints; (c) the hip joints (or just behind); (d) a point just in front of the center of the knee joints; and (e) a point just in front of the ankle joints. Muscular activity is called upon to approximate this posture or, if the body is pulled out of the line of gravity, to bring it back into line.

Because sitting and recumbent postures are so variable in time and space, the CG of the whole body is not of much consequence. However, in seated working postures the CG of the parts that are not in equilibrium between the force of gravity and the support surface(s) influences stresses and strains on the bones, joints, and muscles.

The problems of static posture, then, revolve around the truism that the balance or equilibrium of the human body or its articulated parts depends on a fine neutralization of the forces of gravity by counter-forces. These counter-forces may be supplied most simply both internally and externally by a supporting horizontal surface or series of horizontal surfaces that are inert. The "easiest" posture which a human being can achieve is our normal posture for the first year or so of our lives and for about half of our lives thereafter. When we lie down, we bring the center of gravity of the entire body, as well as any or all of its parts, closest to a supporting antigravitational surface.

Healthy persons who do not tense their muscles can sit comfortably and relax in many positions, and can even work in many different manners without pronounced increase in muscular activity. Nervous subjects do not relax completely in more than a few positions, and they cannot change their individual optimal working positions without a markedly increased exertion of muscle power.[1]

Most people do not appreciate that, among mammals, man has the most economical of antigravity mechanisms once the upright posture is attained. The expenditure of muscular energy for what seems to the student of phylogeny to be a most awkward position is actually extremely economical. Most comparative anatomists certainly seem to be ignorant of this fact. A quadruped that is required to maintain the multiple joints of its limbs in a state of partial flexion by means of muscular activity demonstrates a much more wasteful antigravity machinery. An exception to this seems to be the elephant, whose limbs serve as static columns to maintain an enormous weight. On the other hand, the specialization of the elephant's weight-bearing limbs is so great that it cannot produce a true jump for even short distances. Relative to its size, the muscles of its limbs are quite puny compared with man's. The reason for this disproportion is that, unlike the elephant, man is constantly challenging gravity by his continued wide range of postures, and great power is required simply to achieve them. Thus we find that man's so-called antigravity muscles are not so much to maintain normal standing and sitting postures as they are to produce the powerful movements necessary for the major changes from lying to sitting to standing, and running and climbing. Therefore it is wrong to equate the antigravity muscles of man with those of the common domestic animals which stand on flexed joints.

In man, the column of bones that carries the weight to the ground constitutes a series of links. Ideally, these links should be so stacked that the line of gravity passes directly through the center of each joint between them. But even in man this ideal is only closely approached and is never completely reached—and then only momentarily. A completely passive equilibrium is impossible because the centers of gravity of the links and the movement centers of the joints between them cannot be all brought to coincide perfectly with the common line of gravity. In spite of this, Steindler and many others have greatly exaggerated the amount of effort required to maintain the upright posture. The fatigue of standing is emphatically not due to muscular fatigue and, generally, the muscular activity in standing is slight or moderate. Sometimes it is only intermittent. On the other hand, the posture of quadrupeds, which is maintained by muscles acting on a series of flexed joints, is highly dependent on continuous support by active muscular contraction. Of course, the same is true for the human being in any but the fully erect standing posture.

VERTEBRAL COLUMN

Vertebral Bodies and Intervertebral Discs

Each vertebral *body* is a short, cylindrical block of bone flattened at the back and possessing a slight "waist." Many vertical lamellae of spongy bone in its interior enable it to resist compression; its outer covering of compact bone is very thin. Adjacent bodies are firmly united to one another by an *intervertebral disc* roughly one-fifth to one-third as thick as the neighboring bodies. This disc is composed of concentric rings of fibrocartilage and a central mass of pulpy tissue, the *nucleus pulposus*, which represents the remains of the notochord. The disc, being under pressure, bulges, i.e., it is convex at its periphery. Discs are "shock absorbers" giving resilience to the column, and they are relieved of pressure only when the body is recumbent. Being the nonrigid portion of the column, they also give it its flexibility. When the body is erect and in the "normal" position, the various parts of each disc are under uniform pressure, but when the vertebral column is flexed, extended, or bent sideways, one part of the disc is under increased compression whereas another part of the same disc is under tension.

An *anterior* and a *posterior longitudinal ligament* extend the length of the column, one down the fronts, the other down the backs of the vertebral bodies; they are firmly attached to the discs (which they reinforce), and they guard against excessive movement of the flexible column.

Vertebral Arches

A vertebral arch springs from the upper part of the back of its vertebral body (Fig. 4.1), and each half is made up of two parts: (*a*) a very short rounded bar projecting backward from the body and known as the *pedicle*; and (*b*) an oblong plate with sloping surfaces known as the *lamina*. The lamina is continuous with the pedicle and meets its fellow of the opposite side in the midline. The hole thus framed-in behind each vertebral body is the *vertebral foramen*; the succession of foramina make up the *vertebral canal* in which the spinal cord and its coverings reside.

A typical vertebra begins to ossify before birth from three centers of ossification; these ultimately unite to form the adult bone (Fig. 4.2).

Processes

At the angular junction of pedicle and lamina on each side there are three processes, one upward (superior), one downward (inferior), and one lateral-ward (transverse). The *superior* and *inferior processes* meet and form joints with similar processes from adjacent vertebral arches; their chief function is to prevent undesirable movements between adjoining vertebrae (Fig. 4.3). The *transverse process* is chiefly for attachments of muscles, although in the thoracic region a rib abuts against the transverse process and is steadied by it.

Where the two laminae meet in the midline posteriorly, there projects backward a *spinous process* which is for attachment of muscles.

Intervertebral Foramina

Because a vertebral arch springs from the upper part of its vertebral body, a deep notch is visible below the pedicle when the vertebra is viewed from the side. When two adjacent vertebrae are in position, the notch becomes

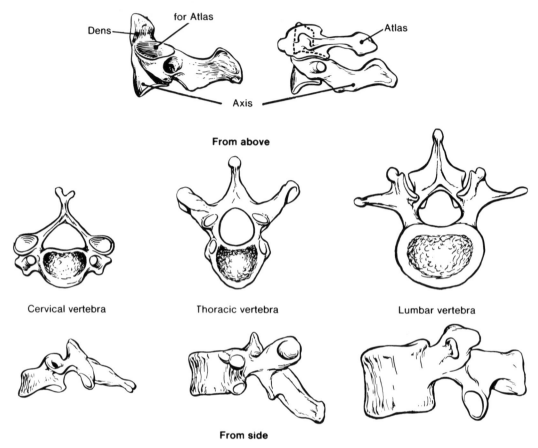

Figure 4.1. Cervical, thoracic, and lumbar vertebrae (from Basmajian[2]).

a hole—the *intervertebral foramen*—which gives exit and entrance to spinal nerves and vessels (Fig. 4.3). The intervertebral foramen is bounded above and below by pedicles; it is bounded in front and behind by joints (intervertebral disc and bodies in front, articular processes and joints behind).

Sacrum

Five vertebral bodies, united by four ossified intervertebral discs, are easily distinguishable on the concave anterior surface of the curved triangular bone that comprises the sacrum. The body of the first of these vertebrae has a prominent, oval, upper surface with a distinctly forward slope. To it is attached a thick disc that unites it to the body of the fifth lumbar vertebra.

Two parallel rows of four pelvic (anterior) *sacral foramina*, in line with intervertebral foramina, serve to separate the sacral vertebral bodies from the parts of the bone lateral to these openings and known as the *lateral masses* (Fig. 4.4). The thick upper part of each lateral mass, smooth above and in front where it is continuous with the side of the first sacral vertebral body, is called the *ala* of the sacrum. On the side of each ala are two areas. In front is a large ear-shaped area by means of which the sacrum articulates with the hip bone on each side. This area is called the *auricular surface* and the articulation is the *synovial sacroiliac joint*. Above it (when the bone is correctly oriented) is an equally large rough area known as the *tuberosity*; it is for a mass of strong, short ligaments that further unite the pelvic girdle to the sacrum and that consti-

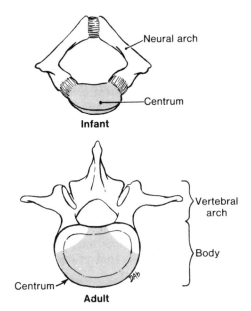

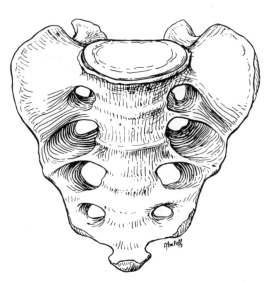

Figure 4.4. Sacrum from front (from Basmajian[2]).

Figure 4.2. Three centers of ossification joined by cartilage form the vertebra in infant. These unite to form an adult vertebra, but the "body" is not the same as the centrum, nor the "vertebral" arch the same as the neural arch (from Basmajian[2]).

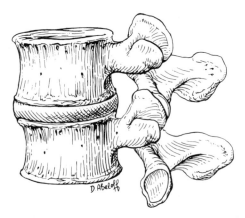

Figure 4.3. Two lumbar vertebrae in articulation. The lower pair of processes grasps the upper and prevents rotation. Note the boundaries of the intervertebral foramen, the exit for a spinal nerve (from Basmajian[2]).

tutes the *fibrous sacroiliac joint*. Below the level of the auricular surface the whole sacrum tapers rapidly since the lower part of the bone bears no weight.

Behind, the bone is convex and much rougher; here the two rows of *dorsal sacral foramina* (in the same vertical plane as the

anterior ones) serve to separate the laminae, which are all fused together, from the lateral mass on each side (Fig. 4.5).

At the upper end of the bone, there projects a pair of large superior articular processes that face one another and embrace the inferior ones of the fifth lumbar vertebra. The triangular upper opening of the sacral canal lies between them and is bounded behind by the paired laminae.

An irregular vertical ridge down the back of the lateral mass of each side represents transverse processes, while a similar ridge medial to the dorsal foramina represents articular processes. Four bony tubercles in the midline represent spinous processes.

At the lower end of the bone, there is a pair of small processes, the *sacral cornua* (horns). Between them is the lower end of the vertebral canal which is closed in life by a tough fibrous membrane.

The extent to which the vertebral (sacral) canal is closed by bone in the lower half of the sacrum is very variable; in other words, the lowest vertebral arches are frequently incomplete or absent.

Coccyx

The irregular coccyx (Fig. 4.5) consists usually of four fused vestigial vertebrae, the first of

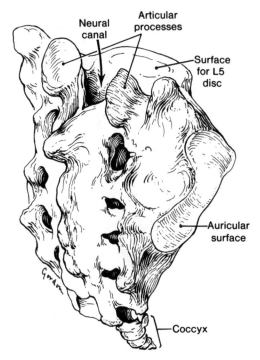

Figure 4.5. Sacrum and coccyx viewed obliquely from behind and right side (from Basmajian[2]).

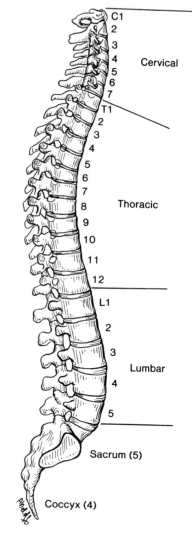

Figure 4.6. Vertebral column from right side. Note intervertebral discs between bodies (from Basmajian[2]).

which is by far the largest. The body of this first coccygeal vertebra is united to the lower end of the sacrum by a fibrocartilaginous intervertebral disc; the vertebral arch is represented by two upwardly projecting horns or *cornua* which meet those of the sacrum. Below this vertebra the bone is nodular and represents the vestigial human tail. It can be felt quite easily in the living person.

FUNCTIONS AND DIFFERENCES IN THE VERTEBRAL COLUMN

Weight-Bearing and Size of Bodies

Weight borne by individual vertebrae increases progressively as the series is descended; vertebral bodies, in consequence, become more massive as they proceed from the cervical to the lumbar region; discs must increase in size in conformity with the bones (Fig. 4.6). (These statements are true only in animals that walk erect; the general tendency among quadrupeds is for vertebrae actually to decrease in size as the column is "descended").

Movements

Movements between individual vertebrae take place (*a*) at the discs and (*b*) at the joints between the (paired) articular processes of the vertebral arches. Movements at the discs are greatest where the discs are thickest; movements at articular processes are greatest where the joint surfaces are largest.

In the lumbar region, both of the above

conditions exist, and here movements are most free. In these lumbar movements, lumbar discs accept considerable strain. If to the normal lumbar movements of flexion, extension, and side-bending, rotary movements were added, the resulting torsion of the discs might be more than they could stand. For this and other reasons, the dispositions of the joints between lumbar articular processes restrict rotation (Fig. 4.3). These joints are "interlocking," i.e., the superior articular processes of the vertebra below grip the outside of the inferior articular processes of the vertebra above. In this region, bending forward and backward can be freely performed; sideways bending is much less free, and rotation is severely limited. Even with this safeguard, lumbar discs rupture more readily than any others.

In the thoracic region, the discs are relatively thin, the opposing surfaces of the articular processes on the vertebral arches are small and flat and face backward and forward; no type of movement is entirely prohibited, yet movements in all planes are slight. Nevertheless, because there are 12 vertebrae in this region, the total mobility between the first and the last is considerably greater than might be thought. The transition from the more mobile lumbar vertebrae to the less mobile thoracic vertebrae is unfortunately rather abrupt, and it is the 11th or the 12th thoracic vertebra that is most commonly fractured.

In the cervical region, the discs are relatively thicker than those in the thoracic region, and the articular surfaces of the processes—facing at first upward and downward but gradually changing to a forward and backward direction—are small but relatively larger also. Thus, the seven cervical vertebrae permit movement in all planes as do the thoracic ones, but the range is considerably greater. In addition to their rather free movements of flexion, extension, and side-bending, the cervical vertebrae engage in movements of rotation (twisting or torsion). It has been observed, however, that such a combination of movements throws excessive strain on the discs. Perhaps this accounts for why the periphery of the upper surface of a typical cervical vertebral body is built-up markedly at the sides and slightly at the back; it slopes away in front (Fig. 4.7).

The first and second cervical vertebrae are very specially modified, for they carry the skull and aid in its movements. They will be discussed separately, below.

Vertebral Foramina

The caliber of the spinal cord varies very little from end to end, but it has two local enlargements associated with the sites of origin of the great nerves destined for the upper and for the lower limbs: these are the cervical and lumbar enlargements. With these facts in mind it is easy to understand why it is that: (*a*) the vertebral foramina are relatively and actually large in the cervical region, where they are also triangular; (*b*) they are small and circular in the thoracic region; and (*c*) they are actually, but not relatively, large in the

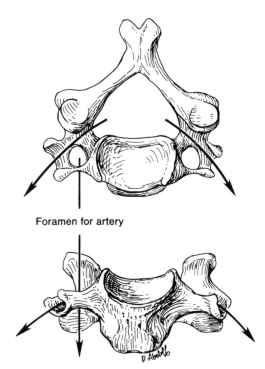

Figure 4.7. A cervical vertebra from above and from in front (see text). Curved arrows lie in gutters for spinal nerves (from Basmajian[2]).

Foramen for artery

lumbar region where, again, they are triangular.

Transverse Processes and Joints for Ribs

A very special feature distinguishes the thoracic vertebrae: they carry the ribs. The head of a rib meets the vertebral column at the side of a disc and at the adjacent edges of two vertebral bodies. In its excursion around the trunk, the rib at first sweeps backward to abut against the front of the tip of a transverse process. The presence, therefore, of little joint surfaces, the one on the body and the other on the transverse process, proclaims a vertebra to be rib-bearing and thoracic.

A special feature distinguishes cervical vertebrae also. Each transverse process has a hole or foramen in it, the bar of bone in front of the foramen being, in effect, an undeveloped rib (Fig. 4.7). This "rib" is in line with the true ribs in the thoracic region, so that the foramen obviously is the space between the rib and the transverse process in the thorax. Through the series of foramina, vessels (vertebral artery and vein) thread their way upward to aid ultimately in the blood supply of the brain. Lateral to the foramen, the issuing spinal nerve rests in a bony gutter formed by the two elements of the compound transverse process.

Sometimes one of the normally undeveloped ribs (usually the seventh) becomes greatly enlarged and like a true rib—a "cervical rib," which may cause symptoms.

Spinous Processes

The "spines" are anchors and levers. They are distinctive for each region: cervical ones have double tips, i.e., they are bifid; thoracic ones are long, slender, pointed, and tend to project more downward than backward; lumbar ones are massive, square-cut, and project straight backward.

Curves of the Vertebral Column

During intrauterine life, the body of the fetus is noticeably flexed, and this applies to the vertebral column as well as to the other structures. Soon, two primary curves, both with their concavities forward, are recognizable, one involving the presacral vertebrae, the other the sacrum itself.

In a structure such as the vertebral column, which is built up of superimposed bodies and discs, these curves must be expressions of differences in thickness between the fronts and the backs of the individual bodies and discs. Furthermore, when it is the bones (bodies) that are chiefly concerned, the curve is likely to be permanent; when the discs also or alone are concerned the resulting curve can be temporarily abolished.

The two permanent or primary curves persist as thoracic and sacral (pelvic). The *secondary curves* develop in the cervical and lumbar regions, and the relatively thick discs that these regions possess take a considerable part in the curves. These secondary curves are convex forward and are subject to temporary elimination. The cervical curve would seem to develop in response to the need for holding the head up. The lumbar curve develops so that the center of gravity of the body will not lie in a plane in front of the hip joints during the sitting or standing positions.

Where the last lumbar vertebra (fifth) meets the sacrum there is an abrupt change; this is provided for by the last lumbar vertebral body and especially by the fact that the last lumbar disc is much thicker in front than behind, i.e., they are wedge-shaped. Occasionally, an accident occurs here, and the lumbar body (fourth and fifth) slips forward—spondylolisthesis; the accident is said to be due to a developmental failure of the neural arch to be fixed to its body, but because the separation is rarely (if ever) at the site of union of arch and body, it seems more probable that it is due to a bilateral fracture of the arch. The fifth lumbar vertebra is often "sacralized" (bodies united by bone) in older persons.

The normal curvatures of the column are rather more pronounced in the female than in the male, and in both sexes there is usually a slight lateral curvature to one side said to be associated with right- or left-handedness. An excessive lateral curvature is known as scoliosis.

ATLAS AND AXIS

The first cervical vertebra, the atlas, has lost its body and consists simply of a ring of bone made up of two *lateral masses* joined in front and behind by the *anterior* and *posterior arches of the atlas* (Fig. 4.8). The upper surface of each lateral mass is elliptical, concave, and articular. The long axis of the ellipse runs mainly anteroposteriorly, but the two ellipses are so placed that they are nearer one another in front than behind, i.e., the anterior arch is shorter than the posterior. On the concave surfaces of the lateral masses, the occipital condyles rock and slide in the nodding movement of "Yes." The lower surface of each lateral mass is circular, flat, and articular and rests on a similar surface of the axis.

Lateral to each lateral mass is the very large and widely set transverse process, containing the foramen previously noted as transmitting the vertebral vessels. This process projects so far laterally that it may be felt on deep pressure behind the mandible just below the ear.

Medial to each lateral mass and encroaching somewhat on the anterior part of the very

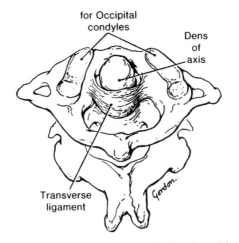

Figure 4.8. Atlas and axis in articulation viewed from behind and above (from Basmajian[2]).

large vertebral foramen, there is a pronounced tubercle to which is attached the very strong *transverse ligament of the atlas* stretching to the tubercle on the other side. The vertebral foramen is divided by this ligament into a smaller anterior compartment and a larger posterior one.

The second cervical vertebra, appropriately named the axis, is distinguished by a blunt, tooth-like process, the *dens* or odontoid process, projecting upward from the body (Figs. 4.1 and 4.8). It is in reality the body of the atlas which has become divorced from the atlas and has joined the body of the axis. This dens projects upward into the anterior compartment of the vertebral foramen of the atlas and provides a mechanism, consisting of a pivot and a collar, whereby the head and atlas can rotate around the dens in the "No" movement. On each side of the dens is a large, flat, and circular joint surface for the support and rotation of the atlas.

The *foramen magnum* in the midline of the base of the skull lies halfway between the posterior edge of the palate and the inion. Its outline is made rather pear-shaped by the encroachment of the paired *occipital condyles* on the sides of its anterior half. These oval lumps of bone have a smooth inferior surface which is convex from front to back and give the impression of a pair of rockers from a rocking chair. They rest in concavities on the upper surface of the first cervical vertebra and by sliding back and forth produce much of the nodding motion of the head signifying "Yes."

JOINTS OF THE VERTEBRAL COLUMN

Two series of joints unite the individual vertebrae of the spinal column: (*a*) the fibrocartilaginous joints (synchondroses) uniting adjacent bodies, and (*b*) the synovial joints uniting adjacent vertebral arches. Because synchondroses are functionally more limited in their movements than synovial joints, it follows that the extent of movement enjoyed by the joints of the vertebral arches is primar-

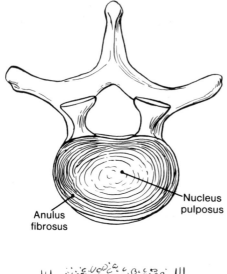

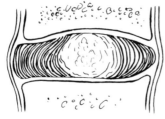

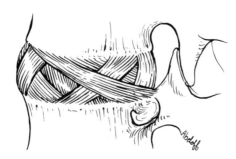

Figure 4.9. Cross-section and vertical cut surface of a lumbar intervertebral disc and a dissection of outer obliquely crossing fibers of annulus fibrosus (from Basmajian[2]).

ily determined by the extent of movement permitted at the discs (Fig. 4.9).

Special Ligaments

The *anterior* and *posterior longitudinal ligaments*, binding the fronts and the backs of the vertebral bodies to one another throughout the length of the column have been noted earlier. The vertebral arches possess restrain-

ing ligaments also. One group consists of the *ligamenta flava*—so called because they are rich in yellow elastic fibers—and they stretch between the adjacent laminae of the vertebral arches; being elastic these ligaments tend to restore the spinal column to a neutral position after it has been flexed. They also serve, with the laminae, to cover the spinal cord posteriorly and so protect the contained spinal cord. A second group unites adjacent spinous processes as *interspinous ligaments*. Contiguous with these posteriorly are longer fibers which stretch the length of several spines and are, in consequence, *supraspinous ligaments*. These have the same effect as the ligamenta flava. Undoubtedly, they relieve the back muscles of considerable work.

In the neck, the supraspinous ligaments are so enlarged as to produce a midline ligamentous partition separating the thick muscles of one side of the back of the neck from those of the other. It is known as the *ligamentum nuchae* (L. = of neck).

JOINTS OF THE RIBS

Synovial joints occur at the heads and the tubercles of the ribs (Fig. 4.10). The capsule of each is thickened in front and is known as a *radiate ligament* because it fans from the rib head (or costal cartilage) to the adjacent vertebral bodies and disc (or sternum). In the interior of each joint is an *intra-articular* ligament that binds the head (or costal cartilage) to the disc (or sternum) and divides the cavity into upper and lower compartments.

The synovial joint at the rib tubercle occurs where the rib, in its backward sweep, abuts against the transverse process of the vertebra with which it numerically corresponds. Each small joint is reinforced, and the rib more firmly bound to the transverse process, by two ligaments, one on each side of the joint. The strong medial one is simply called the *costotransverse ligament* (or *ligament of the neck*); it lies horizontally disposed, and it fills the space between the back of the neck of the rib and front of the adjacent transverse process of the vertebra. The lateral one is the *lateral costotransverse ligament* (or *ligament of*

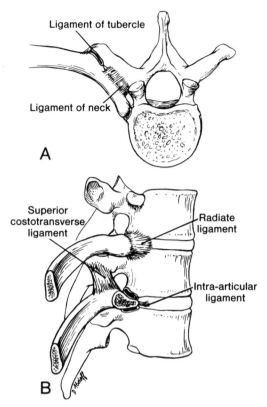

Figure 4.10. Joints and ligaments between ribs and vertebrae **A,** from above; **B,** from side (from Basmajian[2]).

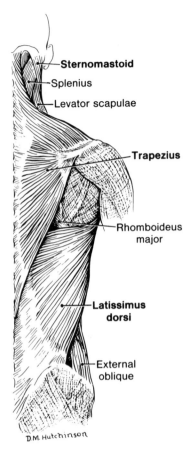

Figure 4.11. These large upper limb muscles (extrinsic muscles of back) cover intrinsic muscles of back (from Basmajian[2]).

the tubercle); it is a short but strong cord that passes horizontally lateralward from the tip of the transverse process to the back of the rib just beyond the tubercle. A third and rectangular ligament stretches vertically from the neck of the rib to the transverse process next above. It often produces a flange on the neck of the rib and is known as the *superior costotransverse ligament.*

The heads of ribs 1, 11, and 12 reach the spinal column not at the side of a disc but at the side of vertebral bodies 1, 11, and 12.

MUSCLES OF THE AXIAL SKELETON
Muscles of the Vertebral Column

Dorsal or Posterior. When the muscles of the upper limb girdle (Fig. 4.11) are removed from the back, the underlying intrinsic muscles are seen to occupy a pair of broad gutters situated one on each side of the vertebral spines and extending laterally as far as the angles of the ribs, the transverse processes of the cervical vertebrae, and the mastoid process. The territory is limited above by the under, horizontal surface of the occipital bone at the back of the head; below it is limited by the back of the sacrum and by the posterior spines of the iliac crests which project somewhat behind the sacrum. The muscles are covered behind by a tough sheet of fascia coextensive with them, and when this is removed the paired muscular columns are exposed (see Figs. 4.12–4.15).

Here, there are scores of muscles or muscle bundles, but they can be organized into more or less definite groups. First of all, the mass of intrinsic muscles is divided into a superficial and a deep group.

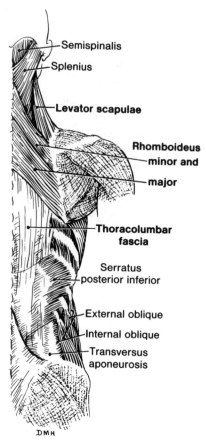

Figure 4.12. Next layer of extrinsic muscles of back. Intrinsic muscles partly revealed (from Basmajian[2]).

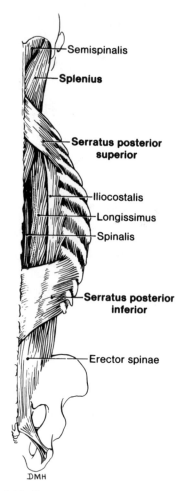

Figure 4.13. Erector spinae and its immediate relations (from Basmajian[2]).

Erector spinae is the name for the *superficial group*. It arises by a strong aponeurosis from the back of the sacrum and adjacent parts of the iliac crest as a single muscle. As the fibers mount the vertebral column, they extend over several segments and in general divide into three columns: (*a*) a lateral one inserted into (and helping to form) the posterior angles of the ribs and, after many overlapping relays of muscle bundles, reaching the cervical transverse processes—*iliocostalis*; (*b*) a middle column inserting into thoracic transverse processes and, after similar relays on cervical transverse processes, reaching the mastoid process—*longissimus* (L. = longest, see Figs. 4.13, 4.14, 4.16); (*c*) confined to the thoracic region is a small column lying medial to the

above-named ones and alongside the tips of the spinous processes to which it attaches—*spinalis*.

The *deep group*, collectively named the *transversospinalis*, lies deep to longissimus along most of the length of the vertebral column. In reality, it consists of a multitude of small muscles in (two or) three layers, whose fibers all run obliquely from the region of transverse processes to the region of spinous processes. Naturally, the muscles of the deepest layer—*rotatores*—have the shortest span, running from one lamina to the next. The most superficial layer, *semispinalis*, is not found below the thoracic region; its bundles have the longest spans (three to six vertebrae), and the upper ones reach the occipital bone. Between these two is a fleshy muscle, *multifidus*, which begins below from the sacrum (deep to the aponeurosis of erector spinae) and, by short relays (two to three vertebrae), it finally reaches the first cervical spinous process (see Fig. 4.15).

Until now we have ignored three superficial muscles, each of which partly covers the large mass of muscle described above: (*a*) *splenius*, (*b*) *serratus posterior superior*, and (*c*) *serratus posterior inferior* (Fig. 4.13; (*a*) is described below; (*b*) and (*c*) are muscles of the thorax.

Muscles at Back of Neck

Just below the skull, several massive muscles fill in the back of the neck where they are separated from their fellows of the opposite side by the *ligamentum nuchae*, already described. The two most important are the *splenius* (L. = a bandage) (Figs. 4.13, 4.15) and the *semispinalis capitis* (Fig 4.14). They arise from lower cervical and upper thoracic verte-

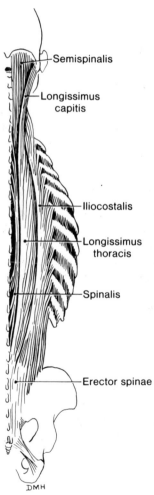

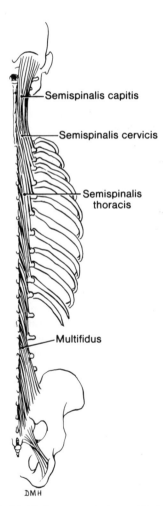

Figure 4.14 Superficial layer of erector spinae splitting into its three columns of muscles as it ascends (from Basmajian[2]).

Figure 4.15. Oblique muscle layers deep to superficial layer. (Rotatores, the deepest layer, not seen.) (from Basmajian[2]).

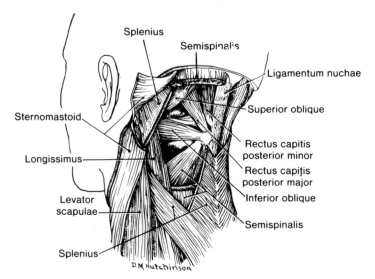

Figure 4.16. Dissection of suboccipital region of the left side (from Basmajian[2]).

bral arches and are inserted on the skull, the splenius running obliquely to the mastoid process and adjacent occipital bone, the semispinalis running vertically to the occipital bone and, with its fellow, covering deeper and smaller muscles now to be noted.

Muscles of Suboccipital Region (Fig. 4.16)

On each side, they are:

1. Obliquus capitis inferior (inferior oblique)—running almost horizontally lateralward from the spine of the axis to the transverse process of the atlas.
2. Obliquus capitis superior (superior oblique)—running almost horizontally backward (in the sagittal plane) from the transverse process of the atlas to the occipital bone.
3. Rectus capitis posterior major—running upward and backward from the spine of the axis to the occipital bone.
4. Rectus capitis posterior minor—insignificant, lying deep and medial to 3, and running from the "spine" (posterior tubercle) of the atlas to the occipital bone.

The first three form a triangle (suboccipital triangle).

Nerve Supply

All of the intrinsic muscles of the back are supplied by posterior branches of the spinal nerves which issue in series from the intervertebral foramina.

Ventral or Anterior Vertebral Muscles

The muscles on the fronts of the vertebral bodies are found only in the neck and in the lumbar region.

On each side of the midline a flat muscle known as the *longus cervicis* clings to the fronts of the bodies of the cervical and upper three thoracic vertebrae; it runs in relays to the atlas (Fig. 4.17). Lateral to the upper part of the longus cervicis, another muscle, the *longus capitis*, runs from the cervical transverse processes to the occipital bone in front of the foramen magnum. Uniting the anterior arch of the atlas to the occipital bone directly above is a pair of short quadrangular muscles on each side, the medial one being the *rectus capitis anterior*, the lateral one, the *rectus capitis lateralis*.

In the lumbar region a powerful muscle, the *psoas major* arises from the sides of the lumbar vertebrae and is inserted on the femur. It is a composite muscle much more concerned with femoral movements than with

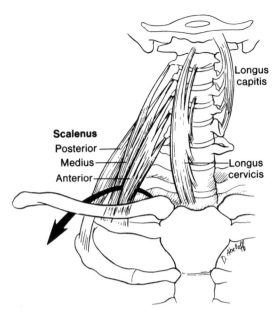

Figure 4.17. Left longus capitis; right longus cervicis; and the right scalene muscles—anterior, medius, and posterior. Arrow indicates course of subclavian artery between scalenus anterior and scalenus medius (from Basmajian[2]).

vertebral, as proved by electromyographic studies.[1]

Nerve Supply. The ventral muscles all are supplied by the anterior branches (rami) of the spinal nerves in their vicinity.

ACTIONS AND FUNCTIONS OF MUSCLES OF THE BACK

It is obvious that the dorsal muscles extend or straighten the column and that their unilateral actions assist in bending the column to the same side.[1]

The *multifidus* and other oblique muscles associated with it are concerned with local movements of the vertebral column, e.g., rotary movement (twisting) of groups of vertebrae. The *splenius* and *semispinalis capitis* extend the head and, if contracting without their fellows of the opposite side, turn the head, tilting the chin up and to the same side. The ventral muscles of the neck flex both the neck and the head. Their unilateral actions help turn the chin down and to the other side.[1]

All of the small suboccipital group extend the head, but the inferior oblique also turns the face to the same side.

A great many other muscles situated far afield also have important actions on the vertebral column. For example, the whole "rectus" group flexes the column; unilateral action of the oblique muscles of the abdominal wall bends the trunk to the same side and twists it to the opposite side. In short, almost any muscle, one of whose attachments is to the axial skeleton, can directly or indirectly influence the vertebral column.[1]

In walking, the vertical muscle masses on the two sides of the vertebral column contract alternately. Those on the same side as the foot that is leaving the ground are contracting while those on the opposite side may or may not also contract; sometimes the imbalance of activity is the reverse, for no apparent reason.[1]

The *posture of the vertebral column,* including the neck, is regulated by the intrinsic muscles of the back, but, contrary to a widely held belief, these muscles are not the prime movers, nor are they necessarily all in constant activity.[3] During relaxed standing most of the muscles are only slightly active most of the time. Individual groups become more active when balance is threatened. When one holds a moderate forward-bending position, the muscles become very active. They relax completely when one bends the back as far forward as possible because the ligaments of the vertebral column assume the load. Muscles are never used where ligaments suffice.[1]

RELATED MUSCLES OF THE NECK

Scalene and Sternomastoid Muscles

There are three scalenes (Gr. = uneven) on each side, *scalenus anterior, scalenus medius,* and *scalenus posterior* (Figs. 4.17, 4.18). The scalenus anterior arises by tendinous slips from the fronts of the transverse processes of the cervical vertebrae (except the highly modified atlas and axis). The slips fuse into a flat muscle which descends obliquely lateralward to be inserted into the upper surface of the first rib.

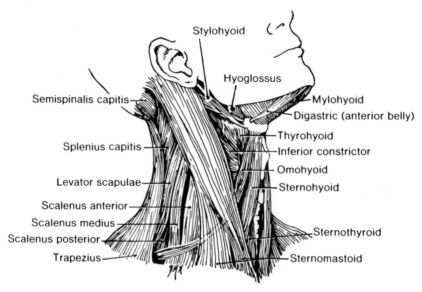

Figure 4.18. Muscles of front and side of neck (from Basmajian[2]).

The *scalenus medius*, rather larger than the scalenus anterior, arises from the backs of the same transverse processes plus that of the axis. It then runs parallel to, but behind, the anterior; it also is inserted into the upper surface of the first rib. The scalenus posterior is but the posterior part of the medius, and its fibers reach the second rib.

Regarding movements of the neck, the scalenes pale into insignificance beside the sternomastoids. Their greatest and most important use is to suspend the thoracic inlet and to maintain its level; they raise the first rib and indirectly the lower ribs during the inspiratory phase of breathing, being particularly active in forced inspiration.[1]

The sterno(cleido)mastoid (Fig. 4.18) runs obliquely down the neck and stands out like a heavy cord when the face is turned to the opposite side. When right and left sternomastoids contract simultaneously, the head and neck are flexed. Unilateral contraction tilts the chin up and to the other side—the position assumed in torticollis (wryneck), due to shortness or spasm of one sternomastoid. The sternomastoid usually does not initiate the simple turning of the head to one side; as a rule it comes into action only during the later part of that movement.

STUDIES OF EMG AND SPINAL MOBILITY

Quantification of back muscle activity in normal subjects was enlarged upon in our study designed to obtain normative back mobility and activity from the erector spinae muscles.[3] It offers clinicians at least one method for assessing dynamic low-back movements in normal or patient populations. A total of 112 adult men and women without histories of chronic low back pain, traumatic back pathology, scoliosis, or degenerative disc disease associated with pain or movement limitations served as normal subjects. They were grouped by sex within decades. Both range of motion and EMG evaluations were performed once per subject. Occasionally, repeated measurements were undertaken when some doubt existed concerning the accuracy or fluidity of dynamic movements.

EMG electrode placements were determined from measurements made on dissected cadaver material. The lower electrode pair rested on the fascial cleft separating the more medial multifidus muscle from the longissimus, while the upper pair were positioned on the longissimus. Therefore, recordings made from the upper electrode pair reflected activity levels of the longissimus muscle, while EMG recorded from the other electrode pair showed the activity from (at least) the longissimus and multifidus muscles.

Range-of-Motion Measurements

Straight Leg Raising (SLR). There was no significant interaction between age and sex during SLR activities; however, women showed more mobility than men across ages for both left (p < 0.02) and right (p < 0.02) legs. Mean active hip flexion measurements indicate that women had greater mobility than their male counterparts, while men in the 30- to 39-year group had bilateral limitation in SLR movements (Fig. 4.19).

Spinal Forward Flexion (Vertebral Separation). Increases in distance between the seventh cervical and first sacral spinal processes were recorded in centimeters during full forward trunk flexion with maintained

knee extension. Analysis of variance by age and sex did not indicate significant interaction, but a sex effect was present, with men showing a significantly greater increase in intervertebral distance during flexion (p < 0.008). As seen in Fig. 4.20, men showed larger changes than women, and the oldest subjects showed the least amount of intervertebral separation.

Trunk Rotation. Neither a significant sex-age interaction nor a significant main effect could be detected during trunk rotation to the left or right. Figure 4.21 graphically shows that men and women of different ages performed this movement similarly.

Lateral Bending. The mean values for lateral bending to the left and right are plotted in Fig. 14.22. Analysis of variance revealed a significant sex-age interaction. Significant differences between sexes occurred in the 30- to 39-year age groups upon bending to the left (p < 0.05) or the right (p < 0.02).

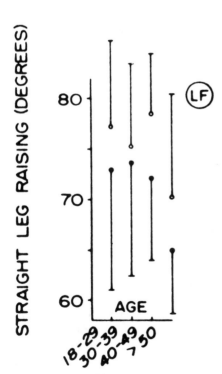

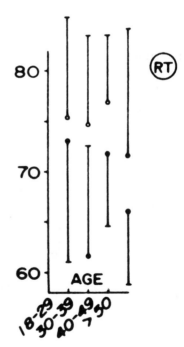

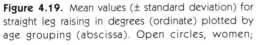

Figure 4.19. Mean values (± standard deviation) for straight leg raising in degrees (ordinate) plotted by age grouping (abscissa). Open circles, women; closed circles, men. Abbreviation: Lf = left; Rt = right (from Wolf et al.[3]).

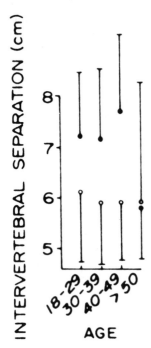

Figure 4.20. Mean values (± standard deviation) for intervertebral separation, measured in centimeters between spinous processes C7-S1 during trunk flexion (ordinate) plotted by age grouping (abscissa). Open circles, women; closed circles, men (from Wolf et al.[3]).

Electromyographic (EMG) Measurements

Repeated measures of EMG activity from specific electrode placements produced no significant trial effect. These findings suggest that the methodology of guiding subjects' movements would result in consistently reproducible integrated EMG readings during multiple trials using the same electrodes.

Trunk Flexion-Extension. Findings for the difference in EMG activity in full-trunk flexion versus extension were consistent among all subjects at each electrode placement. As expected, extension EMG activity always exceeded activity during trunk movements ($p < 0.001$). Additionally, the magnitude of these differences was not the same for each age group, and a significant age-sex interaction was obtained for differences recorded at electrode placements ($p < 0.05$). Multiple comparison tests revealed that for all

electrode placements the magnitude of difference between flexion and extension EMG was significantly greater ($p < 0.05$) in men than in women in the 18- to 29-year age group. EMG silence was observed when 70° of trunk flexion was exceeded and most commonly was seen between 80°–90°. This observation could be made from any electrode placement. EMG activity usually resumed after 20° of extension from the fully flexed trunk position, but occurred anywhere from 90°–30° of flexion.[3]

Lateral Rotation (Standing). At one placement, the differential EMG produced a significantly negative mean score while at the second, left minus right EMG values were significantly positive and at the third and fourth, significant differences in EMG turning were not detected. Furthermore, the differences in EMG during rotation were statistically dissimilar in magnitude for men and women in the 18- to 29-year age group at the first placements ($p < 0.003$) and the second ($p < 0.0001$).

Lateral Rotation (Sitting). The results were mixed among the sex and age groups, showing neither a significant age-sex interaction nor a significant age or sex effect within group.

Bending at the Knees (Stooping). All electrode placements revealed consistent findings. Significant age-sex interactions were observed ($p < 0.005$), and the youngest group of women had significantly higher levels of EMG activity than their male counterparts ($p < 0.01$).

Quiet Sitting. There were no significant differences in EMG activity between men and women within any age group.

Summary of Normative Study[3]

This group was characterized by people whose lifestyle was primarily sedentary (even compared to older men) which might account for lower range-of-motion values (Figs. 4.19, 4.20, 4.22). Hence, consideration of occupation and activity patterns must be incorporated into the establishment of any normative

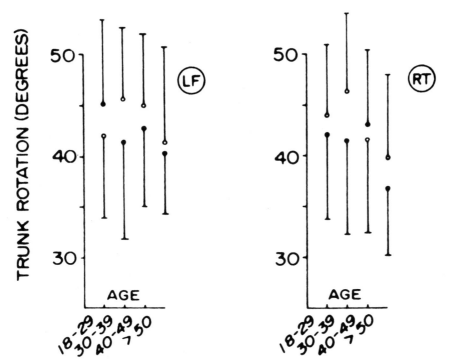

Figure 4.21. Mean values (± standard deviation) for trunk rotation in degrees (ordinate) plotted by age grouping (abscissa). Open circles, women; closed circles, men. Abbreviation: Lf = left; Rt = right (from Wolf et al.[3]).

mobility profile. Generally, our mobility measurements are compatible with standards reported by other clinicians, with women showing slightly greater movement than men. A significant sex effect was found during vertebral separation in trunk flexion, probably attributable to the greater excursion and larger morphology in men. Both straight leg raising and lumbar spinal flexion produced lower values than reported elsewhere. These limitations are probably due to tight (shortened) hamstring muscles which would restrict both movements.

Lateral bending movements produces significant sex-age interactions, and thus men and women should not be grouped within a specific age range. Because significant differences in movement to one side, but not the other, were observed in some groups and because none of our subjects showed a noticeable scoliosis or discrepancy in leg lengths our findings might be attributable to measurement error. Nonetheless, the mean ranges by

sex and age group are in accord with other reports.

Movements during which EMG recordings were made can be divided into dynamic (trunk flexion=extension, lateral rotation-standing, and bending at knees) and static (quiet sitting and lateral rotation-sitting) activities. Significant sex-age interaction were observed for all dynamic activities while such occurrences were not observed during static activities. Therefore, the clinician should not group all subjects when establishing normative EMG data during these dynamic movements. On the other hand, data from men and women can be combined by age groupings during quiet sitting or rotation in a sitting position.

The significantly greater EMG activity observed in trunk extension versus flexion confirms previous EMG studies on the function of the erector spinae muscle group. That the magnitude of differences between flexion and extension EMG was significantly greater in men than women at ages 18–29, might easily be attributed to the selective differences in erector spinae muscle mass for these men. Furthermore, relative quiescence in EMG activity after 70° of trunk flexion, as recorded from all electrode placements, confirms the observations already noted that ligamentous structures, not the erector spinae, support the fully flexed lumbar vertebral column.

During lateral rotation movements while standing and with the hips manually stabilized, the findings suggest that the erector spinae muscles serve to maintain the upright posture, in harmony with the gluteus maximus, and stabilize the back during rotatory movements to the opposite side.

While our subjects necessarily bent at the knees in performing the stooping motion, the posture of the back and trunk varied considerably. This variation might well account for the sex-age interactions. Several members of our youngest women group did stoop with only moderate trunk flexion, perhaps 10°–20°. This positioning will strongly activate the

erector spinae muscle group and might account for the higher EMG levels for women in this age group.

The prospects for expanding the present findings appear promising. Still to be documented are patterns of EMG activity from the hip extensors or abdominal muscles. Differences in EMG levels or patterns from these muscle groups during dynamic movements in a normal population versus a back pain patient population might produce additional treatment strategies.

Comparison of Surface and Inserted Electrodes

Because there are some discrepancies between electrode techniques, Lois Wolf and her colleagues[4] recorded bilateral lumbar muscle activity with both techniques during various movements (flexion, extension, rotations, and side-bends). Ten women with normal backs were the subjects. Both surface and inserted fine-wire electrodes yielded a symmetric ac-

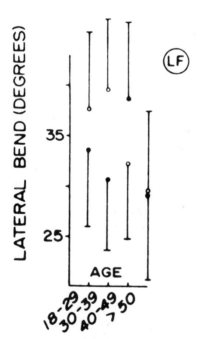
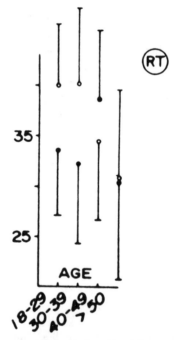
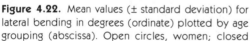

Figure 4.22. Mean values (± standard deviation) for lateral bending in degrees (ordinate) plotted by age grouping (abscissa). Open circles, women; closed circles, men. Abbreviation: Lf = left; Rt = right (from Wolf et al.[3]).

tivity during extension. During rotations, fine-wire electrodes revealed symmetric activity (as shown in earlier studies by Donisch and Basmajian[1]), but surface electrodes recorded bilateral symmetry. The activity of the contralateral side was registered during side-bending. These findings suggest that the "cross-talk" effects from adjacent muscles contaminate some surface-electrode results and must be guarded against.

INTERACTION OF MUSCLES AND FASCIA

A number of provocative new views have been expressed about the dynamics of the spine during the past decade.[5] Bogduk,[6] found that erector spinae components are biomechanically not in a position to extend the spinal column forcefully, and only multifidus could contribute significantly as an extensor. In later work, Bogduk[7] emphasized the role of the thoracolumbar fascia and its closely related aponeuroses of origin of the latissimus dorsi and transversus abdominis. These broad, tough sheets blend with the fascia which split to ensheathe the paravertebral muscles. Gracovetsky and Farfan[8,9] went further to elaborate a mathematical model that depends on the tough but "passive" role during lifting of these sheets of connective tissue attached to the bones.

RECUMBENT POSTURE

Let us now turn to the recumbent posture, which we assume for one-third of our lives. Here, in this pleasantest of postures, the force of gravity is counteracted by mechanisms that are entirely passive. Repeated EMG studies by many investigators have demonstrated beyond the shadow of a doubt that resting muscles exhibit no neuromuscular activity.[1]

MUSCLE TONE AND RELAXATION

Most muscle physiologists now agree that electromyography shows conclusively the

complete relaxation of normal human striated muscle at rest. In other words, by relaxing a muscle, a normal human being can abolish neuromuscular activity in it. This does not mean that there is no "tone" (or "tonus") in skeletal muscle, as some enthusiasts have claimed. It does mean, however, that the definition of "tone" should include both the passive stiffness of muscular (and fibrous) tissues

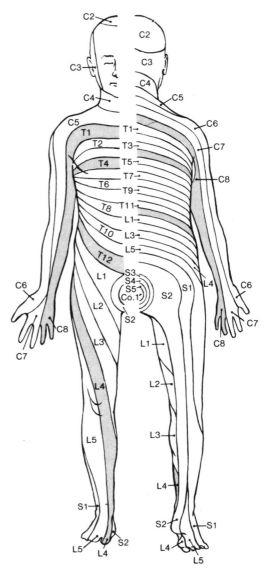

Figure 4.23. Dermatomes: the strips of skin supplied by the various levels or segments of the spinal cord (from Basmajian[2]).

and the active (although not continuous) contraction of muscle in response to the reaction of the nervous system to stimuli. Thus, at complete rest, a muscle has not lost its tone, even though there is no neuromuscular activity in it.[1]

In the clinical appreciation of tone, the more important of the above two elements is the reactivity of the nervous system. One can hardly palpate a normal limb without causing such a reaction. Therefore, the clinician soon learns to evaluate the level of "tone," and it may seem of little consequence to him that the muscle he is feeling is, in fact, capable of complete neuromuscular inactivity. In spite of this, he would be surprised to learn that an experienced subject can simulate hypotonia or even atonia of lower motor neuron disease and successfully deceive—if only for a brief period—the most astute physician.

DERMATOMES AND MYOTOMES

The human torso shows evidence of its segmental development in that its nerve supply is by an orderly series of spinal nerves. The strip-like area of skin supplied by one pair of spinal nerves is known as a dermatome (Gr. = skin-slice), and these dermatomes have been mapped by different investigators by varying techniques and with somewhat varying results. In Figure 4.23, it will be noted that there is a regular sequence of dermatomes on the

limbs, too, because the limbs are outgrowths from the torso in the cervical and lumbosacral regions. All clinicians dealing with patients having nerve injuries must be familiar with the general pattern of the dermatomes.

Although the segmental origin of skeletal muscles and their nerves is less apparent, the myotomes (Gr. = muscle slices), which parallel the dermatomes in general distribution, can be traced and are important, too.

REFERENCES

1. Basmajian JV, DeLuca CJ. Muscles alive: their functions revealed by electromyography. 5th ed. Baltimore: Williams & Wilkins, 1985.
2. Basmajian JV. Primary anatomy, 8th ed. Baltimore: Williams & Wilkins, 1982.
3. Wolf SL, Basmajian JV, Russe CTC, et al. Normative data on low back mobility and activity levels. Am J Phys Med 1979;58:218.
4. Wolf LB, Segal R, Wolf SL, Nyberg R. Quantitative analysis of surface and percutaneous electromyographic activity in lumbar erector spinae in normal young women. Spine 1991;18:155–161.
5. Singer KP, Giles LGF, Day RE. Intra-articular synovial folds of thoracolumbar junction zygaphophyseal joints. Anat Rec 1990;226:147–152.
6. Bogduk N. A reappraisal of the anatomy of the human erector spinae. J Anat 1980;131:525.
7. Bogduk N, Twomey LT. Clinical anatomy of the lumbar spine, New York: Churchill Livingstone, 1987.
8. Gracovetsky S, Farfan H. The optimum spine. Spine 1986;11:543.
9. Gracovetsky S. The spinal engine, New York: Springer-Verlag, 1988.

5

Clinical Assessment of the Low Back: History and Structural Evaluation

RICH NYBERG

Inherent in the management of a spinal musculoskeletal condition is the determination of the problem to be treated. To the manual therapy practitioner a functionally oriented approach in evaluation is fundamental to the understanding of the patient's complaint, a fact that will be emphasized throughout this book. The identification of the type of motion disorder found during the evaluation determines the nature of the treatment.

The manual therapy clinician observes and feels for functional status. The assessment process and the events being analyzed are different from the diagnostic methods utilized to identify disease. The detection and labeling of a disease entity is clearly important, but a disease diagnosis is not enough. The guidelines for treatment in a functional approach involve the delineation of the components resulting in movement dysfunction. The emphasis is on determining impairment, the loss or abnormality of the physiologic function, and disability, the lack of ability to perform an activity within the range considered normal.[1]

CLASSIFICATION

The traditional diagnostic categories used to classify low back disorders focus on disease, pathology, or symptoms. The back conditions of patients are typically defined in such terms as degenerative disc disease, spondylolisthesis, facet arthropathy, or muscle strain. Examples of diagnostic labels in the *International Classification of Diseases: Clinical Modification* include simply, low back pain or arm pain. Although these medical diagnoses are accepted by the Health Care Financing Administration and are used as the basis for payment by third party organizations,[2] they do not identify the cause of the problem and therefore do not provide information on how to treat. Moreover, the pathologic entity established by radiographic testing is most likely the result of functional disturbances which have existed before the development of the pathology.

A meaningful diagnosis names the primary dysfunction.[3] Information obtained in an evaluation which emphasizes functional performance establishes the intent and direction of treatment. A diagnosis of degenerative disc disease, although descriptive, is not as informational as spinal motion restriction, which signifies the physiologic impairment and relates directly to the functional activity limitation. Therefore, the manual therapist does not determine treatment strategy on the basis of nominal categorization of a disease or condition but rather on the positions, movements, and activities that affect the signs and symptoms.

Classification of movement disorders of the spine has yet to be operationally developed, defined, or utilized for diagnostic means. The essential features of each type of motion dysfunction need to be identified so that the characteristics of the movement problem can be recognized by the evaluator. Nominal diagnoses may or may not have distinct motion behavior characteristics. For example, sacroiliac strains and lumbar strains may have very similar movement patterns and consequently may be classified in the same movement category. Conversely, a medical diagnosis of disc protrusion may result in very different motion reactions in individuals, depending on the status or severity of the condition. Conceivably, a minor, stable disc protrusion may not affect spinal motion behavior, while an unstable disc protrusion may significantly interfere with many spinal motion activities. In this situation, two different movement dysfunction diagnoses are made despite only one medical label—disc protrusion. More importantly, the signs and symptoms produced for the movement dysfunction identified determine how treatment is rendered.

The development of diagnostic categories for motion disorders of the spine needs to be established by standardized clinical tests. In 1987, the NIOSH Low Back Atlas (issued by the National Institute of Occupational Safety and Health) identified 19 tests and measures with acceptable reliability (<.74 for Cohen's

Kappa and >.79 coefficients for the interclass correlation coefficient [ICC]).[4] The use of the *NIOSH Low Back Atlas* of standardized tests is an important step in defining musculoskeletal low back pain for the clinical practitioner. Tests not considered acceptable according to criteria, but found useful to the clinical examiners were designated to a marginal category. Refinement in testing procedure was considered necessary to improve reliability in marginal tests. The tests and measures regarded as acceptable were mostly related to pelvic and lumbar position, lumbar mobility, and hip mobility (Table 5.1). Further studies standardizing test procedures and substantiating reliability of evaluative techniques are essential to the justification of a functional approach to musculoskeletal disorders.

VALIDITY AND RELEVANCE

Equally important is establishing the validity of clinical tests measuring spinal position or mobility. Measuring how far the fingers reach to the ground may be a highly reliable method to determine forward bending of the spine. However, x-ray studies show that the finger distance obtained to the floor is not an accurate assessment of lumbar flexion range of motion. In fact, one study has shown that some ankylosing spondylitis patients with fused lumbar motion segments are capable of

---

Table 5.1
NIOSH Low-Back Atlas of Standardized Tests and Measures

Standing
Lumbar spine—flexible ruler
Iliac crest (posterior)—crest tester
Posterior superior iliac spine (static)—visual assessment
Iliac crest (anterior)—crest tester
Anterior superior iliac spine—visual assessment
Right side bending—vertical ruler
Left side bending—vertical ruler

Sitting
Iliac crest (anterior)—crest tester
Iliac crest (posterior)—crest tester
Posterior superior iliac spine (static/flexion)—visual assessment
Lumbar spine (relaxed sitting posture)—flexible ruler
Sustained slouched sitting—flexible ruler

Prone
Prone hip rotation range of motion—gravity goniometer
Sustained extension in lying, press-up—flexible ruler/symptom changes
Short hip extension length—visual assessment

Supine
Double straight leg raise ROM—gravity goniometer
Hamstring length—gravity goniometer
Hip flexor length—visual assessment

Side lying
Gluteus medius strength—visual assessment

touching the floor,[5] presumably from motion obtained in the hip joints and the flexibility of the hamstrings.

The information obtained through clinical testing must also be relevant to the problem. Only data that are clinically significant to the problem assist in the decision-making process determining treatment. The identification of a leg length discrepancy or a 20° restriction in hip internal rotation may be reliable and valid information but may be totally meaningless to the patient who complains of lumbosacral pain while sitting. Likewise, the presence of an L5/S1 spondylolisthesis may be unrelated to the low back pain and motion restriction complaints of a 55-year-old man. The x-ray diagnosis of spondylolisthesis may be a valid assessment of bone structure at L5, but the existence of a spondylolisthesis as determined by radiographic tests does not ensure its significance to the patient's pain or mobility problems.[6]

The type, frequency, and duration of motion activity useful for recovery and prevention of spinal pain has not been experimentally specified. The studies related to soft tissue changes to immobilization and movement, however, support the theory that motion, if therapeutically promoted, enhances the reparative process and facilitates functional recovery.

Regardless of the underlying cause, the ultimate consequence of low back disorder is limitation in physical function. The ability of an individual with back pain to move freely or exert force is adversely affected. The justification of biomechanical analysis for understanding the nature and extent of low back pain is therefore obvious. Motion is evidence of and fundamental to life. Patients suffering from back pain commonly report of an interference in some, if not many, aspects of life's activities. The return to full activity status is predicated on the restoration of movement and as a result, the success of a rehabilitation program necessitates a motion focus. The selection of a specific form of motion therapy for a particular dysfunction, however, has to been validated despite the existence of numerous strategies. Perhaps the type of movement activity utilized in the recovery from and prevention of a back condition is not as important as the frequency and duration of the activity.

The relative value of a specific motion therapy approach, however, cannot be assessed until clinical evaluation procedures are determined to be reliable and valid. The following section identifies the most common clinical tests used to evaluate a low back patient's condition with respect to intake information and history, structural alignment, active and passive movement performance, tissue condition, neurovascular status, and functional activity level. An analysis of the test's predictive value, accuracy in measurement, and reproducibility is provided.

INTAKE INFORMATION/HISTORY

The importance of conducting a standardized protocol for evaluating low back pain has been substantiated.[7] An investigation of two standardized methods of evaluating low back pain patients demonstrates the positive impact of a consistent, unbiased clinical approach on the frequency of low back pain, days lost from work and the number of low back surgeries. If the evaluation strategy utilized for assessing a low back condition is organized and practical, the treatment outcomes will likely be favorable regardless of the type of patient. In addition, consistent regularly performed evaluation procedures lead to significant cost savings in industrial low back claims.

The necessity of using a systematic, standard form for obtaining reliable and pertinent clinical information relating to a low back complaint is essential.[8] Careful definition of terms used on an evaluation form decreases error in interpretation. Descriptions such as low back pain and sciatica need to be clarified to avoid misunderstanding. For example, observer reliability is improved if patients point to the area of pain rather than describe the site, suggesting that evaluators have different criteria for discriminating low back from sciatic pain.

PAIN ANALYSIS

Pain Drawings

Pain drawings have demonstrated acceptable evaluator reliability in locating the area of discomfort. The simplicity of pain drawings offers the clinician an efficient tool in evaluating pain as well as assists in predicting response to treatment. Ill-defined, widespread, nonanatomic pain drawings strongly suggest individuals who have nonorganic involvement (Fig. 5.1). An expanded, nondistinct pain drawing is predictive of a poor response to treatment, and the increased probability of developing chronic complaints.[9]

Pain drawings are also predictive of the psychologic profile of a patient with low back pain. Results show a fairly high positive relation between the hypochondriasis and hysteria scores of an Minnesota Multiphasic Personality Inventory (MMPI) test and pain drawing scores.[10] Elevated hypochondriasis and hysteria scores on the MMPI are prognostic of poor treatment results.[11] Pain drawings, although simple to administer, must be carefully analyzed, since as many as 40% of chronic pain patients' markings may be incomplete or anatomically inaccurate regarding the painful site body marking.[12] Therefore, the accuracy of pain drawings must be investigated during the history by having the patient describe and point to the areas of involvement. Although the exact location of pain may help in determining a diagnosis, the evaluator must be aware of the difficulty in obtaining precise pain descriptions due to the multisegemental nature of spinal innervation. Pain drawings, however, appear to forecast a

Where is your pain?
Please mark on the drawings below the areas where you feel your pain.

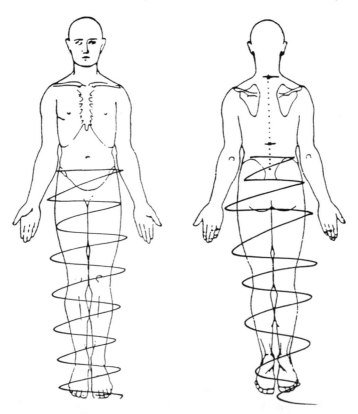

Figure 5.1. Diffuse, nonanatomic pain drawing.

patient's psychologic profile. The use of a pain drawing provides evidence for the necessity of further psychologic assessment, which in turn may offer insight into the success of an intervention program.

Indexes and Questionnaires

Various pain rating indexes have been established in an attempt to evaluate patients' pain experience. The use of pain questionnaires to assess the intensity, sensory nature, and emotional quality of pain provides a mechanism for clinicians to rate pain in a quantitative manner. Utilization of the McGill Pain Questionnaire (Fig. 5.2) provides a calculable means for measuring pain statistically. Patients demonstrate selectivity in choice of pain word descriptors and are reasonably consis-

tent in the words chosen initially upon repeated testing provided the condition had been unchanged.[13]

The number of sensory word descriptors selected does not appear to correlate with the affective nature of one's pain experience. For example, cancer patients with high scores in sensory discrimination have no significant difference in emotional word selection than patients having menstrual pain.[13] The type of pain identified by low back patients seems to vary considerably and does not appear to offer discriminating nor predictive information.[8] For this reason, sole reliance on pain type to differentiate the tissue origin of the problem should be questioned.

The pain rating index determined by the rank value for each word descriptor and the present pain intensity score correlate signifi-

There are many words that describe pain. Some of these words are grouped below. Check (✓) any words that describe the pain you have these days.

1.	2.	3.	4.	5.
Flickering	Jumping	Pricking	Sharp	Pinching
Quivering	Flashing	Boring	Cutting	Pressing
Pulsing	Shooting	Drilling	Lacerating	Gnawing
Throbbing		Stabbing		Cramping
Beating				Crushing
Pounding				

6.	7.	8.	9.	10.
Tugging	Hot	Tingling	Dull	Tender
Pulling	Burning	Itchy	Sore	Taut
Wrenching	Scalding	Smarting	Hurting	Rasping
	Searing	Stinging	Aching	Splitting
			Heavy	

11.	12.	13.	14.	15.
Tiring	Sickening	Fearful	Punishing	Wretched
Exhausting	Suffocating	Frightful	Grueling	Blinding
		Terrifying	Cruel	
			Vicious	
			Killing	

16.	17.	18.	19.	20.
Annoying	Spreading	Tight	Cool	Nagging
Troublesome	Radiating	Numb	Cold	Nauseating
Miserable	Penetrating	Drawing	Freezing	Agonizing
Intense	Piercing	Squeezing		Dreadful
Unbearable		Tearing		Torturing

Figure 5.2 McGill Pain Questionnaire.

cantly with the number of words chosen. Each category in the McGill Pain Questionnaire demonstrates internal consistency in measuring pain as well as significant correlation between categories. Therefore, the effects of therapeutic intervention strategies on pain can be evaluated with reasonable clinical reliability through the use of a pain questionnaire. The most sensitive indicator of change in pain status is reflected in the rank value of the words in the pain rating index, rather than the present pain intensity or the number of words chosen.[13] Patients may indicate that pain has in fact changed by marking less severe word descriptors but at the same time report the pain intensity to be the same and mark the same number of words as before.

Potential chronic pain patients, however, can possibly be identified during the acute stage.[14] The potential chronic pain patient complains of numerous pain locations, has deep musculoskeletal pain, is highly anxious during the acute stage, and typically has a lower activity level allowing a preoccupation with pain. Thus, an argument can be made for the axiom which states, "Those who have something better to do don't hurt as much."[15] Intervention programs which focus on teaching patients active lifestyle behaviors may therefore prevent the development of the pain-prone personality.

Interestingly, severe emotional conflict as indicated by word descriptors or higher pain intensity scores does not seem to correlate significantly with patients receiving compensation.[16] Patients on compensation appear to be similar to noncompensation patients in terms of the frequency of psychologic disturbance and prevalency of nonorganic findings. Compensation intensifies a patient's description of pain only when objective evidence of injury is present. Patients on compensation are therefore probably no more likely to malinger than patients not on compensation. Clearly, other factors are needed to explain why compensation interferes with recovery, since the literature consistently demonstrates the negative relationship between satisfactory therapeutic outcome and compensation.[17–19]

Pain Location and Duration

In regard to pain location, the most common area of complaint is the central lumbosacral region. The presence of lumbosacral discomfort during an episode of low back pain, however, is not predictive for recurrence within the following year. The utilization of symptom diagnosis is likewise not a strong indicator of future risk of low back pain. Sciatica or radiating leg pain, on the other hand, is a significant sign and forecaster of future episodes, particularly if the pain is below the knee.[20] People who experience sciatica tend to have more recurrences and longer periods of discomfort than people with low back pain episodes.[21,22] The presence of pain below the knee correlates strongly with time loss from work.[23] The longer a person remains out of work, the greater is the probability of the individual not returning to the same work responsibilities. In one such study, 50% of the people with a low back condition for over 6 months were not able to resume previous work positions.[24]

People with sciatic pain tend to have longer periods of symptomatology than those with low back pain, although both conditions tend to be self-limiting. Some report that 86% of patients with low back pain will recover in one month regardless of the treatment rendered.[25] Other investigations, however, indicate only a 50% recovery rate within one month for patients with sciatica.[26] The tendency toward improvement over time is therefore evident but not universal.

The concept of pain centralization can be used to predict treatment outcome. Centralization of pain refers to the shifting of distal pain to a more proximal or central location.[27] A patient reporting of lumbosacral pain after initially complaining of pain radiation into the lower extremity below the knee has therefore experienced a centralization phenomenon. The occurrence of pain centralization following initial treatment indicates a favorable prognosis and a successful outcome. In contrast, failure to achieve central or proximal pain relocation when distal pain exists often predicts a poor treatment outcome and a need for surgery.[28]

Pain Intensity

In terms of the intensity of the symptoms, the only parameter of importance in indicating future risk is whether the individual woke up during the night because of the pain. Complete or periodic interference in normal work or house activities does not appear to relate significantly to the development of subsequent problems.[20] The severity of the pain when measured on a pain intensity scale (Fig. 5.3) does not provide discriminating evidence for predictive behaviors.[29] Pain rating scales when used as a sole indicator of the potential outcome for patients with low back pain fail to provide significant prognostic information[30] and therefore should be interpreted with caution.

Onset of Symptoms

Both sudden and gradual onset of symptoms are believed to be associated with the length of disability. Gradual, nontraumatic back pain development has been found to be predictive of increased disability and longer symptoms than acute onsets. In one study 70% of patients with insidious onsets continued to have back pain in a one-year-follow-up after the initial symptoms. In contrast, only 55% of the acute onset patients were still experiencing pain after one year.[20]

Other studies indicate acute onsets to be more likely to prolong symptoms and disability. The reason for acute onset identification, at least in the United States, may relate to the potential for a compensable claim.[31] The greater the chance and the higher the amount of monetary reward also relate to the probability of identifying a compensable low back injury as the causative factor.[32] The involvement of an attorney with low back compensation claims significantly increases the prospects of chronic pain and disability. Psychologic and physical measurements show more improvement in patients without legal proceedings than patients involved in litigation.[33] Further support to this finding is found in another study which showed that 90% of patients with legal claims report chronic pain conditions.[29]

FACTORS IN LOW BACK PAIN

Precipitating Factors

The precipitating event in low back pain has been evaluated in work-related settings. Over 48% of low back episodes investigated in one study related to lifting.[23] Falling and slipping were found to be the second most common injury event. Pulling is found to be more frequently related to the onset of low back pain than pushing.[34] Sudden, unexpected exertion while carrying a heavy object is frequently cited as a precipitating event in low back pain development.[35]

Low back pain patients not receiving workman's compensation, however, are less likely to identify a singular event or injury as the definitive precipitating factor. For exam-

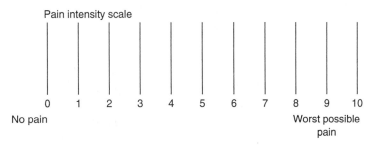

Indicate your pain level now (x) and also at the worst times (✓).

Figure 5.3. Pain Intensity Scale.

ple, in workman compensation back injuries only 16.7% of the patients reported no specific activity precipitation to the problem. This finding differs from the observations made in nonworkman compensation low back patients where approximately 50% report no specific incident factors.[22,36] Since the Workman Compensation System requires a specific incident or injury for eligibility, the likelihood of a singular event cause for low back pain increases. In most cases, therefore, back pain has multifactorial causes and is probably not just related to work requirements.

Related Risk Factors

Repeated loading of the spine is associated with greater risk of back pain as a result of cumulative fatigue and decreased stress-bearing capacity. Cumulative shear and compression loads as measured at the thoracolumbar and lumbosacral discs have been found to be significantly higher in male back pain groups than in a no pain group.[37] The total number of years working was also found to be significantly greater in the pain group than in the nonpain group. The cumulative load exposure for compression and shear, therefore, is likely to be higher for pain groups because of the number of work years.

The process of spinal mechanical derangement which predisposes individuals to back pain is therefore most likely to be gradual. Theories related to cumulative load disorders of the spine suggest that prolonged loading reduces disc height and water content, which in turn decreases imbibition pressure. The loss of disc height also changes ligament rest tension. The mechanical changes within the spine associated with prolonged, repeated loading, aging, and lifestyle behaviors reduce tissue tolerance to stress and predisposes one to back injury. Perhaps this theory of mechanical derangement helps to explain why a worker may develop back pain 1 day while working at a job he/she has performed for many years. The cumulative load theory provides some rationale for why static work postures such as sitting and standing have been

identified as potential risk factors for low back pain.[38]

In a retrospective cross-sectional study of a random sample of 1760 women aged 38 to 64 various work factors were analyzed for their relationship to low back pain.[39] Three physical factors were found to relate to low back pain: increased frequency of forward bending, lifting, and standing. Lifting in particular has been cited as an important risk factor for low back pain and has been related to almost one-half of all compensable low back pain episodes.[40] Weight lifting was found to be a significant predictor of low back pain in a survey done on 1221 men aged 18 to 55. Forty-four percent (44%) of the moderately symptomatic patients and 54% of severe low back pain patients performed repetitive lifting of 20 kgs or more.[41] In addition, the aggravation of low back symptoms from coughing and sneezing seem to relate to the rapid and repeated forward bending of the spine rather than to an increase in intraspinal pressure.[38]

Low back pain is more probable when the physical demands of the job exceed the individual's strength capability. The chance of injury has been found to be three times more likely when the physical job requirements are greater than the worker's strength ability.[42] The incidence of spine pain and the number of days absent from work correlate positively to individuals who perceive the job to be physically demanding.[35,43] A clear relationship also exists between the severity of back pain and the heaviness of the work activities.[44] Documentation also exists to show that workers who lift more than 150 times a day or less than 50 times a day are more prone to work-related low back pain.[45]

Work-Associated Factors

Workers with high-risk occupations associated with low back pain include truck drivers, material handlers, nurses, and nurses's aides. Truck drivers are five times more likely to develop an acute lumbar disc herniation than nontruck drivers.[46] The severity of symptoms and the frequency of low back pain episodes is increased in individuals involved in greater vehicle use.[47] The driving of automobiles, motorcycles, buses, tractors, trucks, and heavy construction equipment is more prevalent in patients with low back pain.

Vibration. The amount of time spent sitting, along with the effects of vibration while driving are indicated as probable causative factors for low back pain. An increase in fatigue failure of the spinal ligaments, faster creep rates in vertebral motion segments, and evidence of muscle fatigue in the abdominal and paraspinal muscles demonstrate the potential adverse effects of constant vibrational load.[48] For example, vertical vibrations of 5 Hz, 3mm peak to peak amplitudes and peak accelerations of less than 2 m/s^2 were found to reduce sitting height from head to sitting surface by an average of 9 mm.[49] The incidence of low back injury has also been demonstrated to be somewhat higher in patients involved in activities that require jackhammers, chainsaws, and rotary cultivators; this further substantiates vibration as an associated factor.

Nursing and Physical Therapy. The increase in work-related incidence of low back pain in nurses and nurse's aides is reported to be a function of frequent patient handling and lifting, which is often performed in awkward positions and with sudden, unexpected exertions.[50,51] Not only is the incidence rate fairly high (46.8%), but the recurrence rate is very high in nurses's aides (82%) complaining of low back pain.[51] In comparison to nurses, who have a 19.9% work-related incidence of low back pain, physical therapists have a 29% frequency of occurrence. The first 4 years of work was found to be the most likely period of initial onset in both groups, presumably because of inexperience in proper patient handling or in assessing a patient's physical ability.[52]

Prognostics. The role of sitting as a sole prognostic indicator for low back pain is less clear. Some studies demonstrate more low back pain in people working predominantly in a sitting position.[38] Other studies do not find sitting to be a risk factor.[53] Nonwork-related weekend sitting, however, has been positively correlated to disc herniation in males.[54] The sitting position more often aggravates than relieves low back pain, particularly in females.[20] Psychologic factors related to an individual's personality, work requirements, and environment may therefore be significant indicators of low back trouble.

Psychologic variables such as dissatisfaction with work activities and job status correlate with low back pain. Descriptions of monotonous or repetitive work tasks are more frequently given by individuals with low back pain.[31,32,55] Low back complaints are also more common among people who report of anxiety, depression, and stress.[47] Individuals who worry and report fatigue and nervousness at the end of a work day are more likely to experience low back discomfort.[53]

Demographic and Lifestyle Factors

Age and Gender. The frequency of low back pain increases from ages 20 to 40, remains relatively stable between 40 and 60, and then seems to decrease slightly after 60, particularly in men.[56] Symptoms tend to first develop between the 25th and 30th years. Although the occurrence of back pain in children is relatively low, the significance should be considered serious with respect to a underlying spinal pathology.[57]

The frequency rate of sciatica is greatest from age 30 to 40.[20] Patients older than 40 who have no prior history of low back pain and work at physically demanding jobs miss more time from work than sedentary workers with back pain.[23] The effect of age as a single factor in predicting disability is not clear. Some report that age is not an important factor in determining outcome of an episode of back pain[58] while others show that age is a predictor of disability.[59,60] A tendency exists for younger patients to report less severe back pain than older patients.[41,61] Whereas women demonstrate an increase in back pain prevalence with age, men show a peak incidence at age 40.[62]

Although men are more likely to be involved in compensable low back injuries, the overall incidence of back pain in women is slightly greater (4%). The reasons offered include: biologic tissue changes from pregnancy and childbearing, physical stress of child rearing, multiple role obligations, anatomical and biomechanical differences, response to stress, and increased likelihood of reporting symptoms.[63] Less certainty is found with respect to whether men or women are more apt to be disabled or less likely to return to work after a compensable low back injury.[60,64]

Although the effect of age alone in regard to the prevalence of back pain is not highly significant, the interaction of age and marital status, on the other hand, demonstrates a strong relationship to back pain. A high correlation exists between back pain and women over 35 who are no longer married, especially in the 50–64 age range. The necessary increase in involvement in all activities of daily living, along with changes in social activity and support may increase physical and emotional stress which in turn causes or aggravates back pain. In married groups no relationship is found between age and back pain.[63]

Educational Level. The association of back pain with educational level has also been studied. Investigations into this relationship demonstrate less reported low back pain, absenteeism, and disability in married individuals with higher education. The ability to adjust a work situation or job task is likely to be greater for people with more education, since they are probably involved in professional, managerial, or skilled occupations. To the contrary, people with less education are typically involved in work activities which require greater physical demand. Time off from work and the possibility of reinjury is therefore more probable in persons with lower educational attainment. The relationship of back pain to people with less than a high school education is especially high in younger age groups (35–49). Education beyond high school is associated with a lower rate of reported back pain.[65]

Body Height, Weight and Mass. Body height and weight are independent risk factors for low back pain as well as for lumbar disc herniation. The risk of lumbar herniation is two times greater in men over 180 cm (> 6 ft) and three times greater in women over 170 cm (> 5 ft 6½ in).[66] With respect to body mass a consistent trend is present between increased back pain prevalence and increased weight. A significant increase in low back complaints is found in the most obese subjects. Individuals in the top 20% weight category have a 1.7 times higher incidence of back pain than subjects in the lowest 20% weight category.[67] While one study finds a stronger association between body mass index and back pain for women[67] another study demonstrates the body mass index to be a predictor of herniated lumbar discs in men, but not women.[66]

Smoking. Back pain frequency increases with increased levels of smoking.[67] The occurrence of low back pain rises especially in smokers with over 50 years of smoking and for those who smoke more than a pack a day. Some suggest that the correlation of low back pain and smoking is due to increased cough symptoms which result in repeated, forceful trunk flexion and an increase in intradiscal pressure. The presence of chronic cough, bronchitis, and emphysema, however, have been found to be independent risk factors to back pain and not just associated to smoking. Some authorities theorize that the nicotine content in cigarettes interferes with vertebral body blood flow as well as the diffusion of nutrients through the vertebral endplates into and out of the disc. The adverse impact on disc metabolism makes the disc more vulnerable to injury. Moreover, the risk of back pain is the same for individuals who stopped smoking over ten years ago and people who have never smoked, indicating that lifestyle behavior changes have a positive effect.

Recreational Activities. Participation in recreational activities seems to have a marginal relationship to low back pain. Asymptomatic individuals as well as people with severe low back pain tend to be less involved in sports activities such as jogging and cross-country skiing than those who participate.[41] On the other hand, people who become less active in sport activities between adolescence and later years are more likely to develop severe low back pain than people who continue with their sport activities. The intensity of low back symptoms tends to be mild in patients who are currently exercising.

Family History. A strong familial predisposition to discogenic low back pain appears to exist. In one study 35% of patients with presumed disc conditions were found to have at least one family member with discogenic problems.[68] In contrast, only 12% of asymptomatic subjects reported to have near relatives with discogenic back problems. Thirty-seven percent (37%) of patients who had lumbar disc surgery had at least one family member with a history of disc-related back pain. Ten percent (10%) of the surgical patients had family members who had also undergone disc surgery, as opposed to only 1% of asymptomatic subjects. The predisposition of family members to back pain is probably related to both genetic and environmental factors.[68]

Pregnancy. Women in the later stages of pregnancy or in early postpartum are susceptible to back pain. In two separate studies a 49% and a 54% incidence of low back pain was found during pregnancy.[69,70] Of the women who experience symptoms, as many as 50% may report sciatica,[69] while 12% complain of severe low back pain which causes significant limitation in daily activities.[70] Women most likely to develop back-related complaints during pregnancy are 30 years or older and have already had one or more children. The severity of the symptoms, therefore, tends to increase roughly 5% every 5 years and after the first pregnancy. The risk of low back problems increases during pregnancy, presumably because of the stress on the spine from the increased weight of the uterus. The increase in stress on spinal structures from the additional load occurs simultaneously with a weakening of the ligamentous support system brought about by the release of relaxin hormone.[71] The ability of

spinal tissues to resist mechanical deformation during pregnancy is therefore compromised.

Balance of Rest and Activity. The most common factors identified by back pain patients for relief of symptoms were lying down or walking around. In one study, pain relief was found by 52–54% of low back patients when lying down and by 34–39% when walking around.[20] On the basis of these findings an argument can be made for establishing a balance between rest and activity for recovery from a back pain episode. Since 2 days of bedrest appears to be as effective as 1 week's rest from a back condition involving sciatic symptoms,[72] resumption of some form of activity is reasonable even during the early stages of the problem.

Summary of Factors

To summarize, the relationship of a number of factors to low back pain has been analyzed. The most established factors relating to low back pain are presented in Table 5.2. Awareness of the various influences and possible causes of low back pain may enable the im-

Table 5.2

Symptomatic, Risk, Work, Demographic and Lifestyle Factors Related to Back Pain Incidence or Recovery

1—Standardization of evaluation strategy
2—Pain drawings
3—Stress resulting in anxiety or depression
4—Workman's compensation
5—Sciatic pain
6—Duration of work time loss
7—Night pain
8—Legal claim filed
9—Materials handling—bending, lifting (Less than 50 or more than 150 x's/day)
10—Number of years worked (<4 years)
11—Standing for more than 4 hours/day
12—Jobs perceived to be physically demanding
13—Driving
14—Nonmarried women over 35
15—High percentile categories for height and weight
16—Smoking, especially with chronic cough symptoms
17—Familial incidence
18—Women in later stages of pregnancy, particularly those over 30 years with two or more previous full term pregnancies.

plementation of successful preventive measures or may assist in providing information that will enhance recovery.

PHYSICAL EVALUATION

Reliability and Validity

Before establishing definitive categories of back pain, reliable and valid clinical methods of assessment must be determined. The use of advanced technology in the form of radiographic, computerized axial tomography (CAT), and magnetic resonance imaging has provided further anatomical insight into the nature of back pathology. The relevance of radiographic abnormalities, however, with respect to functional performance as well as to symptoms is less clear. The documentation of a degenerative spinal condition, for example, correlates poorly with symptomatology.

In one study, CAT scans were interpreted to be positive in 50% of the asymptomatic subjects over 40 on the basis of the degenerative findings.[73] X-ray studies demonstrate no significant difference in the incidence of spondylosis and disc degeneration between patients with and without low back pain.[74] The value of radiographic signs for predicting low back or associated leg pain is therefore minimal.

Furthermore, the reliability of examiners in interpreting x-rays is poor for most variables studied. In one study, only six out of 56 variables analyzed by three examiners were considered reliable measures (short leg, sacral base angle, Ferguson's weight-bearing line, lumbarization, spondylolysis, and spondylolisthesis).[75] The lack of agreement in interpreting imaging tests as well as the nonrelevance or questionable significance of the findings emphasizes the importance of the physical evaluation in determining a diagnosis. Although certain aspects of the physical examination of a low back condition have not shown clinically acceptable reliability, other components have demonstrated consistency. The lack of agreement in some tests for low back dysfunction is not unique to the spinal orthopedic evaluation. High levels of agreement between cardiologists in interpreting auscultated sounds were not demonstrated in Raftery and Holland's study.[76] In another study, the clinical estimation of liver size as determined by a number of physicians did not show consistency.[77] Furthermore, no relationship was found between palpable assessment and radiologic measures of liver size in 25 patients when examined by 3 physicians.[78] The reliability of interpreting respiratory signs was also found to vary considerably among physicians.[79]

The objective of the following section is to assess the reliability, validity, sensitivity, and predictability of various components of the low back physical examination. Certain aspects of the low back physical evaluation have been demonstrated to correlate with myelogram findings.[80] Other parts of the examination offer predictive information regarding low back pain development and recurrence.[22,81] Some clinical tests of the spine may therefore be helpful in assessing treatment or surgical outcomes, while other tests have not shown reliability in testing or sensitivity to the nature of the low back impairment. The manual practitioner must be aware of the diagnostic value of each test utilized in the clinical examination of a back patient to make judgments regarding the nature of the problem as well as determine prognosis. Clinical decisions should be based on tests which demonstrate consistency, accuracy, and sensitivity to the problem.

Standardization—a Necessity

Information received from the clinical exam needs to be obtained under controlled circumstances, otherwise observer error will be significant. Independent test procedures for neuromusculoskeletal conditions performed by multiple examiners result in low interrater reliability.[82] Standardization of test procedures commonly utilized in a low back evaluation requires further delineation in order to establish criterion-based testing protocol. Without specific guidelines for the performance of evaluative tests, the findings will be interpreted differently.

Testing Interaction. The effects of testing interaction must also be considered as a source of disagreement.[83] The effects of a random-ordered examination may lead to disagreement in test findings. Spinal motion test results, for example, may differ, depending on whether neurologic tests are performed before or after the motion exam. Provoking of symptoms in prior tests is likely to alter the findings in successive tests. If a patient's leg pain has been exacerbated by a straight leg test, a subsequent lumbar flexion motion test may be adversely affected. The *importance of a fixed sequenced examination* is apparent when evaluating for examiner reliability of test outcome.

Consistency. Another factor affecting the reliability of test procedures concerns the consistency of the findings. A stable finding with repeated testing will most likely improve reliability within and between examiners. In contrast, a transient finding changes from test to test and can interfere with examiner agreement. Neuromuscular events, occurring between or during test procedures commonly alter the degree of muscle activity and sensitivity, leading to disagreement in findings. Consequently, tests that rely on evaluating transient signs should be interpreted with caution by manual practitioners.

STRUCTURAL EVALUATION

Trunk Length/Body Height

Trunk length as obtained by subtracting leg length from total height or measuring trunk height in sitting is significantly greater in adults and teenagers with back pain.[84,85] When the relationship of sitting to standing height is equal, as found in a study on 116 top Swedish male athletes, the frequency of back pain is the same.[86] Diurnal changes in body height are well-documented and are apparently the result of disc height reduction in response to loading.[87,88] An average height loss of 1% has been calculated from morning to evening in a sample population of over 1200[87] with the highest rate of shrinkage occurring in the first hour after rising.[89] The

rate of height loss decreases during the day and decreases with age.[87,90]

Diurnal body height changes are influenced by the amount, type, and duration of load as well as the amount of height recovery when unloaded. Increasing spinal load increases the rate of creep within the disc, which results in faster shrinkage.[90] If the load varies during a day's activities the rate of creep and subsequent height loss also changes. For example, a significantly greater height loss is found after 1 hour of running than during 7.5 hours of relatively static activities.[91]

Postural Effects. Chair type and design have been shown to affect trunk shrinkage. For example, trunk shrinkage rates are higher for stools than for easy chairs with a full-sized backrest inclined at 110° and a 4 cm lumbar support. Conversely, recovery corresponds to the type and amount of unloading. Although, some recovery is possible with relatively low loading, as in the case of an ergonomically designed easy chair, the fastest return of body height occurs when lying down.[90] In one study, 70% of body height was restored within the first half of sleep at night (Fig. 5.4A). A 0.2% recovery or about a 4.5 mm increase in height is possible during a day by resting 1 hour in a lying position at noon (Fig. 5.4B). In addition, height increases are accelerated during rest periods if the lumbar spine is in a flexed position.[89]

The clinical measurement of body height may therefore be used to evaluate the effects of loading and unloading on spinal structures. The type, amount, and duration of loading and unloading can be analyzed with respect to trunk height. Recommendations regarding loading influences and recovery periods can be made in part by body height changes. The method of measurement is noninvasive, reliable, and inexpensive.

Sagittal Alignment

Normal anatomic spinal curves give the vertebral column flexibility while maintaining stiffness and stability.[92] Sagittal curves also provide a mechanism for improving the force

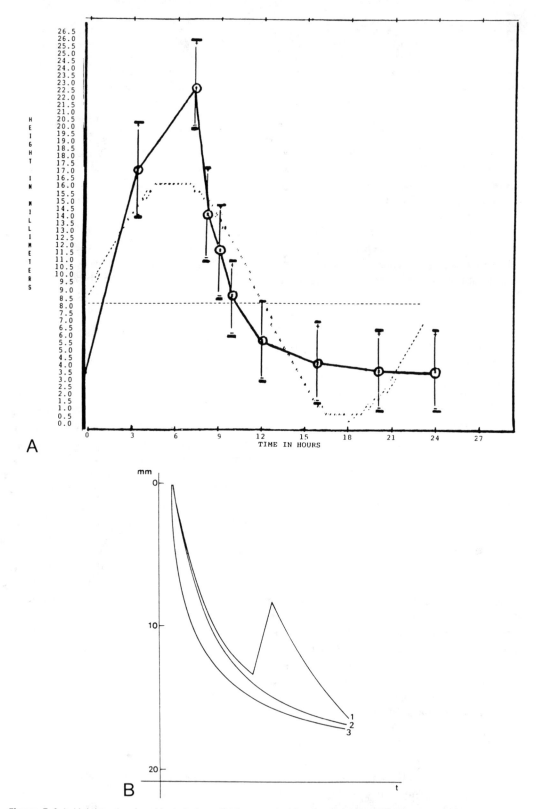

Figure 5.4.A Height gained and lost during a 24-hour period from a midnight-baseline set at 3.5 mm. Unbroken line indicates observed mean values. The dashed line represents the cosinor curve fitted to the data.

Figure 5.4.B The influence on body height by loading and nonloading (age groups: 16–50 years). **1:** After one hour's rest at midday, **2:** after one day's normal loading, **3:** additional loading for one hour in the morning with 10 kg.

attenuation capacity of the spine. The determination of the adequacy or significance of spinal curve formation in regard to back pain is a subject of concern to practitioners. Since the preservation of normal spinal curves is required for load bearing, a substantial loss or increase in curve formation may contribute to back pain development.

Radiographic analysis of lumbosacral angles as measured from L2 to the top of the sacrum was found to be $45° \pm 22°$ at 2 standard deviations around the mean. Lumbosacral angles less than 23° and greater then 68° were considered hypolordotic and hyperlordotic, respectively (Fig. 5.5).[93] Women were found to have a 4.4° larger mean lumbosacral angle than men, but no significant difference exists between black and white populations.[93] The apparent increase in lumbosacral angle of blacks is related to a more prominent buttocks.[94] The degree of gluteal prominence may interfere with clinical calculations of the actual lumbar lordosis. Clinicians, therefore, must be careful to observe and assess lumbar curve formation and not buttock prominence.

Twomey has shown a significant decrease in lumbar lordosis with increasing age after adolescence by 32% in females and 20% in males.[95]

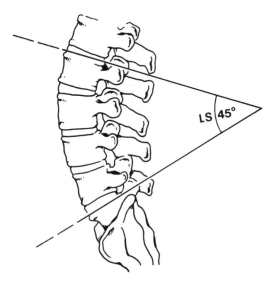

Figure 5.5. Measurement of lumbosacral angle.

Clinical Effects. The relationship of low back pain and lumbar lordosis is not clear. Some authorities suggest that an exaggerated lumbar lordosis increases anterior shear stress at the lumbosacral angle and causes postural back strain.[96] Support for this claim is provided in a study on female gymnasts which shows a significant correlation between increased lordosis and low back pain.[97] Others have found no relationship between the lumbosacral angles of asymptomatic individuals and low back pain patients along with a wide variation in angles.[98,99] In contrast, evidence from x-ray studies by Splithoff[100] and Magora and Schwartz[101] show that a loss of lumbar lordosis is related to low back pain. These x-ray findings support the contention of some clinicians who claim that acute disc prolapses or herniations often flatten or reverse the lumbar lordosis.[27,102,103]

Clinical Measures of Spinal Curves. Visual observation and determination of sagittal spine curves have not been tested for reliability or validity. The consistency and accuracy of clinical judgments must therefore be questioned with respect to evaluating the lumbar lordosis. Noninvasive measurements of lumbar curves using inclinometers, kyphometers, pantographs, and flexirules have been investigated. Intra- and interobserver reliability was demonstrated with inclinometer, kyphometer, and pantograph measures while intraobserver reliability was found with the flexirule.[104-107] Spinal pantograph examination of spinal saggital curves when compared to x-ray shows accurate measures for thoracic kyphosis but a tendency for slight underestimation for lumbar lordosis.[105] Although external testing of lumbar curves correlates poorly with roentgenograph measurements, the clinical value of noninvasive measuring tools may still be warranted on the basis of clinically acceptable intra- and interrater reliability.[108,109]

Radiograph measures, despite their offering of an actual measure of lumbosacral angle, are more expensive and time-consuming, and they are potentially hazardous. This adds to the value of reliable, valid, inexpensive, time efficient and easy to use clinical techniques in evaluating spinal curvature for detecting changes in alignment. The relationship of spinal position to movement and pain can then be investigated in a clinically meaningful manner.

Pelvic Inclination

The influence of pelvic inclination in the sagittal plane on the degree of lumbar lordosis is significant. Lateral radiographs demonstrate considerable positive correlations between the angle of declivity of the sacrum and the amount of lordotic curvature. The direct effect of pelvic position on lumbar curvature alters the distribution of compressive stress within the spine as well as the activity status of the musculoligamentous tissues in order to balance the load. Adjustments in pelvic inclination, according to mathematical models, allow for changes in lumbar lordosis and result in minimizing compressive stress on the spine.[111]

Is the degree of anterior or posterior inclination of the pelvis different in patients with low back pain? The evidence is not clear. Pelvic tilt angles did not show a significant difference between low back patient and healthy groups in a study using a noninvasive computerized method for determining external body landmarks.[112] In the study, pelvifemoral angles (degree of hip flexion) were found to be significantly greater in the patient group. Lateral x-rays of 33 patients with an L5 spondylolysis, demonstrated a 12.9° increase in the declivity angle of the sacrum when compared to normal subjects.[110] Small sacro-horizontal angles (4.7° or less), however, where also found to correlate significantly with back pain in top Swedish male athletes (Fig. 5.6).[86] These findings suggest that clinical assessment of both hip and pelvic position should be included as part of a low back evaluation.

Pelvic Tilt. Clinical determination of standing pelvic tilt angles using a noninvasive technique involving a depth caliper and meter sticks[113] has shown to be reliable.[114,115] The means for standing pelvic tilt angles on nor-

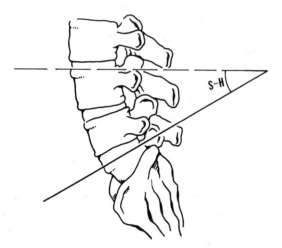

Figure 5.6. Sacro-horizontal angles.

mal subjects were calculated to be 8.35° and 9.2° in the two studies. The standard deviations (4.17° and 6.4°), although comparable to other clinical goniometric methods of evaluating the lumbar spine or pelvis, are slightly higher for goniometric measures of extremity joints. In addition to providing objective information, this clinical method of measurement for assessing pelvic tilt angle in the sagittal plane was found to be relatively quick.

Palpatory Analysis

Palpatory analysis of pelvic position has not been shown to be highly reliable. In one study, iliac crest height comparison in the standing and sitting positions demonstrated only 35 and 41° intertester agreement respectively.[116] In another study, intra- and interrater agreement for determining iliac crest height in standing among experienced physical therapists ranged roughly between 60% and 70%.[117] Position assessment and comparison of the anterior and posterior superior iliac spines (ASIS, PSIS) were also found to exhibit poor intertester reliability with percent agreements of approximately 35–44%. Through the use of rasterstereography and surface curvature analysis the dimple impressions observed on the pelvis have been shown to accurately correspond to the position of the PSISs.[118] Observational analysis alone may therefore provide a more consistent method for evaluating PSIS position than observing and palpating. The inability to reliably palpate pelvic landmarks is most likely due to differences in testing methods.

A low correlation exists for palpatory determination of iliac crest height and radiographic findings of pelvic position. Iliac crest position as judged by palpation was within 5 mm of the radiograph measurement in only 17 out of 50 cases. Palpatory assessment of pelvic position needs further study and refinement in test methodology in order to obtain clinically meaningful information. The relevancy of pelvic position findings by palpation study must be questioned until reliability in measurement and validity in testing is established. In view of the contention by many clinicians that positional disturbances within the pelvic articulations cause low back, pelvic, and possibly lower extremity pain the importance of improving clinical palpatory skills is essential.

LEG LENGTH DISCREPANCY AND PELVIC OBLIQUITY

Leg length differences are common among individuals who appear to have normal skeletal configuration and therefore are considered standard variants. Asymmetric growth of the lower extremities is the result of an out-of-phase growth process during skeletal development of the long bones of the lower limbs.[119] The significance of a leg length difference to back pain relates to the mechanical changes in pelvic and lumbar position. Postural scoliosis and pelvic obliquity have been associated with leg length discrepancies. Alterations in stress distribution within the spine along with compensatory tissue responses for maintaining an asymmetric position may be responsible for back pain development.

Measurement

Tape Measure. With the exception of one tape measure method,[120] clinical tests for determining leg length have been shown to be inaccurate when compared to radiographic measurements. Tape and block correction measures of leg lengths depend on palpating bony landmarks such as the ASIS or greater trochanters which are not easily nor reliably located. In addition, the bony landmarks used are sometimes asymmetric in osteologic development and not reflective of true position on each side. Observer error of up to ± 10 mm has been found in clinical methods for assessing leg lengths.[121-123] When using the tape measure method for determining leg length an average of two tests may improve validity estimates to .79.[120]

Radiologic methods for measuring leg length are reasonably reliable (0—2 mm)[124,125] but cannot be justified for routine clinical use because of radiation exposure, time required for proper set-up, and the necessity of special equipment. One clinical radiography study of leg length demonstrates a higher prevalence of low back pain in individuals with leg length discrepancies of 5 mm or more.[126] Table 5.3 illustrates the percent incidence of leg length disparity in chronic back pain patients and in an asymptomatic group according to Friberg's study.[126] The results of Friberg's study are consistent with previous investigations which show a higher frequency of leg length inequality of 10 mm or more in patients with low back pain than in normal populations.[125-128]

Sciatica and hip pain are more common on the side of the longer extremity when leg length discrepancies of 5 mm or more exist.[125] The laterality of symptoms supports the biochemical influence of a leg length discrepancy on the lumbar spine, pelvis, and hips. A leg length difference will typically cause pelvic tilt to the side of the short leg, lumbar side bending towards the long leg, and rotation toward

Table 5.3
Friburg's Radiographic Findings[126]

Leg Length Inequality	Low Back Pain Group (%)	Asymptomatic Group (%)	Ratio (LBP%:A%)
<5 mm	24.6	56.5	0.43
5 mm or more	75.4	43.5	1.73
10 mm or more	30.1	15.6	1.93
15 mm or more	11.7	2.2	5.32

the convexity of the curve. The lumbar motion segments are therefore subjected to increased mechanical stress from combined bending and torsion loads (Fig. 5.7). The pelvic tilt toward the side of the short leg causes a varus position of the hip on the side of the longer leg (Fig. 5.8). The increased weight-bearing stress in the hip joint of the long leg typically results in arthrotic change and is possibly the cause of hip discomfort.

The effect of a short leg on spinal alignment has been examined with standing x-rays.[129] Of the 545 subjects studied, 45% demonstrated lumbar convexity toward the side of the short leg, 23% had no lateral deviations, and 32% exhibited lumbar convexity to the side of the long leg. Ipsilateral lumbar convexity associated with a short leg is considered a normal compensatory mechanism designed to minimize mechanical stress at the lumbosacral juncture by distributing load more evenly throughout the curve. Nonadaptive lumbar responses to a short leg such as a straight or contralateral lumbar convexity result in abnormal concentrated stress at L5–S1 (Fig. 5.9A,B). Presumably, the ability of the lumbar spine to accommodate for a leg length discrepancy depends upon the inherent mobility at each motion segment. Whereas segmental restriction interferes with positional adjustment, normal motion function allows adaptive response, which in turn helps to reduce localization of force at any one particular vertebral level.

Muscular Causes of Pelvic Obliquity

Pelvic obliquity is also alleged to be caused by muscle imbalances or contractures about the hips, pelvis, and spine.[130] Hip abductor and/or adductor muscle imbalances or contractures have been reported to lead to pelvic tilting, toward the side of the tight abductors and away from the side of the tight adductors[131,132] (Fig. 5.10A,B). Sufficient research to document this relationship, however, is lacking. Similarly, the influence of hip flexor and extensor muscle imbalances on pelvic inclination or rotation has yet to be determined. The presumption that hip flexion tightness

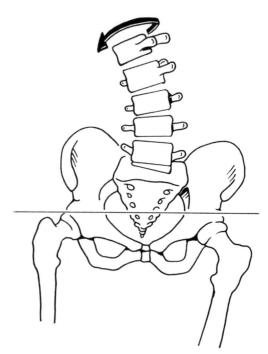

Figure 5.7. Bending and torsional loads to the lower lumbar motion segments associated with a significant leg length discrepancy.

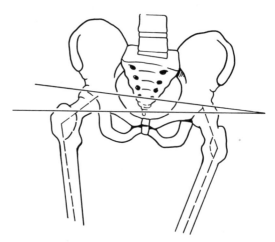

Figure 5.8. Varus hip angle of the longer lower extremity.

leads to anterior pelvic tilt or unilateral anterior rotation was not found to be true in one study.[133] In fact, no correlation was demonstrated between hip extension range of motion and pelvic tilt. Low back pain may occur in

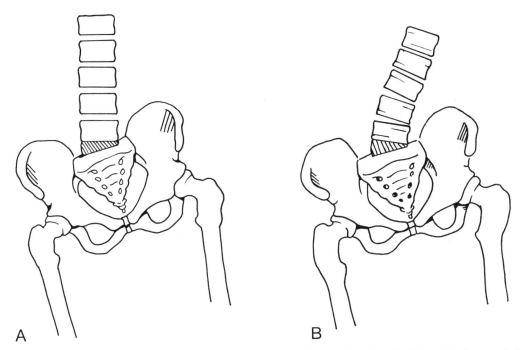

Figure 5.9A,B. Nonadaptive lumbar responses to a short leg (**A**—straight spine, **B**—Contralateral convexity).

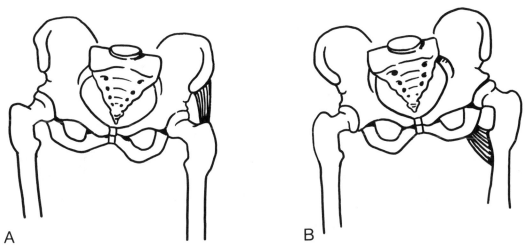

Figure 5.10A. Pelvic tilt toward the side of tight hip abductors.

Figure 5.10B. Pelvic tilt away from side of tight hip adductors.

cases where hip flexor tightness restricts hip extension range-of-motion and a hip flexor contracture develops without pelvic or lumbar position change. This may relate to the inability to tilt the pelvis anterior or to extend the lumbar spine sufficiently when needed, such as in terminal stance phase of gait. Conversely, a hip extension range of motion restriction may bring about a compensatory anterior pelvic tilt and increase in lumbar lordosis which overstresses the posterior structures of the lumbar spine.

Muscle imbalance or contracture in the lateral lumbopelvic musculature involving the iliopsoas, quadratus lumborum, and internal and external oblique abdominals reportedly can cause lateral spinal deviations or scoliotic curves as well as pelvic obliquity.[130] Postural or developmental tendencies for tightness in muscles such as the iliopsoas and quadratus lumborum combined with predisposition of other muscles such as the abdominals toward weakness[134] could result in a lateral spinal deviation as well as a pelvic obliquity. Research relating muscle contracture or imbalances to lumbopelvic position alteration is not substantial, despite the many clinical observations regarding the apparent relationships.[135–137]

LATERAL SPINAL DEVIATION

Lateral trunk deviations or lists observed in the standing position were recorded in 100 out of 1776 back pain patients (5.6%) (Fig. 5.11).[138] One x-ray study[139] demonstrated scoliosis or tilt of the lumbar spine in 9 out of 100 persons without backache and 16 of 100 with backache, indicating a greater incidence of lateral spinal deviation in low back pain patients.[139] The association of trunk list and back pain is commonly recognized by clinicians, but not clearly understood nor verified by controlled prospective studies. In a study involving 43 patients with radicular and nonradicular lumbar symptoms and a control group of 10 nonsymptomatic subjects no significant differences in measured lumbosacral list were found.[140] In a previous x-ray study, lateral spinal deviations of more than 5° were observed in 39% of the subjects tested. No relationship was demonstrated between lateral deviation and low back symptoms. Some degree of lateral spinal deviation is therefore common in nonpain and pain groups. Consequently, the existence of a lateral trunk list is not always significant or relevant to a back condition.

When a trunk list is associated with symptoms, the symptoms strongly suggest a disc lesion. In Porter's study,[138] almost half of the

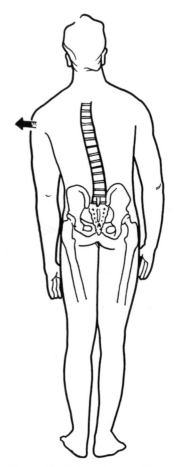

Figure 5.11. Lateral trunk shift.

patients with gravity-induced lateral shifts satisfied the criteria of a symptomatic disc condition, ("unilateral leg pain in a typical sciatic root distribution below the knee, specific neurologic symptoms incriminating a single nerve, straight leg raise limitation of at least 50%; at least two neurologic changes of muscle wasting, muscle weakness, sensory change of hyporeflexia; and radiculographic evidence of disc protrusion").[141] Lateral trunk shifts are frequently predictive of a poor outcome for conservative therapy. Forty percent (40%) of the patients fulfilling the criteria for a disc problem required surgical disc excision.[138]

The direction of the lateral trunk shift does not appear to relate to the side of the symptoms nor to the position of the disc protrusion in relationship to the nerve root.[138,142]

Table 5.4
Structural Findings Relevant to Back Problems

1—Increased trunk length
2—Increase in hip flexion (or pelvi-femoral angle)
3—Reduced and accentuated sacro-horizontal angles
4—Leg length differences of 10 mm or more

Unsupported is the hypothesis that disc protrusions lateral to the nerve root cause trunk shifting away from the symptomatic side, while disc protrusions medial to the nerve root cause shifting toward the side of symptoms. Left lateral trunk lists were found to be more than two times more common than right trunk lists.[138] While right-hand dominance was associated with a tendency toward left trunk shifts, left-hand preference may relate to right trunk listing. Further evidence demonstrating a correlation between handedness and lateral spine deviation is provided in a study by Goldberg and Dowling.[143] In their study, low thoracic scoliotic curve patterns matched handedness in 82% of the 254 girls with idiopathic scoliosis.[142] The lateralization of human functional activities therefore seems to be an influencing factor in spinal position in the frontal plane.

The degree of spinal curvature in the sagittal plane may determine the likelihood of deviations in the frontal plane. Thoracic kyphosis and lumbar lordosis in patients with scoliotic curves are significantly less than non-scoliotic groups.[144] Apparently, adequate sagittal curve configuration protects the spine from significant coronal plane deviation.

Structural findings most relevant to low back problems are presented in Table 5.4. Noteworthy is the fact that relatively few structural conditions correlate with or predict low back trouble. Dependency on structural differences alone for determining the nature of a problem is therefore discouraged.

REFERENCES

1. Jette A. Diagnosis and classification by physical therapists: a special communication. Phys Ther 1989; 69:967–969.
2. Sahrmann S. Diagnosis by the physical therapist—a prerequisite for treatment. Physical Therapy, A Special Communication 1988; 68:1703–1706.
3. Nelson R, Nestor D. Standardized assessment of industrial low-back injuries: development of the NIOSH low-back atlas. Top Acute Care Trauma Rehabil 1988; 1:16–30.
4. Waddell G, Main C, Morris E, et al. Normality and reliability in the clinical assessment of backache. Br Med J 1982; 284:1519–1523.
5. Moll JM, Wright V. The pattern of chest and spinal mobility in ankylosing spondylitis. Rheum Rehabil 1973; 12:115.
6. Macnab I. Backache. Baltimore: Williams and Wilkins, 1977; 51.
7. Weisl SW, Feffer HL, Rothman RH. Industrial low-back pain, a prospective evaluation of a standardized diagnostic and treatment protocol. Spine 1984; 9:199–203.
8. Nelson MA, Allen P, Clamp SE, DeDombal FT. Reliability and reproductibility of clinical findings in low back pain. Spine 1979; 4:97–101.
9. Uden A, Astrom M, Bergenudd H. Pain drawings in chronic back pain. Spine 1988; 13:389–393.
10. Ransford AO, Cairns D, Mooney V. The pain drawing as an aid to the psychologic evaluation of patients with low back pain. Spine 1976; 1:127–134.
11. Wiltse LL, Rocchio PD. Preoperative psychological tests as predictors of success of chemonuleolysis in treatment of the low back syndrome. J Bone Joint Surg 1975; 57:478–483.
12. Cummings GS, Routan JL. Accuracy of the unassisted pain drawings by patients with chronic pain. J Ortho Sports Phys Ther 1987; 8:391–396.
13. Melzack R. The McGill Pain Questionnaire: major properties and scoring methods. Pain 1975; 1:277–299.
14. Murphy KA, Cornish RD. Prediction of chronicity in acute low back pain. Arch Phys Med Rehabil 1984; 65:334–337.
15. Fordyce WE. Behavioral methods for chronic pain and illness. St Louis: Mosby, 1976.
16. Leavitt F, Garron DC, McNeill TW, Whisler WW. Organic status, psychological disturbance, and pain report characteristics in low back pain patients on compensation. Spine 1982; 7:398–402.
17. Beals RK, Hickman NW. Industrial injuries of the back and extremities. J Bone Joint Surg 1972; 54A:1593–1611.
18. Hammonds W, Brana SF, Unikel IP. Compensation for work-related injuries and rehabilitation of patients with chronic pain. South Med J 1978; 71:664–666.
19. White AW. Low back pain in men receiving workmen's compensation. Can Med Assoc J 1966; 95:50–56.
20. Sorenson FB. A prospective study of low back pain in a general population. Scand J Rehabil Med 1983; 15:81–88.

21. Pedersen PA. Prognostic indicators in low back pain. J R Coll Gen Pract 1981; 31:209–216.

22. Troup JD, Martin JW, Lloyd DC. Back pain in industry. A prospective study. Spine 1981; 6:61–69.

23. Goertz MN. Prognostic indicators for acute low back pain. Spine 1990; 15:1307–1310.

24. McGill CM. Industrial back problems. A Control Program. J Occup Med 1968; 10:174–178.

25. Fry J. Back pain and soft tissue rhuematism. Advisory Services Colloquium Proc. London: Advisory Services (Clinical and General) Ltd., 1972.

26. Andersson GJ, Svensson HO, Oden A. The intensity of work recovery in low back pain. Spine 1983; 8:880–884.

27. McKenzie RA. The lumbar spine: mechanical diagnosis and therapy. Waikanae, New Zealand: Spinal Publications, 1981.

28. Donelson R, Silva G, Murphy K. Centralization and phenomenon, its usefulness in evaluating and treating referred pain. Spine 1990; 15:211–213.

29. Waddell G, Main CJ. Assessment of severity in low back disorders. Spine 1984; 9:204–208.

30. Roland M, Morris M. A study of the natural history of low-back pain. Part II: development of guidelines for trials of treatment in primary care. Spine 1983; 8:145–150.

31. Damkot DK, Pope MH, Lord J, Frymoyer JW. The relationship between work history, work environment and low back pain in men. Spine 1984; 9:395–399.

32. Robertson LS, Keeve JP. Worker injuries: The effects of worker compensation and OSHA inspections. J Health Polit Policy Law 1983; 8:581–597.

33. Trief P, Stein N. Pending litigation and rehabilitation outcome of chronic back pain. Arch Phys Med Rehabil 1985; 66:95–99.

34. Snook SH, Campanelli RA, Ford RJ. A study of back injuries at Pratt and Whitney Aircraft. Hopkinton, MA: Liberty Mutual Insurance Co. Research Center, 1980.

35. Magora A. Investigation of the relation between low back pain and occupation. Ind Med Surg 1970; 39:504–510.

36. Bergquist-Ullman M, Larsson U. Acute low back pain in industry. ACTA Orthop Scand Suppl 1977; 170:1–117.

37. Kumar S. Cumulative load as a risk factor for back pain. Spine 1990; 15:1311–1315.

38. Magora A. Investigation of the relation between low back pain and occupation -3, physical requirements: sitting, standing and weight lifting. Ind Med Surg 1972;41:5–9.

39. Svensson HO, Andersson GB. The relationship of low back pain, work history, work environment, and stress. A retrospective cross sectional study of 38 to 64-year old women. Spine 1989; 14:517–522.

40. Snook SH, White AH. Education and training. In: Pope M, Frymoyer J, Andersson G, eds. Occupa-tional Low Back Pain. New York: Praeger Press, 1984.

41. Frymoyer JW, Pope MH, Clements JH, et al. Risk factors in low back pain. J Bone Joint Surg 1983; 65-A(2):213–218.

42. Chaffin DB, Herrin GD, Keyserling WM. Pre-employment strength testing: an updated position. J Occup Med 1978; 20:403–408.

43. Vallfors B. Acute, subacute and chronic low back pain, clinical symptoms, absenteeism and working environment. Scand J Rehabil Med 1985; 1–97.

44. Videman T, Nurminen M, Troup JD. Lumbar spine pathology in cadaveric material in relation to history of back pain, occupation and physical loading. Spine 1990; 15:728–739.

45. Chaffin D, Park K. A longitudinal study of low back pain as associated with occupational weight lifting factors. Am Ind Hyg Assoc J 1973; 34:513–525.

46. Kelsey JL, Hardy RJ. Driving of motor vehicles as a risk factor for acute herniated lumbar intervertebral disc. Am J Epidemiol 1975; 102:63–73.

47. Frymoyer JW, Pope MH, Rosen JC, et al. Epidemiologic studies of low back pain. Spine 1980; 5:419–423.

48. Wilder DG, Woodworth BB, Frymoyer JW, Pope MH. Vibration and the human spine. Spine 1982; 7:243–254.

49. Sullivan A, McGill SM. Changes in spine length during and after seated whole-body vibration. Spine 1990; 15:1257–1260.

50. Cust G, Pearson J, Mair A. The prevalence of low back pain in nurses. Int Nurs Rev 1972; 9:169–178.

51. Dehlin O, Hedenrud B, Horal J. Back symptoms in nursing aids in a geriatric hospital. Scand J Rehabil Med 1976; 8:47–53.

52. Molumphy M, Unger B, Jensen GM, Lopopolo RB. Incidence of work-related low back pain in physical therapists. Phys Ther 1985; 65:482–486.

53. Begqvist-Ullman M, Larsson U. Acute low back pain in industry. Acta Orthop Scand Suppl 1977; 170:1–117.

54. Kelsey JL. An epidemiological study of the relationship between occupations and acute herniated lumbar intervetebral disc. Int J Epidemiol 1975; 4:197–205.

55. Magora A Investigation of the relation between low back pain and occupation. Ind Med Surg 39(11):31–37, 1970.

56. Hay MC. The incidence of low back pain in Busselton. Symposium: Low Back Pain. Twomey LT, ed. Perth: Western Aust Inst Tech, 1974.

57. Turner PG, Green JH, Galasko CS. Back pain in childhood. Spine 1989; 14:812–814.

58. Magora A, Taustein I. An investigation of the problem of sick leave in the patient suffering from low back pain. Ind Med Surg 1969; 38:398–408.

59. Biering-Sorensen F. A prospective study of LBP in

a general population. II. Location, character, aggravating and relieving factors. Scand J Rehabil Med 1983; 15:81–88.

60. Cairns D, Mooney V, Crane P. Spinal pain rehabilitation: Inpatient and outpatient treatment results and development of predictors of outcome. Spine 1984; 9:91–95.

61. Hult L. Cervical, dorsal and lumbar spinal syndromes. Acta Orthop Scand 1954; 24:174–175.

62. Biering-Sorenson F. Low back trouble in a general population of 30, 40, 50 and 60 year old men and women. Dan Med Bull 1982; 29:289–297.

63. Reisbord LS, Greenland S. Factors associated with self-reported back-pain prevalence: a population-based study. J Chron Dis 1985; 38:691–702.

64. Klein BP, Jensen RC, Sanderson LM. Assessment of worker's comp claims for back strains/sprains. J Occup Med 1984; 26:443–448.

65. Haber LD. Disabling effects of chronic disease and impairment. II. Functional capacity limitations. J Chron Dis 1973; 26:126–151.

66. Heliovaara M. Body height, obesity, and risk of herniated lumbar intervertebral disc. Spine 1987; 12:469–472.

67. Deyo RA, Bass JE. Lifestyle and low-back pain, the influence of smoking and obesity. Spine 1989; 14:501–506.

68. Postacchini F, Lami R, Pugliese O. Familial predisposition to discogenic low-back pain. An epidemiologic and immunigenetic study. Spine 1988; 13:1403–1406.

69. Mantle MJ, Greenwood RM, Currey HL. Backache in pregnancy. Rheum Rehabil 1977; 16:95–101.

70. Fast A, Weiss L, Ducommun J, Medina E, Butler JG. Low back pain in pregnancy, abdominal muscles, sit-up performance, and back pain. Spine 1990; 15:28–30.

71. Abramson D, Roberts SM, Wilson PD. Relaxation of the pelvic joints in pregnancy. Surg Gynecol Obstet 1934; 58:595–613.

72. Deyo RA, Diehl AK, Rosenthal M. How many days of bedrest for acute low back pain? A randomized clinical trial. N Engl J Med Vol. 315 1986; 17:1064–1070.

73. Weisl SW, Tsourmas N, Feffer HL, et al. A study of computer-assisted tomography: I, the incidence of positive CT scans in an asymptomatic group of patients. Spine 1984; 9:549–551.

74. Witt I, Vestergaard A, Rosenklint A. A comparative analysis of x-ray findings of the lumbar spine in patients with and without lumbar pain. Spine 1984; 9:298–300.

75. Frymoyer JW, Phillips RB, Newberg AH, MacPherson BV. A comparative analysis of the interpretations of lumbar spinal radiographs by chiropractors and medical doctors. Spine 1986; 11:1020–1023.

76. Raftery EB, Holland WW. Examination of the heart: An investigation into variation. Am J Epidemiol 1967; 85:438–444.

77. Castell DO, O'Brien KD, Muench H, et al. Estimation of liver size by percussion in normal individuals. Ann Intern Med 1969; 70:1183–1189.

78. Blendis LM, McNeilly WJ, Sheppard L, et al. Observer variation in the clinical and radiological assessment of hepato-spelenomegaly. Br Med J 1970; 1:727–730.

79. Gudfrey S, Edwards RH, Campbell EJ. Repeatability of physical signs in airways obstruction. Thorax 1969; 24:4–9.

80. Spangfort E. Laseque's sign in patients with lumbar disc herniation. Acta Orthop Scand 1971; 42:459–460.

81. Biering-Sorenson F. Physical measurements as risk factors for low back trouble over a one year period. Spine 1984; 9:106–109.

82. McConnell DG, et al. Low agreement of findings in neuromusculo-skeletal examinations by a group of osteopathic physicians using their own procedures. J Am Osteopath Assoc 1980; 79:441–450.

83. Beal MC, Goodridge JP, Johnston WL, McConnell DG. Interexaminer agreement on long-term patient improvement: an exercise in research design. J Am Osteopath Assoc 1982; 81:322–328.

84. Fairbank JC, Pynsent PB, Poortvliet JA, Phillips H. Influence of anthropometric factors and joint laxity in the incidence of adolescent back pain. Spine 1984; 9:461–464.

85. Burwell RG, Fraser MA. An anthropometric study of patients with low back pain syndromes. Presented at the International Society for the Study of the Lumbar Spine Meeting, Paris, France, May 1981.

86. Sward L, Eriksson B, Peterson L. Anthropometric characteristics, passive hip flexion, and spinal mobility in relation to back pain in athletes. Spine 1990; 15:376–382.

87. DePukys P. The physiologic oscillation of the length of the body. Acta Orthop Scand 1935; 6:338–347.

88. Markolf KL, Morris JM. The structural components of the intervertebral disc. J Bone Joint Surg 1974; 56A:675–687.

89. Tyrrell AR, Reilly T, Troup JD. Circadian variation in stature and the effects of spinal loading. Spine 1985;10:161–164.

90. Eklund JA, Corlett EN. Shrinkage as a measure of the effect of load on the spine. Spine 1984; 9:189–194.

91. White TL, Malone TR. Effects of running on intervertebral height. J Orthop and Sports Phys Ther 1990; 12:139–146.

92. White AA, Panjaba MM. Clinical biomechanics of the spine. 2nd ed. Philadelphia: J. B. Lippincott Co., 1990.

93. Fernand R, Fox DE. Evaluation of lumbar lordosis:

A prospective and retrospective study. Spine 1985; 10:799–803.

94. Mosner EA, Bryan JM, Stull MA, Shippee R. A comparison of actual and apparent lumbar lordosis in black and white adult females. Spine 1989; 14:310–314.

95. Twomey LT. Age changes in the human lumbar spine. [PhD Thesis] University of Western Australia, Nedlands, Western Australia, Australia, 1981.

96. Williams PC. The diagnosis and conservative management of lesions of the lumbosacral spine. In: Regional Orthopedic Surgery and Fundamental Orthopedic Problems. Ann Arbor: Edwards Brothers, 1948:AAOS 2:103–116.

97. Ohlen G, Wredmark T, Spangfort E. Spinal sagittal configuration and mobility related to low-back pain in the female gymnast. Spine 1989; 14:847–850.

98. Torgerson WR, Dotter WE. Comparative roentgenographic study of the asymptomatic and symptomatic lumbar spine. J Bone Joint Surg 1976; 58A:850–853.

99. Hansson T, Bigos S, Beecher P, Wortley M. The lumbar lordosis in acute and chronic low back pain. Spine 1985; 10:154–155.

100. Splithoff CA. Lumbosacral junction, roentenographic comparison of patients with and without backaches. JAMA 1953; 152:1610–1613.

101. Magora A, Schwartz A. Relation between low back pain syndrome and x-ray findings. Scand J Rehabil Med 1978; 10:145–145.

102. Stoddard A. Manual of Osteopathic Practice. London: Hutchinson, 1969.

103. Cyriax J. Textbook of orthopaedic medicine. Vol. One: Diagnosis of soft tissue lesions. Baltimore: Williams and Wilkins Co., 1975.

104. Mellin G. Measurement of thoracolumbar posture and mobility with a myrin inclinometer. Spine 1986; 11:759–762.

105. Ohlen G, Spangfort E, Tingvall C. Measurement of spinal sagittal configuration and mobility with DeBrunner's Kyphometer. Spine 1989; 14:580–583.

106. Willner S. Spinal pantograph—A non-invasive technique for describing kyphosis and lordosis in the thoraco-lumbar spine. Acta Orthop Scand 1981; 52:525–529.

107. Lovell FW, Rothstein JM, Personius WJ. Reliability of clinical measurements of lumbar lordosis taken with a flexible rule. Phys Ther 1989; 69:96–102.

108. Bryan JM, Mosner EA, Shipee R, Stull MA. Investigation of the flexible ruler as a noninvasive measure of lumbar lordosis in black and white adult female sample populations. J Orthop Sports Phys Ther 1989; 11:3–7.

109. Burdett RG, Brown KE, Fall MP. Reliability and validity of four instruments for measuring lumbar spine and pelvic positions. Phys Ther 1986; 66:677–684.

110. During J. Goudfrooij H, Keesen W, Beeker ThW, Crowe A. Towards standards for posture characteristics of the lower back system in normal and pathologic conditions. Spine 1985; 10:83–87.

111. Gracovetsky S, Kary M, Pitchen I, Levy S, Said RB. The importance of pelvic tilt in reducing compressive stress in the spine during flexion-extension exercises. Spine 1989; 14:412–416.

112. Day JW, Smidt GL, Lehmann T. Effect of pelvic tilt on standing posture. Phys Ther 1984; 64:510–516.

113. Sanders G, Stravrakas P. A technique for measuring pelvic tilt: Suggestion from the field. Phys Ther 1981; 61:49–50.

114. Gajdosik R, Simpson R, Smith R, Dontigny RL. Pelvic tilt, interatester reliability of measuring the standing position and range of motion. Phys Ther 1985; 65:169–174.

115. Alviso DJ, Dong GT, Lentell GL. Intertester reliability for measuring pelvic tilt in standing. Phys Ther 1988; 68:1347–1351.

116. Potter NA, Rothstein JM. Intertester reliability for selected clinical tests of the sacroiliac joint. Phys Ther 1985; 65:1671–1675.

117. Mann M, Glasheen-Wray M, Nyberg R. Therapist agreement for palpation and observation of iliac crest heights. Phys Ther 1984; 64:334–338.

118. Drerup B, Hierholzer E. Movement of the human pelvis and displacement of related anatomical landmarks on the body surface. J Biomech 1987; 20:971–977.

119. Taylor JR, Halliday M. Limb length asymmetry and growth. J Anat 1978; 126:634–635.

120. Beattie P, Isaacson K, Riddle DL, Rothstein JM. Validity of derived measurements of leg length differences obtained by use of a tape measure. Phys Ther 1990; 70:150–157.

121. Clarke GR. Unequal leg length, an accurate method of detection and some clinical results. Rheum Phys Med 1972; 11:385–390.

122. Morscher E, Figner G. Measurement of leg length. Prog Orthop Surg 1977; 1:21–27.

123. Nichols PJ. The short leg syndrome. Br Med J 1960; 1:1863.

124. Gofton JP, Trueman GE. Studies in osteoarthritis of the hip. Part II, Osteoarthritis of the hip and leg length disparity. Can Med Assoc J 1971; 104:791–799.

125. Giles LG, Taylor JR. Low back pain associated with leg length inequality. Spine 1981; 6:510–521.

126. Friberg O. Clinical symptoms and biomechanics of lumbar spine and hip joint in leg length inequality. Spine 1985; 8:643–651.

127. Fisk JW, Baigent ML. Clinical and radiological

assessment of leg length. NZ Med J 1975; 81:477–480.

128. Rush WA, Steiner HA. A study of lower extremity length inequality. Am J Roentgen 1946; 56:616–623.

129. Bailey HW, Beckwith CG. Short leg and spinal anomalies. J Am Osteopath Assoc 1937; 36:7.

130. Winter RB, Pinto WC. Pelvic obliquity, its causes and its treatment. Spine 1986; 11:225–234.

131. Steindler A. Kinesiology of the human body under normal and abnormal conditions. Springfield, IL: Charles C Thomas, 1977.

132. Irwin CE. The iliotibial band: its role in producing deformity in poliomyelitis. J Bone Joint Surg 1979; 31A:141–146.

133. Heino JG, Godges JJ, Carter CL. Relationship between hip extension range of motion and postural alignment. Jour of Orthopedic and Sports Physical Therapy 1990; 12:243–247.

134. Twomey LT, Taylor JR. Physical therapy of the low back. New York: Churchill Livingstone Inc., 1987:253–278.

135. Kendall HO, Kendall FP, Boynton DA. Posture and pain. Melbourne, FL: Robert E. Krieger Publishing Co., Inc., 1981:125–135.

136. Kendall HO, Kendall FP, Wadsworth GE. Muscles testing and function. Baltimore: Williams and Wilkins, 1971:201–239.

137. Steindler A. Kinesiology of the human body, under normal and pathologic conditions. Springfield, IL: Charles C Thomas, 1973:306.

138. Porter RW, Miller CG. Back pain and trunk list. Spine 1986; 11:596–600.

139. Splithoff CA. Lumbosacral junction roentgenographic comparison of patients with and without backaches. JAMA 1953; 152:1610–1613.

140. Arangio GA, Hartzell SM, Reed JF. Significance of lumbosacral list and low back pain. A controlled radiographic study. Spine 1990; 15:208–210.

141. McCulloch JA. Chemonucleolysis. J Bone Joint Surg 1977; 59B:45–52.

142. Tenhula JA, Rose SJ, Delitto A. Association between direction of lateral lumbar shift, movement tests, and side of symptoms in patients with low back pain syndrome. Phys Ther 1990; 70:480–486.

143. Goldberg C, Dowling FE. Handedness and scoliosis convexity: A reappraisal. Spine 1990; 15:61–64.

144. Ohlen G, Aaro S, Bylund P. The Sagittal configuration and mobility of the spine in idiopathic scoliosis. Spine 1988; 13:413–416.

6

Clinical Assessment of the Low Back: Active Movement and Palpation Testing

RICH NYBERG

ACTIVE MOVEMENT TESTING

Objectives

The objectives of active motion testing (AMT) are numerous. Since AMT requires voluntary effort on the part of the patient, a patient's willingness to move is assessed. To some degree, pain tolerance can then be determined. During AMT a patient with a high pain tolerance may exhibit greater range despite pain than a patient with a low pain tolerance. Information related to pain tolerance obtained from active motion tests helps to guide the examination and treatment plan.

Active motion tests identify movements which reproduce a patient's symptoms. Establishing which movements increase, decrease, or do not affect the patient's pain is prerequisite for deciding if and what kind of motion therapy program is desirable. For example, if forward bending of the lumbar spine is painful, though backward bending is not, then instruction to avoid forward bending and promote backward bending may be therapeutic.

Active movement test results are related to structural findings to determine the effect of position on motion. Just as a hip flexor contracture limits hip extension range of motion, an accentuated lumbar lordosis may restrict forward bending of the spine. Likewise, a lumbar spine positioned in right side bending due to a left lumbar convexity may have a left side bending motion limitation. Consequently, the influence of alignment on functional mobility often necessitates postural intervention strategies.

The assessment of active movements provides knowledge about motion behavior with respect to range, direction, control, and velocity. The amount of movement in forward bending, backward bending, side bending, and rotation may indicate the type of problem as well as the severity of the condition. An alteration of motion direction suggests a biomechanical movement asymmetry such as a vertebral motion restriction or hypermobility on one side. Optimal spinal motion control is exhibited when spinal movement occurs at a smooth, even, uninterrupted constant rate.

Evidence of a change in motion velocity which produces a hesitation or acceleration in movement activity (clinically referred to as a spinal hitch or judder) implies a motion-related dysfunction. The degree of resistance offered during recruitment of motion at each spinal level is determined by biomechanical and neurophysiologic functions which affect motion control or quality. Impairment of all aspects of spinal motion, range, direction, control, and velocity has more pathokinesiologic significance than interference of just one parameter. Analysis of active movements requires attention to all components of motion performance.

The relation of movement performance to low back pain has been the subject of clinical and experimental research. Numerous studies have focused on the effect of pain on range of motion, but only a few have investigated movement quality changes as a result of pain and dysfunction. Clinical reports of the tendency and significance of compensatory behavior in the spine relate to influence of one movement area or segment to others (i.e., hip-pelvic complex to the lumbar spine; thoracic spine to lumbar spine; one vertebral motion segment to adjacent segments; left sided motion performance to right).

REGIONAL LUMBAR MOTION

The following section begins with a review and analysis of regional lumbar motion behavior. The understanding and relevancy of abnormal movement performance in the presence of pain can be placed in appropriate context with knowledge of normal movement activity. A study of normal spinal motion with respect to age, sex, height, and weight is presented first. The parameters of AMT such as range of motion (ROM), coupling behavior, and velocity are discussed and then followed by an analysis of the reliability, validity, and practicality of clinical methods used by manual practitioners to assess spinal motion performance. The objective is to assist the clinical specialist in identifying the motion-related problems which are significant to the patient's pain complaints.

Age, Sex, Height, Weight Influences

A wide range of normal mobility exists for each movement plane within all age groups.[1] Not only is the regional lumbar motion variable, but a wide scatter of segmental mobility is also found within age categories.[2] A reduction in total lumbar motion is observed with age;[1-4] however, the most marked loss of lumbar mobility occurs after the age 35.[1,5] Loss of lumbar ROM motion with age occurs in all planes of measurement and can be as much as 23 to 52%.[1] One study demonstrated a consistent decrease in mobility at L5–S1 with

age along with a tendency for the remaining lumbar segments to exhibit an increase in movement.[2]

In regards to sex influence on lumbar motion, clinical studies have shown males to exhibit greater sagittal mobility, and females to have more lateral flexion.[1,4,6] The larger body size and greater weight in males creates additional preloading of the spine which tends to increase sagittal mobility.[7] The narrower waist and wider pelvis in the female may account for the increased movement found in the coronal plane in comparison to men.[1] Knowledge of motion performance differences between male and female is important in interpreting functional ability. Clinical evidence has not established a correlation between weight or height and spinal mobility.[4]

Parameters of Active Mobility Testing

The lumbar spine is most mobile in the sagittal plane and the least mobile in the horizontal plane. The greatest amount of lumbar motion is in flexion, followed by lateral flexion, extension, and rotation. Rotation flexibility in the lumbar spine is 27% of flexion, except at L5–S1 where rotation range increases to 55% of flexion.[8] In a cadaveric study, left and right lumbar motions were notably similar in range and did not show significant differences.[5] Considerable variation in the values obtained for lumbar movements reflect differences in measurement methods as well as failure to consider occupation and activity status. Clinicians need to be aware of the amount of motion range in each plane tested as well as of the fact that mobility in left and right directions should be closely symmetrical.

Curve Contour. From a clinical standpoint, many evaluators of spinal range of motion assess the degree and continuity of regional curve contour during active bending tests. For forward bending, a smooth, continuous posterior curve is presumed to indicate satisfactory range in flexion. An irregular curve formation with straightened segments is believed to represent restriction in motion.

Furthermore, some clinicians watch for sharp angles in the curvature to determine the presence of vertebral instability. A tendency for sharp angle formation adjacent to straight areas may suggest spinal compensatory behavior (Fig. 6.1). Discontinuity in spinal curve contour was found to be slightly higher in back pain patients (41%) than continuous curve formation (34%); however, the differences were not statistically significant.[9] Spinal curvatures in extension demonstrated more variability than the curve patterns in flexion.[9] The variability seen in extension curve contour may reflect disproportionate vertebral mobility among segments during backward bending.

Coupled Motion. Coupled motion response to primary or intentional movement is also analyzed during active lumbar mobility testing. For the clinician, evaluation of coupled motion behavior is difficult, since coupling in the lumbar spine varies in direction and magnitude according to segmental level, spinal posture, and intervertebral disc height. For example, biplanar radiographic studies show increases in primary or intentional movements as well as coupled motions in the lower lumbar spine when intervertebral disc height decreases.[10]

Direction of Coupled Motion. In regard to direction, flexion always accompanies rotation or side bending in the lumbar spine, and therefore some degree of sagittal displacement should be expected during an intentional frontal or horizontal plane movement. Bending in the frontal and sagittal planes should also be expected during a primary rotation motion, whereas horizontal and sagittal plane displacement occurs with lateral bending. While an opposite direction rotation results during lateral flexion of the lumbar spine, the direction of lateral flexion displacement during rotation varies within the lumbar spine. In the upper lumbar spine lateral flexion is the opposite of a primary rotation movement, but in the lower lumbar spine lateral flexion is in the same direction as the intentional rotation.[11] The clinical determination of coupled motion behavior in the lum-

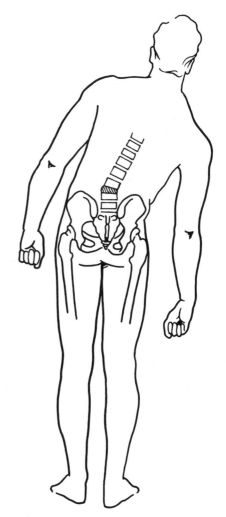

Figure 6.1. Discontinuity in spinal contour during side bending suggestive of compensatory behavior (Sharp angle formation indicates instability, straight areas reveal restriction.)

bar spine by observational analysis is therefore limited. Perhaps the use of spinal motion analyzers will reveal the presence of coupled motions and help the clinician with biomechanical assessment of spine function.

Relative Degrees of Coupled Motion. Manual practitioners judging active motion coupling performance of the spine should bear in mind that coupled motions are generally less than half of the main motion. If a patient's total lumbar forward bending range of motion is 40°, a lateral flexion displacement during forward bending is expected to be less than 20°. Similarly, if side bending right of the lumbar spine is measured to be 20°, the amount of coupling in left rotation is not to exceed 10° and most likely will be much less. As a general rule, the clinician is to regard minor motion deviations (<3°) from the primary movement plane to be within normal limits of coupling behavior.

Velocity. Velocity of movement is typically reduced during back pain episodes and must be evaluated to help determine patient status. Motion velocity may in fact be a more sensitive parameter of back impairment than restriction in range of motion or changes in strength.[12] As a result, an early indicator of improvement from a back condition may be noted by increases in motion velocity rather than an increase in total mobility or trunk strength. Measurements of velocity during trunk motion activities have only recently received attention in clinical low back evaluations with the development of spinal dynomometers. Some suggest that routine back examinations also include assessment of velocity during active mobility testing to more fully understand the effect of back pain on motion activity.[13]

Assessment of Pelvic Mobility

The relationship of low back, gluteal, or lower extremity pain to disorders of the sacroiliac joints is not understood. Research devoted to the role of sacroiliac joint motion disturbance in lumbar-pelvic pain conditions has focused on the relaxation of the pelvic articulations during pregnancy. The frequency of pain complaints during pregnancy is believed to be related to the stretching of supportive ligaments of the pubic symphysis and sacroiliac joints due to widening of the joints or excessive mobility.

The existence of sacroiliac joint mobility has been established by many sources.[14–18] The amount of mobility within the sacroiliac joints is generally agreed to be small when compared to other synovial joints, and as a result the functional role is debated. The irregularity of the joint surfaces, strength of the

ligamentous system and wedge shape configuration of the sacrum enable the pelvic girdle to support high load. The weight-bearing function of the pelvis is widely accepted by biomechanical authorities. However, the role of movement within the sacroiliac joints in providing force attenuation or shock absorption[19] is generally neither understood nor recognized. If sacroiliac mobility is necessary for shock absorption, any limitation or fixation in the joint mechanism could contribute to accelerated and/or possibly greater force distribution into the lumbo-sacral spine, thereby increasing the risk of injury at L5/S1.

The evidence for pelvic instability or motion restriction as a source of a low back condition is not conclusive from a research perspective, yet many clinicians consider pelvic mechanical disturbance to be significant (Chapter 12). The amount of relative movement between the sacrum and ilium is reviewed for further understanding of pelvic mechanics. Knowledge of expected motion within the sacroiliac joints may enable clinicians to relate motion findings to pain complaints.

Sacral Movement

In regard to sacral mobility between the two ilia, one experimental study using stereophotogrammetry demonstrates up to 2° of sacral rotation (flexion/extension) about a transverse axis.[16] Accompanying anterior sacral rotation (flexion) is 2 to 5.6 mm of anterior translation, while posterior sacral rotation (extension) is coupled by 1 to 2 mm of posterior translation.[16,18] Manual pressure on the apex of the sacrum has been radiologically confirmed to produce sacral extension and therefore is a valid method for testing sacral posterior displacement (Fig. 6.2).[16]

Some support exists for asymmetric sacral motion in the form of side bending and rotation.[16] Antagonistic iliac rotations such as what occurs in gait have been theorized to cause posterior and inferior displacement of the sacrum on the side of posterior iliac rotation while iliac anterior rotation is followed by anterior and superior movement of the

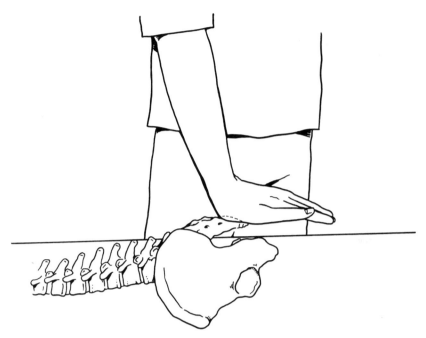

Figure 6.2. Sacral extension produced by manual pressure at the sacral apex.

adjacent articular surface of the sacrum.[19] The amount of asymmetric sacral mobility during unilateral stance has been measured but found to be very small (≤1.3° and 1.0 mm).[16] Further study is necessary to establish mechanical interrelations between the sacrum and ilium.

Ilial Movements

The relative displacement of the ilia with respect to the sacrum has also been investigated by x-ray photogrammetry.[15] The types of displacement observed when antagonistic ilial movements were induced by 60° of hip flexion on one side and 15° of hip extension on the opposite side were found to be identical in 5 subjects studied. Rotation is accompanied by translation on all axes. Anterior/posterior ilial rotation and translation were measured to be 10–12° and 6 mm, respectively. Wilder's study supports the association of ilial translation with rotation on the basis of the position for the axes of rotation.[20] He further states that ilial translation may serve to tighten ligaments and absorb energy, thus fulfilling an important role of the sacroiliac joint (Fig. 6.3). The clinical practitioner must recognize the

significance of associated motion behavior within the sacroiliac joints as well as the degree of movement to effectively determine the nature of a mechanical pelvic problem and the possible effect on the lumbosacral spine.

Although experimental studies of sacroiliac mobility generally agree that consistent three-dimensional movement exists, the degree of motion measured varies somewhat among studies. A recent roentgen stereophotogrammetric analysis of sacroiliac joint mobility[21] found considerably less ilial rotation and translation in the sagittal plane (2.5° and .7 mm, respectively) than previous studies. Differences in test positions may explain the variation in measurements observed. The clinician should understand that sacroiliac movements are normally small. Therefore, detection of significant motion in the pelvic articulations during a physical examination should alert the evaluator to the possibility of mechanical instability.

Pubic Mobility

Mobility of the pubic symphysis has been investigated by electromechanical and stereo-

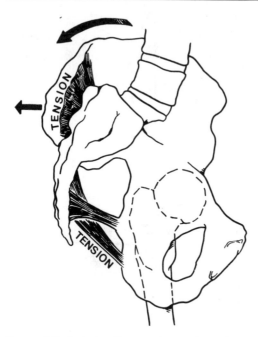

Figure 6.3. Posterior iliac rotation and translation causing tension in the deep posterior sacroiliac ligaments.

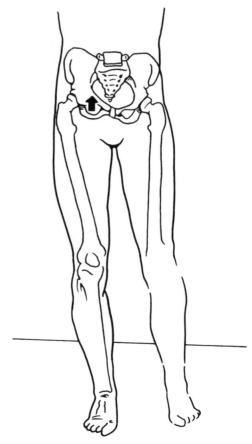

Figure 6.4. Superior translation at the pubic symphysis with unilateral standing.

photogrammetry methods.[22] Both measurement techniques reveal small movements. Translations not exceeding 2 mm and rotations up to 3° were found at the pubic symphysis in all two axes on two subjects. The same study confirmed the validity of hip flexion and unilateral standing tests for assessing vertical translation at the pubic symphysis (Fig. 6.4).

Several researchers of pelvic motion indicate that instability exists if vertical symphyseal mobility exceeds 2 mm. One such investigator stated that when vertical symphyseal mobility exceeds 2 mm, sacroiliac symptoms result.[23] Other researchers report pelvic instability when symphyseal width exceeds 10 mm and vertical motion is more than 5 mm.[24,25] The diagnosis of pelvic instability, however, has not been shown to be consistently associated with increased symphyseal mobility, but has been related to a high incidence of osteoarthritic change in the sacroiliac joints.[26] The cause of pelvic instability is most frequently connected to hormonal influences

and trauma during pregnancy and parturition.[27,28] Hypermobility of pelvic articulations may also result from pelvic fractures or postural strains.[29]

Evaluation of Clinical Testing of Pelvic Mobility

Clinical tests for detecting pelvic movement typically involves palpation and/or measurement of PSIS displacement. Total pelvic tilt range of motion was recorded to average 14.3° with a standard deviation of 5.2° using the depth caliper-meter stick method. Posterior pelvic tilt ROM was calculated on the average to be 6.5°, while anterior pelvic tilt averaged 7.9°. The test measurement method was reliable across examiners (Fig. 6.5).[30]

Inferior and medial displacement of the PSIS has been demonstrated in 30 subjects standing with one leg supported in 120° of hip flexion. Using a millimeter plexiglass grid for measurement, the mean inferior and medial PSIS position changes were 6.85 mm (±1.88 mm) and 4.58 mm (±1.88 mm), respectively. Intra- and interrater reliability of the plexi-grid measurement method was within 1.5 mm for inferior movement and within 1 mm for medial movement (Fig. 6.6).[31]

In a subsequent clinical study of sacroiliac mobility the effects of passive hip abduction and external and internal rotation on PSIS movement were measured with the plexiglass technique. Tendencies for ipsilateral PSIS excursion in lateral and inferior directions during hip abduction and internal rotation were established at approximately a 90% level. Lateral PSIS displacements of 3.37 ± 1.64 mm and 3.28 ± 1.39 mm were calculated for hip abduction and internal rotation, respectively (Fig. 6.7). Inferior PSIS movement was usually less than 2 mm. Hip external rotation produced significant PSIS position changes in an inferior direction but not for medial movement, although tendencies for inferior and

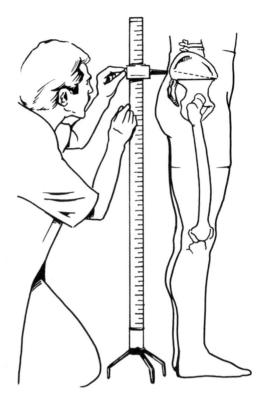

Figure 6.5. Pelvic inclination measurement.

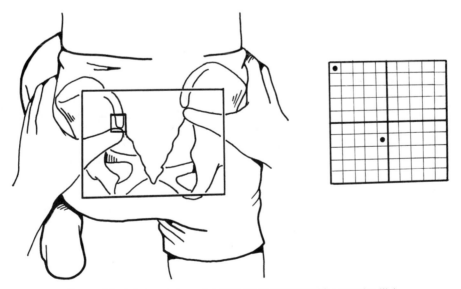

Figure 6.6. Inferior and medial PSIS displacement with posterior ilial rotation secondary to 120° of hip flexion.

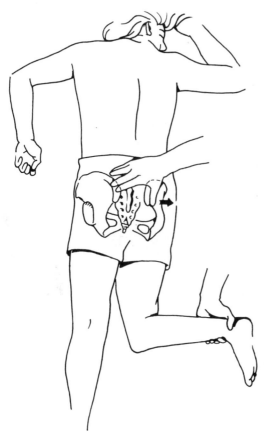

Figure 6.7. Lateral PSIS displacement with ilial internal rotation secondary to hip abduction and internal rotation.

experience. Both studies demonstrate the importance of standardizing test procedures for assessing sacroiliac movement so that meaningful information regarding pelvic function can be obtained. Perhaps other tests for sacroiliac mobility need to be considered and examined for reliability. In addition, the use of plexiglass grids and depth caliper-meter sticks should be encouraged for measuring sacroiliac mobility, since reliability for these clinical instruments has been shown to be satisfactory. Still to be investigated is the accuracy of clinical measures for sacroiliac motion when compared to x-ray study.

Lumbo-Pelvic Mechanical Relations

The effect of sacroiliac position and mobility on the lumbar spine also requires additional study. Tilting and rotation of the ilia along with a corresponding reaction by the sacrum may alter the transmission of force into the lumbosacral spine. Capsular and ligamentous support tissues may receive abnormal tension as a result of changes in pelvic alignment or mobility. In addition, mechanical stress imparted to the intervertebral discs is asymmetric. Figure 6.8 illustrates the influence of a left sacral tilting and rotation, left ilial posterior rotation and right ilial anterior rotation on an L5/S1 segment which remains stationary.

In this example, compression loading increases on the right side of the L5–S1 motion segment, while tension loading increases on the left side. Capsular-ligamentous tension is therefore uneven on each side of the segment, possibly resulting in adaptive tissue shortening on the right and stretch-elongation on the left. Sagittal shear stress and horizontal plane torsional force is imparted to the intervertebral disc at L5–S1 as a consequence of antagonistic ilial rotations and sacral rotation. The annular fibers are stressed in the same direction of the shear and torque forces. Internal disc deformation also results from alterations in compression and tension loading. L5–S1 may eventually become vulnerable to injury through several possible mechanisms: left

medial PSIS displacement exist. Accuracy in assessment of PSIS position was less than or equal to 2 mm.[32] Results from the two clinical studies of pelvic mobility indicate that small movements in specific directions exist within the sacroiliac joints with passive hip motions.

Clinical evaluation of sacroiliac mobility using standing and sitting flexion tests demonstrated poor reliability in one study.[33] The same study also reported a 47% level of agreement for the Gillet (marching) test (a measure of posterior ilial rotation). A more recent investigation of the Gillet marching test, however, demonstrated a 68% intraexaminer agreement and a 65% agreement among examiners.[34] For positive test findings, interestingly, lower intraexaminer agreement was found for the evaluators with greater levels of

facet capsular stretch irritation, right facet joint compression, posterior longitudinal ligament irritation from abnormal tension development, and/or annular tensile/torsional stress. Although the illustration provided is clinical theory, the biomechanical basis for lumbosacral pain from pelvic position or motion disturbance is rational.

CLINICAL INSTRUMENTATION FOR EVALUATING LUMBAR ACTIVE MOVEMENTS

Numerous noninvasive clinical methods have been used and advocated to study lumbar active range of motion for the purpose of providing objective measurements. Use of instrumentation for analyzing spinal motion is recommended by some researchers in favor of clinical eyeball estimate which has been shown to detect only gross loss of movement.[35] Reliability, utility, or ease in application and validity of a measurement method are important factors to consider when selecting a tool for assessing spinal motion. An appraisal of the various clinical methods for examining lumbar mobility is presented.

Finger Tip to Floor Method (Fig. 6.9)

Measuring finger tip distance to the floor while subjects maintain a fully flexed or laterally flexed spinal posture has been found to be a reliable method.[36,37] A modification in the finger tip to floor technique positions the subject standing on a stool. Forward bending measurements can then be obtained on subjects who otherwise would touch the floor. Intra- and intertherapist reliability for the modified finger tip to floor method was .98 and .95 respectively.[38]

Although reliability and utility of the finger tip to floor measurement technique is acceptable, the validity of the method for assessing lumbar flexion range of motion must be questioned. Since finger tip to floor distance is also a function of hamstring length, hip and thoracic flexion, as well as upper extremity flexibility, assessments of lumbar forward bending range must be made with dis-

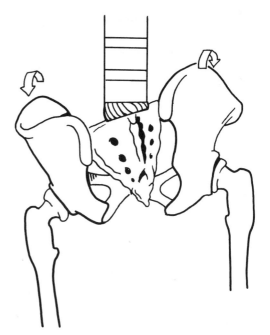

Figure 6.8. Mechanical stress alteration at a nonadaptive L5–S1 segment. The L5–S1 motion segment is positionally unresponsive to the changes in pelvic alignment.

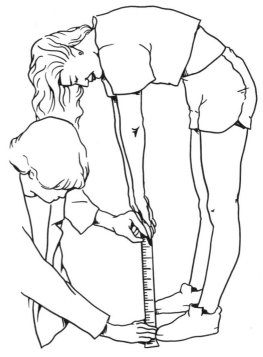

Figure 6.9. Finger tip to floor measurement of spinal flexion.

cretion. In addition, differences in arm, trunk, and leg length (i.e., long arms and trunk, short legs) may mislead examiners to believe that lumbar flexion is more than what actually exists. Anthropometric differences also make comparisons among patients difficult. Another disadvantage of the finger tip to floor distance method is the fact that a neutral starting position is not defined. Information regarding actual total range of lumbar motion is therefore limited.

Tape Measure Methods (Fig. 6.10)

Lumbar Flexion. Tape measure methods of measuring spinal motion have been based on a skin distraction technique developed by Schober.[39] A modified Schober method for assessing lumbar flexion or extension involves skin marking 10 cm above and 5 cm below the lumbosacral juncture on subjects in erect position.[40] After full flexion the distance between the marks is measured with a tape. Any increase in distance between skin marks represents a measure of lumbar flexion mobility. Mean skin distraction for a sample population of 195 females and 147 males was found to

be 6.27 cm. Ninety percent of the population studied were able to distract skin marks at least 5 cm during full flexion.[40] As noted previously, spinal range of motion measured by the Schober technique was determined to be age-dependent.

Intra-[41] and interexaminer[42] reliability of the modified Schober method for measuring lumbar flexion has been demonstrated in some studies but not in others.[43–45] Similarly, correlation comparison studies between radiologic and the modified Schober technique for measuring lumbar flexion are inconclusive. While one investigation indicates a correlation coefficient of .97[40] between radiologic and clinical methods, another study demonstrates an r = .43, suggesting that the clinical measurement gives only an index of true spinal mobility.[45] The importance of having a reliable clinical means for evaluating lumbar motion should not be dismissed despite the possibility of external lumbar angles not being identical to internal lumbar angles as measured by x-ray.

The Schober method[39] is simple to perform and is capable of measuring spinal flexion independent of hip movement. Clini-

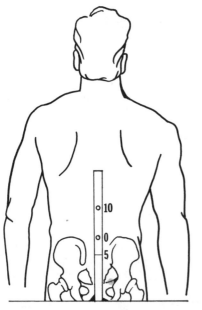
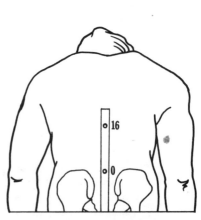

Figure 6.10. Tape measure method of assessing skin distraction in forward bending.

cal identification of the lumbosacral junction, however, may err by 2 cm which causes a 3° to 5° difference in range of motion. Anthropometric characteristics such as trunk length will determine the number of motion segments involved in a forward bending test. Measurement of some individuals may include lower thoracic intervertebral motion, while in others only lumbar movement is measured. The tape measure method of Schober is unable to identify a starting position of the spine and can only analyze flexion.

Lateral Flexion. Tape measurements of lateral flexion have also been studied by measuring the distance between two marks on the lateral aspect of the trunk (Fig. 6.11) before and after side bending. Distraction of skin marks on the opposite side or approximation of skin marks on the same side of lateral flexion can be measured. Skin mark approximation during lateral flexion decreases with age, demonstrating loss of flexibility and is greater for females than males (4.8 cm).[46]

Intra- and interobserver repeatability for the lateral flexion tape measure method is fair, suggesting that an improvement in technique is necessary. When compared to internal angles of lateral flexion measured radiologically the approximation of skin marks revealed a good correlation (r=.79).[46] The importance of an objective clinical method for evaluating lateral flexion relates to the possible differen-

tial diagnosis of spinal conditions such as ankylosing spondylitis which tends to limit side bending mobility before flexion ROM.[47]

Backward Bending. Except for one indirect method, measurement of backward bending is the least reliable. Measuring the horizontal distance to a wall from the suprasternal notch on subjects yielded satisfactory reliability between two evaluators (r=.83–.89) (Fig. 6.12).[48] Although repeatability in measurement appears good for this tape measure method of assessing trunk extension, the actual lumbar curvature is not analyzed. As a result, hip extension range of motion is unaccounted and could in fact be partly responsible for the distance calculated.

Flexirule (Figs. 6.13A,B)

Measurement of back surface contour with use of a flexible ruler has been demonstrated to be a reliable and valid method for calculating total lumbar flexion and extension range of motion. Intraobserver reliability for flexirule analysis of lumbar sagittal mobility has revealed correlation coefficients greater than .95 with measurement variability of 3–4°.[49–51] In addition, the flexirule external calculations of lumbar sagittal mobility approximate radiographic measurements within 6° and can also be used to accurately compare upper and lower lumbar sagittal mobility.[50,51] As a result, the flexirule offers a potential

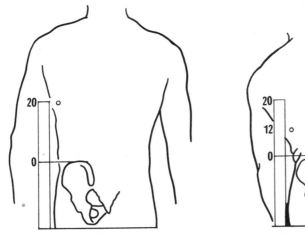

Figure 6.11. Tape measure method of assessing skin distraction in side bending.

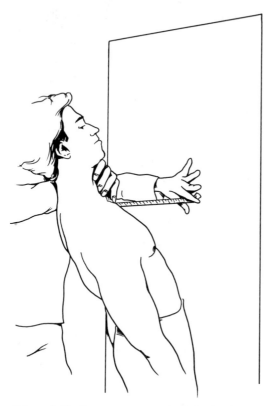

Figure 6.12. Tape measure method for backward bending.

means for analyzing the distribution of lumbar sagittal mobility by differentiating upper from lower lumbar range of motion. Flexirule measurements of lumbar curves may enable detection of regional differences in mobility.

In another flexirule study no correlation was found between surface flexirule and radiograph measures of lumbar intersegmental motion.[52] Measurements of intersegmental movement by the flexirule method are inaccurate due to the errors in calculating the differences between small angles. Therefore, although total and regional lumbar mobility can be assessed with the flexirule technique, intersegmental mobility cannot be determined accurately.

Spondylometers, Inclinometers, Goniometers

Spondylometer. Other instruments have also been utilized and studied for measuring

spinal mobility in the sagittal plane. The spondylometer, first described by Dunham and tested by Sturrock,[53] consists of two brass rods connected at a hinge with a protractor containing a moveable pointer at one end. The protractor end is placed at the base of the sacrum, and the other end is placed on the spinous process of C7 in the erect, flexed (Fig. 6.14) and extended positions.[53] In a comparison study of three clinical methods for measuring spinal mobility, the spondylometer was found to be the easiest method to use. Interrater reliability for spondylometer measures ranged from .76 for flexion to .87 for extension.[43]

In Sturrock's spondylometer study, total spinal range of motion in the sagittal plane decreased with age as expected. Extension range of motion was found to be greater in women in the childbearing years than in men of the same age. Extension range in patients with ankylosing spondylitis was markedly reduced even when flexion and total sagittal mobility was within normal limits. Measurement of backward bending mobility therefore may be the most sensitive active motion indicator of ankylosing spondylitis.[53]

Kyphometer. A similar instrument to the spondylometer is the Kyphometer designed by DeBrunner.[54] The Kyphometer places the protractor at the hinge between the two arms instead of at one end. Like the Spondylometer, the Kyphometer allows quick (approximately 1 minute) noninvasive measurement of sagittal spine position and movement. Measurement reproducibility in terms of variability coefficients is very good for position and mobility of the thoracic and lumbar spines. Variability in measures was also found to be good, even among inexperienced testers. Ohlen et al. point out the importance of explicity, standardized instructions to obtain consistency in starting position and movements to be measured.[54]

Inclinometer. This device consists of a degree dial attached to two plastic buttons which are placed onto the section of the spine to be measured. A weighted needle which remains vertical indicates the angle of spinal

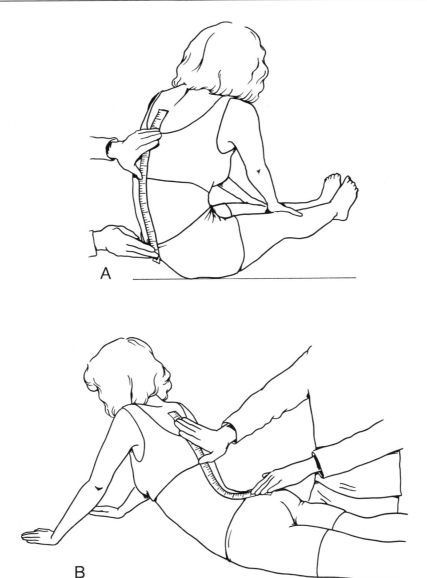

Figure 6.13A. Flexirule measurement of lumbar forward bending.

Figure 6.13B. Flexirule measurement of maximum lumbar lordosis.

incline (Fig. 6.15). In two studies,[45,55] inclinometers were shown to have variability coefficients of approximately 14–16° when measuring total sagittal or lumbar range.[45,55] Repeatability in measures was found in two other investigations using inclinometers,[40,44] but, when compared to the flexirule or spondylometer, inclinometer technique is less accurate, particularly for spinal flexion.

Loebl's inclinometer study supports the clinical observation of increased thoracic kyphosis development with age in both males and females.[55]

Inclinometer correlation studies with radiographs of spinal mobility vary in results depending on whether a one- or two-inclinometer method is used. While one study reports no significant difference between a

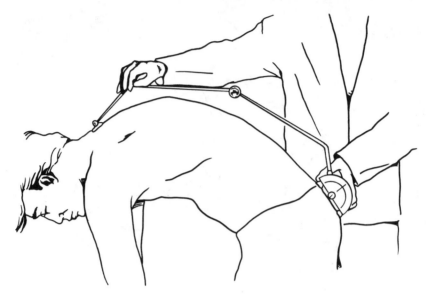

Figure 6.14. Spondylometer measurement of forward bending.

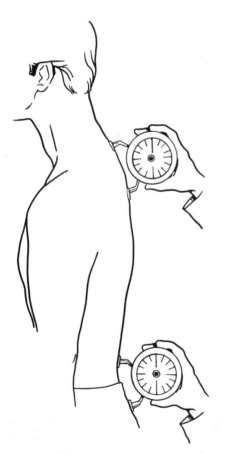

Figure 6.15. Dual inclinometer measurement of forward bending.

two-inclinometer method and the motion findings from radiographs,[56] another study using the one-inclinometer method described by Loebl demonstrates large disparity in measures with x-ray.[45] The difficulty in conforming the straight edge of the inclinometer base to the curvature of the spine may necessitate use of the two-inclinometer method which involves subtracting sacral inclinometer measures from an upper spinal inclinometer measure.

Goniometry. Goniometric measurements of spinal flexion/extension movements obtained by calculating the difference between femoral-trunk angles and hip range of motion have shown consistency in repeated testing (r=.85).[57] With respect to usability, however, this goniometric technique takes longer, since four measurements are required (hip flexion and extension, femoral-trunk flexion and extension). In addition, the test positions are difficult to maintain and often become uncomfortable.

Although standard and parallel goniometer (Figs. 6.16**A,B**) measures of lumbar curves offer reasonably reliable assessment of spinal flexion[44,58] more difficulty is encountered with extension due to skin motion and folding which tilts the goniometer platform. The ex-

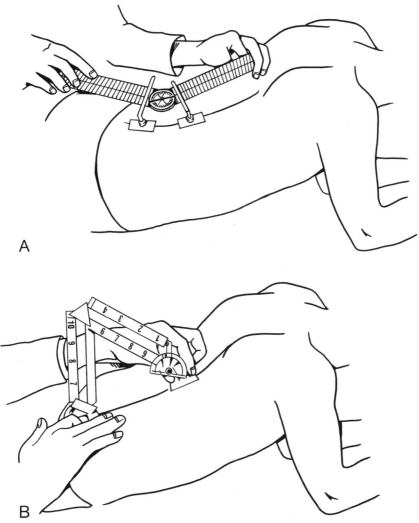

Figure 6.16A. Standard goniometric measure of lumbar curve.

Figure 6.16B. Parallel goniometric measure of lumbar curve.

ternal measurements obtained by goniometric technique also differ significantly from internal measures acquired from roentgenograms.[44] As a result, the goniometric methods do not offer any significant advantage over other noninvasive techniques.

Compass Method for Thoracolumbar Rotation

By attaching a compass containing a 2° division scale to a wooden auxiliary tool with two parallel arms, one fixed to the compass based arm and another capable of sliding, thoracolumbar rotation was measured (Fig. 6.17). Average intertester and intratester correlation coefficients of .79 were obtained by Mellin for repeated testing of thoracolumbar rotation.[59] Total thoracolumbar rotation was determined by using the jugular notch of the sternum and the spinous process of T1 as reference markers. Lower thoracolumbar rotation can be ascertained by a xiphisternum and a horizontally corresponding vertebral

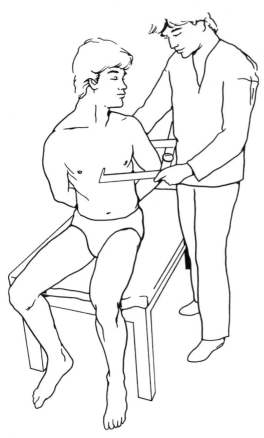

Figure 6.17. Compass measurement of thoracolumbar rotation.

spinous process. By subtracting lower from total thoracolumbar rotation measures Mellin calculated upper thoracolumbar rotation.[59,60]

The mean total rotation of the thoracolumbar spine on 39 nonpainful subjects was 94.6°, which compares closely with other studies measuring spinal rotation. Lower thoracolumbar rotation range was 72.9°, while upper thoracolumbar range was 20.8°. Although no left or right differences were found for lower thoracolumbar rotation, significant differences in right (12.8° ± 5.4°) and left (8.0° ± 4.9°) rotation were identified for upper thoracolumbar rotation.[60] Reliable measures of spinal rotation are necessary in situations where horizontal plane mobility is impaired, particularly when other motion planes are less affected by the condition.

DISADVANTAGES OF CLINICAL INSTRUMENTATION

Despite the objectivity of clinical instrumentation in measuring spinal range of motion, a number of disadvantages exist. For some instruments such as the flexirule, the position of measurement must be maintained while the back surface contour is determined. The information obtained relating to spinal flexion range may not only be irrelevant with respect to the nature of the problem or how to manage the patient, but the position sustained during measurement could possibly aggravate the condition.

Many of the clinical instruments are capable of only measuring sagittal movement. In certain low back pain conditions, sagittal mobility may be less predictive of the problem than side bending or rotation.[60] Calculation of spinal forward and backward bending mobility by clinical instrumentation could therefore have less meaning than other movements in assessing a low back problem. Since other movements aside from spinal flexion and extension are important to evaluate, the need for one clinical measurement device to assess multiple planes is apparent. Otherwise, the clinician is required to use as many as three instruments to assess each motion plane.

Neuromuscular and biomechanical performance *during* spinal movements cannot be ascertained through clinical devices which examine end range of motion. Parameters such as motion control, velocity, and direction offer information regarding neuromuscular behavior, such as muscular contraction-relaxation responses and efficient sequencing, timing, and coordination of muscular activity. Guarded spinal motion behavior, as determined by EMG calculations, show significant correlations with partial movement and pain behavior.[13]

In other investigations[61,62] abnormal flexion-relaxation responses in chronic low back pain patients, such as the inability of the lumbar paraspinals to deactivate around 40° of trunk flexion, were not just related to limitation in spinal mobility. Low back pain may therefore interfere with the dynamics of motion activity irrespective of the range obtained. The ability of a clinician to detect decreases or increases in spinal flexion-relaxation responses without use of back surface EMG analysis is limited, due to the subjectivity of observational assessment and the need for further definition of motion control parameters.

The use of *computerized spinal dynometers* enables assessment of motion velocity, torque production during movement, and range of motion. Improvements in the development of such instruments are needed to demonstrate reliability.[63] The potential of evaluating the dynamics of spinal motion performance using such instrumentation, however, is unlimited, particularly if interfaced with EMG analysis of muscle activity. Conversely, the limitations of clinical measurement tools for calculating only range of motion are evident.

RELATIONSHIP OF STRUCTURE TO ACTIVE MOVEMENTS

The correlation of spinal position and mobility has been a subject of interest and confusion among clinical investigators. Despite an apparent association between structural alignment of the spine and spinal movement, few studies have explored the relationship from a research standpoint. If alignment does affect spinal motion, then determination of appropriate motion responses must consider the structural make-up of the individual.

One study on 64 young female gymnasts (mean age, 12 years)[64] found a positive correlation between the degree of lumbar lordosis and the amount of lumbar forward bending range of motion. Conversely, a negative correlation was revealed between lumbar lordosis and backward bending. For every degree of lumbar lordosis, lumbar flexion increased .5° and lumbar extension decreased 1.5°. As a result, for every 1° of lordosis there is a 1° loss in total lumbar sagittal mobility.

A study on 476 low back pain patients[60]

supports the same findings and also revealed greater lateral flexion with increased lumbar lordosis. Consequently, lumbar flexion and side bending appear to increase with the amount of lordosis, whereas extension range decreases. Knowledge of tendencies for motion loss in certain directions based on the degree of sagittal curvature may help the clinician determine which type of motion activities to promote in the development of a therapeutic exercise program.

The degree of thoracic kyphosis or lateral spine deviation, as determined by Cobb angle measures, on 127 patients with idiopathic scoliosis also appears to correlate with thoracic spinal mobility.[64,65] The greater the Cobb angle or thoracic kyphosis the less sagittal mobility there is in the thoracic spine. Total side bending and rotation mobility of the thoracic spine was significantly reduced when scoliotic deformities increased. Likewise, minor scoliotic curves in the lumbar spine also negatively influenced total lateral bending and rotation.

A relationship between lateral lumbar shifts and side bending range of motion was confirmed in a study on 24 low back pain patients.[66] In this study, contralateral side bending movement was restricted or painful in 71% of the patients observed to have obvious lateral trunk shifts. Patients demonstrating left lateral shifts, therefore, are most likely to have difficulty with right side bending. In regard to management of patients with propensities toward lateral trunk shifts, perhaps movement activities which safely promote contralateral side bending should be considered.

HYPOMOBILITY

Spinal motion limitation is presumed to be related to low back pain. Some studies seem to establish a definitive relationship between restriction in spinal movement and back pain, while other studies do not. In one study, for example, the range of spinal motion offered clear evidence of improvement in spinal function, but correlated poorly with the patient's problems.[67] Additional support to the contention that spinal flexibility is not significantly related to the incidence of back pain is provided in a study on 3020 employees of Boeing Aircraft.[68] Lumbo-sacral flexion, sit and reach measures of overall forward bending, and lateral flexion ranges were evaluated and then re-evaluated approximately 3 years later. No association was found between any of the flexibility measures and back pain reports. The premise that spinal inflexibility is predictive of back pain may not be substantiated, at least in an industrial work setting. Moreover, the assumption that greater spinal mobility reduces the frequency of back pain is without universal scientific support.

Although spinal flexibility measures may not be predictive for low back pain, an association between previous or current low back pain and spinal range of motion does exist. Whether the restriction in spinal movement is a cause of the problem or a protective response to pain, however, is not clear. As a result, uncertainty remains as to whether an improvement in mobility helps to resolve the pain or the increase in range occurs once the symptoms subside.

Lateral Flexion and Rotation

Spinal motion restrictions in lateral flexion and rotation have been found to correlate significantly with the degree of low back trouble in a study on 151 men aged 54–63 years.[69] Forward bending mobility, despite being a most commonly used spinal active movement test, was not a specific indicator of back disability. In another study, forward bending range of the lumbar spine was not limited in top Swedish athletes with back pain.[70] Furthermore, increases in lateral bending and rotation ROM have been found to be positively related to improvements in the degree of low back trouble. However, since the subjects tested did not suffer from acute pain, the improvements in mobility were thought to indicate true changes in spinal function and not just reflect a reduction in pain.

Further evidence for the apparent relationship between lateral flexion restriction in the spine and low back pain is established from Weitz's findings[71] from lateral flexion roentgenograms: 28 out of 34 patients with myelographic or surgically confirmed disc protrusions had impaired lateral bending toward the side of the disc bulge (Fig. 6.18). The use of lateral bending x-rays rather than static films on patients suspected of having a lumbar disc protrusion may, therefore, be warranted.

In a follow-up study of 301 men and 175 women having chronic or recurrent low back pain, rotation and lateral flexion range of motion was found to correlate with low back pain chronicity and frequency more than flexion and extension.[60] A biplanar radiographic study of lumbar segmental mobility revealed that lateral bending and rotation at L4–5 were less in patients experiencing leg numbness.[72] Stiffness in side bending and rotation is therefore a sensitive indicator of chronic or episodic low

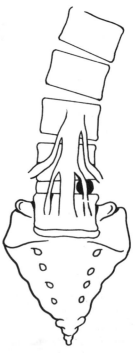

Figure 6.18. Restricted side bending toward the side of disc bulge.

back pain. The relevancy of testing active movements of the spine in nonsagittal planes is therefore evident.

Why nonsagittal spinal motions are affected by low back pain more than sagittal movements is unclear. The tendency for low back problems to be unilateral may account for the restrictions noted in left and right side bending/rotation. Perhaps nonsagittal movements in chronic low back pain individuals stiffen more than flexion because flexion mobility is a requirement for most daily activities, whereas side bending and rotation are less essential.

Extension Range

Loss of extension range has also been found to be more closely related to low back pain than flexion. In a study using pre-employment screening tests on a volunteer population of 1741 men and 1150 women, backward bending range decreased more markedly in individuals reporting low back pain than flexion.[73] In a previous study, pain on passive lumbar extension was found to be of value as a clinical sign for predicting episodes of low back pain.[74] A subsequent study demonstrated a significant relief of low back pain during active lumbar extension after intra-articular injection of the L4–5 and L5–S1 facet joints.[75] Spinal movement examination should therefore include backward bending tests, since loss of extension motion or pain on backward bending is associated with or predictive of low back pain. Perhaps just as important is the maintenance of extension range of motion through exercise activities to reduce the risk of low back problems.

Caution for Clinicians

Noteworthy is the fact that limitation in spinal flexion mobility is not always related to low back pain, except in current conditions where flexion is extremely limited.[76] Despite the lack of association between flexion range of motion and low back trouble, most clinical examinations of the spine tend to concentrate on lumbar flexion motion performance. In a

similar vein, the value of exercise programs for low back patients which only promote spinal flexion is of question, particularly if flexion range is not significantly affected. The inclusion of multi-plane motion testing and treatment of the spine for low back pain patients would seemingly be important.

In Mellin's study,[60] restrictions in thoracic mobility were found to correlate more strongly with chronic or recurrent low back pain than lumbar motion limitations.[60] This finding is of considerable interest to clinicians and researchers who maintain that spinal segments and regions show compensatory tendencies. Studies showing relationships between one segment or area of the spine and another lend support to the contention of spinal compensatory behavior. Additional support to the spinal compensatory theory is established in a study by Burton on 545 working adults.[77] In this study, women who participated in school sport activities and also maintained upper lumbar flexibility had reduced chronicities of low back pain. Apparently, motion performance in the thoracic and upper lumbar spinal segments influences the amount or distribution of mechanical stress in the lumbosacral spine. Management of low back pain conditions may subsequently require evaluation and treatment of upper lumbar, thoracic, or possibly cervical spinal segments.

CLINICAL INSTABILITY

Hypermobility of the spine or a spinal motion segment simply means increased motion. Hypermobility is not necessarily symptomatic and therefore does not always indicate a pathophysiologic motion state. Symptomatic hypermobility of clinical instability involves increased abnormal motion resulting in sufficient mechanical tissue deformation to cause considerable pain.[78]

By definition alone, clinical instability would seem to be associated with certain types of symptomatic back conditions. Repeated injury or one substantial traumatic blow to a spinal segment may result in clinical instability causing periodic or constant pain from irritated tissue. Clinical detection of increased spinal motion activity, either segmentally or regionally, using noninvasive measures or radiographs taken in different bending positions has helped to establish some evidence relating clinical instability to low back problems. Presumably, the unstable motion segment(s) cause(s) increase stress to facet capsules/articular surfaces and supporting ligaments as well as the annular fibers of the disc and the cartilaginous endplates.

Hypermobility and low back difficulty was investigated and reported in 1971 by Howes and Isdale.[79] Spinal and peripheral joint hypermobility was identified during clinical examination on 19 out of 25 female low back patients who had been ruled-out for disc lesions, spondylosis, spondylolysis, sacro-ilitis, and posterior joint syndrome. The number of back-ache patients determined to be hypermobile accounted for more than the 4% and 10% incidence rates of hypermobility found in general populations in two separate studies.[80,81] Hypermobility was therefore considered to be a significant factor related to the low back problem.

More recently, the modified Schober method for measuring spinal flexion revealed that men with the greatest lumbar mobility were most prone to experience low back difficulties over a one year period.[82] In further support of the clinical instability theory for low back pain is a study by Lankhorst et al. on the natural history of idiopathic low back pain.[83] Patients possessing greater spinal mobility had less functional recovery than patients who continued to have restricted range of motion. Functional improvement in patients with range of motion limitations was thought to be related to the stabilization of hypermobile spinal segments.

A study with anteroposterior lateral bending and lateral flexion-extension x-ray views of 7 patients with various low back problems demonstrated abnormal increased motion at either L4–5 or L5–S1 in one or more planes.[78] Increased segmental motion was evident in abnormal vertebral tilt angles and excessive translation mobility. In the case of an L4–5

hyperflexion instability, for example, anterior sagittal plane rotation of L4–5 is greater than 20°, and anterior sagittal plane translation is more than 4.5 mm (Fig. 6.19).[8] With respect to the intervertebral space abnormal disc closure on the side to which the patient bends is observed along with abnormal opening on the side away. Excessive translation and tilt is also evident in the facet joints.

Others support the relevance of clinical instability to lower back problems on the basis that the majority of lumbar disc symptoms derive from L4–5 and L5–S1 intervertebral levels which are the most mobile lumbar segments.[8,84] Potential development of unstable motion segments at the two lower lumbar intervertebral levels exists in light of the high load-bearing responsibilities. Characteristic of clinically unstable motion segments is increased movement in normal and/or abnormal directions.[79] From a clinical standpoint the examiner looks for abnormal out-of-plane motion activity with tendencies for displacement toward the stiffer side of the motion segment(s)[78] or away from the more mobile side. Clinically unstable motion segments will also typically move asymmetrically. Free motion will occur in one direction and restricted motion in the opposite direction. Clinical determination of unstable motion segments through observation of active movements re-

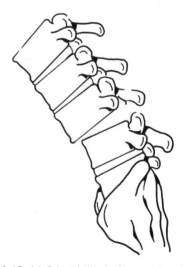

Figure 6.19. L4–5 instability in forward bending.

quires establishing specific criteria for what constitutes instability. Manual practitioners consider clinical instability by observing one or more of the following events during active movement tests:

1. Hinging or fulcruming at one or more spinal levels on one or both sides (Fig. 6.20**A**),
2. A momentary catch (typically during flexion) causing directional change,
3. Tendencies to maintain a lumbar lordosis during flexion (Fig. 6.20**B**),
4. Grasping and/or pushing on the thighs for support when returning from flexion (Fig. 6.20**C**),
5. An increase in pain or delayed pain if extreme ranges of motion are maintained for 20 sec or more,
6. Guarded, hesitating motion performance.

Inherent to the nature of clinical instability is the propensity for unstable segments to become temporarily restricted in one or more directions. The spinal segment catches or temporarily binds in a given position and is unable to unlock unless moved or repositioned in a precise manner so as not to induce muscle contraction. In the situation of a temporarily locked unstable motion segment active movement testing may actually reveal restricted range in one or more planes. Mobilization therapy, under these circumstances, is appropriate for the purpose of realignment and restoration of motion activity.

In summary, both hypomobility and hypermobility to the extreme range appear to be related to low back problems. The need to test multiple planes of motion has been established. The clinical methods for reliably assessing motion problems require further investigation. Support for clinical evidence of motion abnormalities through mobility x-ray films is also essential for verification of the problem.

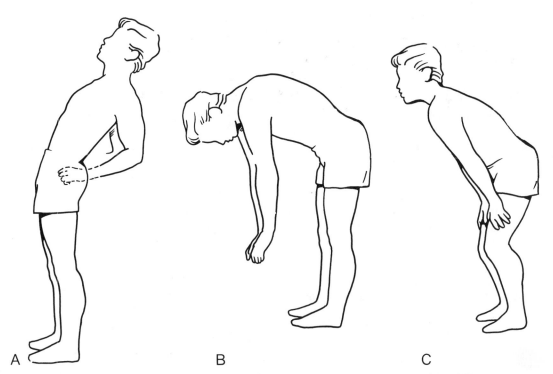

A   B   C

Figure 6.20A. Fulcruming observed during backward bending, suggestive of instability.

Figure 6.20B. Maintenance of lumbar lordosis during forward bending.

Figure 6.20C. Holding and/or pushing on thighs when returning from flexion.

HIP RANGE OF MOTION

Correlations between hip mobility and low back trouble indicate the importance of testing hip ROM. Correct assessment of abnormal hip mobility requires knowledge of expected hip motion performance. Radiographic analysis of sagittal hip ROM on 95 normal subjects was found to vary between 107 and 178°, with decreasing range noted with age.[85] Clinical measures of active hip range of motion are given in Table 6.1.[86]

In an investigation on 230 active, young, healthy adults, females were shown to exhibit more hip flexion and extension than men.[57] Although no significant left/right bias was observed, mean differences of 3.5° in females and 4.2° in males were found between sides. Clinicians should account for normal differences in hip range of motion between sides when analyzing hip mobility. Hip mobility seems to be less affected by age than lumbar spine mobility. Perhaps physical activity has a greater influence on hip range than lumbar range of motion.[57]

Hip mobility has been shown to correlate with low back problems and recovery.[69] Hip flexion and extension range of motion measures were found to be inversely related to the degree of low back difficulty. Subjects with greater pain complaints demonstrated more restriction in hip flexion and extension range. Treatments consisting of heat, electrotherapy, massage, exercise, and back education for 3 weeks resulting in increases in hip flexion and external rotation correlated with progress.[69] Questions remain as to whether the increase in hip mobility facilitates recovery or the reduction in pain allows hip range to improve.

Further indication of a significant relationship between hip mobility and the degree of low back pain was established in a study involving 476 working men and women who suffered from chronic or recurrent low back pain.[87] For women, hip flexion and extension range of motion was significantly less in subjects having higher levels of pain and disability. For men, restrictions in hip internal rotation as well as flexion and extension correlated with a higher lower back pain index. The most significant correlation between hip range of motion and low back pain difficulty was with hip extension. Considerable restrictions in hip extension were strongly associated with greater low back pain and disability scores. The significance of using the Thomas test to determine hip flexor tightness and/or joint restriction is clear when considering the relationship of hip extension range to low back trouble.

In the same study,[87] hip flexion and extension also correlated with lumbar spinal mobility in all planes, but particularly in rotation. A tendency for greater spinal mobility was evident in subjects with more hip flexion and extension. Spinal rotation seemed to be especially associated with sagittal hip mobility. Consequently, the results of hip range of motion tests may coincide with the mobility of the lumbar spine.

Less femoral and tibial rotation was found in students aged 13–17 years with low back pain than in students without back pain.[88] The theory suggesting that reduced lower extremity range of motion places additional or altered mechanical strain on the lumbo-pelvic complex is supported by this study and others. Clinical observation of exaggerated or abnormal spine and pelvic movements in patients with hip joint osteoarthritis has been substantiated by motion analysis.[89] A group of 19 patients with unilateral osteoarthritis of a hip joint had significant restrictions in hip range of motion when compared to the unaffected side and to a control group of 10 subjects. Using a television-computer motion analysis

Table 6.1
Normal ROM Values of Active Hip Movements

Active Hip Movement	ROM Values
Flexion	110°–120°
Extension	0°–15°
Abduction	30°–50°
Adduction	30°
External Rotation	40°–60°
Internal Rotation	30°–40°

system, patients with unilateral hip osteoar-thritis were shown to have an increase in both sagittal and coronal plane movements of the pelvis. In subjects with more severe hip motion restrictions, the pelvic tilt increased to a maximum tilt forward during stance phase on the affected leg. As sagittal movement of the pelvis increased in response to hip joint restriction, sagittal and coronal plane movements of the spine also increased. Increased pelvic and spinal motion associated with a loss in hip joint mobility is thought to be a compensatory mechanism. The deviation in lumbo-pelvic movement alters and possibly magnifies spinal stress. As a result, individuals with less adaptive potential within the spine may be susceptible to back pain problems when hip mobility is impaired.

The relatedness of hip motion disturbance to low back pain is further substantiated by clinical accounts of back pain relief following hip arthroplasty procedures. Aggravation of spine symptoms by deformity of the hip is called a secondary hip-spine syndrome by some investigators.[90] Evaluations must recognize the problems in both areas to identify the full nature of the problem.

The specific characteristics of hip motion disturbances in patients with low back pain were examined by Ellison et al.[91] In this study, 48% of the low back pain patients compared to 27% of the asymptomatic subjects had more external hip rotation than internal hip rotation. Although the exact relationship between back pain and restricted internal rotation of the hip is unknown, imbalances in hip rotation range should be noted in evaluation. Whether restoration of hip internal range of motion can influence the degree of back pain remains to be seen.

Summary of Active Movement Testing

The results from active movement tests have been examined with regard to an association with lower back problems. A number of significant findings are reported to relate to either the degree or frequency of low back trouble. Table 6.2 establishes significant active

movement test information which is most likely relevant to low back problems.

PALPATION TESTS

As the heading denotes, manual practitioners rely on palpatory analysis of soft tissue and skeletal structures to help identify problems related to the lumbar spine. Palpatory evaluation typically involves three aspects of study—a) condition, b) position, and c) segmental mobility. The condition of tissues is determined by palpatory testing of temperature, moisture, tension or resistance, and tenderness. Palpatory positional assessment of spinal skeletal structures is performed to identify alignment. Segmental mobility testing involves palpation analysis of intervertebral movement by passive maneuvers of the spine or extremities. Palpatory evaluation attempts to further define the stage of the condition and nature of the problem.

The next section investigates the significance, reliability, and accuracy of common palpatory examination methods used in the clinical evaluation of a low back problem.

TISSUE CONDITION

Temperature and Moisture

Evaluation of temperature differences in the body is utilized to determine the stage of the condition. Presumably increased temperature in an area is a function of vasodilation or inflammation.[92-94] Decreased temperature as measured cutaneously may suggest vasocon-

Table 6.2
Active Movement Test Findings Relevant to the Presence of Low Back Problems

---

—Significant restrictions in lateral flexion and rotation
—Asymmetric lateral bending range
—Restriction and pain upon backward bending
—Significant thoracic motion limitations
—Extreme hypermobility in forward bending or lateral bending
—Limitations in hip flexion and extension (particularly hip extension)
—Imbalance between hip internal and external range of motion (I.R. < E.R.)

---

striction, vascular interference, or fibro-fatty infiltration.[95] Skin temperature changes are believed to reflect the existence, acuteness, or chronicity of a somatic dysfunction. Instrumental methods of recording body temperature include thermocouples and infrared thermography.

Thermocouple Devices. These record from probes that make direct contact with the skin. Typically, two probes are placed on each side of the spinous processes. Sharp deflections to one side signify localized temperature alterations from either vasoconstriction or vasodilation. Reliable manual evaluation of paraspinal temperature differences requires even pressure delivery, consistent angular contact, and standardized gliding rates for probing. Therefore, the sensitivity as well as reliability of thermocouple devices for measuring paraspinal skin temperature are questionable.

Infrared Thermography. This technique measures radiant heat loss from the body in the infrared ranges. The images produced by thermography are the result of emissions and reflections from not only the skin, but from deeper tissue layers as well. Thermography, therefore, does not just measure body surface temperature. Testing of asymptomatic subjects shows bilateral symmetrical thermograms of the back. Paravertebral warm areas have been identified in erect posture thermograms with the lumbar spine exhibiting a widened area over the upper one third of the sacroiliac joints. Investigators report the normal back thermogram to appear "tadpole" in appearance (See Fig. 6.21).[96]

Interpretation of the significance of warm or cool areas depends on what constitutes normal variation. In one study, a 2°–3.5° variation in back skin temperature was determined in 35 pain-free subjects without history of major illness or surgery.[97] Although temperature patterns were relatively constant within subjects, no uniform variation in temperature among subjects was established from the recorded mean temperature of 31.4°C. Despite inconsistent temperature patterns between

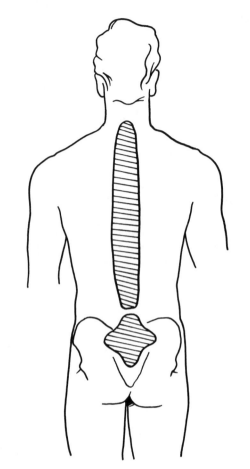

Figure 6.21. Tadpole appearance of a normal back thermogram.

subjects, evaluators reported that warm and cool areas could be determined. Further study to establish normal variants in back temperature is needed for interpretation of meaningful findings in patients with back problems.

Asymmetric discontinuous distributions of hypothermic and hyperthermic areas on the back have been reported in patients with myelographic confirmed disc disorders. Lateral positioned disc herniations at L5–S1, for example, have been shown to correlate with an ipsilateral increase in temperature at the same level and slightly medial to the sacroiliac joint.[98] The gluteal areas in eight individuals with back pain were found to exhibit cold patches which were not observed in 14 pain-free subjects used as controls. The possibility of muscle spasm produced vasoconstriction accounting for the temperature decrease was considered since strong, sustained, isometric gluteal contractions produced cold patches also.[96]

Liquid Crystal Thermography (LCT). The use of LCT to substantiate nerve root compression due to lumbosacral lateral spinal stenosis was evaluated and compared to the findings of clinical assessment, myelography, computerized tomography, electromyography, and surgery.[99] The level of agreement was: 53%, clinical assessment; 45%, myelography; 46%, CAT scan study; 41%, EMG; and 53%, surgery. In addition, each test was analyzed against the surgeon's overall assessment. A 48% agreement was demonstrated using LCT in contrast to agreement rates of 65% for clinical assessment, 71% for myelography, 71% for CAT scans, and 70% for EMG. LCT was therefore the least reliable method of investigation for diagnosing nerve root compression.

Is Thermography Practical? Although the use of thermography for differential diagnosis of specific back conditions is limited, a potential exists for its use as a diagnostic aid for confirmation of back pain. Question arises, however, as to the necessity of an expensive method of testing for validation of a back problem, particularly when information as to the specific nature of the condition is not obtained. Despite no documented evidence as to the reliability and validity of palpatory determination of temperature-related changes, manual methods to evaluate temperature are commonly used in physical examinations. Experienced manual practitioners involved in evaluating musculoskeletal problems may be capable of reliably detecting temperature deviations which reflect somatic dysfunction. Thermographic measures to determine or substantiate the existence of a back problem is therefore questionable, especially when considering the accuracy of non-health-trained parents in identifying temperature elevations of a few degrees in their sick children.

Sweat Gland Activity

Analysis of sweat gland activity by palpation is routinely used by manual therapists and physicians to evaluate sympathetic nerve activity. Palpatory exploration of the skin for areas of moisture indicates greater sweat gland activity from an increase in sympathetic nerve activity. Conversely, dry areas represent reduced sweat gland activity from a decrease in sympathetic nerve activity. The consistency and accuracy of manual practitioners to determine variations in sweat gland activity of the back has not been established.

Sudomotor studies[100–102] have utilized an electrical skin resistance method for measuring sweat gland activity. Low levels of electrical skin resistance are found in areas of increased sweat gland activity, while high skin resistant areas relate to decreased sweat gland activity. Investigations on hundreds of asymptomatic, resting subjects have shown electrical skin resistance of the back to exhibit a diversity of patterns.[100] Repeated testing of normal subjects at different dates demonstrates a high degree of reproducibility in the distribution of low resistance areas. Although statistical support is not provided, the investigators report that in each subject the probability of finding low resistance values in certain areas, segmental levels and sides is greater than the average value recorded during a given period of time. Two- to thirty-fold differences were reported in areas of low resistance. The lumbar spine, for example, is normally a lower resistant area than other parts of the spine, indicating larger amounts of present or residual moisture from increased sweat gland activity.

Electrical skin resistance recordings of sudomotor activity in paravertebral areas were found to decrease in 15 subjects after a .3 ml injection of 6% saline into the erector spinae or intercostal musculature produced referred pain[101] (Fig. 6.22). Additional areas of low electrical skin resistance also appeared after myofascial injection in dermatomal related regions. The lowering of skin resistance follow-

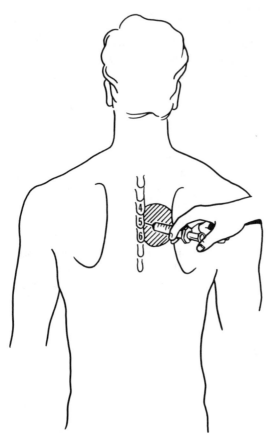

Figure 6.22. Areas of low skin resistance after injection of .3 ml of 6% saline into the left paraspinals adjacent to the spinous process of T5.

authors reported frequent correlations between low skin resistance regions and areas of musculoskeletal disturbance. The lowering of electrical skin resistance associated with increased sweat gland activity in select areas of chronic cases appears to reflect a sustained hyperactivity (augmentation) of efferent sympathetic nerve pathways. The areas of increased sweat gland activity, therefore, reflect a distortion in existing patterns of efferent sympathetic activity caused by chronically altered or intensified afferent activity from somatic or visceral structures. Korr et al. suggest that affected segments are unable to function in a coordinated manner, due to hyperactive sympathetic outflow.[102]

Sympathetic manifestations of myofascial or visceral irritation such as temperature and moisture alteration may provide useful information to the clinician with respect to spinal segmental dysfunction. According to Korr's vasomotor and sudomotor studies,[100–106] the affected segment is in or nearly in a constant state of alarm. As a result, the segmentally related areas actually present in a "cold sweat." Even during rest conditions "emergency" sympathetic activity may be sustained[103] adversely affecting the tissues derived from the involved spinal segment.

ing injection occurred as quickly as two minutes and lasted as much as 24 hours or more. In the same study, spinal postural stress induced by creating a lateral pelvic tilt or leg length discrepancy also exaggerated existing low resistance areas and established new areas.

In a follow-up study,[102] electrical skin resistance testing was performed on 130 individuals with different back problems. The types of conditions included pain of varying intensity, motion limitations, and structural asymmetries such as leg length inequalities and abnormal spinal curves. The existence of musculoskeletal disturbance was established by radiographic, electromyographic, and clinical evaluations; however, specific criteria defining conditions were not reported. Although no statistical information was provided, the

Red Response

Cutaneous vascular responses of the trunk are utilized by clinicians to evaluate vasomotor tone regulated by the sympathetic division of the autonomic nervous system. Observation of vasodilating responses of the skin during and after manual pressures or friction offers a clinical means of evaluating vasomotor activity. Intense, prolonged, red responses indicate areas of low vasodilatation threshold, whereas weak, briefly appearing red responses represent areas of high vasodilatation threshold. For evaluative purposes, the clinician observes the red response elicited after one or two finger firm pressure (others use the back edge of the thumb nails) on the paraspinal areas of each side of the spine from T1 to the sacrum. The accuracy of the technique depends upon consistent pressure stimulation in regard to intensity of force used and velocity. Reliability in manual performance of the evaluative procedure and in interpreting the red response has not been investigated.

Comparative intensity and duration of red responses to standardized frictional stimuli to the back were studied by using a device called the mechanical "skin stroker."[104] Regional differences in red responsiveness have been identified. The lumbar area is typically less red responsive than the thoracic paraspinal area.[104,105] Criteria for the differentiation and significance of red responses were not established. However, Wright et al.[104] reported that weak, quick-fading responses approximated 30 seconds or less, whereas persistent red responses often lasted 5 minutes or longer. To investigate the significance of variations in red response of the paraspinals to mechanical stimuli their subjects were tested at different ambient temperatures. The strength and duration of red responses were increased when subjects were tested at warm temperatures (28°C). Red responses were weaker or absent despite strong stimuli at cooler temperatures of 21°C. Temperature changes influencing vasomotor tone, therefore, also appear to affect red response. Segmental differences in red response found on a patient in a room with constant temperature may therefore suggest local changes in vasomotor tone.

The results of vasomotor and sudomotor studies seem to indicate that sympathetic hyperactivity reflects cutaneously. Local or generalized cutaneous signs of lowered temperature, hyperhidrosis, and a weakened, short-duration red response have been noted in normal subjects as well as in patients with various musculoskeletal disturbances. Stimuli to abnormal spinal segments appear to result in exaggerated and/or prolonged responses through the sympathetic pathways. The lesioned spinal segment has been described as a "neurologic lens" which focuses and augments impulses from multiple tissue sources upon the tissues innervated from that spinal level.[106]

The *sensitivity* and *relevancy* of skin manifestations to aberrant segmental behavior needs further experimental validation particularly in regard to statistical analysis. Furthermore, the reliability of examiners in detecting significant skin-related changes has yet to be determined. Possible detection or support for the existence of abnormal spinal segmental behavior through cutaneous evaluative procedures, however, may help in functional diagnosis. Unfortunately, evaluative techniques such as skin drag commonly used to identify skin temperature and moisture changes are not amenable to multiple examination protocol due to test interaction problems.[107]

Myofascial Tension

According to Travell and Simons, normal muscles do not possess taut bands of muscle fibers.[108] Abnormal tension in myofascial tissue suggests protective guarding of a painful or dysfunctional area. The tissue origin of pain or dysfunction is sometimes the myofascia. The tension in the myofascia may also represent a protective response to deeper tissue injury. Despite clinical claims relating myofascial tension to various musculoskeletal problems, the predictive relationship is not well established. Questions regarding the relevancy of myofascial tension states to painful conditions must be addressed in view of the presence of myofascial tension areas in asymptomatic individuals.

The term *fibrositis* was used first by Gowers[109] in 1904 to mean palpable hardness of muscles due to inflammation of the fibrous tissues. Evidence of inflammatory hyperplasic areas in the connective tissue of muscle was demonstrated in the same year by Stockman.[110] Characteristic of palpable nodules in what is now called *myofibrositis* is the histologic demonstration of massive amounts of metachromatic mucoid substance in the interfascicular and intercellular spaces.[111,112] Verification of connective tissue changes in paraspinal musculature is provided in an immunohistologic study of collagen types and fibronectin on patients with lumbar disc herniations.[113]

Although the distribution of type one and type three collagen and fibronectin in 24 patients with lumbar disc herniations was similar to 9 cadavers without known back problems, marked fibrosis and thickening was evident in the endo- and perimysial areas of the multifidi at the L4–5 and L5–S1 levels in the biopsies of the patient population.

Palpatory identification of swelling or tissue bogginess in areas of myofascial tension is supported by Awad's findings[112] of localized edema associated with herniation of muscle fascicles just beneath the deep fascia. According to Strange,[114] palpable, localized muscle bundles in spasm are verified by the following clinical features: (*a*) the tissue thickening is spindle shaped; (*b*) the indurated tissue lies parallel to the fibers of the involved muscle; (*c*) the affected muscle bundles can be moved at right angles to the line of muscle fibers; and (*d*) pressure evokes a reflex muscle contraction.

Kellgren[115] clearly demonstrated the potential of paraspinal myofascia to evoke a painful response after injection of hypertonic saline. Local as well as referred pain patterns were identified. By stroking or pinching the superficial fascia of the infraspinatus muscle during a muscle biopsy, Travell[108] was also able to produce referred pain. Less clear is the relationship of myofascial tension areas to the painful condition. Are myofascial regions of tension more frequently associated with painful musculoskeletal conditions than in asymptomatic individuals? Are the myofascial sites of induration more numerous, extensive, concentrated, extreme, etc. in patients with back pain?

Investigations. The existence of tension in myofascia found by palpatory analysis has not been extensively examined to determine test sensitivity and observer reliability. Using graphic representation of test observations instead of statistical measures, one group of investigators[116] found superficial and deep paraspinal tissue compression tests to be sensitive to initial complaints and changes in con-

dition. Tissue compression tests also showed good long-term interexaminer agreement with repeated testing during patient improvement. Results of this study suggest the potential of manual methods for detecting myofascial tension.

Paraspinal fingerpad palpation was found to be helpful in identifying general areas of tissue tension associated with a regional dysfunction in the thoracic spine.[107] Agreement levels among four examiners testing 30 subjects ranged between 80 and 86%. Although wide areas of tissue tension could be detected with reasonable consistency, the distribution of paraspinal tightness was not specifically related to one spinal segment. The use of palpatory procedures to detect the degree of soft tissue tension as determined by shear and compression tests may provide useful information regarding (a)symmetrical distribution of tissue tightness. The relevancy of tissue tension findings in the paraspinal areas to spinal dysfunction and pain requires further investigation. Quantification of myofascial tension levels with the use of palpatory methods also presents a challenge to researchers of manual evaluative procedures.

Myofascial Tenderness

Knowledge of normal pressure thresholds and tolerance to soft tissue structure is requisite to determining the significance of myofascial tenderness in patients. *Pressure threshold*, defined as the minimum force needed to cause discomfort, has been studied in asymptomatic subjects. *Pressure tolerance* is the maximum force that can be withstood and is the point at which subjects say "stop."

Controversy exists regarding pain threshold levels between men and women. Some studies do not demonstrate significant differences between sexes,[117] whereas other studies show males to have higher pain thresholds.[118] Pain thresholds appear to be relatively constant in the body, varying by less than 20%. In asymptomatic subjects pain thresholds to electrical stimuli are below 1 mA. Thresholds above 1 mA or threshold differences of .2 mA between related dermatomes were considered significant of pathology, according to Noterman[119] who suggested that fear and fatigue may also decrease pain threshold. The possibility of lowered pain thresholds from fear of reinjury and fatigue response from pain is noteworthy since both conditions seem to be commonly related to chronic low back problems.

Pressure Tolerance. This is greater in males than in females. In one study pressure tolerance over the deltoid muscle in women was 10.2 ± 3.2 kg, whereas men had values of 11.8 ± 2.6 kg.[120] No differences were demonstrated between sides with respect to pressure tolerance. Although evaluative consideration must be given to the difference in pain tolerance between men and women, the similar values obtained from side to side provide an opportunity for comparative analysis. The clinical significance of myofascial tenderness to palpation pressure can be established with greater certainty when further documentation of normal pressure threshold and tolerance is obtained.

Tender Points in Muscle. These are defined locations which, when palpated with approximately 4 kgs of pressure, elicit a pain response. The pain elicited often results in a jump response and an outcry from the patient. The frequency of tender points in muscle associated with low back pain has not received substantial attention in research. In one study, an unmeasured "slight-to-heavy" pressure elicited a small tender point in the paraspinal tissue ½ inch to 2 inch away from the midline in 85% of the 239 back pain patients evaluated.[121] The relation of tender points to hyperaesthetic areas (as determined by a sharp response to a 45° angled pin pressure) was found to be very constant, and the frequency of tender points increased from the cervical to lumbar spine. The existence of tender points was considered to correlate directly with the extent of the back condition.

Likewise, patients with criteria-based fibromyalgia syndrome will identify pain in specific tender points. Included among the 14 sites listed as tender points in fibromyalgia syndrome are the low lumbar paraspinal areas and buttocks.[122] Muscle biopsy examination has not revealed any significant fiber type changes in muscle tender spots; however, lower levels of ATP and ADT and higher levels of ADM and creatine have been found in fibromyalgia patients.

Motor Points. Tender motor points may have diagnostic and prognostic value in back pain conditions. Motor points are fixed anatomical sites characterized by high electrical conductance and low skin resistance. The motor point of a muscle possesses the greatest density of sensory end organs due to the presence of a neurovascular hilus. As a result, a muscle is most easily excitable as well as most susceptible to palpable tenderness at the motor point.[123] Using thumb or one finger palpation pressure sufficient to compress the neurovascular hilus and motor endplate against underlying bone the motor points of the paravertebral muscles (generally located 2.5 cm lateral from the midline) and posterior aspect of the lower extremity were examined in 100 patients with two types of low back symptoms (groups (a) and (b)), and 50 patients without back complaints (group c).[124] Of the 50 patients in group (a) diagnosed with low back strain/sprain secondary to muscle or ligamentous injury, 52% had tender motor points and were disabled for an average of 19.7 weeks as compared to group (b)'s average of 6.9 weeks for low back strain/sprain in patients who did not have tender motor points. Forty-nine out of 50 patients in (a) with radicular signs and symptoms suggesting disc involvement had tender motor points and were disabled for an average of 25.7 weeks. The tender motor points were located in the muscle or myotome which corresponded to the probable segmental level of involvement. In contrast, only 7 out of 50 subjects in (c) without back problems had tender motor points. In this study[124] and in a subsequent study by Gunn and Milbrandt,[125] the presence of tender motor points served to delineate the nature of a back condition (*strain/sprain* versus *nerve involvement*), identify the location of segmental injury, and predict the degree of disability.

Recommendation. The use of palpation pressure to determine the existence of tender motor points in the paravertebral, buttock, and posterior lower extremity musculature is therefore recommended as part of a standard back examination.

Myofascial Trigger Points. These are defined by Travell and Simons[108] as a hyperirritable locus within a taut band of muscle and/or associated fascia which can also exhibit tenderness to firm palpation when active. The immediate muscle area about a trigger point is tense and often feels ropey, nodular, or band-like upon palpation. Passive or active stretching as well as strong contraction of the affected muscle or moderate pressure to an active, irritable trigger point causes local and/or referred pain. Zohn and Mennell,[126] among others,[127] suggest that trigger points are hyperactive or irritable muscle spindles. Although the location and pain distribution patterns of paravertebral trigger points have been identified, the relationship of trigger points to low back trouble is not substantially established. However, the literature does report studies investigating the relationship of joint disorders to trigger points. In one study,[128] for example, the frequency of tender points and jump responses in 14 women with rheumatoid arthritis was about twice that found in a control group of 18 subjects, but the frequency of trigger points was not different. In contrast, earlier studies[129,130] suggested a trigger point association with articular disease.

Facet Syndrome. Evidence exists for a possible correlation between facet joint irritation and well localized paravertebral tenderness. A retrospective analysis of 22 facet syndrome patients diagnosed and selected for facet injection according to conventional criteria was conducted by Hilbig and Lee.[131] Four clinical evaluative criteria were used to establish a facet problem—back, buttock, and groin pain, well localized paraspinal tenderness, pain reproduction with extension and rotation toward the symptomatic side, and

significant radiographic evidence of facet arthrosis on the involved side. They strongly correlated to a positive response from facet injection. Sixty-seven percent of the patients with well-localized paravertebral tenderness had relief of symptoms for more than 6 months after facet injection. Despite the authors' caution against using any one single evaluative finding to diagnose a facet disorder or predict response from facet injection, the results indicate the importance of including palpation for tenderness in a back examination.

Reliability. Reliability in assessing soft tissue tenderness as related to back pain has not been demonstrated. Despite 79% agreement on the presence or absence of localized paravertebral (within 5 cm of the midline) or gluteal tenderness, only a 30% agreement was found regarding the specific anatomical site of tenderness.[35] Further question as to the reliability in detecting soft tissue tenderness in the paravertebral and gluteal musculature is raised in a subsequent study by McCombe.[132] Two orthopedists and one physical therapist were found to be unreliable in assessing paravertebral and gluteal tenderness in two independent groups of low back pain patients. Defining exact soft tissue locations to be tested as well as consideration regarding the degree and velocity of pressure applied is essential in establishing reliability in assessment of soft tissue tenderness. Neither of the two studies cited above[35,132] reported specificity in evaluative procedure for determining sensitivity to palpation pressure. Nonetheless, discretion must be used in identifying the specific nature of a back problem when evaluative findings show poor reproducibility.

Electromyography. Palpable evidence of myofascial tension must not be related to myoelectrical activity status. No evidence exists to support a positive relationship between EMG activity and the existence of trigger points, nodular areas, and tension palpated in muscle. The presence of palpable changes in muscle tension seems to occur in the absence of electrical activity.[133]

Methods of Myofascial Palpation

Compression Testing

—A perpendicular directed palpation pressure utilized to evaluate tension state, resistance, or responsiveness to load, tenderness, or pain.

—Consideration must be given not only to direction of load, but to the velocity imparted. Quickly applied compressions are most likely to induce a reflex muscle twitch and/or pain response.

Shear Testing

—A parallel directed gliding force used principally to evaluate extensibility of the myofascial tissues.

—Shear tests should be conducted systematically in all directions to detect changes in extensibility.

Pincer Testing

—Involves gentle squeezing and rolling of a muscle belly between thumb and fingers to assess transverse mobility, tension state, and tenderness. Pincer testing of the paraspinals is best accomplished by using thumb contact on the medial border adjacent to the spinous processes and finger contact along the lateral border at the tip of the transverse processes.

Need for Studies. The specific methods of myofascial palpation have not been evaluated or compared for reliability, validity, or sensitivity to low back problems. Attention should be given to further defining each procedure so that consistency in performance is obtained among clinicians. Use of clinical instruments such as dolorimeters for analyzing myofascial compliance or tenderness requires additional study to determine clinical usefulness.

Trunk Muscle Function

A thorough analysis of trunk muscle function is provided in Chapter 15, *Spinal Exercise.* Clinical evaluation of trunk muscle performance should involve isometric strength, dynamic strength, coordination, and endurance tests since evidence exists to show possible impairment in any or all of these parameters.

The use of isokinetic or isodynamic back machines can provide objective measurement of trunk flexor and extensor strength.

Most studies[134,135] show reduced trunk strength in back pain patients when compared to controls, particularly in chronic back cases. Some studies[136] report greater loss of trunk flexor strength, while others indicate a greater reduction in trunk extensor strength.[137] Consideration is given to the fact that under normal conditions trunk extensor strength is more than flexor strength. Additional precaution regarding interpretation of trunk muscle strength is necessary since isolation of trunk musculature performance from the hip and pelvic muscles is difficult despite attempts to fixate the lower extremities and pelvis.

In a study on 500 chronic low back pain patients Janda found that 80% demonstrated poor movement control.[138,139] He observed over-activation of muscles not required during a given motion, motor incoordination in the form of mass, uneven movements, difficulty in fine motor coordination skill, and a tendency to mirror movements performed with one side on the opposite side. The quality and control of motion activity in chronic low back patients with musculoskeletal dysfunction seems to directly impair the central nervous system's motor functioning. In turn, the abnormal movement patterns which develop in association with painful dysfunctions perpetuate the condition and may lead to stress in other parts of the spine.

Recommendation. The clinician should include motor coordination and control tests such as a dynamic trunk curl to assess movement patterns and recruitment. Inability to hold a trunk curl position, observation of an anterior pelvic tilt and/or lumbar extension, and early activation of the hip flexors most likely indicate a poor working relationship between the iliopsoas, back extensors, and abdominals. The functional inefficiency of the trunk and pelvic musculature as observed during a trunk curl may interfere with normal stress distribution and mechanical activity in the lumbar spine.

Fatigue. Trunk muscle endurance also

seems to be affected in back pain conditions. Trunk flexor fatigue in response to isokinetic contraction activity is greater in back patients than in control subjects, whereas back extensor fatigue remains unchanged. Sustained contraction testing of trunk musculature to determine endurance is a more sensitive indicator of trunk muscle performance than testing by repeated contractions. Clinical assessment of abdominal strength should therefore include an evaluation of prolonged contraction ability.

Vertebral Palpation for Position

Some manual practitioners palpate bony processes to evaluate vertebral position. Both spinous and transverse processes are utilized in the thoracic and lumbar regions while the articular processes of facet joints can be used

in the cervical spine. However, detection of vertebral positional changes by palpation of bony processes has not been tested for reliability, validity, or sensitivity. The results of in vitro and in vivo experiments using AP radiographs and CAT scans indicate that deviations in spinous processes do not necessarily indicate vertebral rotation or asymmetry of the neural arch. Instead, the deviation can be created within the spinous process itself.[140]

Recognition of the existence of asymmetrically formed and/or deviated spinous processes is necessary when analyzing by palpation. Examples (Figs. 6.23 **A,B,C,D**) of possible vertebral positional faults are provided with precaution taken in interpretation of findings. Figures 6.23**A** and **B** show the relative spacing of spinous processes to differ between T5–6 and T6–7. In Fig. 6.23**A**, T6 has forward bent on T7 resulting in a small

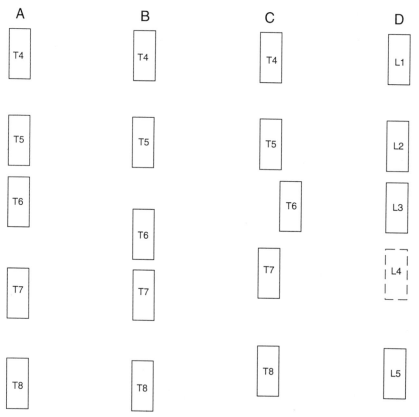

Figure 6.23. A, T6 Forward bent on T7; **B,** T6 Backward bent on T7; **C,** T6 Left rotated on T7; **D,** L4 Anterior to L5 producing a step between L4 and L5 suggestive of a spondylolisthesis.

interspinous space at T5–6 and a large interspinous space at T6–7. Figure 6.23**B** shows T6 backward bent on T7 causing a large space between T5–6 and a small space at T6–7. Figure 6.23**C** demonstrates a possible left rotation at T6–7 as a result of the spinous process of T6 deviated to the right. Figure 6.23**D** represents a possible spondylolisthesis at L5 secondary to a step found at L4–5 with L4 being anterior to L5.

Spondylolisthesis. Identification of a vertebral positional fault is suggestive of spinal segment mechanical impairment but is not an absolute indicator of a problem. Even the confirmation of a spondylolisthesis does not ensure relevancy to the problem[141] nor indicate the extent of movement available at the motion segment.[142] In a study by MacNab the incidence of spondylolisthesis in back pain patients of 3 age groups was examined. The group over 40 had an incidence rate of spondylolisthesis about the same as the whole white population in North America (6%). The incidence of spondylolisthesis in the 26–39 age group of back pain patients was 7.6%, whereas under 25 the incidence is 18.9%. Therefore in a patient under 25 the defect is most likely related to the symptoms. A patient over 40 is less likely to have back pain from the spondylolisthesis.

The presumption that symptomatic spondylolisthesis results in instability in the form of increased forward and backward translation may not be true in cases of grade one or two slips. Results from one study[142] using biplanar radiography on patients with grade one and two symptomatic spondylolisthesis show reduced mobility at the involved segment as well as throughout the lumbar spine.

Experienced manual clinicians tend to use positional analysis with caution. Manual detection of vertebral positional faults provides possible incriminating evidence of dysfunction which should be corroborated with other findings, particularly motion discoveries.

Reliability in palpation of spondylolisthesis or other vertebral position changes has not been studied. However, six cases with palpable

shelf were noted during clinical examination of 64 female gymnasts.[64] In all six gymnasts, a spina bifida was determined radiographically. Since a high correlation is reported between spina bifida and pars defect, a revealing of spondylolisthesis by palpation of bony processes is a distinct possibility.

Bony Tenderness

Tenderness of spinous processes, the sacroiliac joint, and iliac crest are reported to be potentially reliable findings in patients with low back pain.[132] In comparison to soft tissue tenderness, bony tenderness was a more reliable finding. The relationship of bony tenderness to back pain, however, was not investigated.

Anterior spinal tenderness may relate to low back pain according to a study by O'Brien.[143] Definite sensitivity to palpation of the anterior aspect of the L5 and S1 vertebrae was reported in over 75% of patients with current complaints of low back pain, as opposed to only 4% of asymptomatic subjects. Pain upon palpation of the anterior aspect of L5–S1 may not be incriminatory for an L5–S1 problem but is highly suggestive of a lumbar abnormality.

Segmental Mobility Testing

Purpose. The purpose of segmental mobility testing is to assess specific movements at each spinal motion segment. Segmental mobility testing is evaluated passively by digital palpation or direct pressure to facet joints, spinous processes, transverse processes, or interspinous spaces. Passive intervertebral motion testing (PIVM) attempts to determine the potential and possibly actual movement at individual motion segments without interference from muscle activity. Theoretically, therefore, if active spinal movements are observed to be limited and passive segmental testing reveals normal excursion, then the active motion restriction probably has a neuromuscular basis.

Since the objective of segmental motion testing is to examine passive mobility, patient relaxation is critical. Difficulty in relaxation interferes with evaluator assessment of passive segmental motion and invalidates the test.

Judgment of spinal motion at a segmental level requires knowledge of expected ranges at each spinal level. Degree values of spinal segmental mobility are presented in Figure 6.24.[8] To accurately determine spinal mobility at a specific segment an evaluator must consider sex, body type, and age. A qualitative analysis of resistance to passively induced motion is also important to consider. A grading scale commonly utilized to assess segmental mobility of the spine is presented in Table 6.3. Note that criteria for grading segmental motion involves both quantitative and qualitative factors (range and resistance).

Recommendation. Regardless of whether direct pressures are delivered or digital palpation is used, the pressures or contacts for spinal segmental mobility testing should be light. Sensory discrimination of small movements between vertebrae requires not only concentration, but gentle active or passive reception of the motion event. Repetitive testing of spinal segmental motion may result in an increase, decrease, or inconsistency in movement. An increase may suggest a slight restriction is improving with repeated movement, whereas a decrease may indicate an increase in segmental irritability. Inconsistent findings with repetitive testing of spinal segments is likely to relate to changes in patient relaxation.

Variables. In testing segmental mobility by direct pressure on spinous processes, Denslow found variability in spinal reflex thresholds.[144] Thresholds for reflex paraspinal

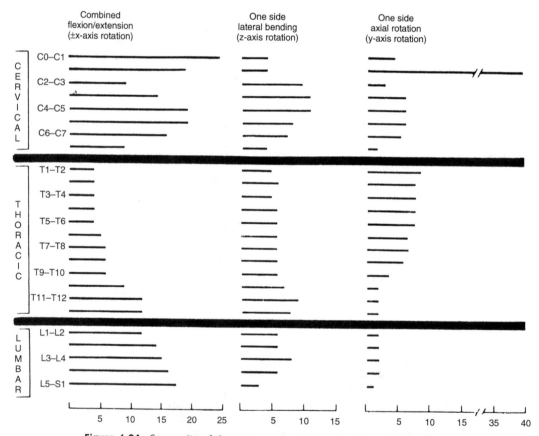

Figure 6.24. Composite of the most representative values for spinal segmental mobility in the traditional planes of motion within each region.

Table 6.3
Passive Intervertebral Motion (PIVM) Grading Scale

Grade	Description	Criteria
0	Ankylosed	No detectable motion in the segment. Use motion x- ray to confirm.
1	Considerable restriction	Significant decrease in range and/or significant resistance.
2	Slight restriction	Partial decrease in range and/or some resistance.
3	Normal	Expected range and resistance.
4	Slight hypermobility	Some increase in range and/or decrease in resistance.
5	Considerable hypermobility	Significant increase in range and/or significant decrease in resistance.
6	Unstable	Excessive, abnormal range without restraints.

muscle contraction and pain to pressure stimuli applied to spinous processes were found to be relatively constant within subjects over time unless a change in condition occurred, but vary among segments, sides, and between subjects. Motor reflex thresholds varied 1–7 kg between segments. Upper thoracic segments demonstrated lower thresholds (typically 1–2 kg), whereas the highest thresholds (6–7 kg) were recorded from L1–L4. Threshold changes between adjacent spinous processes were usually within 1 kg, indicating gradual differences are the rule. A reflex paravertebral muscle contraction secondary to pressure stimulus at one spinous process and not to adjacent spines, therefore, has significance in regards to the level of excitability at the reactive segment.

Confirmation of mean threshold differences between left and right sides of the same spinal segments was provided in a follow-up study.[145] The discovery of a unilateral reflex contraction to spinous process pressure signifies a lower threshold to stimuli on that side. Low threshold spinal segments show tendencies for hyper-responsive behavior to not only direct pressure stimulation but to indirect stimulation. As a result, pressures delivered at a high threshold segment may cause reactivity at a distant low threshold segment. Apparently electrical impulses generated from pressure stimuli to a high threshold spinal segment bypass motoneurons in intervening high or normal threshold segments to activate motoneurons in the anterior horn of a distant low threshold segment.

Facilitation. Pain was not typically produced in spinal segments having high reflex thresholds. At low threshold segments pain often resulted and tended to continue even after the stimulus was removed. Not only does a low threshold segment appear to be in state of facilitation (hyper-excitability leading to exaggerated responses) but it also tends to exhibit a wind-up phenomenon (continued abnormal firing after withdrawing stimulus). Manual practitioners evaluating spinal segmental mobility also note the level or irritability to palpation pressures. Detection of facilitated segments[103] in the spine becomes a routine part of the evaluation helping the clinician identify with levels and degree of vertebral dysfunction.

Accuracy in identifying facilitated segments was reported in the study by Denslow, Korr and Krems.[145] By palpation facilitated segments were felt to have "doughy and boggy" supraspinous tissues, corresponding paravertebral muscles with less resiliency to compression tests, and paraspinal ropy bundles. Palpation determination of facilitated segments by one examiner was in agreement with EMG findings of lower motor reflex thresholds in 35 out of 40 vertebrae tested (87.5%). Although further work in establishing reliability and validity of palpation assessment methods is essential, the findings in this study offers promise to the advancement of manual therapy.

Palpation Skills

Palpation skills of skilled manipulative therapists and untrained subjects have been studied using a palpation simulator.[146] Both groups were instructed to palpate and report the point of initial resistance to downward movement of a plunger controlled by an electromagnet. Manipulative therapists detected resistance earlier in the range and demonstrated greater accuracy in locating the resistance as measured by smaller deviations from the mean than untrained subjects. The reliability of manipulative therapists in perceiving the onset of resistance was measured to be within ± .16 mm. The use of palpation methods to examine lumbar intervertebral sagittal motions, which averages 15° of flexion/extension and 2 mm of anterior shear,[8] would appear to be well within the level of sensory discrimination and precision of a trained manipulative therapist.

Using a four grade movement scale (1—bony block, no movement; 2—stiffness present; 3—normal; 4—hypermobile) 9 instructors in manipulative therapy tested 4 subjects for passive intervertebral motion at various levels.[147] Results were compared to the principal instructor's findings. An 86% agreement was reported among examiners. The differences found in test scores among instructors varied only one motion grade. Authors felt the reproducibility of passive intervertebral motion testing to be remarkably good even though the test findings were not statistically analyzed. Although authors agree that the acquisition of manual sensitivity skills requires years of training, the study demonstrates the potential of trained practitioners to feel small differences in movements between spinal motion segments.

Consistency in grading spinal segmental motion was also examined by physical therapists in a later study. The reliability within and between 5 physical therapists using a 0–6 grading scale on 5 normal subjects was investigated.[148] Data were analyzed descriptively by means of means and standard deviations, since the grading scale is not continuous. Intratherapist reliability between blind and normal conditions as well as among different test directions was considered reasonably good. Most deviations in test scores were within one grade with repeat testing by one examiner. Intertherapist

reliability, however, was not found to be consistent. Factors which may influence interrater reliability among therapists using passive intervertebral motion tests include differences in: interpretation of the grading scale; levels of experience among examiners; training method of therapists; degree of subject relaxation or sensitivity.

The above study suggests the need for further standardization of passive intervertebral motion testing with respect to definition of the grading scale and actual procedures used to improve inter-rater reliability. Acceptable and less variable findings for intratherapist reliability is consistent with the results of other studies.[149,150]

Relevancy, Reliability, Validity

The next question regarding manual detection procedures of spinal motion segments relates to relevancy. If passive segmental motion testing is a potentially reliable clinical tool for identifying movement differences between vertebral levels, then are the findings relevant to the specific problem? A study on 20 patients determined either to have or not have a symptomatic cervical facet joint by means of radiologically-controlled nerve blocks was performed to rate the ability of a manipulative therapist to identify symptomatic facet joints.[151] Eleven patients were first evaluated by diagnostic nerve blocks and then examined by the physical therapist. Nine other patients were examined by the physical therapist first and then by means of nerve blocks. Symptomatic joints were determined with nerve blocks when complete pain relief was obtained and the pain provoking movement was asymptomatic. The criteria used in manual examination for specifying symptomatic joints included abnormal resistance and end feel to passive intervertebral motion tests as well as the reproduction of pain. All 15 patients with proven symptomatic facet joints were identified by the physical therapist. The segmental level of the symptomatic joint was also established by the manual examination in every patient verified by nerve blocks to have a facet joint syndrome.

Accurate assessment of specific spinal motion segments is requisite for reliability in passive intervertebral motion testing and in locating exact vertebral levels in dysfunction or pain. Although additional study is required to demonstrate reliability and validity of manual procedures for determining segmental problems, the results of studies to date show the potential of skillfully trained manual practitioners in utilizing palpation methods of assessment. The accuracy of the instrument can be criticized for lack of measurement preciseness, but the exactness of an evaluative tool is only meaningful when the findings are relevant or sensitive to the problem. A patient's preference for manual examination versus radiological investigation can be clearly understood should the results of the manual tests be diagnostic of the problem.

Biplanar Radiography. The use of biplanar radiography has also provided evidence for the diagnostic value of evaluating segmental motion. By measuring angular and translation movements during lumbar flexion and extension, investigators found significantly reduced shear-flexion ratios at symptomatic vertebral levels in 78 patients.[152] Palpatory analysis of spinal segmental mobility routinely uses flexion and anterior translation tests to evaluate individual vertebral motion status. Validation studies of palpation techniques for measuring segmental flexion-anterior translation could therefore conceivably utilize biplanar radiography for verification.

Motion symmetry at segmental levels of the lumbar spine was the subject of another biplanar radiography study.[153] Twelve patients with known herniated discs, as determined by clinical examination, myelography and in 11 patients by surgery, were found to have significantly greater motion asymmetry at the involved level during lateral flexion than at uninvolved levels. The results of this study suggest that passive segmental mobility testing be specific for direction since motion loss to one side may signify a problem.

Furthermore, the concept of segmental motion compensation within or among spinal segments of the lumbar region must be considered during passive motion testing. Radiographic studies have observed tendencies for the L3–4 spinal level to exhibit relatively hypermobility in flexion-extension range of patients with L4 to sacrum fusions.[154] Lateral flexion and translatory movements have also been noted to increase at L3–4 vertebral levels located above fused lower segments.[10] Results of these segmental motion studies suggest an interdependency in mechanical behavior among spinal segments.

If spinal segments demonstrate functional interdependency then the specific amount of motion at each level may be less important than the relative movement between segments. Individuals determined to have greater motion discrepancies from level to level perhaps may be more vulnerable to back injury than individuals with less segmental variation. Given this assumption, subject two with lumbar segmental motion findings as shown in Table 6.4 is possibly at more risk for low back pain than subject one. Likewise, a spinal segment which has significant restriction on one side and considerable hypermobility on the opposite side may tend to be more symptomatic than a spinal segment which has equal, but slight hypermobility on both sides.

Summary of Palpation Testing

Palpation findings that are probably meaningful to the existence of a lumbar pain condition are presented in Table 6.5. Findings determined by palpatory methods to have reasonable clinical reliability as well as sensitivity to the problem are identified. The need for further substantiation of palpatory findings through research is recognized.

Table 6.4
Lumbar Segmental Motion Findings in Two Individuals Using a 0–6 Grading Scale

Segment	L5–S1	L4–5	L3–4	L2–3	L1–2
Subject One	2	3	2	2	2
Subject Two	5	5	2	1	1

Table 6.5
Palpatory Findings Most Likely Related to a Low Back Condition

1) Paravertebral tissue tension
2) Tender paravertebral and posterior lower extremity points
3) Bony tenderness (spinous process, ilium, anterior aspect of L5 and S1 vertebral bodies)
4) Local or distant reflex muscle contraction to spinous process pressure
5) Pain upon spinous process or facet joint pressure
6) Facilitated segmental tissue
7) Abnormal segmental mobility

TESTING FOR NERVE INVOLVEMENT

Straight Leg Raising

Passive straight leg raising is considered to be an important clinical test for nerve irritability. Under normal circumstances passive straight leg raising causes tension in the neuromeningeal pathway (sciatic nerve, lumbo-sacral plexus, related nerve roots, and meningeal investments) which is transmitted from distal to proximal until the tension is constant throughout the length of the system.[155] Tension transmission of the neuromeningeal pathway is sufficient to cause movement of lumbo-sacral nerves when the lower extremity is raised 20° to 30°. In cadaveric subjects 35–55-years-old the fifth lumbar nerve root and the first sacral nerve moved 3 mm and 4 to 5 mm, respectively in response to passive straight leg raising. After 70° little additional movement was observed.[156] By simulating a disc prolapse, Brieg and Troup[155] were able to demonstrate limitation to straight leg raising in fresh cadaveric specimens. The simulated disc prolapse increased the resting tension in the associated nerve root as well as the lumbo-sacral plexus. The basis for clinical identification of a disc protrusion by straight leg raise testing is related to this "tissue borrowing phenomenon" described by Brieg and Troup.

Specificity. How conclusive is straight leg raise testing for a lumbar disc condition? In a prospective study on 403 patients with lumbar disc herniation, confirmed by myelographic and operative findings, 94% tested positive to straight leg raising.[157] Although nonspecific in determining exact level of involvement, when straight leg raising was positive under 30°, herniations of lower lumbar discs were more common. In another study pain and limitation in passive straight leg raising was associated with lower lumbar disc conditions in 98.2% of the 113 patients who underwent surgery.[158] The distribution of pain induced by straight leg raising predicted the location of the disc protrusion in 88.5% of the sample population. All 4 patients with low back pain produced by straight leg raise had central disc protrusions. When back and leg pain occurred the disc protrusion occupied an intermediate location (protrusion contact with cord dura and spinal nerve) in 67 out of 74 patients, whereas lateral disc protrusions caused lower extremity pain only during straight leg raise in 28 out of 30 patients. An earlier study by Edgar and Park[159] supports the relationship of the location of pain produced by straight leg raise and the position of the disc protrusion. The size of the protrusion and the degree of straight leg raise also appears to correlate. Protrusions greater than 20 mm resulted in a 20° or less restriction in straight leg raise. Protrusions of 11–20 mm resulted in straight leg limitations of 21–40° in 74% of the patients studied while protrusions of 10 mm or less limited straight leg raise 41–70° in 75% of those patients.

Tests which reinforce the probability of nerve irritation established by straight leg raising include dorsiflexion of the ankle, head and neck flexion and internal rotation of the hip.[155] The qualifying tests of dorsiflexion, internal hip rotation, and cervical flexion are performed at the limit of pain free range of straight leg raising in attempts to stretch neural tissues from below and above the site of primary pain. Knowledge of additional test movements which influence neural tension may help to substantiate nerve involvement. Confirmation of nerve irritability may also be observed in standing postures. Patients with acute sciatic nerve pain typically stand with the heel raised and knee flexed, the hip externally rotated and the head in backward bending to reduce nerve tension.

Lateral Recess. When straight leg raise is not related to disc protrusion, nerve entrapment in the lateral recess may be implicated. Eleven of 15 patients with intense sciatic pain and positive straight leg raise findings, but no evidence of disc herniation at the time of surgery, were relieved of symptoms during a 5-year study by surgical unroofing and decompression of an entrapped nerve root in the lateral recess.[160]

The experienced clinician is aware of the effects of straight leg raise to other structures aside from nerve. Interpretation of a positive straight leg raise sign must consider tight hamstrings, posterior hip capsulitis, sacroiliac dysfunction, lumbar facet irritation, and thoraco-lumbar myofascial tightness to be possible sources of painful limitation. The specific sign of nerve irritation on straight leg raising is therefore limited to the reproduction of radiating leg pain.[159]

Diurnal Effects. Another consideration when performing a straight leg raise exam is time of day tested. Diurnal changes in straight leg raise were found in 20 out of 28 patients who satisfied clinical criteria for a lower lumbar disc protrusion.[161] A 10° or more increase in straight leg raise occurred during a 3-hour upright period of time following a night of recumbency. The mean repeatability in measurement was 1.6° for one examiner using a precision oil-filled goniometer.[161] The study explains the reduction in straight leg raise after a period of recumbency on the imbibition of fluid within the disc and the subsequent bulging of the annulus. As the patient assumes an upright position the fluid is gradually expressed from the disc reducing the amount and degree of tension of the bulge and so improving straight leg raise ability.

Related Tests

Cross Leg Pain. Positive crossed or contralateral straight leg raising is highly indicative of a poor response to conservative man-

agement. Although the topographic position of a disc lesion is not predictable in patients with cross leg pain during straight leg raising a high incidence of sequestration or extrusion (16 out of 17 patients) has been noted in operated patients.[162] Positive cross leg pain was present in only 30% of patients studied, but is highly indicative of nerve irritation.

Great Toe. Quantitative measurement of extensor hallucis strength is considered an excellent screening test for disc lesions. Of 26 patients known to have evidence of nerve root pressure, 15 had weakness and 10 showed fatiguability of the extensor hallucis longus muscle. Eight of the 11 who underwent surgery had involvement of the L5 nerve root.[163] Since the first sign of motor involvement is muscle fatigue, evaluators are advised to test for prolonged muscle effort instead of testing singular, short duration isometric performance which may still show full power. A comparable muscle strength study for S1 nerve involvement was not found in the literature.

Reflexes

A depressed or absent ankle jerk is a very reliable sign for S1 nerve involvement. In contrast, individuals with fifth lumbar nerve conditions typically have normal knee and ankle jerks.[164] Repeated testing of tendon reflexes is also suggested to determine fading responses which may signify a developing nerve root problem.

As a general rule, nerve tests for lumbar pain conditions are quite sensitive. Positive test results from straight leg raising, cross leg straight leg raising, and qualifying or confirmation tests for straight leg raising are indicative of nerve involvement. Weakness of the extensor hallucis muscle and depressed or absent ankle reflexes incriminate L5 and S1 nerve problems, respectively.

REFERENCES

1. Moll JM, Wright V. Normal range of spinal mobility. An objective clinical study. Ann Rheum Dis 1971; 30:381–386.
2. Hilton RC, Ball J, Benn RT. In-vitro mobility of

the lumbar spine. Ann Rheum Dis 1979; 38:378–383.

3. Lindahl O. Determination of the sagittal mobility of the lumbar spine. Acta Orthop Scand 1966; 37:241–254.

4. Macrae IF, Wright V. Measurement of back movement. Ann Rheum Dis 1969;28:584–589.

5. Twomey L. The effects of age on the ranges of motions of the lumbar region. Aust J Physiother 1979; 25:257–263.

6. Wolf SL, Basmajian JV, Russe TC, Kutner M. Normative data on lowback mobility and activity levels. Amer J Phys Med 1979; 58:217–229.

7. Panjabi MM, Krag MH, White AA, Southwick WO. Effects of preload on load displacement curves of the lumbar spine. Orthop Clin North Am 1977; 8:181–192.

8. White AA, Panjabi MM. Clinical biomechanics of the spine. 2nd ed. Philadelphia: J.B. Lippincott Co., 1990.

9. Anderson JA, Sweetman BJ. A combined flexirule/hydrogoniometer for measurement of lumbar spine and its sagittal movement. Rheum Rehabil 1975; 14:173–179.

10. Stokes IA, Wilder DG, Frymoyer JW, Pope MH. Assessment of patients with low-back pain by biplanar radiographic measurement of intervertebral motion. Spine 1981; 6:233–240.

11. Panjabi MM, Yamamoto I, Oxland TR, Crisco JJ. How does posture affect the coupling in the lumbar spine? Spine 1989; 14:1002–1011.

12. Marras WS, Wongsam PE. Flexibility and velocity of the normal and impaired lumbar spine. Arch Phys Med Rehabil 1986; 67:213–217.

13. Ahern DK, Hannon DJ, Goreczny AJ, Follick MJ, Parziale JR. Correlation of chronic low back pain behavior and muscle function examination of the flexion-relaxation response. Spine 1990; 15:92–95.

14. Frigero NA, Stoew RR, Howe JW. Movement of the sacroiliac joint. Clin Orthop Rel Res 1974; 100:370–377.

15. Lavignolle B, Vital JM, Senegas J, Destandau J, Toson B. An approach to the functional anatomy of the sacroiliac joints in vivo. Anat Clin 1983; 5:169–176.

16. Egund N, Olsson TH, Schmid H, Selvik G. Movements in the sacroiliac joints demonstrated with roentgen stereophotogrammetry. Acta Radiol 1978; 19:833–846.

17. Weisl H. The articular surfaces of the sacro- iliac joint and their relation to the movements of the sacrum. Acta Anat 1954; 22:1–14.

18. Weisl H. The movements of the sacroiliac joint. Acta Anat 1955; 23:80–91.

19. Pitkin HC, Pheasant HC. Sacrarthogenetic telalgia, II. A study of sacral mobility. J Bone Joint Surg 1936; 28:365–374.

20. Wilder DG, Pope MH, Frymoyer JW. The func-

tional topography of the sacroiliac joint. Spine 1980; 5:575–579.

21. Sturesson B, Selvik G, Voen A. Movements of the sacroiliac joints. A roentgen stereophotogrammetric analysis. Spine 1989; 14:162–165.

22. Walheim GG, Selvik G. Mobility of the pubic symphysis, in vivo measurements with an electromechanic method and a roentgen stereophotogrammetric method. Clinical Orthop Rel Res 1984; 191:129–135.

23. Chamberlain WE. The x-ray examination of the sacroiliac joint. Del Med J 1932; 4:195–201.

24. Hagen R. Pelvic girdle relaxation from an orthopaedic point of view. Acta Orthop Scand 1974; 45:550–563.

25. Lindsey RW, Leggon RE, Wright DG, Nolasco DR. Separation of the symphysis pubis in association with childbearing. A case report. J Bone Joint Surg 1988; 70A:289–292.

26. Walheim GG, Olervd S, Ribbe T. Motion of the pubic symphysis in pelvic instability. Scand J Rehabil Med 1984; 16:163–169.

27. Abramson D, Roberts SM, Wilson PD. Relaxation of the pelvic joints in pregnancy. Surg Gynecol Obstet 1934; 58:595–613.

28. Goldthwait JE, Osgood RB. A consideration of the pelvic articulations from an anatomical, pathological and clinical standpoint. Boston Med Surg J Cl 1905; II:593–601.

29. Pennal GF, Massiah KA. Nonunion and delayed union of fractures of the pelvis. Clin Orthop 1980; 151:124–129.

30. Alviso DJ, Dong GT, Lentell GL. Intertester reliability for measuring pelvic tilt in standing. Phys Ther 1988; 68:1347–1351.

31. Cantrell M, Keith-Watts K, Mallet L, Rosch J, Schuster C, Nybert R, Catlin P. A study of the difference in the position of the posterior superior iliac spine at zero degrees versus 120° of unilateral hip flexion. Unpublished Master's Thesis, Atlanta: Emory University Department of Physical Therapy, May, 1989.

32. Nyberg R, Catlin PA, Cappelli S, Ibach K, Parker M, Wickson T. The effect of passive hip abduction, external rotation and internal rotation on posterior superior iliac spine excursion. Unpublished Master's Thesis, Atlanta: Emory University Department of Physical Therapy, May, 1990.

33. Potter NA, Rothstein JM. Intertester reliability for selected clinical tests of the sacroiliac joint. Phys Ther 1985; 65:1671–1675.

34. Herzog W, Read LJ, Conway JW, Shaw L, McEwen MC. Reliability of motion palpation procedures to detect sacroiliac joint fixations. J Manipulative Physiol Ther 1989; 12:86–92.

35. Waddell G, Main C, Morris E, et al. Normality and reliability in the clinical assessment of backache. Br Med J 1982; 284:1519–1523.

36. Frost M, Stuckey S, Smalley LA, et al. Reliability of measuring trunk motions in centimeters. Phys Ther 1982; 62:1431–1437.

37. Broer MR, Galles NR. Importance of the relationships between various body measurements in performance of the toe touch test. Res Quart 1958; 29:253–363.

38. Gauvin MG, Riddle DL, Rothstein JM. Reliability of clinical measurements of forward bending using the modified finger-tip-to-floor method. Phys Ther 1990; 70:443–447.

39. Shober P. The lumbar vertebral column and backache. Meunchener Medizinische Wochenschrift 1937; 84:336.

40. Macrae IF, Wright V. Measurement of back movement. Ann Rheum Dis 1969; 28:584–589.

41. Gill K, Krag MH, Johnson GB, Haugh LD, Pope MH. Repeatability of four clinical methods for assessment of lumbar spinal motion. Spine 1988; 13:50–53.

42. Miller BH, Lee P, Smythe HA, Goldsmith CH. Measurement of spinal mobility in the sagittal plane: new skin contraction technique compared with established methods. J Rheumatol 1984; 11:507–511.

43. Reynolds PM. Measurement of spinal mobility: a comparison of three methods. Rheum Rehabil 1975; 14:180–185.

44. Burdett RG, Brown KE, Fall MP. Reliability and validity of four instruments for measuring lumbar spine and pelvic positions. Phys Ther 1986; 66:677–685.

45. Portek I, Pearcy MJ, Reader G, Mowat AG. Correlation between radiographic and clinical measurement of lumbar spine movement. Br J Rheum 1983; 22:197–205.

46. Moll JM, Liyanage SP, Wright V. An objective clinical method to measure lateral spinal flexion. Rheum Phys Med 1972; 11:225–239.

47. Barnes CG. The differential diagnosis of backache. Br J Hosp Med 1971; 5:219.

48. Maihaffer GC, Echternach JL. Reliability of a method of measuring backward bending of the thoracolumbar spine. J Orthop Sports Phys Ther 1987; 8:574–577.

49. Hart DL, Rose SJ. Reliability of a noninvasive method for measuring the lumbar curve. J Orthop Sports Phys Ther 1986; 8:180–184.

50. Burton AK. Regional lumbar sagittal mobility: measurement by flexicurves. Clin Biomech 1986; 1:20–26.

51. Tillotson KM, Burton AK. Noninvasive measurement of lumbar sagittal mobility, an assessment of the flexicurve technique. Spine 1991; 16:29–33.

52. Stokes IA, Bevins TM, Lunn RA. Back surface curvature and measurement of lumbar spinal motion. Spine 1987; 12:355–361.

53. Sturrock RD, Wojtulewski JA, Hart FD. Spondylometry in a normal population and in ankylosing spondylitis. Rheum Rehabil 1973; 12:135–142.

54. Ohlen G, Spragfort E, Tingvall C. Measurement of spinal sagittal configuration and mobility with DeBrunner's kyphometer. Spine 1989;14:580–583.

55. Loebl WY. Measurement of spinal posture and range of spinal movement. Ann Phys Med 1967; 9:103–110.

56. Mayer TG, Tencer AF, Kristoferson S, Mooney V. Use of noninvasive techniques for quantification of spinal range of motion in normal subjects and chronic low back dysfunction patients. Spine 1984; 9:588–595.

57. Troup JD, Hood CA, Chapman AE. Measurements of the sagittal mobility of the lumbar spine and hips. Ann Phy Med 1968; 9:308–321.

58. Dillard J, Trafimow J, Andersson GB, Cronin K. Motion of the lumbar spine, reliability of two measurement techniques. Spine 1991; 16:321–324.

59. Mellin G. Method and instrument for noninvasive measurements of thoracolumbar rotation. Spine 1987; 12:28–31.

60. Mellin G. Correlations of spinal mobility with degree of chronic low back pain after correction for age and anthropometric factors. Spine 1987; 12:464–468.

61. Ahern DK, Follick MJ, Council JR, Laser-Wolston N, Litchman H. Comparison of lumbar paravertebral EMG patterns in chronic lowback pain patients and nonpatient controls. Pain 1988; 34:153–160.

62. Triano JJ, Schultz AB. Correlation of objective measure of trunk motion and function with lowback disability ratings. Spine 1987; 12:561–565.

63. Dillard J, Trafimow J, Andersson GB, Cronin K. Motion of the lumbar spine, reliability of two measurement techniques. Spine 1991; 16:321–324.

64. Ohlen G, Wredmark T, Spangfort E. Spinal sagittal configuration and mobility related to low-back pain in the female gymnast. Spine 1989; 14:847–850.

65. Ohlen G, Aaro S, Bylund P. The sagittal configuration and mobility of the spine in idiopathic scoliosis. Spine 1988; 13:413–416.

66. Tenhula JA, Rose SJ, Delitto A. Association between direction of lateral lumbar shift, movement tests, and side of symptoms in patients with low back pain syndrome. Phys Ther 1990; 70:480–486.

67. Million R, Hall W, Nilsen KH, Baker RD, Jaysow MI. Assessment of the progress of the back pain patient. Spine 1982; 7:204–212.

68. Battie MC, Bigos SJ, Fisher LD, Spengler DM, Hansson TH, Nachemson AL, Wortley MD. The role of spinal flexibility in back pain complaints within industry. A prospective study. Spine 1990; 15:768–773.

69. Mellin G. Chronic low back pain in men 54–63 years of age, correlations of physical measurements

with the degree of trouble and progress after treatment. Spine 1986; 11:421–426.

70. Sward L, Eriksoon B, Peterson L. Anthropometric characteristics, passive hip flexion, and spinal mobility in relation to back pain in athletes. Spine 1990; 15:376–382.

71. Weitz EM. The lateral bending sign. Spine 1981; 6:388–397.

72. Stokes IM, Wilder DG, Frymoyer JW, Pope MH. Assessment of patients with low-back pain by biplanar radiographic measurement of intervertebral motion. Spine 1981; 6:233–240.

73. Troup JD, Foreman TK, Baxter CE, Brown D. The perception of back pain and the role of psycholphysical tests of lifting capacity. Spine 1987; 12:645–657.

74. Lloyd DC, Troup JD. Recurrent back pain and its prediction. J Soc Occup Med 1983; 33:66–74.

75. Jackson RP, Jacobs RR, Montesano PX. Facet joint injection in low back pain. A prospective clinical study. Spine 1988; 13:966–971.

76. Burton AK, Tillotson KM, Troup JD. Variation in lumbar sagittal mobility with low-back trouble. Spine 1989; 14:584–590.

77. Burton AK, Tillotson KM, Troup JD. Prediction of low-back trouble frequency in a working population. Spine 1989; 14:939–946.

78. Kilkaldy-Willis WH, Farfan HF. Instability of the lumbar spine. Clin Orthop Rel Res 1982; 165:110–123.

79. Howes RG, Isdale IC. The loose back: an unrecognized syndrome. Rheum Phys Med 1971; 11:72–77.

80. Sutro CJ. Hypermobility of bones due to "overlengthened" capsular and ligamentous tissues. Ann Surg 1947; 21:67–76.

81. Grahme H. Hypermobility syndrome: benign condition or indicator of a hereditary connective tissue disorder? Intern Med 1983; 4:141–147.

82. Biering-Sorenson F. Physical measurements as risk factors for low back trouble over a one year period. Spine 1984; 9:106–109.

83. Lankhorst GJ, Van de Stadt RJ, Van der Korst JK. The natural history of idiopathic low back pain. Scand J Rehabil Med 1985; 17:1–4.

84. Allbroo D. Movements of the lumbar spinal column. J Bone Joint Surg 1957; 39B:339–345.

85. Ahlback SO, Lindahl O. Sagittal mobility of the hip joint. Acta Orthop Scand 1964; 34:310–322.

86. Magee DJ. Orthopedic physical assessment. Philadelphia: W. B. Saunders Co., 1987:241.

87. Mellin G. Correlations of hip mobility with degree of back pain and lumbar spinal mobility in chronic low-back pain patients. Spine 1988; 13:668–670.

88. Fairbank JC, Pynsent PB, Poortvliet JA, Phillips H. Influence of anthropometric factors and joint laxity in the incidence of adolescent back pain. Spine 1984; 9:461–464.

89. Thurston AJ. Spinal and pelvic kinematics in osteoarthrosis of the hip joint. Spine 1985; 10:467–471.

90. Offierski CM, Macnab I. Hip-spine syndrome. Spine 1983; 8:316–321.

91. Ellison JB, Rose SJ, Sahrmann SA. Patterns of hip rotation range of motion: a comparison between healthy subjects and patients with low back pain. Phys Ther 1990; 70:537–541.

92. Duensing F, Becker P, Rittmeyer K. Thermographic findings in lumbar disc protrusions. Arch Psychiatr Nervevenkr 1973; 217:53–70.

93. Agarwal A, Lloyd KN, Dovey P. The dermography of the spine and sacroiliac joints in spondylitis. Rheum Phys Med 1970; 10:349–355.

94. Huskisson EC, Berry H, Browett J, Wykeham Balme H. Measurement of inflammation. Ann Rheum Dis 1973; 32:99–102.

95. Jones C. Physical aspects of thermography in relation to clinical techniques. Bibl Radio 1975; 6:1–8.

96. Tichauer ER. The objective corroboration of back pain through thermography. J Occup Med 1977; 9:727–731.

97. Kelso AF, Grant RG, Johnston WL. Use of thermograms to support assessment of somatic dysfunction or effects of osteopathic manipulative treatment: Preliminary report. J Am Osteopath Assoc 1982; 82:182–188.

98. Edeiken J, Wallace JD, Curley RF, et al. Thermography and herniated lumbar disc. Am J Roent Radiol Ther Nucl Med 1968; 102:790–796.

99. Mills GH, Davies GK, Getty CJ, Conway J. The evaluation of liquid crystal thermography in the investigation of nerve root compression due to lumbosacral lateral spinal stenosis. Spine 1986; 11:427–432.

100. Korr IM, Thomas PE, Wright HM. Patterns of electrical skin resistance in man. Acta Neuroveget 1958; Bd XVII Wein 17:77–96.

101. Korr IM, Wright HM, Thomas PE. Effects of experimental myofascial insults on cutaneous patterns of sympathetic activity in man. Acta Neuroveget 1962; Bd XXIII, Wein 23:329–355.

102. Korr IM, Wright HM, Chace JA. Cutaneous patterns of sympathetic activity in clinical abnormalities of the musculoskeletal system. Acta Neuroveget 1962; Bd XXV, Heft 4:589–606.

103. Korr IM. IV. Clinical significance of the facilitated state. J Am Osteopath Assoc 1955; 54:277–282.

104. Wright HM, Korr IM Thomas PE. Regional or segmental variations in vasomotor activity. Federation Proceedings 1953; 12:161.

105. Di Palma JR, Foster FI. Segmental and aging variations of reactive hyperemia in human skin. Am Heart J 1942; 24:332–344.

106. Korr IM. Neural basis of the osteopathic lesion. J Am Osteopath Assoc 1947; 47:191–198.

107. Johnston WL, Allan BR, Hendra JL, et al. Inter-

examiner study of palpation in detecting location of spinal segmental dysfunction. J Am Osteopath Assoc 1983; 82:839–845.

108. Travell JG, Simons DG. Myofascial pain and dysfunction, the trigger point manual. Baltimore: Williams and Wilkins, 1983.

109. Gowers WR. Lumbago: its lessons and analogues. Br Med J 1904; 1:117–121.

110. Stockman R. The causes, pathology and treatment of chronic rheumatism. Edinburgh Med J 1904; 15:107–116, 223–235.

111. Brendstrup P, Jespersen K, Asboe-Hansen G. Morphological and chemical connective tissue changes in fibrositic muscles. Ann Rheum Dis 1957; 16:438–440.

112. Awad EA. Interstitial myofibrositis: hypothesis of the mechanism. Arch Phys Med Rehabil 1973; 54:449–453.

113. Lehto M, Hurme M, Alaranta H, Einola S, et al. Connective tissue changes of the multifidus muscle in patients with lumbar disc herniation, and immunohistologic study of collagen types I and III and fibronectin. Spine 1989; 14:302–309.

114. Strange FG. Debunking the disc. Proc R Soc Med 1966; 59:952–956.

115. Kellgren JH. Observations on referred pain arising from muscle. Clin Sci 1938; 3:175–190.

116. Beal MC, Goodridge JP, Johnston WL, McConnell DG. Interexaminer agreement on long-term patient improvement: An exercise in research design. J Am Osteopath Assoc 1982; 81:322–328.

117. Procacci P, et al. Pain threshold measurements in man. In: Bonica JJ, Procacci P, Pagni CA, eds. Recent advances on pain—Pathophysiology and clinical aspects. Springfield, IL: Charles C Thomas, 1974:105.

118. Notermans SL, Tophoff MM. Sex difference in pain tolerance and pain apperception. In: Weisenberg M ed. Pain:clinical and experimental perspectives. St. Louis: CV Mosby, 1975:111.

119. Notermans SL. Measurement of the pain threshold determined by electrical stimulation and its clinical application. In: Weisenberg M ed. Pain: clinical and experimental perspectives. St. Louis: CV Mosby, 1975:72.

120. Fischer AA. Pressure tolerance over muscles and bones in normal subjects. Arch Phys Med Rehabil 1986; 67:406–409.

121. Glover JR. Back pain and hyperaesthesia. Lancet, May 1960; 1165–1169.

122. Kaplan RO, Maier WP. Fibromalgia syndrome, a clinical review. Emory Univ J Med 1991; 5:36–41.

123. Gunn CC. Motor points and motor lines. Am J Acupuncture 1978; 6:55–58.

124. Gunn CC, Milbrandt WE. Tenderness at motor points: a diagnostic and prognostic aid for low back injury. J Bone Joint Surg 1976; 58A:815–825.

125. Gunn CC, Milbrandt WE. Early and subtle signs in low back sprain. Spine 1978; 3:267–281.

126. Zohn DA, Mennell JM. Musculoskeletal pain. Boston: Little Brown and Co., 1976:190.

127. Tarsy JM. Pain syndromes and their treatment. Springfield, IL: Charles C Thomas, 1953:274.

128. Reynolds MD. Myofascial trigger point syndromes in the practice of rheumatology. Arch Phys Med Rehabil 1981; 62:111–114.

129. Good M. Five hundred cases of myalgia in British Army. Ann Rheum Dis 1942; 3:118–138.

130. Kelly M. Fibrositis and common pains of daily practice. Med J Aust 1946; 2:480–485.

131. Helbig T, Lee CK. The lumbar facet syndrome. Spine 1988; 13:61–64.

132. McCombe PF, Fairbank JC, Cockersole BC, Pynsent PB. Reproducibility of physical signs in low back pain. Spine 1989; 14:908–918.

133. Kraft GH, Johnson EW, LaBan MM. The fibrositis syndrome. Arch Phys Med Rehabil, March 1968; 49:155–162.

134. Nachemson A, Linoh M. Measurement of abdominal and back muscle strength with and without low back pain. Scand J Rehabil Med 1969; 1:60–65.

135. Smidt G, Herring T, Amundsen L, et al. Assessment of abdominal and back extensor function. Spine 1983; 8:211–219.

136. Thortensson A, Arvidsson A. Trunk muscle strength and low back pain. Scand J Rehabil Med 1982; 14:69–75.

137. Addison R, Schultz A. Trunk strengths in patients seeking hospitalization for chronic low-back disorders. Spine 1980; 5:539–544.

138. Janda V. Muscles, central nervous system regulation and back problems. In: Korr IM, ed. The neurobiologic mechanisms of manipulative therapy. New York: Plenum Press, 1978:27.

139. Jull GA, Janda V. Muscles and motor control in low back pain: Assessment and management. In: Twomey and Taylor, eds. Physical therapy of the low back. New York: Churchill Livingstone, 1987:259.

140. Van Schaik JP, Verbiest H, Van Schaik FD. Isolated spinous process deviation. A pitfall in the interpretation of AP radiographs of the lumbar spine. Spine 1989; 14:970–976.

141. MacNab I. Backache. Baltimore: Williams and Wilkins, 1977:51.

142. Pearcy M, Shepherd J. Is there instability in spondylolisthesis. Spine 1985; 10:175–177.

143. O'Brien JP. Anterior spinal tenderness in low-back pain syndromes. Spine 1979; 4:85–88.

144. Denslow JS. An analysis of the variability of spinal reflex thresholds. J Neurophysiol 1944; 7:207–215.

145. Denslow JS, Korr IM, Krems AD. Quantitative studies of chronic facilitation in human motoneuron pools. Amer J Physiol 1947; 150:229–238.

146. Evans DH. Accuracy of palpation skills. Thesis,

South Australian Institute of Technology, 1982. In: Grieve GP. Modern manual therapy. New York: Churchill Livingstone, 1986:501–502.

147. Kaltenborn F, Lindahl O. Reproducibility of the results of manual mobility testing of specific intervertebral segments. Swed Med J 1969; 66:962–965.

148. Gonnella C, Paris SV, Kutner M. Reliability in evaluating passive intervertebral motion. Phys Ther 1982; 62:436–444.

149. Hellebrandt FA, Duvall EN, Moore ML. The measurement of joint motion. Part III, Reliability of goniometry. Phys Ther Rev 1949; 29:302–307.

150. Boone DC, Axen SP, Lin CM, et al. Reliability of goniometric measurements. Phys Ther 1978; 58:1355–1360.

151. Jull G, Bogduk N, Marsland A. The accuracy of manual diagnosis for cervical zygapophysical joint pain syndromes. Med J Aust 1988; 148:233–236.

152. Stokes IA, Frymoyer JW. Segmental motion and instability. Spine 1987; 12:688–691.

153. Stokes IA, Medlicott PA, Wilder DG. Measurement of movement in painful intervertebral joints. Med Biol Eng Comput 1980; 18:694–700.

154. Frymoyer JW, Hanley E, Howe J, Kuhlmann D, Matteri R. A comparison of radiographic findings in fusion and nonfusion patients ten or more years following lumbar disc surgery. Spine 1979; 4:435–440.

155. Brieg A, Troup JD. Biomechanical considerations in the straight leg test, cadaveric and clinical studies of the effects of medial hip rotation. Spine 1979; 4:242–250.

156. Goddard MD, Reid JD. Movements induced by straight leg raising in the lumbo-sacral roots, nerves and plexus, and in the intrapelvic section of the sciatic nerve. J Neurol Neurosurg Psychiatry 1965; 28:12–17.

157. Kortelainen P, Puranen J, Koivisto E, Lahoe S. Symptoms and signs of sciatica and their relation to the localization of the lumbar disc herniation. Spine 1985; 10:88–92.

158. Shiqing X, Quanzhi Z, Dehad F, Anhui H. Significance of the straight-leg-raising test in the diagnosis and clinical evaluation of lower lumbar intervertebral-disc protrusion. J Bone Joint Surg 1987; 69-A:517–522.

159. Edgar MA, Park WM. Induced pain patterns on passive straight leg-raising in lower lumbar disc protrusion. J Bone Joint Surg 1974; 56-B:658–557.

160. Epstein JA, Epstein BS, Rosenthal AD, Carras R, Lavine LS. Sciatica caused by nerve root entrapment in the lateral recess: the superior facet syndrome. J Neurosurg 1972; 36:584–589.

161. Porter RW, Trailescu IF. Diurnal changes in straight leg raising. Spine 1990; 15:103–106.

162. Khuffash B, Porter RW. Cross leg pain and trunk list. Spine 1989; 14:602–603.

163. Finsterbush A, Frankel U, Pharm B, Arnon R. Quantitative power measurement of extensor hallucis longus: a simple objective test in evaluation of low-back pain with neurological involvement. Spine 1983; 8:206–210.

164. Yates DA. Unilateral lumbo-sacral nerve compression. Ann Phys Med 1964; 7:169–179.

7

Dynametric Testing of the Trunk

ANDREW J. TATOM, III

IMPORTANCE OF DYNAMETRIC TESTING

Low back pain is one of the most prevalent and costly benign medical conditions in industrialized societies, particularly in the United States.[1–13] It is therefore alarming that only 10–15% of the patients' complaints of low back pain have a certain, diagnosed cause for their symptoms.[14]

ALTERNATIVE TO RADIOGRAPHIC EXAMINATION

Radiographs do not give the evaluator needed information on patient functional performance. Based on the limited usefulness of traditional radiographic study, an alternate method of documentation of low back function is indicated.

DYNAMIC TESTING WITH A DYNAMOMETER

The first alternate method of documentation of low back function was measurement of lumbar force with a spring balance dynamometer. This started the evolution of dynametric testing of the trunk.

The term "dynamometer" is a popular term for devices that measure human performance. A more accurate description of these devices would be an **actuator** coupled with a **transducer.** An actuator is a mechanism for moving or controlling something indirectly.[15] A transducer is a device that is actuated by

power from one system and supplies power to a second system,[15] such as a potentiometer, accelerometer, or force transducer. As it relates to dynamic testing of the trunk, the actuator controls the performance. The transducer converts the energy of that performance into a signal that can be directly related, usually with the aid of a computer, to units of measure, i.e., degrees per second, pounds-feet, and/or degrees of motion. These units of measure can then be used to describe and document performance.

REALITY VERSUS CLINICAL (TECHNOLOGICAL) LIMITATIONS

In the quest for accurate human performance testing, the type of information collected has been limited by the technology of the devices available to collect it. Consequently, even the National Institute for Occupational Safety and Health (NIOSH) standards for lifting tasks are based on static biomechanical considerations.[16,17] The validity of NIOSH standards relies on the evidence which suggests that the amount of weight lifted during a particular job task is the cause of some low back injuries.[18–20] However, the ability to predict injuries using the isometric model is limited to jobs which require the worker to use a high percentage of his strength potential.[21,22] The use of isometric testing to describe human performance is widespread. However, there are very few "real-life" situations that would require an individual to sustain a maximal static contraction. Therefore, the information derived through traditional isometric testing is limited.

Most back injuries are associated with dynamic conditions such as bending or twisting.[19,23-25] Investigators explored the relationship of dynamic testing and real-life situations, and studies showed that the trunk muscle response to movement and the resulting forces imposed on the spine significantly change when the trunk is tested dynamically.[26] In an effort to measure and evaluate the dynamic aspects of trunk function, the first early dynamic trunk testing devices were modified isokinetic extremity devices that measured trunk motion with controlled velocity.[27-33] Early researchers found that torques generated by the trunk extensors appear to be velocity-dependent.[34,35]

Although preferable to static measures, isokinetic measures of human performance are limited because very few "real-life" situations require an individual to move at a constant velocity. This is not to say that isokinetic devices do not accurately measure trunk performance as well as any other device. To date, no research has been performed attempting to determine if one measuring method is more accurate than another.

Continuing toward measuring "real-life" functional trunk capabilities, researchers have measured *acceleration* and its effects on spinal loading. It has been shown that as the acceleration of the trunk increases, there is a corresponding increase in the load at the L5/S1 level.[36] *Velocity changes* have also been shown to be sensitive measures for confirming complaints of low back pain.[37,38] Taking the premise of acceleration one step further, several investigators have used *isoinertial measures* to evaluate the effort during human performance testing.[17,39,40]

ROLE OF COUPLED MOVEMENTS DURING TESTING

When discussing human performance testing, it is important to question the validity of restricting the motion of the low back to the sagittal plane. The spine is a three-dimensional structure and has been shown to exhibit accessory motion.[41-45] It has also been shown that the coupling of forces due to accessory movement change as the result of fatigue or injury.[44,45] Finally, since it is clinically acknowledged that bending and twisting have a significant association with the increase in incidents of low back pain,[19,23-25] it is reasonable to speculate that evaluation of trunk performance should include all planes of motion of the trunk to allow measurement of the accessory movements that occur in "real life." Examples of accessory movements will be discussed later on in this chapter.

TYPES OF SPINAL DYNAMOMETERS

To understand the types of spinal dynamometers, one must understand the variables each controls and measures.

External Measurement Versus Internal Function

Variables of actual muscular displacement, velocity, acceleration, force, work, and power exist on the muscular level. For most clinicians, access to this level of testing is not available. Therefore, all of our tests are indirect. For example, "knee strength" is usually measured at the interface of the distal tibia and dynamometer. In isokinetic knee extension, the angular speed of the tibia in relation to the femur is kept constant. However, one cannot assume that the shortening of the quadriceps muscle itself is constant due to the change in the instantaneous axis of rotation as the tibia moves on the femur. The actual change in muscle length is not directly proportional to the speed of the leg. This illustrates the discrepancy between external measurements and actual internal function.

Compressive Forces

Regarding the trunk, both internal and external forces load the spine. External forces are those that are applied from the outside of the body (i.e., gravity or weight of the limb or weight of the object). Internal forces are those forces supplied internally by the body musculature to counterbalance or exceed the external forces. Because they are working at a mechanical disadvantage and may become excessive, internal forces usually far exceed the external forces. A very simplified example is as follows: if a simple system in equilibrium is described where the fulcrum is the spinal column and a weight of 10 lbs. is being held 2 feet in front of the fulcrum, the torque generated by the weight is 20 lbs/ft.

A simple definition of torque is: *torque = force × perpendicular distance* from the axis of rotation. The erectores spinae, which are (for purpose of illustration) 1 inch behind the fulcrum, need to counter balance 20 lbs/ft of torque to keep the system in equilibrium. Since the erector spinae is closer to the fulcrum by $1/24$ the distance when compared to the weight held by the extremity, to keep the system in balance the erector spinae must generate 240 lbs/ft. torque. The net compressive force on the spine is the combination of both the 20 lbs/ft force held by the extremity plus the 240 lbs/ft force generated by the erector spinae for a total of 260 lbs/ft compressive force. In the case of spinal compression, the internal forces become the primary source of spinal loading.[46]

Therefore, the evaluator must realize that the data the machine delivers are not a direct representation of actual occurrence within the body. The best the evaluator can do is make judgments about internal forces based on indirect measures utilizing external devices. Therefore, careful selection of experimental variables is necessary to avoid artifacts which may lead the evaluator to erroneous conclusions. For clarification, it is necessary to define the variables also involved in human performance testing.

DEFINITIONS AND VARIABLES

Variables

Independent Variable. Purposely manipulated to generate the experimental conditions (i.e., force, resistance, or degrees per second).

Dependent Variable. Observed/recorded to provide information about the effects of the manipulation of the independent variables (i.e., recorded torque, velocity, range of motion, etc.).

Controlled Variables. Purposely maintained at defined conditions so that they do not interfere with the relationships between the independent and dependent variables (e.g., only "healthy" subjects are tested of the same sex, age, etc.).

Confounding Variables. Can or do interfere with the relationships between independent and dependent variables, (i.e., learning effect, secondary gain issue(s), environmental conditions, etc.).

Physical Measures

Acceleration. The rate of change of velocity with respect to time.

Displacement. The change in the angular or linear position of a body.

Duration. The time during which something exists or lasts.

Force. A vector quantity that describes the action of one body on another. Force either tends to cause motion or causes motion.

Mass. The quantity of matter in an object, representing the resistance to a change in acceleration or deceleration. ("Moment of inertia" is the rotational equivalent of mass.)

Repetition. One action or duplication of a specific action.

Velocity. A measure of a body's motion in a given direction, a vector quantity that has both magnitude and direction.

TYPE OF TRUNK ASSESSMENTS: ISOMETRIC, ISOKINETIC, ISOINERTIAL, AND FREE DYNAMIC[47] (SEE TABLE 7.1 AND FIG. 7.1)

These types of test modes are available commercially and have been well described in the literature.

Table 7.1
Independent and Dependent Variables in Several Techniques to Measure Motor Performance Adapted from[47]

Names of Techniques	Isometric		Isokinetic		Isoinertial		Freedynamic	
Variables	Ind /	Dep	Ind /	Dep	Ind /	Dep	Ind /	Dep
Duration	C	X	C	X	C	X	C	X
Displacement linear/ang	O		C	X	C	X		X
Velocity linear/ang	O		C			X		X
Acceleration linear/ang	O		O			X		X
Force/Torque	C	X	C	X		X		X
Resistance mass moment of inertia	C		C		C		C	X
Repetition	C	X	C	X	C	X	C	X

C = Variable can be controlled.
O = Variable is not present.
X = Can be dependent variable.

Isometric Assessment

Isometric (static) testing requires a constant length of the muscle involved. This sets displacement as the controlled variable, and its value is 0. All motion-related variables (velocity and acceleration) are also 0. The recorded dependent variables could be duration, force, and repetitions.

Isokinetic Assessment

Isokinetic (dynamic) testing requires controlled movement of the body segment at a constant velocity greater than 0. Velocity is now the controlled variable, which means there is no acceleration, so acceleration equals 0. Dependent variables could be duration, displacement, torque, and number of repetitions.

Isoinertial Assessment

Isoinertial (dynamic) testing requires the resistance (mass, moment of inertia) to be set to a constant. The dependent variables could then be duration, displacement, velocity, acceleration, force, and repetitions (Acceleration is not directly measured but can be calculated from the velocity).

Free Dynamic Assessment

Free dynamic testing requires no control over variables because the task becomes the test. Due to the lack of independent variables, changes of the dependent variables are difficult to explain. In other words, the subject is allowed to move freely without any restriction imposed by attachment to external devices in any way. Free dynamic activity is "real-life," but it is difficult to explain why a change in the dependent variable occurred without being able to control the independent variable.

EVALUATION FACTORS—THEORY, PURPOSE, AND DISCREPANCIES

Several factors must be considered when selecting the testing condition appropriate for evaluation:

1. The *ultimate purpose* of measurement must be established, i.e., monitoring progress through a rehabilitation program only, or testing certain aspects of whether a worker is capable of performing particular job functions, or simply documentation of a patient's function at one particular point in time;

2. A *sound theoretical base* on how the human body functions i.e., how does the back move in real-life;

3. Realization of the *discrepancies* between real-life performance and subject performance in your dynamometer; i.e. restricted to one plane of movement, stabilization of pelvis, alignment of machine axes;

4. An understanding of the *different theoretical models* that back dynamometers are based on, according to available information.

UNBALANCED FORCES

Return to the definition of *Isoinertial Testing* where the resistance (mass, moment of inertia) is set to a constant, and movement occurs only when the resistance is exceeded. The unbalanced force (unbalanced force = the total recorded torque minus resistance) causes the movement and acceleration.

This follows Newton's second law of motion (law of acceleration). This law states that *when an object is acted on by a force, its resulting acceleration is directly proportional to the force and inversely proportional to its mass and takes place in the direction of the acting force.*[48] This means a subject's velocity in an isoinertial dynamometer is dependent upon the magnitude of the unbalanced force. The same principle applies to free dynamic tests.

Available Information

Our methods of testing range from very simple, (isometric), to complicated, (free dynamic). Our knowledge about what occurs within the body is the greatest for the isometric tests since isometric instrumentation has been available the longest. Our research body of knowledge decreases as the tests become more complicated because the instrumentation required to record more complex movements has not been available as long as isometric testing and because less research has been completed using more sophisticated techniques. As testing technology improves by allowing us to test "real life" situations more accurately, our body of knowledge will increase. However at present, there is an inverse proportional relationship between the "realness" of the test and our accumulated body of knowledge as the result of limited technology (see Fig. 7.1). Simple isometric tests were the standard until recently, and the bulk of our knowledge is based on their limitations.

A greater degree of accuracy and reliability

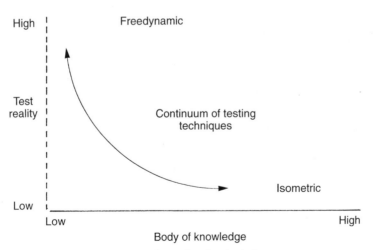

Figure 7.1. Flow of testing techniques.

is our goal in measuring the actual trunk function. The evolving state-of-the-art testing equipment is making the needed level of accuracy attainable, and as this occurs more research will be performed. Eventually our body of knowledge will increase and more information will be available for "real life" tests rather than isometric tests.

KNOWING WHY TO TEST

The first and most important indication for trunk dynametric testing is to know why the test is being performed and what benefit testing will be to the patient or the subject. Trunk dynametric testing gives insight into a patient's function at one point in time. Rarely, if ever, should a clinician judge a patient's condition on the basis of only a single dynametric test. Although currently the emphasis is on objective data, rather than on a clinician's subjective descriptions of a patient's functional condition, the physical exam which includes patient complaint, mechanism of injury, course, and nature of condition are vital information too. Dynamic testing gives the clinician a mechanism to support clinical judgments with "hard numbers," and, in some cases, it helps the clinician to maintain objectivity.

Clinical motion tests, including functional capacity evaluations, have been an attempt to measure overall function. However, until the advent of trunk dynametric testing, there were few objective methods utilizing devices to specifically document motion function of the trunk. Historically, our frame of reference was based upon the extremity model, i.e., following injury or surgery, the involved extremity is different when compared to the contralateral side. Girth measurements are affected, test grades of manual muscle strength change, and endurance and coordination of the limb are also affected. Tests of the non-affected extremity establish a criterion test for comparison. However, in trunk testing following an injury, there is no opposite back member to use as a comparison test. Pre-injury data are invaluable, but rarely available. However,

test results are very helpful even without pre-injury data, as will be described.

INFORMED CONSENT

It is important to realize that any type of testing, from isometric to free dynamic, carries a risk of injury. The clinician should follow the model that has been established by medical ethics and tradition, i.e., the potential benefits from the testing procedure should outweigh the potential for risks of injury/reinjury during testing. A process of informed consent should be instituted to describe to the patient the risks, benefits, and procedures of trunk dynametric testing.

INDICATIONS FOR TESTING

Indications include but are not limited to:

1. Documentation of Function

1. Range of motion in the dynamometer
2. Force production in the dynamometer
3. Velocity in the dynamometer

The measurement tool chosen will determine the variables to which the clinician is limited in data collection.

2. Monitoring Rehabilitation Progress

Pretesting is necessary throughout the rehabilitation period to document patient progress. This gives the clinician, 1) a tool to give the patient feedback on progress through rehabilitation, and, 2) the ability to modify the rehabilitation program, based on comparative test data.

3. Third Party Documentation

These make available objective information on patient function for insurance companies, independent medical evaluations, attorneys, workers' compensation, etc.

CONTRAINDICATIONS FOR MAXIMUM EFFORT TESTING

Contraindications include, but are not limited to:

1. Acute herniated nucleus pulposus with either:
   (a) Sciatica
   (b) Neurological deficits
2. Moderate and severe osteoporosis or osteomalacia
3. Gross mechanical instability, i.e., unstable vertebral fracture or unstable spondylolysthesis
4. Pregnancy—unless cleared by the patient's OB-GYN physician

RELATIVE CONTRAINDICATIONS FOR MAXIMUM EFFORT TESTING

These include, but are not limited to:

1. Mild osteoporosis or osteomalacia
2. Acute phase of injury (i.e., sprain or strain)
3. Early postoperative laminectomy
4. Spinal tumors
5. High grade spondylolisthesis
6. Retained internal fixation (e.g., Harrington rod)
7. Advanced rheumatoid arthritis
8. Infections of the spinal area
9. Paget's disease
10. Hypoparathyroid
11. Abdominal aortic aneurysm
12. Abdominal hernia
13. Stable angina
14. Congestive heart failure
15. Respiratory insufficiency
16. Anticoagulant therapy
17. History of intracranial hemorrhage
18. Status post sternotomy
19. Claustrophobia
20. Potential power failures

INTERRUPTION OF TESTING

The clinician must also be aware that it may be necessary to stop a test in progress. Reasons to discontinue testing may include, but not be limited to:

1. dizziness/syncope
2. shortness of breath
3. nausea
4. chest pain
5. neck pain
6. arm pain
7. rib pain of sharp, sudden onset which increases with inspiration—may indicate a rib fracture
8. incapacitating claustrophobia

General Caution

Overall, if the subject has a condition where testing would weaken the spine, the clinician should exercise caution with testing. The overall decision on testing is based on good clinical judgment.[49]

CHOOSING A TESTING DEVICE

To choose a testing device, the clinician must:

1. understand how the trunk functions;
2. know what functions to measure;
3. Examine the published research and determine any existing prejudice regarding test protocols;

(The information previously presented in this chapter will facilitate the choice of one of the four testing techniques that best satisfies the above three criteria.)

4. examine independent reliability studies of the equipment being considered;[50–52] and
5. examine the available devices and determine which comes closest to the preferred testing technique, bearing in mind the business aspect, (i.e., cash flow, cost, space, return on investment, amortization, etc.) before making the purchase.

INTEGRATION OF DYNAMETRIC INFORMATION AND CLINICAL FINDINGS

Integration of dynametric testing information with clinical findings from a manual exam requires a sound theoretical knowledge of back function. The function of the low back has been described using:

1. *biomechanical models*, in relation to the physics of the osseous elements of the spine and their relation to one another;
2. *dynamics models*, based on action of muscles in relation to their attachments;
3. *functional models* proposed by clinicians, based on the previous two models.

For the purposes of this chapter, the functional definition of the low back (lumbar trunk) is a section of the body that comprises the pelvis and the lumbar vertebrae and discs from L5/S1 through T12/L1, and the corresponding soft tissue.

However, when measuring the function of the lumbar spine, or trunk, the clinician must bear in mind that the trunk does not function independently, but as a part of the whole body.

Functions of the Trunk

In reality, almost every activity involves the low back, which:

1. supports the upper torso
2. protects the spinal cord and its nerve roots
3. provides a platform to support the functions of the upper extremities
4. houses and protects the viscera
5. connects the upper and lower extremities

"REAL LIFE" OBSERVATIONS

Observe the trunk in "real life": how it moves; what it does; its functional patterns in 1, 2 or 3 planes. Then choose the variables or combinations of variables that should be measured: torque, range of motion, velocity.

Torque

Observation of the torque produced during a particular movement is one method to measure function. Angular torque, as used to measure angular limb movement is measured in pounds-feet.

In normal movement, torque must precede motion, since force must first be generated to move the body part or an object. Torque recordings vary depending on the type of machine used to measure them. For example, with isokinetic and isometric devices, torque is not controlled, and therefore is a dependent variable. The magnitude of the measured torque is in direct proportion to the effort exerted by the subject. In contrast, free dynamic and isoinertial devices control resistance, mass, and moment of inertia. There-

fore, the total measured torque readout is the sum of the resistance plus the unbalanced force. Since high velocities are created by relatively small unbalanced forces (Newton's Second Law of Motion), the total recorded torque is to some extent (loosely) dependent upon the resistance set on the device. Consequently, recorded torques are only slightly higher than the set resistance against which the subject is tested.

Range of Motion

Observation of range of motion (displacement), produced during a particular movement is one method to measure function. (Technically, angular motion should be described in radians, not in degrees or revolutions. However, conventionally, angular range of motion is recorded in degrees.[48]) Range of motion allows us to describe where the body is in space, usually related to a constant, such as anatomical zero, or machine neutral.

Velocity

Observation of velocity produced during a particular movement is one method to measure function. Angular velocity is measured in degrees per second. (Technically, velocity should be described in radians per second, not in degrees per second.[48] However, conventionally, angular velocity is recorded in degrees per second.)

Velocity appears to be emerging as one of the most sensitive measures of spinal motion performance. Velocity not only quantifies the performance, it qualifies the performance.

Example. Two individuals of the same arm length, one a power lifter and the other an average man, both have the same task of bench pressing 100 pounds. The average man struggles and takes 3 seconds to complete the lift, but the power lifter takes less than 1 second.

Both lifters have the same arm length, which eliminates the range of motion as a discriminating factor, because the distance the weight traveled was identical. The load is the same for both lifters, eliminating force as the discriminating factor, since both lifters had to generate a force in excess of 100 pounds to move the weight. The factor that appears to differentiate the performances of the two lifters is the time (duration) required to complete the lift, which is the *overall velocity* (degrees per second).

However, if the overall velocity of the two lifts happens to be the same for both lifters, the changes in velocity during the lift allow us to qualify the control of the lift. Picture the average man struggling and jerking (a series of accelerations and decelerations) throughout the lift and the power lifter moving smoothly, well-controlled during the lift. Both lifters completed the lift in the same amount of time. Therefore, neither range of motion, force, nor overall velocity are discriminating factors. The difference was the control, ("jerkiness"), or the changes in velocity throughout the lift.

Hence, changes in velocity are the factors that allow us to compare and **qualify** the performances of the two lifters.[53,54] Clinical observation has been validated with research in regard to velocity; as the load or resistance increases the velocity at which a subject moves decreases. This is a phenomena that has been observed but not documented. Several descriptive studies have been completed that supply the reference tables of "normal" subject performance with regard to range of motion torque and velocity. These are available for the clinician to use as a reference point with which to compare their patients' performance.[55,56]

In summary, definition of the function(s) to be measured facilitates the choice of variable(s), e.g., in measurement of spinal joint capsular patterns, range of motion appears the most sensitive. In measurement to determine fitness to perform a particular job, torque may be the most sensitive. Velocity appears the most sensitive measurement in determining effort. While all of the above are measurements of function, some are more sensitive to particular applications than others.

ISOSTATION B-200 (FIG. 7.2)

A dynametric testing device should reasonably document normal functions that have been explained in detail in previous chapters of this book, such as pure and combined spinal movements and force couples. The Isotechnologies IsoStation B-200 is such a device.

The IsoStation B-200 from IsoTechnologies of Hillsboro, N.C., is a three-dimensional isoinertial trunk testing unit. It measures **force** through torques in pounds-feet, position in degrees, and **velocity** in degrees-per-second about all three axes simultaneously. This delivers continuous data on **force, position,** and **velocity** in **three dimensions,** yielding **nine channels** of data. The B-200 software allows one to compare any combinations of the nine channels of data.

NORMAL CONDITION

Studying the dynamic models of spinal motion, one must examine the lines of force created by the three major muscle groups of the trunk. The posterior muscles include the transversospinalis, interspinalis, longissimus, iliocostalis, serratus posterior inferior, and the latissimus dorsi. The lateral muscles include the quadratus lumborum and the psoas. The muscles of the abdominal wall, which

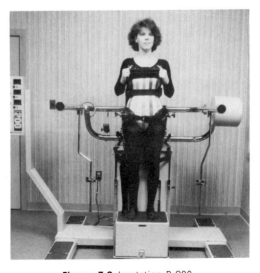

Figure 7.2 Isostation B-200.

include the two rectus abdominis muscles, transversus abdominis, and the internal and external obliques. Each muscle group is responsible for primary movements of the trunk, but their lines of force allow for more than one direction of pull on the spine. The way the muscle groups work in synergy determines the way the spine moves.

When the pelvis is fixed, the posterior muscles of the spine cause backward bending of the trunk. The lateral muscles of the trunk cause lateral flexion. (Note: The psoas contributes some slight lateral flexion to the ipsilateral side and rotation toward the contralateral side and is a minor trunk flexor.)

Rotation of the trunk is caused by the paravertebrals, the lateral muscles of the trunk, and the muscles of the abdominal wall. Forward bending of the trunk is caused by the muscles of the abdominal wall. The muscle groups of the trunk have overlapping synergistic functions. As a result, coupled motions of the trunk occur.[57] Coupled motions

are defined as patterned torques and movements noted in the secondary axes that coincide with torques and movements produced in the primary axis of a given repetitive test.[58]

Documentation of normal force couples has been well described. Fatigue also appears to play a significant role in the movement of the trunk.[45] It has been shown that as the flexors and extensors fatigue during repetitive trunk flexion and extension, the total arch of flexion and extension decreased and their movement was slower. At the same time there was greater range of motion and less motor control recorded on the coronal and transverse planes. With these data, one could cautiously postulate that as primary muscles of flexion and extension fatigued, the secondary muscle group activity increased to complete the required task. With this increase in secondary muscle group activity the spine may be loaded with more injury-prone patterns and place a person at greater risk of injury when the primary muscles are fatigued.[45,46]

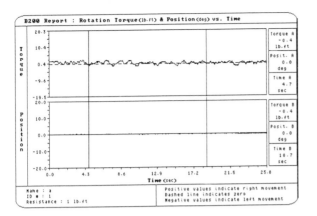

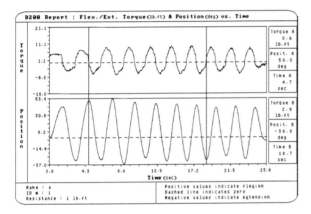

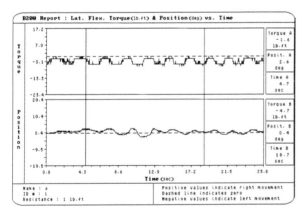

ISOSTATION B-200 PRINTOUTS

These are acutal test result printouts allowing interpretation of spinal motion patterns and measured on the IsoStation B-200. They are interpreted thus:

In the flexion/extension axis, positive values indicate flexion (forward bending). Negative values indicate extension (backward bending).

In the lateral flexion and rotational axes, positive values indicate right movement; negative values indicate left movement. In all graphs, the dashed line indicates 0, where there is no recorded motion, torque, or velocity.

For the sake of illustration in this context, the torque graph will appear on the top, and the position graph on the bottom. The primary movement/effort occurs in the primary axis. For example, when the subject is asked to side bend, lateral flexion becomes the primary axis, and flexion/extension and rotation become the secondary axes.

Units of measure are indicated along the vertical axis. With time as the constant, represented by the horizontal axis, the solid vertical bar line is a "snapshot in time" that describes the patient's instantaneous performance in all three dimensions, as depicted in the photographs below each graph.

1. TEST

Range of motion, flexion/extension: the primary axis is the flexion/extension axis, which is the center graph. The first line at 4.7 seconds is full flexion for that repetition at 50.0°. The second line is at 18.7 seconds and is full extension for that repetition −30.8°. (Note that there are recorded torques on the vertical axis. This is the force required to overcome the mass of the machine during the range of motion test). There is nil recorded on the rotational axis and only slight motion recorded on the lateral flexion axis. The photographs at the bottom of the graph represent the position the subject is in during the described

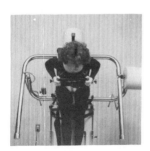

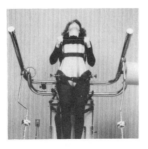

(continued)

(1. TEST continued)

movement in time. Note, accessory
movements are under voluntary control of
the subject and can thereby be controlled.
Many times accessory movements are not
recorded until the subject is acclimated to
the testing device and then will move in a
more "normal" fashion.

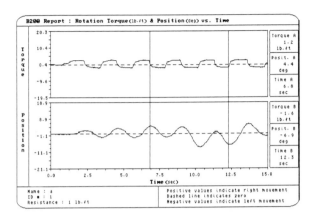

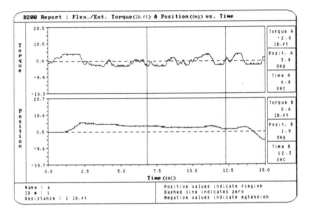

2. TEST

Range of motion: lateral flexion in the erect posture: the primary axis is lateral flexion which is the bottom graph. The first line at 6.8 seconds. The subject is laterally flexed left to −15.6° with a combined rotation of 4.4° to the right and combined flexion of 3.8°. The second line is at 12.4 seconds. The subject is laterally flexed to the right to 22.1° with a combined rotation of −6.9° and combined flexion of 1.9° to the left. (To more clearly demonstrate the coupled movement between lateral flexion and rotation, the cursors are set to where the maximum amount of rotation occurs during the lateral flexion movement and **not** at the end-points of lateral flexion.) The photographs at the bottom of the graph represent the position the subject is in during the described movement in time.

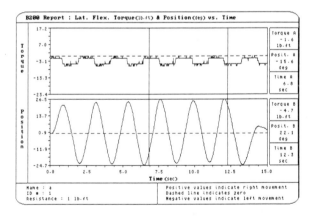

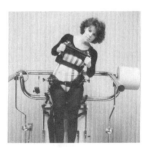
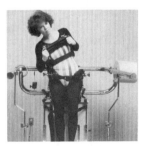

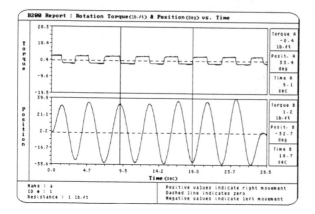

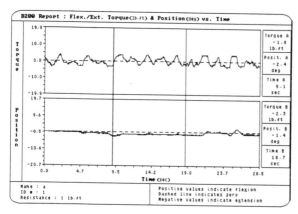

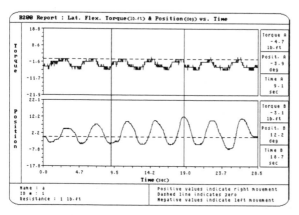

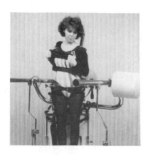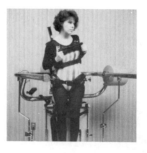

3. TEST

Range of motion test for rotation in the erect position: the primary axis is rotation, which is the top graph. The first line at 9.1 seconds. The subject is rotated to the right 33.4° with a side bend lateral flexion of −3.9° to the left and −2.4° extension. The second line at 18.7 seconds. The subject is rotated −32.7° to the left with a combined movement of 12.2° to the right and −2.3° extension. The photographs at the bottom of the graph represent the position the subject is in during the described movement in time. Note even though flexion and not extension is the expected coupled movement during rotation, the deviation of the flexion/extension tracing away from the baseline is minimal, particularly when compared to the significant amount of flexion recorded on Test 2 during lateral flexion. This illustrates the point that in human performance testing the researcher must take into account individual subject variation and look at overall patterns. Research has been conducted (not performed on the Isostation B-200) that documents the presence of accessory movements in the secondary axis during primary movements.[59] Examples of accessory movements will be discussed later on in this chapter. This supports what has been found with the B-200.

When rotation is the primary axis being measured in the B-200, there is approximately 9.5° of accessory motion measured in the flexion/extension axis and 8.9 of motion measured in the lateral flexion axis; when flexion extension is the primary axis there is approximately 2.3° of accessory motion measured in lateral flexion and 2.3° measured in rotation. When lateral flexion is the primary axis there is approximately 4.0° of accessory motion measured in rotation and 5.8° measured in flexion extension.

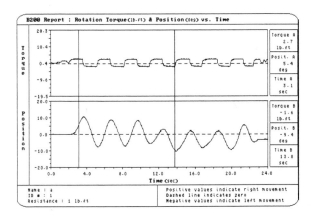

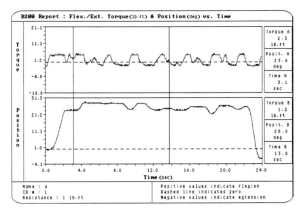

4. TEST

Range of motion test for lateral flexion in the flexed posture: the primary axis is lateral flexion, which is the bottom graph. The first line at 3.1 seconds: the subject is flexed forward 23.6°, laterally flexed 10.4° to the right, with a combined rotational movement of 5.4° to the right. The second line at 13.8 seconds: the subject is flexed forward to 25.0°, laterally flexed −8.7° to the left with a combined rotational movement of −9.4° to the left. The photographs at the bottom of the graph represent the position the subject is in during the described movement in time.

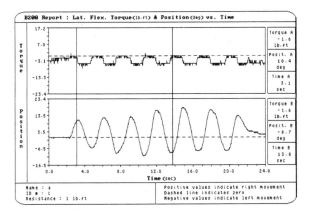

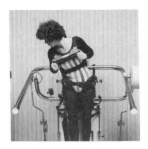
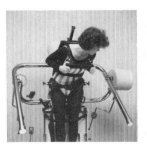

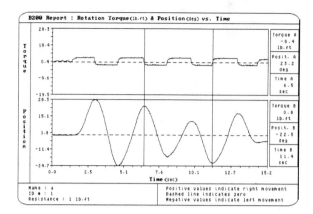

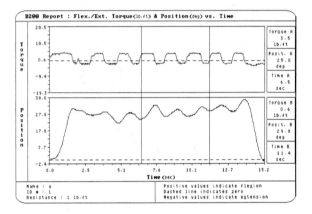

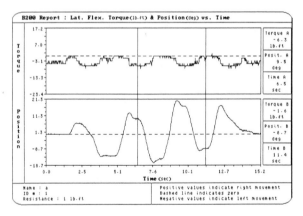

5. TEST

Range of motion test for rotation in the flexed posture, the primary axis is rotation, which is the top graph. The first line is at 6.5 seconds: the subject is flexed forward to 25.0°, rotated right to 23.2° with a combined right lateral flexion to 9.5°. The second line at 11.4 seconds: the subject is flexed forward to 29.8°, rotated left to −22.5° with a combined left lateral flexion movement of −8.7°. The photographs at the bottom of the graph represent the position the subject is in during the described movement in time.

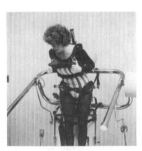
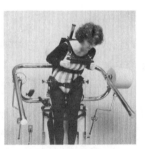

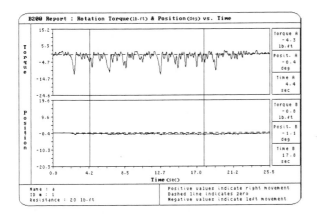

Name : a
ID # : 1
Resistance : 20 lb-ft

Positive values indicate right movement
Dashed line indicates zero
Negative values indicate left movement

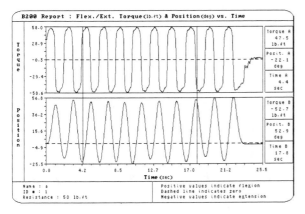

Name : a
ID # : 1
Resistance : 50 lb-ft

Positive values indicate flexion
Dashed line indicates zero
Negative values indicate extension

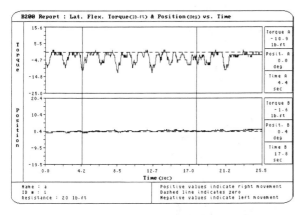

Name : a
ID # : 1
Resistance : 20 lb-ft

Positive values indicate right movement
Dashed line indicates zero
Negative values indicate left movement

6. TEST

Dynamic testing against resistance 50 lb/ft in flexion/extension and 20 lb/ft of resistance for rotation and lateral flexion. The primary axis is flexion/extension which is represented by the middle graph. The first line at 4.4 seconds is the start of the flexion movement (which begins at full extension) with a recorded torque of 47.5 lb/ft. The maximum recorded torque for flexion occurs during the midrange and is 58 lb/ft. The second line at 17.8 seconds is the start of the extension movement (which begins at full flexion) with a recorded torque of −52.7 lb/ft. The maximum recorded torque for extension occurs during the midrange and is −58.6 lb/ft. It has been documented that the maximum recorded torque occurs for flexion and extension when the subject is in the flexion portion of the movement.[27,60] (Note that a regular pattern of torque spikes appears in rotation and lateral flexion. These appear to be present for all subjects, but direction and magnitude vary with each individual.)

The photographs at the bottom of the graph represent the position the subject is in during the described movement in time.

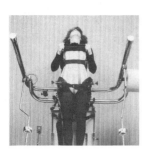
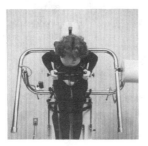

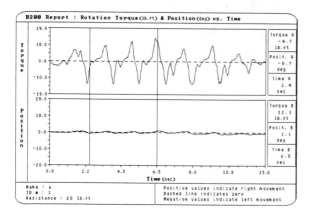

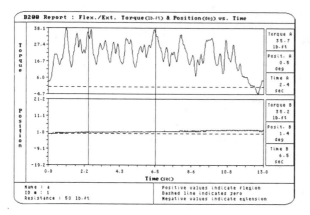

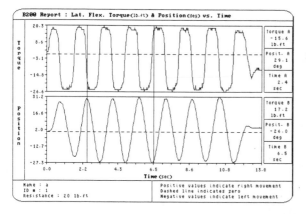

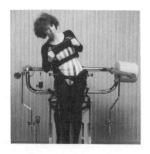 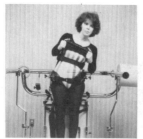

7. TEST

Dynamic testing against resistance of 20 lb/ft in lateral flexion and rotation and 50 lb/ft in flexion/extension axis. The primary axis is lateral flexion, which is the bottom graph. The first line at 2.4 seconds: the subject is laterally flexed 29.1° to the right (the starting point of left lateral flexion). Generating −15.6 lb/ft of torque to the left while generating a coupled −4.7 lb/ft of rotational torque and 35.7 lb/ft of flexion torque. The second line at 6.5 seconds; the subject is laterally flexed −26.5° to the left, (the starting point of right lateral flexion) generating a 17.2 lb/ft of torque to the right and 35.2 lb/ft of flexion torque and a coupled rotational torque of 12.1 lb/ft to the right. Overall, there is little movement in the rotation or flexion/extension axes. It is important to note that when working against resistance, movement patterns change when compared to movement against no resistance or very low resistances. As demonstrated here, when working against resistance in the upright posture, lateral flexion and rotational torques are in the same direction instead of opposite, as seen in only range of motion studies with no resistance. The reason that this occurs concerns the lines of pull of the primary muscles. The primary muscles for lateral flexion are the quadratus lumborum, psoas major, internal and external obliques. The quadratus lumborum ipsilaterally side bends the trunk. The psoas major ipsilaterally side bends the trunk and causes contralateral rotation. The internal oblique is a strong ipsilateral rotator, and the external oblique causes contralateral rotation. Because of the internal oblique working to assist in lateral flexion it also causes ipsilateral rotation.[57] There is a large flexion torque produced which could be explained by the mechanical advantage the trunk rotators possess because their line of pull is so far anterior to the axis of rotation of the trunk that when they contract they cause a flexion movement.

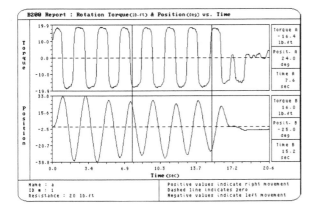

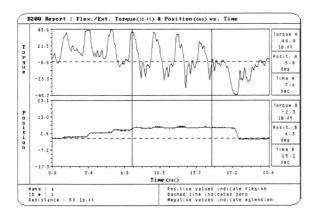

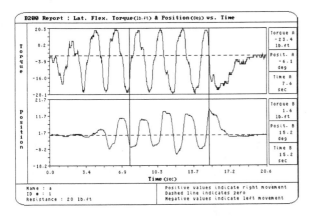

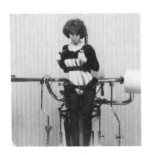
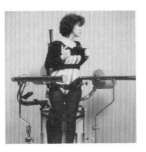

8. TEST

Dynamic testing for rotation against 20 lb/ft resistance and lateral flexion and 50 lb/ft for flexion/extension in the upright position: the primary axis is rotation—the top graph. The first line is at 7.6 sec. The subject is rotated to the right at 24.0° generating a −16.4 lb/ft of torque to the left (left rotation is the primary movement). The primary muscles responsible for trunk rotation left are the right external oblique and the left internal oblique.

There is a coupled-motion torque of side bending left of −23.4 lb/ft which occurred at −6.1° which would be produced by the left psoas major and quadratus lumborum.[57,61] There is also a flexion-coupled motion torque of 40.4 lb/ft which occurred at 5.8° flexion. The explanation for the coupled-flexion torque is this: because of the mechanical advantage that is obtained by the trunk rotators having their line of pull so far anterior to the axis of rotation of the spine that a large flexion torque is generated when they contact during rotation. The second line is at 15.2 seconds—the subject is rotated to the left at −25.0° generating 16.0 lb/ft of torque to the right (right rotation is the primary movement).

The primary muscles responsible for trunk rotation right are the left external oblique and the right internal oblique; there is a coupled-motion torque of side bending torque of 1.6 lb/ft which occurred at 15.2° which would be produced by the right psoas major and quadratus lumborum. There is also an extension-coupled motion torque of −2.3 lb/ft which occurred at 6.3° of flexion. It has been shown that when the spine is laterally flexed or rotated it has a tendency to go to the upright posture.[62,63] At this point in time the spine is flexed, which could explain the extension torque, however, if you look at the flexion/extension torque pattern as a whole when compared to the rotational torque pattern, the subject generates a high flexion torque during left rotation and a relatively low flexion torque or extension torque when rotating right. This may be explained by individual variation in muscle recruitment patterns. (Note: the pattern's consistent throughout the test and further research must be performed to answer these questions.)

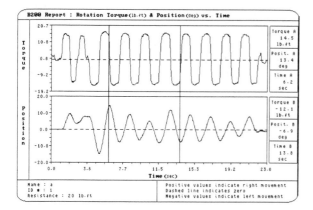

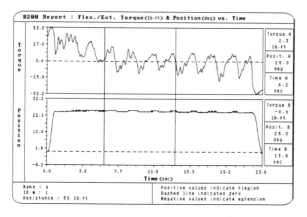

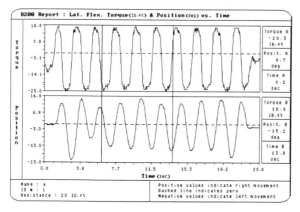

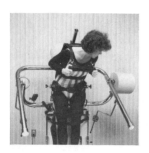
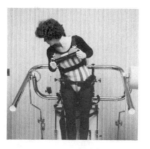

9. TEST

Dynamic testing of lateral flexion in the flexed position against 20 lb/ft of resistance in lateral flexion and rotation and 50 lb/ft in flexion/extension: the lateral flexion axis is the primary axis—the bottom graph. The first line is at 6.2 seconds; the subject is flexed forward 25° and generating a 2.3 lb/ft flexion torque, laterally flexed 8.7° to the right (where left lateral flexion movement begins) and generating a left lateral flexion torque of −20.3 lb/ft, with a coupled rotational movement of 14.5 lb/ft to the right. The second line is at 13.8 seconds. The subject is flexed forward to 25.0° generating −0.6 lb/ft of extension torque, laterally flexed to −15.2° to the left (where lateral flexion movement to the right begins) and generating a lateral flexion torque of 10.9 lb/ft to the right, with a coupled rotational torque of −6.9 lb/ft to the left. The major differences between testing lateral flexion in the erect and flexed position are: there is a decreasing amount of flexion torque which turns into extension torque when testing in the flexed position, and it appears rotation torque and movement lag slightly behind lateral flexion, for their actions are opposite at the beginning of a movement but in the same direction during the bulk of the movement. The primary muscles for lateral flexion are the quadratus lumborum, psoas major, internal and external obliques. Ipsilateral lateral flexion is caused by the quadratus lumborum, psoas major, and the obliques. The contralateral rotational force is supplied by the psoas and the external oblique.

The ipsilateral rotational movement is supplied by the internal oblique. It also appears that as the subject progressed through the test the torque activity on the flexion/extension axis moved from flexion to extension. An explanation may be that as the subject begins to move more "naturally" in the B-200 (not concentrating on how the movement occurs) the subject should move to a more erect posture. This is because during axial rotation or lateral flexion the spine has a tendency to straighten to a more neutral posture. Note that there is a regular appearance to the flexion/extension torque pattern even as it moves from flexion torques to extension torques. They may be explained by individual muscle recruitment patterns and could vary from subject to subject.

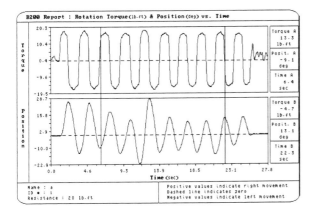

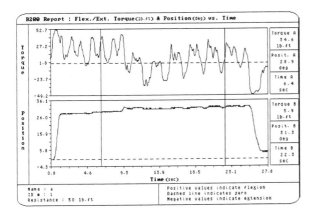

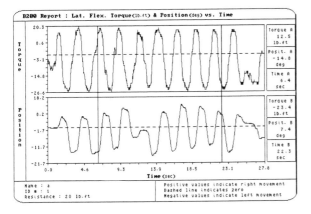

10. TEST

Dynamic testing of rotation in the flexed position against 20 lb/ft of resistance for rotation and lateral flexion and 50 lb/ft for flexion/extension. Rotation is the primary axis—the top graph. The first line is at 6.4 seconds. The subject is flexed forward to 28.9° and generating a flexion-coupled motion torque of 34.6 lb/ft. The subject is rotated −9.1° to the left (where rotation right begins) and is generating a torque of 13.3 lb/ft to the right. The primary muscles responsible for right rotation are the left external oblique and right internal oblique. There is a combined lateral flexion torque of 12.5 lb/ft to the right, which is produced by the right psoas major and quadratus lumborum. The coupled flexion torque of 34.6 lb/ft could be explained by the mechanical advantage that the trunk rotators have because their line of pull is so far anterior to the axis of rotation of the trunk that when they contract they cause a flexion movement. In general, however, you would expect to see coupled extension torques recorded because during rotation or lateral flexion the spine has a tendency to move toward neutral, which is not seen with this subject. The mechanical advantage of the trunk rotators with their strong flexion component overpower the extensors, and the net effect is flexion. It should be noted, however, that the pattern of a flexion torque during left rotation and a low flexion torque or extension torque during right rotation is the same pattern the subject produced during testing in the erect position and is probably this individual's muscle recruitment pattern. The second line is at 22.3 seconds. The subject is flexed forward to 31.3° generating a torque of 5.9 lb in flexion. The subject is rotated 13.1° to the right (where rotation left begins) generating −4.7 lb/ft of torque to the left. The primary muscles responsible for left rotation are the right external oblique and the right internal oblique. There is a combined lateral flexion torque of −23.4 lb/ft to the left which is produced by the left psoas major and quadratus lumborum. Again the combined flexion torque would be explained by the mechanical advantage that the trunk rotators have because their line of pull is so far anterior to the axis of rotation of the trunk that when they contract they produce a flexion movement.

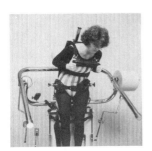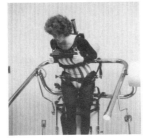

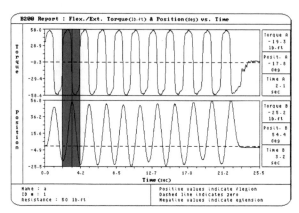

GRAPH #1

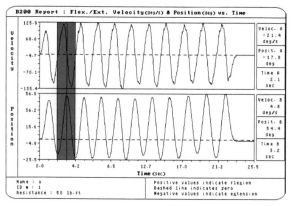

GRAPH #2

11. TEST

Dynamic testing includes use of velocity studies. Velocity studies can be performed on any test that involves movement. The first half of the shaded area represents a movement from full extension of −17.8° to full flexion of 54.4°. The second half of the shaded area represents a movement from full flexion of 54.4° to full extension of −23.1°. Both the first and second graphs (Torque versus Position and Velocity versus Position) are of the same test, and the position tracing is a constant for each. Compare the torque readout with the velocity tracing. As expected, there is an increase in torque prior to the increase in velocity. This is because torque must occur prior to movement, and movement must occur for velocity to be present. This is better illustrated with an enlargement of part of the graph. The third and fourth graphs are "zoom" graphs. It is an enlargement of a graph section for closer study and comparison, the first line the subject is fully flexed to 54.4° (the start of the extension movement). There is no velocity (Graph #4), for the subject is changing direction from flexion to extension, but notice there is approximately −30.0 lb/ft extension torque being generated.

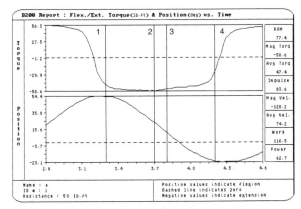

GRAPH #3

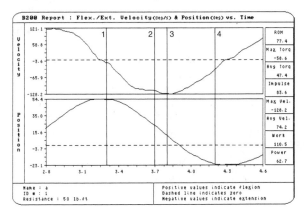

GRAPH #4

(Graph #3) (Remember all values regarding extension are preceeded with a minus sign) Movement can not start until the generated subject torque exceeds the resistance (in this case 50 lb/ft). As the subject increases torque unbalanced forces are created, so movement and velocity develop. The second line represents the point at which maximum extension torque of –58.6 lb/ft is reached at a position of instantaneous 23.6° (Graph #3) of trunk flexion (still while the subject is extending) with velocity of approximately –116°/sec. (Graph #4) the third line represents where maximum velocity of –128.2°/sec (Graph #4) is reached at an instantaneous position of 11.5° of trunk flexion with an extension torque of –55.1 lb/ft. (Graph #3) The fourth line is full extension of –23.1° where velocity is approximately zero. (Graph #4) As the subject is changing direction from extension to flexion note the 22.9 lb/ft torque (Graph #3) that is being generated to start flexion. As with extension the subject will not move until the resistance is overcome. This is the cycle that is repeated when a change of direction is made in any axis.

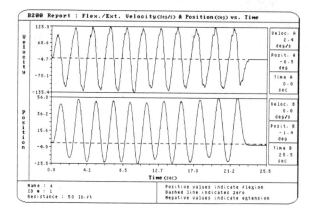

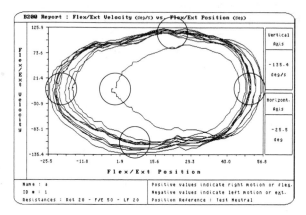

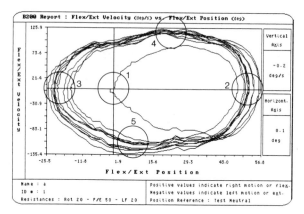

11A. TEST

Graph IIA is generated from the same data collected during test 11. The top graph is the velocity and position versus time graph; the bottom graph (ovoid) is velocity versus position. The constant of time has been eliminated; therefore, the graph continuously inscribes over itself, producing an ovoid graph. The horizontal axis represents position, with full flexion to the right and full extension to the left. The vertical axis represents velocity with maximum velocity in flexion at top and maximum velocity in extension at the bottom. The circle labeled #1 is where the subject is in the upright position and not moving.

This is why the graph starts and stops here. Circle #2 represents full flexion of 56.8°.

Also note: velocity (represented by the horizontal axis) is at 0°/sec because the subject must stop and reverse motion to move from flexion to extension. The circle #3 represents full extension at −25.5°. Note that velocity is at 0°/sec because the subject has to stop moving from full extension to flexion. Circle #4 represents maximum velocity of 125.9° per second during the flexion movement and is reached at 18° of flexion. Then there is a rapid deceleration to prepare to reverse the movement to extension. Circle #5 is where the maximum velocity of −135.4° per second is reached during the extension movement at 7.9° of flexion. Then there is a rapid deceleration to prepare to reverse the movement to flexion. Due to the orientation of the graph, with flexion being positive and extension being negative, this graph is inscribed in a clockwise direction.

PRESENTATION OF ABNORMAL CONDITIONS

Several studies have demonstrated the ability of the B-200 to discriminate between populations with and without back pain.[58,64,65] However, to date, an effective testing protocol to determine severity or the degree of motion impairment against an accepted standard of low back pain has not been developed.

The following section will present documentation and description of abnormal conditions as recorded by the IsoStation B-200.

CAPSULAR PATTERN

As discussed in previous chapters, the capsular pattern for a segmental restriction on the right side is:

    a. lateral flexion restriction to the left;

    b. rotation restricted to the right;

    c. a slight deviation right during the forward bending of the trunk.[66]

Please note: The machine can not document what **level** the restriction is, only which **side.** The clinician must determine the level of restriction through clinical motion testing.

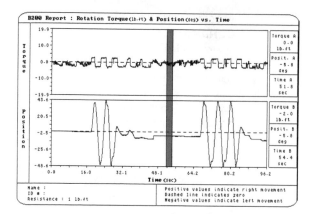

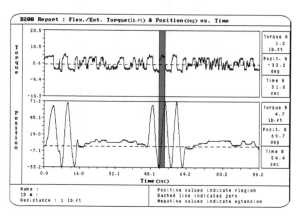

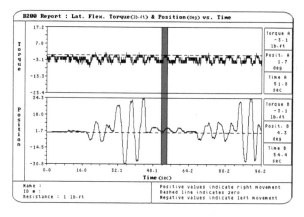

12. TEST

Documentation of a capsular pattern. Note: when examining three dimensions with the IsoStation B-200, the subject must complete a series of repetitions to achieve as close to "natural" movement in the machine as possible. Graph #12 is range of motion documentation of a capsular pattern with a right side restriction. Rotation right is 43.6°, left is −48.6°. Lateral flexion right is 34.3°, left is −30.8°. The shaded area represents a full flexion movement starting at −33.2° extension and moving to 71.2° flexion with a coinciding lateral flexion movement to the right starting at 1.7° and ending 4.3°. This was consistently measured for each flexion movement during the second set of flexion/extension movements. The lateral flexion positional changes are small; however, they are consistent and easily documented. B-200 documentation can support clinical impressions by providing hard data findings to a third party, such as insurance companies, attorneys, physicians, etc.

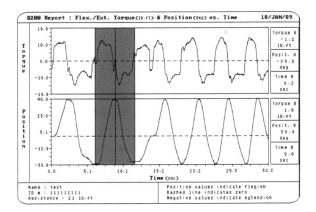

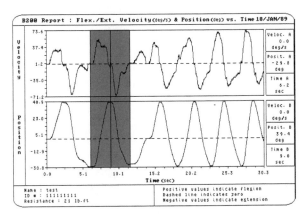

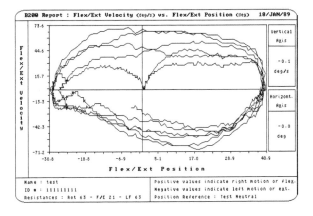

13. TEST

Dynamic testing using velocity studies of low back pain patient. The first half of the shaded area represents a full flexion movement from −29.8 extension to 39.4° flexion. The second half of the shaded area represents a full extension movement from 39.4° flexion to −26.9° extension. Both the Torque versus Position and Velocity versus Position graphs represent the same test, and the position tracing is constant for each. The torque signatures, (a "signature" is the general characteristic shape of one repetition's tracings, regardless of magnitude or location) are not the same. The Velocity versus Position graph demonstrates the variance of the signatures. The flexion portion of the movement shows the greatest variation. The overall velocity at which an injured person moves is much slower than a normal subject,[67-69] as demonstrated here (73.6°/sec in flexion as opposed to the normal subject in test 11 of 125.9°/sec). The inscribed (ovoid) velocity position graph demonstrates slow movement, which is more consistent during extension than flexion.

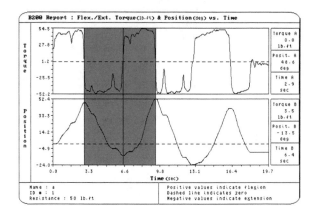

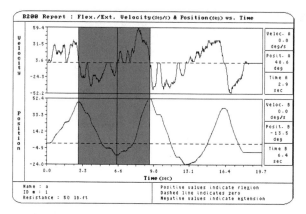

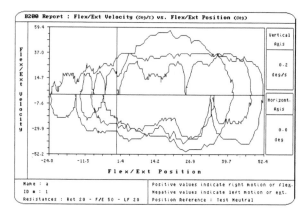

14. TEST

Dynamic testing using velocity studies of a subject feigning a low back dysfunction. The first half of the shaded area represents a full extension movement from 48.6° flexion to −13.5° extension. The second half of the shaded area represents a full flexion movement from −13.5° extension to 52.4° flexion. Both the Torque versus Position and Velocity versus Position graphs represent the same test, and the position tracing is constant for each. Examination of the torque signatures for flexion and extension reveals greater differences than the torque signatures. Examination of the velocity signatures for flexion and extension reveals significant differences. Examination of the Velocity versus Position (ovoid) graph reveals overt performance inconsistencies. Motion tracings of velocity performed show little if any reproducibility, which is typical of a subject attempting to manipulate the outcome of a test.[70]

LATERAL SHIFT

It is possible to document a lateral shift or lateral bending signs. This would allow you to document patient list and restricted side bending movement. For example, if a patient has a disc herniation medial to the nerve root on the right or a lateral disc herniation to the nerve root on the left or nerve root entrapment on the right, the patient may stand straight or with a list to the right. Decreased left side bending may also exist.[71] This can be documented with the B-200, but several extra steps must be taken if the patient has a list. First, align the connecting rod that holds the back pack to the patient so if the patient is side bent you are not forcing the patient to stand straight. Second, prior to range of motion testing go into set up and change position reference to machine neutral.

By making these two simple changes you can document the degree of list compared to the orthogonal machine neutral position (which would allow you to retest and document change over time) and have a constant to compare left and right side bending too. If you do not use machine neutral, the position the patient starts in, even if with a significant list, will be reported as 0° and may give you misleading information. The B-200, to document the lateral bending sign, should be used in conjunction with your orthopedic exam.

DOCUMENTING CLINICAL EXAMINATION OF THE TRUNK

Clinical examination should include, but not be limited to, history, postural evaluation, active and passive spinal movement tests, neurological exam, and palpation testing.

The active movement exam may indicate a hypomobility on the right side. (Manual examination is designed to determine the level(s) of the restriction.) Both these active and passive movement patterns, however, can be documented utilizing a three-dimensional measuring device. Documenting abnormal motion patterns through the use of spinal dynametric testing will support clinical observations with objective data.[41-44]

REHABILITATION WITH SPINAL DYNAMOMETERS

Identification of specific motion deficits in a patient from manual and mechanical evaluation, plus a thorough understanding of the capabilities of a back machine make establishing a graduated rehabilitation program relatively straightforward. Clinicians should apply their knowledge of rehabilitation to the back the same as for an extremity. If a deficit is identified during testing, rehabilitation for correction of the deficit is planned, i.e., high repetition protocols for decreased endurance, range of motion protocols for decreased flexibility, progressive resistance protocol for decreased strength, etc. The versatility of the testing device determines the limits of its use in rehabilitation.

Some devices offer feedback during the workout, a feature important for certain patients, specifically those who have difficulty understanding exertion levels or who are in need of an external stimulus to maintain a predetermined exercise level, etc. Most devices restrict movement to a single plane. In reality, however, people do not move in single planes. One device, the IsoStation B-200, allows controlled rehabilitation utilizing functional diagonals movements, i.e., modified PNF patterns for the trunk. The B-200 allows a closer simulation of job-specific trunk movements than a single axis dynomometer. However, the B-200 does not offer an eccentric mode, and eccentricities are a normal part of trunk function.

Therapists can tailor rehabilitation activities and focus specific trunk exercise programs based on the measured demands of the job. The therapist must also include rehabilitation of the upper and lower extremities, for the whole body is involved in work tasks and rehabilitation should not be only limited to the trunk.

Spinal dynamometers can be useful as one of many elements in a complete, integrated low back rehabilitation program, along with other tools such as educational programs, flexibility, cardiovascular fitness, strengthening, job simulation, work hardening, and psychological evaluation and treatment.[72–74]

Spinal dynamometers in low back rehabilitation can involve: 1) monitoring patient progress and 2) conditioning.

1. Monitoring Patient Progress

The use of dynamometers to monitor patient progress in a rehabilitation program provides objective data. Once the appropriate test procedures and protocols have been chosen for a particular patient condition, they can be repeated at established time intervals throughout the rehabilitation process. Data obtained from spinal dynomometers allows for the establishment of goals. Time frames can be set to achieve set goals. The data give the clinician another tool to help the patient throughout the rehabilitation program.

Data provide direct feedback to the patient on the progress or lack of progress in the program. A series of tests provide documentation that demonstrates patient improvement to third party payers which can expedite reimbursement for treatment. Test documentation furthermore offers quantifiable data that can support clinical judgments in a court of law.

2. Conditioning

Most dynamometers allow patients to travel through a range of motion. The use of range of motion during a workout is appropriate for the patient who experiences pain with exertion, but may have little pain with motion, or as a flexibility activity for individuals with restricted motion. Range of motion is also a good exercise when a patient is apprehensive of exercise in a spinal dynamometer and needs to be acclimated to the machine. Most dynamometers also allow the patient to work in the isometric mode. The isometric effort need not always be a maximal voluntary contraction. In cases where spinal compression loads

need to be limited, i.e., acute disc conditions, it could be 25%, 50%, or 75% of the patient's perceived maximal effort. This allows a gradual controlled increase in patient activity.

Increasing trunk strength isometrically benefits patients who have pain with movement but little pain with force production. It is useful at the beginning of the rehabilitation process to acclimate the patient to the dynamometer.

Because of certain conditions, maintaining strength is possible while motion is limited, e.g., in cases where the patient has an internal fixation devices.

Dynamic rehabilitation is movement against a set resistance (or load), or movement at a predetermined speed. Rehabilitating patients who are at a low functional level or a high pain level requires working against a low load or at a slow speed. Lower loads, or slower speeds help prevent exacerbation of symptoms, but build patient's confidence and tolerance. Slower speeds permit the patient to catch up to the machine, which allows the patient to generate force against the dynamometer. As the patient tolerance to dynamic testing improves, resistance and speeds can be increased along with repetitions. Variations on all of the above can be designed by the clinician for developing limited range of motion protocols to avoid movement or risk injury, i.e., limited rotation, for a patient with an unstable spine recovering from a discectomy. The schedule and speed of progress in the rehabilitation program can be guided by serial testing throughout the rehabilitation program.

The dynamometer is an important tool in back rehabilitation programs. Programs and dynamometers should be flexible, allowing therapists to adapt them to many different types of patient situations.

USE OF SPINAL DYNAMOMETERS FOR EMPLOYMENT DECISIONS

The main goal of screening is matching the worker to the job. Screening decreases the risk of job-related injuries and associated costs.

Industry is now bearing a significant financial burden for low back pain. Industries constantly seek controls to increase profitability by prevention of injuries. Screening, including back testing, can decrease lost time due to injuries, Workers' Compensation and insurance costs, direct medical expenses, rehabilitation and retraining costs, and down time. Productivity, morale, and profits all increase when injuries are prevented and people are matched up to suitable jobs according to their physical capabilities.

The federal government has developed and enforces certain guidelines for the formation of screens. Therefore, the legal aspects of screens must be considered.

According to the Uniform Guidelines on Employee Selection Procedure (UGESP),[75] which have been adopted by the Equal Employment Opportunity Commission (EEOC) and other federal departments, the guidelines are based on Title VII of the Civil Rights Act of 1984 (as amended by the EEOC act of 1972), executive order #11246 (as amended by executive order #11375), the Age Discrimination and Employment Act of 1967 and the Rehabilitation Act of 1973. Employment discrimination based upon race, color, religion, sex, national origin, age, or handicap is prohibited.

The courts have made it clear that jobs requiring physical strength must be made available to all applicants on an individual basis, regardless of race, color, religion, sex, national origin, age, or handicap, hereinafter referred to as "protected groups." This means that any member of a protected group may not be excluded from testing by an employer.

All tests that determine employment decisions, pencil and paper tests, as well as tests of physical strength, must comply with federal guidelines. Employment decisions are defined by the guidelines as including hiring, promotion, demotion, referral, retention, etc. A test may yield an "adverse impact" on the hiring rate, or the percentage of total hires, of protected groups. An "adverse impact" is defined by the percentage of "protected group" hires compared to total hires. Federal agencies have adopted a rule of thumb under which they will generally consider a "substantially different rate of selection" to be the selection rate of any protected group of less than 80% of the selection rate of the group with the highest selection rate.

If the screen causes an "adverse impact" on a protected group, it must be validated and proven to be based on the essential, documented requirements of the job, that is, a legitimate business necessity, substantially related to the successful performance of the job. Otherwise, use of the test results in employment decisions could be deemed unlawful.

For example, if in the tester's mind a particular job is deemed to require a high degree of trunk strength to perform it safely, the B-200 could measure an applicant's trunk strength to see if it is greater than the standard set by the tester. Research has shown that males typically generate more trunk torque than females. This screen would have an adverse impact on females, and it could be considered unlawful if the standard could not be validated because the "standard" was not based on essential requirements of the job. However, if a statistical relationship is found between scores on B-200 testing and job performance, a standard could be supported through criteria validity. Then the screen would be lawful even with an adverse impact regarding the number of females hired when compared to the number of males hired.

TYPES OF VALIDITY STUDIES

Criterion validity is the statistical relationship between scores on a selection procedure(s) and job performance of a sample of workers.

Content validity demonstrates that the content selection procedure is representative of important aspects for performance on the job.

Construct validity must demonstrate that selection procedure(s) measures a construct (underlying human trait) and that this construct is important for successful job performance.

Validation Strategies

Validation strategy or strategies should be:

1. Appropriate for the type of selection procedure and the employment situation,
2. Technically and administratively feasible. Whatever method of validation is used, the basic logic is one of prediction, i.e., the presumption that the level of performance on the selection procedure will, on the average, be indicative of performance on the job after selection.[75]

Therapists utilizing back testing machines in screening should be aware of governmental requirements regarding testing procedures and protocols related to EEOC guidelines when the results of such tests are used in making employment decisions. Testing that has no impact on employment decisions does not require compliance with federal guidelines, such as testing as an element of a wellness program, or general screening.

TRUNK DYNAMOMETER TESTING CRITERIA

Performing strength tests using trunk dynamometers or other functional tests should meet six criteria: 1) safety, 2) reliability, 3) validity, 4) practicality, 5) predictive value, and 6) legality.[76]

Methods for designing pre-employment screens are outlined as follows:[77,78]

1. Job relatedness to testing only on the critical job components;
2. Rationale for using only critical job components when making placement decisions;
3. Methods for determining criteria of job tasks;
4. Development of an integrated job assessment.

For employment decisions, using only trunk dynametric testing for pre-employment screens is, in most cases, inadequate. However, the data from all trunk dynamometers gathered prior to an injury will serve as a base line. If an employee is tested and later injured on the job, having a record of his "good back" will provide invaluable data in determining the effect the injury has on his performance, if any. Having this information will facilitate his rehabilitation and eventual return to work.

The use of spinal dynamometers in pre-employment screening is limited because criterion validity studies have not as yet been performed. Once these studies have been performed, dynametric testing of the spine will have a significant role in pre-employment screening.

TESTING FOR CONSISTENCY OF EFFORT

It is not valid to assume that inconsistent test results indicate malingering. Variables such as lack of understanding of test procedures, easy fatiguability, unidentified impairment, fear of reinjury or pain, test anxiety, or symptom magnification syndrome[79] can produce inconsistent effort, and should not be construed as willful manipulation of test results.

Malingering?

The definition of malingering is the willful, deliberate, and fraudulent feigning or exaggeration of the symptoms of illness or injury, done for the purpose of a consciously desired end,[80] such as to influence or alter medical or legal opinion.

The emphasis of the definition is on **conscious effort of a patient to mislead.** Few medical practitioners are trained and licensed to deal with peoples' conscious will (the psychological aspect of the patient). If a therapist tries to fill this role in a court of law without proper credentials, the testimony will be discounted. However, information that physical therapists can provide for medical and legal professionals can add significant strength to the testimony.

Trunk dynamometers are not lie detectors. They are tools that measure some aspect of function and the repeatability of function. There has been some research utilizing coupled movements in the determination of how much effort a patient is putting forth during trunk testing.[68,81] For example, an inconsistency emerges if during a three-dimensional test a patient asked to give a best effort during a side bending test produces a low amount of torque recorded in the primary side-bending axis, and then during the rotational test a greater amount of side-bending torque is recorded when the patient is not consciously thinking about side bending. If enough inconsistencies are present you can make the statement that, for whatever reason, the patient did not give his or her best effort.

Studies have shown that under certain conditions, human performance should be consistent.[82–84] Inconsistency indicates, for whatever previously-cited reason, the patient is not putting forth a best effort each time. Therapists can document the inconsistencies of the performance. Inconsistencies may have a statistical basis, i.e., coefficient of variation or a "logical" basis, i.e., intertest velocity against a lower resistance should be greater than velocity against a higher resistance, or torque intertest generation should be greater when pushing against a slower speed than a higher speed. Maximum isometric force generation should be greater than dynamic force generation. Erratic and inconsistent position, torque, and velocity signatures (for an example refer to Test 14); this information, along with the supporting information from the physical exam and other functional tests, will give a trained psychologist objective data on which to base an opinion.

Fortunately, there are few malingerers. Some people tested fall into the category of *symptom magnification syndrome*.[85] Nevertheless, therapists should plan and prepare complete, concise, easily-understood documentation as though the results of each series of tests would be presented in a court of law. Requests for consistency of effort tests indicate a question in the referring physician's mind regarding the validity of the patient's subjective complaints, and often the conflicting opinions are settled in a court of law.

Therefore, physical therapists should use extreme caution in making definitive statements about patients' performance, unless they can substantiate their opinions with published research. This foundation in research and fact gives credibility to the testimony.

Physical therapists involved in consistency of performance situations should prepare for a court appearance understanding that they are considered to be experts. They should thoroughly educate themselves in court procedures, terminology, and cross-examination tactics. Preparing before the need arises will allow them to present information in a professional manner.[86,87]

CONCLUSION

In closing, the future for trunk dynametric testing is bright. However, as with all new technologies, trunk dynametric testing must be thoroughly researched, and statements of patient function can only be made based on research studies. A trunk dynamometer is a tool only as good as the clinician using it. This tool should be integrated into rehabilitation programs and not be expected to be the panacea for low back pain. However, spinal dynamometers do provide information that has been unavailable in the past and are a significant addition to any program dealing specifically with low back disorders.

REFERENCES

1. Hult L. Cervical, dorsal and lumbar spinal syndromes. Acta Orthop Scand 1954; 24:174–175.
2. Horal J. The clinical appearance of low back disorders in the city of Gothenburg, Sweden. Comparison of incapacitated probands with matched controls. Acta Orthop Scand 1969; 118(suppl):1–109.
3. Kellgren JH, Lawrence JS. Osteo-arthrosis and disk degeneration in an urban population. Ann Rheum Dis 1958; 17:388–397.
4. National Center for Health Statistics. Prevalence of Selected Impairments, United States—1977, Series 10, No. 134. DHHS Publication (PHS) 81-1562. Hyattsville, Maryland, 1981.
5. Deyo RA, Tsol-Wu YJ. Descriptive epidemiology of low-back pain and its related medical care in the United States. Spine 1987; 12:264–268.
6. Nagi SZ, Riley LE, Newby LG. A social epidemiology of back pain in a general population. J Chron Dis 1973; 26:769–779.
7. Frymoyer JW, Pope MH, Clements JH, et al. Risk factors in low-back pain: an epidemiology study. J Bone Joint Surg 1983; 65A:213–218.
8. Kelsey JL. Epidemiology of musculoskeletal disor-

ders. New York: Oxford University Press, 1982:145–167.

9. Frymoyer JW, Pope MH, Clements JH, et al. Risk factors in low-back pain: an epidemiological study. J Bone Joint Surg 1983; 65A:213–218.

10. Andersson GBJ, Pope MH, Frymoyer JW. Epidemiology. In: Pope MH, Frymoyer JW, Andersson G, eds. Occupational low back pain. New York: Praeger, 1984:101–114.

11. Morris A. Identifying workers at risk to back injury is not guesswork. Occup Health Saf 1985; 55:16–20.

12. Spengler DM, Bigos SJ, Martin NA, et al. Back injuries in industry: a retrospective study. I. Overview and cost analysis. Spine 1986; 11:241–245.

13. Matheson LN. Prevention of disability induced retirement. Ind Rehabil Quart 1988; 1:1–5.

14. Dillane JB, Fry J, Kolton G. Acute back syndrome: a study from general practice. Br Med J 1966; 2:82–84.

15. Websters Ninth New Collegiate Dictionary. Springfield, MA: Meriam-Webster Inc, 1987.

16. Rodgers SH. The NIOSH work practices guide to manual lifting. The physiological basis. Paper presented at AIHA conference, June 6, 1982.

17. Ayoub MM. Psychophysical techniques. Paper presented at AIHA conference, June 1982.

18. Troup, JDG. Relation of lumbar spine disorders to heavy manual work and lifting. Lancet 1965; 1:857–861.

19. Chaffin DB, Park KS. A longitudinal study of low-back pain as associated with occupational weight lifting factors. Am Ind Hyg Assoc J 1973; 34:513–525.

20. Anderson, GBJ. Epidemiologic experts on low back pain in industry. Spine 1981; 6:53–60.

21. Chaffin DB. Human strength capability and low-back pain. J Occup Med 1974; 16:248–254.

22. Chaffin DB, Herrin GD, Keyserling WM. Pre-employment strength testing: an updated position. J Occup Med 1978; 20:403–408.

23. Magora A. Investigation of the relation between low back pain and occupation: 4. Physical requirements. Bending, rotation, reaching and sudden maximal effort. Scand J Rehabil Med 1973; 5:186–190. J Occup Med 1978; 20:403–408.

24. Magora A. Investigation of the relation between low back pain and occupation: 5. Psychological aspects. Scand J Rehabil Med 1973; 5:191–196.

25. Bergquist-Ulman M, Larssou U. Acute low back pain in industry: a controlled prospective study with special reference to therapy and confounding factors. Acta Orthop Scand 1970; 170(suppl):1–117.

26. Marras WS, Reilly CH. Networks of internal trunk loading activities under controlled trunk motion conditions. Spine 1988; 13:661–667.

27. Langrana N, Lee C, Alexander H, et al. Quantitative assessment of back strength using isokinetic testing. Spine 1984; 9:287–290.

28. Mayer TG, Smith SS, Kondrask G, Gatchel RJ, Carmichael TW, Mooney V. Quantification of lumbar function. Part 3: preliminary data on torso rotation testing with myoelectric spectral analysis in normal and low-back pain subjects. Spine 1985; 10:911–920.

29. Smith SS, Mayer TG, Gatchel RJ, Becker TJ. Quantification of lumbar function, Part 1: isometric and multispeed isokinetic trunk strength measures in sagittal and axial planes in normal subjects. Spine 1985; 10:757–764.

30. Mayer TG, Smith SS, Keeley J, Mooney V. Quantification of lumbar function, Part 2: sagittal plane trunk strength in chronic low-back pain patients. Spine 1985; 10:765–772.

31. Kishino, ND, Mayer TG, Gatchel RJ, Parrish MM, Anderson C, Gustin L, Mooney V. Quantification of lumbar function. Part 4: isometric and isokinetic lifting simulation in normal subjects and low-back dysfunction patients. Spine 1985; 10:921–927.

32. Marras WS, Rangarajuly SL. Trunk force development during static and dynamic lifts. Hum Factors 1987; 29:19–29.

33. Nordin M, Kahanovitz N, Verderame R, et al. Normal trunk muscle strength and endurance in women and the effect of exercises and electrical stimulation. Spine 1987; 12:105–111.

34. Thorstensson A, Nilsson J. Trunk muscle strength during constant velocity movements. Scand J Rehab Med 1982; 14:61–68.

35. Marras WS, King AI, Joynt RL. Measurements of loads on the lumbar spine under isometric and isokinetic conditions. Spine 1984; 9:176–187.

36. Freivalds A, Chaffin DB, Garg A, Lee KS. A dynamic biomechanical evaluation of lifting maximum acceptable loads. J Biomech 1984; 17:251–262.

37. Marras WS, Wongsam PE. Flexibility and velocity of the normal and impaired lumbar spine. Arch Phys Med Rehabil 1986; 67:213–217.

38. Deutsch SD, Litchman HM. A comprehensive system to evaluate back function. Presented at the Isotechnologies Users Application Seminar, Dallas, TX, June 1988.

39. Jiang BC. Psychophysical capacity modeling of individual and combined manual materials handling activities. Unpublished dissertation. Lubbock, TX: Texas Tech University, 1984.

40. Jiang BC, Smith JL, Ayoub MM. Psychophysical capacity modeling of individual and combined manual materials handling capacities using isoinertial strength variables. Hum Fac 1986; 28:691–702.

41. Dumas GA, Poulin MJ, Roy B, Gagnon M, Javanonic M. Quantitative anatomy of trunk muscles. Proceedings of North American Congress on Biomechanics, 1986:81–82.

42. Parnianpour M, Buchalter D, Nordin M, Kahanovitz N. A non-invasive in-vivo measurement technique for assessment of the six degrees of freedom of trunk motion. In: Lanta SA, King JA, eds.

Advances in bioengineering. New York: American Society of Mechanical Engineers, 1986:28–29.

43. Seeds RH, Levene J, Goldberg HM. Normative data for IsoStation B100. J Orthop Sports Phys Ther 1988; 9:141–155.

44. Seeds RH, Levene JA, Goldberg HM. Abnormal patient data for the IsoStation B100. J Orthop Sports Phys Ther 1988; 10:121–133.

45. Parnianpour M, Nordin M, Frankel V, Kahanovitz N. The triaxial coupling of torque generation of trunk muscles during isometric exertions and the effect of fatiguing isoinertial movements on the motor output and movement patterns. Spine 1988; 13:982–992.

46. Frankle VH, Nordin M. Basic biomechanics of the skeletal system. Philadelphia: Lea and Febiger, 1980.

47. Kroemer KHE, Morris WS, McGlothin JD, McIntyre DR, Harvey M. Toward understanding human dynamic motor performance. Submitted for publication.

48. Barham JH, Wooten EP. Structural kinesology. New York: MacMillian Publishing Co., Inc. 1973:99–100.

49. B-200 Users Manual Revision 200. Iso Technologies, Inc. Hillsborough, NC, June 1988.

50. Tatom A. The reliability of the static torso lift and the IsoStation B-200, relationship between the performance measures from each device and the effects of mood on performance. Presented at the 6th Annual Conference of the Virginia Physical Therapy Association, Inc. Arlington, VA, March 1988.

51. Parnianpour M, Nordin M, Cartas O, Kahanovitz N. The validity and reliability of the B-200 IsoStation: a triaxial system for functional assessment of the trunk. Presented at B.A.C.K.S., Utah, March 1987 and Musculoskeletal Disease in the Workplace—from Pre-Employment to Disability, AAOC, Dallas, TX, September 1987.

52. McIntyre D. The stability of isometric trunk flexion measurements. J Spin Dis 1990; 2:80–86.

53. McIntyre D, Glover L, Seeds R, Leven J. The characteristics of preferred low-back motion. J Spin Dis 1990; 3:147–155.

54. Parnianpour M, Nordin M, Sheikhzadeh A. The relationship of torque, velocity, and power with constant resistance load during sagittal trunk movement. Spine 1990; 15:639–643.

55. Leven J, Seeds R, Goldberg M, Frazier M, Fuhrman G. Trends in isodynamic and isometric trunk testing on the Isostation B-200. J Spin Dis 1989; 2:20–35.

56. Nelson J, Johnston J. B-200 sample population data. Hillsborough, NC: Isotechnologies, 1988.

57. Kapandiji IA. The physiology of the joints. Vol 3. The trunk and the vertebral column. New York: Churchill Livingstone, 1974:73–120.

58. Deutsch S. Comprehensive evaluation of back function. Pawtucket, RI: Occupational orthopaedic Cen-

ter, Inc. Presented at the Isotechnologies 1988 User Applications Seminar, Dallas, TX, June 1988.

59. Buchalter D, Parnianpour M, Viola K, Nordin M, Kahanovitz N. Three-dimensional spinal motion measurements. Part 1: a technique for examining posture and functional spinal motion. J Spin Dis 1989; 1:279–283.

60. Campello M, Parnianpour M, Cartas O, Sheikhzadeh A, Nordin M. The effect of trunk flexion angle on the triaxial isometric trunk muscles strength. Presented APTA Annual Conference June 1990 and MASS Fifth Annual Meeting Aug. 1990.

61. Farfan H. Mechanical disorders of the low back. Philadelphia: Lea and Febiger, 1973:182–186.

62. Panjabi M, Yamamota I, Oxland T, Crisco J. How does posture affect the coupling? Spine 1989; 14:1002.

63. White A, Panjabi M. Clinical biomechanics of the spine. Philadelphia: J.B. Lippincott, 1978:103–109.

64. Seeds R, Levene D, Goldberg H. Abnormal patient data for IsoStation B-100. J Orthop Sports Phys Ther 1988; 10:121–133.

65. Spengler D, Frazer M, Regan K, Guy D, Ross A. Objective assessment of low back function. Presented at the Association of Bone and Joint Surgeons 39th Annual Meeting, Kiawah Island Resort, SC, April 1987.

66. Paris SV. Course Notes . . . the spine etiology and treatment of dysfunction. Copyright Stanley V. Paris, 1979:100–101.

67. Szepalski M, Federsprel C, Paty S, Hayez J, Debate J. Reproducibility of trunk isoinertial dynamic performance in patients with low back pain. J Spin Dis 1992; 5:78–85.

68. Deutsch S, Litchman H. A comprehensive system to evaluate back function. Presented Fourth Annual Meeting of the North American Spine Society 1989.

69. Seeds R, Levene J, Goldberg H. Abnormal data for the IsoStation B-200. Accepted for publication in J Orthop Sports Phys Ther.

70. Spengler D, Szpanski M. Newer assessment approaches for the patient with low back pain. Contemp Orthop 1990:21.

71. Weitz E. The lateral bending sign. Spine 1981; 6:388–397.

72. Gatchel RJ, Mayer TG. Functional restoration for spinal disorders: the sports medicine approach. Philadelphia: Lea & Febiger, 1988.

73. Berryhill BH. Industrial Rehabilitation Manual. Waco, TX: Work Comp, Inc, 1986.

74. Commission on Accreditation of Rehabilitation Facilities, Standards Manual for Organizations Serving People with Disabilities. Tucson, Arizona; 1989.

75. Uniform Guidelines on Employee Selection Procedures. See 43 FR 38240, et seq. (Aug. 25, 1978) and 43 FR 40223 (Sept. 11, 1978).

76. Equal Employment Opportunity Commission. Of-

fice of Personnel Management. Department of Justice. Department of Labor. Department of the Treasury; Adoption of questions and answers to clarify and provide a common interpretation on employee selection procedures. FR Vol. 44, No. 43, March 2, 1979.

77. Hogan JC, Bernacki EJ. Developing job related preplacement medical examinations. J Occup Med 1981; 23:469–475.

78. Matheson LH. Functional capacity evaluation 1988. Presented at: Industrial Medicine; An Introductory Course for Therapists. Boston, MA, October 2, 1988.

79. Matheson LH. How do you know that he tried his best? The reliability crisis in industrial rehabilitation. Ind Rehabil Q Vol. 1, No. 1, Spring 1988.

80. Dorlands Illustrated Medical Dictionary. New York: W.B. Saunders Company, 1974.

81. Spengler DM. Spinal dynametric testing; state of the art. Vanderbilt University Medical Center. Presented 2nd Annual BACKS Symposium, Hilton Head Island, SC, May 1988.

82. Chaffin DB, Herrin GD, Keyserling WM, Foulke JA. Pre-employment strength testing. NIOSH Technical Report, DHEW (NIOSH) Publication No. 77-163, 1977.

83. Zeh J, Hansson T, Bigos S, Spengler D, Battie M, Wortley M. Isometric strength testing: recommendations based on statistical analysis of the procedure. Spine 1988; 11:43–46.

84. Harber P, SooHoo K. Static ergonomic strength testing in evaluation of occupational back pain. J Occup Med 1984; 26:872–884.

85. Matheson LN. Symptom magnification syndrome. Presented at Industrial medicine: an introductory course for therapists. Boston, MA, Oct. 2, 1988.

86. Brimer MA. Depositions: the physical therapist as witness. Clin Man 1987; 7:30–32.

87. Fields A, Home DF. Adequate office records in medicolegal problems, Postgrad Med, 1963.

8

Biofeedback for Assessment and Treatment of Low Back Pain[a]

RICHARD A. SHERMAN and JOHN G. ARENA

This chapter is designed to give readers a basic understanding of what biofeedback is, as well as how it is generally utilized as part of the overall assessment and treatment of low back pain. It reviews virtually all of the published studies and many of the clinical reports, providing an analysis of how well-demonstrated the techniques are along with the strengths and weaknesses of the literature. Recommendations based on this analysis are made for further study and immediate application of the techniques.

BIOFEEDBACK

Biofeedback is a dynamic combination of learning processes and procedures in which the patient and the therapist receive objective information about the immediate status of a physiological parameter. They can use this information to determine abnormalities in the parameter's level, reactivity, and way of functioning, and to correct any abnormalities identified. Figure 8.1 illustrates the typical arrangement and components of an EMG biofeedback system designed for recording patients with low back pain. Surface sensors are mounted over the central bellies of the

paraspinal muscles with the references at the level of L4. Signals from the muscles are amplified and processed to produce visual and auditory cues, which generally change in proportion to changes in muscle tension.

Technical choices have to be made to determine the correct bandwidths to record, methods to avoid movement artifacts during recording, and optimal ways to process the signals to produce a useful feedback display. These choices would require an entire book to discuss adequately, so they cannot be covered here in sufficient detail. Any attempt to gloss over complex, but vital, considerations would lead therapists to make recordings which could provide very misleading information. These topics have been covered in several excellent books including Schwartz's *Biofeedback: A Practitioner's Guide*[1] and the Association for Applied Psychophysiology's *Revised Applications Standards and Guidelines for Practitioners of Biofeedback.*[2]

Biofeedback has been shown to be an effective adjunct to therapies for a wide range of problems including headaches, anxiety disorders, and neuromotor rehabilitation.[3,4] However, the literature on the usefulness of biofeedback as an adjunct in treatment of low back pain is mixed and confusing. Virtually all of the significant research on treatment of low back pain with biofeedback has emphasized the use of surface electromyographic

---

[a]The opinions and assertions contained in this chapter are the private views of the authors and are not to be construed as official or as reflecting the views of the United States Departments of Veterans Affairs, Army, or Defense.

Biofeedback

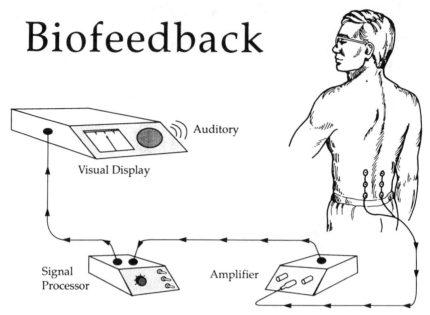

Figure 8.1. Typical system for recording and feeding back signals from the low back paraspinal muscles.

(EMG) signals recorded from a variety of sites, combined with various types of home practice using a variety of muscle tension awareness and control techniques. The mixed results of attempts to apply biofeedback to generic low back pain are probably due more to both (*a*) lack of understanding of the relationships between low back pain and muscle tension and (*b*) inability to determine which factors are causing most of an individual's pain, than to defects in the individual studies.

ETIOLOGY OF BACK PAIN

Low back pain has an incredible complex of overlapping etiologies involving a constantly changing mix of nerve, spinal, muscular, postural, and emotional processes.[5,6] Attempts to relate the level of paraspinal muscle tension to diagnosis and pain intensity during recording have had mixed results.[7–10] While our environmental recordings[11–13] and some of our in-laboratory studies[7] have indicated a general relationship between the amount of muscle tension and the intensity of low back pain diagnosed as being due to muscle tension problems, other literature does not support

these findings.[10] There are no consistent relationships between paraspinal muscle tension of subjects standing still and the diagnosis of low back pain.

There should be a relationship between the effectiveness of EMG biofeedback and the cause of the patient's low back pain. If the pain is almost entirely unrelated to muscle tension, then EMG biofeedback should not be a direct help for the condition. For those patients where muscle tension is a leading cause of the pain, the devices should at least show abnormal readings. However, if the muscle tension patterns are abnormal because of an underlying physical problem, the patterns of tension may only be minimized, but not removed, through the use of self-control and awareness strategies. The situation is rarely simple when an actual patient is being evaluated because of the overlapping problems which combine and interact to produce the momentary perception of pain intensity. For example, a patient who has back pain primarily due to arthritis may also show asymmetries between the left and right paraspinals because one set is kept abnormally tense due to guarding. The muscles on that side may be kept sufficiently tense for a long enough time to cause considerable pain. At the same time, the stress due to experiencing pain for which no cure is apparent is likely to cause an increase in muscle tension among many people. People who respond to stress with their muscles as their primary physiological system are characterized as musculo-skeletal stress responders. They tend to show greater increases in muscle tension when under physical and psychological stress than do people who have other physiological systems which primarily respond to stress (e.g., cardiovascular responses among stress labile hypertensives). The increased muscle tension causes even more pain, which, in turn, causes more stress, so a vicious cycle is established. This cycle is complicated by the tendency for depression and anxiety to magnify the perceived intensity of pain.[14] The theoretical, cyclic relationships between stress, anxiety, depression, sustained elevated muscle tension, and pain are illustrated in Fig. 8.2. Thus, when a biofeedback device indicates an abnormally high level of tension in a paraspinal

muscle, it might be from stress responses; guarding; abnormal muscle use in which one muscle takes over another's tasks; or a primary, muscular, cause of the back pain. Since these causes of pain change with time and activity, they are not likely to be the same at two different recordings, so the recordings are not likely to be consistent. Nouwen and Bush[15] recently reviewed the literature relating paraspinal EMG to chronic low back pain. They concluded that "there is no consistent evidence that low back pain patients have elevated paraspinal EMG or that its reduction is likely to be an active ingredient in biofeedback therapy." They also stated that "research on paraspinal EMG patterns is still preliminary and, therefore, treatment based on their modification is experimental."

Adequate assessment of the contribution of paraspinal muscle tension to a particular individual's low back pain is further complicated by both temporal and movement factors. Since pain caused by muscle tension occurs mainly after muscles have been "too tense for too long," the muscles may no longer be tense by the time a person is re-

Psychophysiologic Pain Cycle

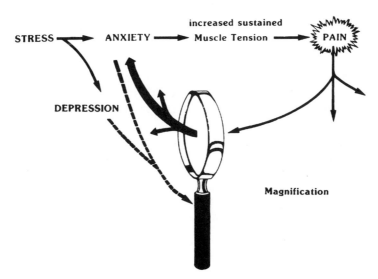

Figure 8.2. Cyclic relationships between stress, muscle tension, and pain, as complicated and magnified by depression and anxiety.

corded, even though the pain still persists. Trial recordings[11–13] of 18 subjects diagnosed as having back pain due to muscle-related problems were performed in the subjects' normal work environments over periods of 6 to 12 hours per session with each subject being recorded for between two and four sessions. Subjects were recorded with an ambulatory two-channel surface EMG which could hold over 20 hours of data and contained both movement sensors and a key pad for entering pain intensity and type of behavior. Every subject showed a very high predictive correlation between change in level of paraspinal EMG and change in low back pain. Muscle tension increased between half an hour and several minutes prior to back pain increasing. Many instances were recorded in which back pain was still rated as relatively high, but the EMG had already decreased prior to a subsequent decrease in reported pain intensity. This device is pictured in Fig. 8.3.

We have not analyzed these data yet for relationships between movement and muscle tension. However, it is already well-recognized that muscles behave abnormally in many conditions causing low back pain. For example, when a patient twists sideways, the paraspinals may not show much change in tension if accessory muscles are taking over their jobs. Thus, an adequate evaluation of muscle tension components has to include movement. None of our studies,[7–10] which attempted to relate immediate changes in pain intensity with overall pain, produced consistent results. In our studies, paraspinal activity was recorded while patients were bending directly forward from the waist to 30° of flexion. This means that interpretation of the data is open to question since it is not related to immediate pain intensity. Wolf et al.[16] found that surface EMG recording techniques tend not to be as sensitive as percutaneous recordings to various movements, so the techniques themselves may have to be refined.

Many people have attempted to work out replicable ways to record the back muscles in the clinical setting. This should optimize the chances of recognizing abnormal patterns

which can be corrected. Both Headley[17] and Cram[18] have published books giving clinical directions for identifying abnormal patterns. Headley[19] has developed a system for monitoring the paraspinal muscles of subjects who are bending and twisting while in the clinic. She reports consistent results which are useful in both diagnosis and treatment. Middaugh and Kee's work can be reviewed for an excellent assessment of relationships between the use of biofeedback equipment for assessment and its use for treatment of low back pain.[20] However, much more research needs to be done in examining the reliability of recording back muscles.

POSSIBLE MECHANISMS OF ACTION

Since biofeedback is rarely used alone without some form of home practice involving increased muscle tension awareness training, it is very difficult to tease out the major ways biofeedback actually helps patients with low back pain. This task is made significantly more complex by the lack of generally accepted, clear-cut ways to recognize abnormal paraspinal muscle tension patterns and use them as guides to training toward normality. For example, biofeedback may disrupt the pain-muscle-tension-stress cycle either by (a) increasing awareness of when muscles are beginning to tense abnormally so they are relaxed before causing additional or primary pain, or by (b) dampening the entire cycle by helping patients learn to recognize and control their stress responses. Biofeedback may have direct effects on abnormal muscle tension patterns, even though they are not clearly defined by either the clinicians or the patients. This occurs when patients become so aware of the relationships between patterns of tension and subsequent onset of pain that they use their new knowledge of control strategies to modify these patterns. Thus, biofeedback may directly enable patients to see abnormal patterns. The patients may then work toward correcting these patterns during the feedback session. This last possibility is, ideally, how biofeedback is supposed to be working, but

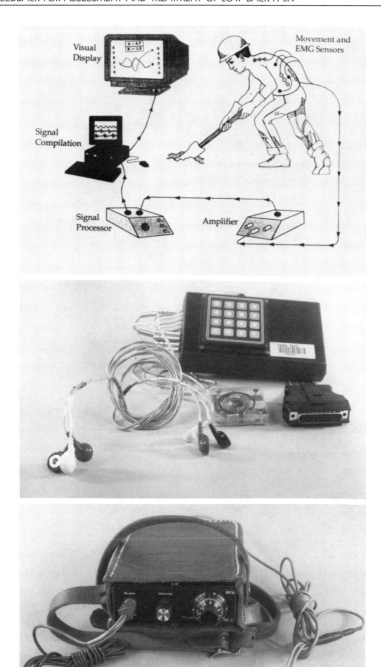

Figure 8.3. A future system capable of providing an individualized feedback signal, derived from a composite of many sources shown to contribute to the patient's back pain. The system would be based on such current technology as the computer-based ambulatory recorder (depicted below the futuristic system) and the ambulatory feedback device (depicted at the bottom of the illustration).

demonstrating that this is its major mechanism is beyond our reach at this time.

Difficulties in Interpretation of the Clinical Literature

Clinical reports indicating the usefulness of biofeedback for the treatment of low back pain are common. However, very few good, controlled studies have been done which actually demonstrate its effectiveness. Problems common among the published studies include: tiny sample sizes (less than 10), brief follow-ups (less than 6 months), no carefully defined diagnostic categories, no differentiation between acute and chronic (over 6 months duration) low back pain, lack of reports of pain intensities during evaluation, lack of reports of abnormalities seen upon evaluation (used to set criteria to work toward), a frequent lack of recording subjects while in motion, lack of standardized placement of sensors, and no record of the bandwidths recorded. This means that it is exceedingly difficult to evaluate the literature in a meaningful way.

CRITERIA FOR EVALUATING STUDIES

The primary purpose of this chapter is to present a scholarly review of the available literature on the biofeedback treatment of low back pain. In order for a study to provide an adequate test of the researcher's hypotheses (i.e., to be "valid"), however, it must be essentially free of methodological and conceptual shortcomings. As an aid in this review, we have delineated a number of "pivotal points" which we feel are necessary for any low back pain biofeedback study to have both internal and external validity.[21] We have used as our guide the two basic concepts of experimental design and control because they pertain directly to controlling secondary variance and minimizing error variance. Internal validity relates to the study's ability to control for individual differences and outside influences, i.e., subject factors and environmental factors. External validity refers to how generalizable

the study is to other populations. Some of the criteria we have specified are necessary for any scientific study to have validity, while others are specific only to biofeedback studies or even only to low back pain research. The specific criteria used, as well as the rationale for them, is as follows:

A. Subjects

The basic issue in this section is, "Was an adequate description of the subjects given?" For a study to have internal validity, that is, in order for another clinician or researcher to replicate the outcome of a particular study, a clear description of the subjects must be given. Moreover, if an adequate description of the subject factors is not given, then external validity cannot be determined.

1. Diagnosis. Accurate and reliable diagnosis is the keystone of both good clinical research and good clinical care. Therefore, the lack of clearly-defined diagnostic categories (that is, simply combining all low back pain subjects into a single diagnostic grouping) is a serious methodological limitation. Unfortunately, in the low back pain arena, this is often the case. This is surprising, for in no other area of pain is it assumed that different types of pain in the same region and/or pain that is believed to be caused by differing pathophysiologies can be lumped together. For example, in headache literature, the importance of clearly defined inclusion and exclusion criteria for the different diagnostic categories has been repeatedly stressed,[22,23] as it has in the spinal cord and amputee[24] literature. To illustrate, we have used the criteria set forth by the American Academy of Orthopedic Surgery[25] in our low back pain research.

2. Inclusion and Exclusion Criteria. It is important for researchers to *a*) specify in detail the criteria used to diagnose and select subjects and *b*) provide descriptive information regarding the population studied.[26] This information will enable other researchers to determine if their subjects are comparable to those employed in the study, and it will allow clinicians to better determine whether a particular treatment has a high probability of leading to fruition with a particular patient.

The criteria used to preclude participation in a study must also be described. For example, a clinician attempting to form a treatment plan for a low back pain patient should know that the patients who were excluded from a particular biofeedback treatment outcome study were taking narcotics and had prior back surgery. Likewise, a clinician-researcher attempting to replicate the study may obtain differing results if such exclusion criteria were not specified and the replication included such subjects.

3. Acute versus Chronic. Although this point is covered somewhat in the above criterion, we feel that it is so important that it deserves a specific category. Every study of low back pain should describe if the subjects were acute or chronic low back pain sufferers. In addition, a brief definition of what the investigators considered chronic or acute (e.g., pain lasting greater/less than 6 months) should be given.

B. Basic Experimental Design Issues

1. Number of Subjects. Psychophysiological measures show large variability, both between and within subjects.[27-30] Moreover, we[31,32] have shown quite a large variability within various diagnostic categories of low back pain subjects on surface EMG measures of paraspinal muscles. In some instances, the standard deviation was larger than the mean of the group. One traditional way to reduce variability is to increase sample size.[33] Therefore, treatment outcome studies employing psychophysiological measures in the area of low back pain are limited in the usefulness and generalizability of their findings if they employ a limited number of subjects. We have arbitrarily selected a number of 10 or more per experimental group as the cut-off point for meeting this criterion.

2. Control Group. If an experiment is to possess internal validity, one must first be sure that the treatment outcome, or the difference found between the experimental groups, is due to the manipulation of the independent variable (i.e., treatment) rather than uncontrolled variables (differences between the experimental groups). It is not our purpose here to go into a detailed explanation of the importance of a control group in scientific studies.[34] Obviously, we feel that the addition of a control group would be preferable to no control group. Even a basic waiting list control group at least controls for the effect of temporal factors. Also, one must determine beforehand that the experimental groups are evenly matched on important variables which could potentially affect the dependent measure. See Sturgis and Arena[33] for a description of these parameters.

C. Methodological Issues Concerning Biofeedback

1. Adaptation Period. An adaptation period is defined as the period of time the subject spends in the experimental situation before the onset of the experimental condition (typically the feedback condition) occurring. The importance of an adequate adaptation period in psychophysiological research has long been a topic of discussion. Unfortunately, there has been little empirical research to help the researcher or clinician decide what duration an adequate adaptation period should consist of.[35-38]

The function of an adaptation period in psychophysiological research is twofold. First, it allows the subjects to familiarize themselves with the novel, experimental situation (many people are not used to having electrodes attached to various parts of their anatomy while they sit in a sound and light attenuated room with their eyes closed). Second, it allows the psychophysiological responses being measured to stabilize. If these responses were fluctuating prior to the onset of feedback, one could not be certain that it was the feedback that led to the findings, or if the findings could better be attributed to random fluctuations in the psychophysiological measures due to the lack of a sufficient period of stabilization. On the basis of the admittedly sparse research, we have assigned an arbitrary cut-off of 5 or more minutes as an adequate baseline/adaptation period.

2. Pretreatment Psychophysiological Assessment. The conceptual logic underlying the use of biofeedback with chronic low back pain sufferers[15] is that (*a*) the pain is either caused (in the case of unspecified musculoskeletal back pain) or exacerbated by (in the case of spondyloarthritis or intervertebral disc disorders) elevated levels of muscle activity in the paraspinal region, and biofeedback works specifically on reducing these muscle tension levels; or (*b*) the pain is exacerbated by high overall levels of psychophysiological arousal, and biofeedback reduces arousal. Therefore, if elevated levels of muscle tension or other signs of psychophysiological arousal are not present in the low back pain sufferer, then biofeedback should not be effective. Conversely, those individuals with high muscle activity or psychophysiological arousal should benefit from biofeedback for their low back pain. It therefore follows that a pretreatment psychophysiological assessment to evaluate these assumptions is essential.

3. Instrumentation and Procedural Issues. If experimenters or clinicians are going to replicate the results of a biofeedback treatment outcome study, it is important that the details involving the parameters of the biofeedback instrumentation and procedural issues be specified. We feel that four rules are essential: (*a*) specify the equipment used (i.e., name of manufacturer, exact unit number, etc.); (*b*) describe the electrode placement exactly. (It is not sufficient to simply state "the paraspinal region" or "frontal EMG." Give the exact specifications or a reference to a standard text on site placement, as in Lippold;[39] (*c*) Give the specific EMG bandpass because the reader must know whether a bandpass was adequate for a particular muscle site. For example, for frontal EMG a bandpass of 100–200 Hz is adequate, but for paraspinal or trapezius EMG a much wider bandpass—we use 90–1000 Hz—is necessary; (*d*) detail any site preparation (e.g., did the

experimenters simply place the electrodes on the subject, without checking for resistance or swabbing down the site with alcohol and an abrasive pad?).

4. Learning to Criterion/Number of Biofeedback Sessions. The determination of whether or not a patient has learned a specific biofeedback response has long been an issue in biofeedback. Some argue that a criterion should be set before treatment, based either on preexisting norms or the baseline measure of the subject/patient (e.g., 50% reduction in paraspinal activity from session 1 baseline), and treatment should continue until the subject or patient has met the learning criterion. Others argue that in a research study such a criterion confounds the results, for when some subjects have five sessions and others have 24, that could lead to a possible temporal rather than treatment effect. Moreover, they argue, there are no data to support that learning the biofeedback response to one criterion is any more efficacious than learning to a lesser criterion or learning to a fixed number of sessions. Although we prefer a combination (learning to a specific criterion and a minimum and maximum number of biofeedback sessions), but, not wishing to enter the argument, we have decided to score a study as meeting this criterion if (*a*) learning to criterion did occur or (*b*) at least eight biofeedback sessions occurred.

5. Description of Biofeedback Procedures. In order to replicate a biofeedback study, the experimenters must give a detailed description of the procedures. Did the experimenters stay in the room and coach the subjects, or did they leave the room and let them explore the biofeedback responses on their own? Was feedback auditory, visual, tactile, etc.? Were subjects in a sound and light attenuated room? Was room temperature kept constant? Were subjects asked to attempt to achieve a specific attitude (e.g., a passive, "let the response occur" attitude, etc.)?

6. Generalization. Generalization involves a determination of whether or not the subject will carry the learning that may have occurred during the biofeedback session into the "real world." There are many ways to test for generalization. The most common, by far, is a "self-control" condition which is interspersed between a baseline and a feedback condition. The self-control condition involves asking the patient to control the desired psychophysiological response (e.g., "Please try to lower your back muscle tension") without any feedback. If the subject can control the response, the experimenter may assume that between session learning (i.e., generalization) has occurred. Another method of testing for generalization is to present a pre- and post-treatment stressor to the subject and, if there is less arousal during and after a stressor in the post-test, the experimenter may infer that generalization has occurred.

7. *Practice.* Biofeedback is a learned response, involving active participation on the part of the subject/patient; thus, home exercise should be an essential component of any biofeedback regimen. Since biofeedback is a learned response, the more one practices the better should be one's treatment outcome. (Vladimir Ashkenazy didn't become an expert pianist by playing a piano only once a week for an hour.) Interestingly, there have been only two experimental tests of the role of home practice, one involving community volunteers for a stress management program,[40] the other involving the relaxation treatment of headache.[41] In the first study, there was no significant effect of practice on improvement. In the second, there was a trend at the .056 level for those who were instructed to practice at home to reduce their headache activity. Although the research is mixed, the concept of practice makes such intuitive sense that we feel it is an essential criterion.

D. Methodological Issues Specific to Biofeedback for Low Back Pain

1. EMG Measurement during Postures and Movements. One of the important predictions which follows from the two primary theories regarding the psychophysiological etiology of chronic low back pain[15]—the reflex-spasm and stress-causality models—is

that the paraspinal EMG levels of low back pain subjects during various postures and movements will be higher than those of non-pain controls. Given this important postulate, results of studies failing to evaluate and treat their patients in multiple postures and/or movements would be especially troublesome. Most psychophysiological low back pain assessment studies measure EMG levels when subjects are in only one position, usually prone, or, in some few instances, standing.[31]

2. Measurement of Paraspinal Muscle Activity. As previously stated, the logic underlying the use of biofeedback with chronic low back pain sufferers is that the pain is either caused or exacerbated by elevated levels of muscle activity in the paraspinal region. Thus, even if one is following a general arousal theory and is using frontal EMG and/or hand surface temperature as the feedback response, it would be prudent to measure (not necessarily give feedback from) the paraspinal muscles.

E. Outcome Measures, Clinical Significance, and Follow-Up

1. Pain Diary. If an experiment is to rise above the scientific sophistication of an anecdotal report, it is important to have objective outcome measures. Perhaps the most commonly used measure of "pain" relief is the pain diary. In this diary, the subjects/patients record their pain levels on a predetermined scale a specified number of times a day (typically either once a day, four times a day, or hourly). The lack of a pain diary is a grave methodological limitation which vitiates the results of any study. To meet this criterion, it is necessary for the pain diary to be kept for some period by the subject (e.g., simply asking the subject to rate his pain level on a particular scale before and after each biofeedback session is inadequate).

2. Multiple Outcome Measures. Pain is a complex phenomenon. Thus, the use of multiple outcome measures, in addition to the pain diary, is required. For example, one could use significant other ratings of pain improvement;[42] measures of psychological distress such as the Minnesota Multiphasic Personality Inventory (MMPI) or the Millon Clinical Multiaxial Inventory (MCMI); measures of physical and psychosocial disability such as the Sickness Impact Profile[43] which consists of 136 items designed to assess illness-related dysfunction in 12 categories such as recreation, communication, and ambulation, and also yields a physical and psychosocial dysfunction score, as well as a total dysfunction score; and behavioral measures such as the Pain Behavior Checklist[44] which has subjects rate on a 5-point scale the frequency in which they have engaged in 20 common pain behavior categories over the past week; or more strict behavioral observation scales such as that of Keefe and Block,[45] in which they describe an observation system for measurement of "concomitant behaviors such as guarded movement, bracing, rubbing, grimacing, and sighing displayed by chronic low back pain patients during activity" (p. 363). To meet this criterion, an experiment has to include at least one outcome measure in addition to the pain diary. (Note: Measures of changes in EMG levels are not sufficient to meet this criterion. Rather, they would count for meeting the "learning to criterion," mentioned above.)

3. Measures of Medication Usage. Some mention of medication usage must be included in every low back pain biofeedback study. Medication usage is an important and objective outcome measure that all health care professionals would agree on as a crucial determinant of successful outcome. As well as being a factor in treatment outcome, medications may affect the psychophysiological responses themselves. For example, in the headache literature, Blanchard and his colleagues[46,47] have demonstrated that high medication usage is an indicator of poor prognosis. Unfortunately, we know of no scale that rates the relative value of analgesic medications used in low back pain research, although there is one commonly used in headache research.[48]

4. Statistical and Clinical Significance. To the average researcher, statistical tests are the "proof" that a treatment achieved the desired effect. This is characterized as, "statistical significance." To the average clinician, a statistical test tells nothing of importance. The typical "on-line" clinician wants to know if the patients in a study significantly improved, and if his/her patient will improve using similar procedures. This is defined as "clinical significance."[49] The cogent argument the clinician may present to the researcher is as follows: "I don't care if you achieved an effect statistically significant at the .001 level, if the difference in your treated group is only a 5% reduction in pain. If you have enough subjects in a group, everyone knows that even a small effect can be significant." These different views of significance are simply restatements of the "group versus individual subject experimental design" dichotomy, which itself is a restatement of the nomothetic versus idiographic way of viewing science. As one of us is a research physiologist (RAS), and the other a clinician-researcher (JGA), we of necessity take a compromise position. We feel that the dichotomy is artificially created because for adequate treatment outcome studies one must present measures of both statistical and clinical significance. For example, in our treatment outcome studies,[50–53] we have always presented the group data, followed by the percentage of those subjects significantly improved. Moreover, when the sample size is less than 25 per group, we also present the data individually. Thus, to meet this criterion, studies must present both statistical (where applicable) and clinical (e.g., percentage of subjects who have achieved at least a 50% reduction in pain) significance.

5. Follow-Up. Finally, the long-term (greater than 6 months) maintenance of treatment effects are an essential factor in evaluating the efficacy of any intervention: What good is a treatment if its effects begin to dissipate after only 3 months? Unfortunately, in behavioral medicine in general, and biofeedback especially, there is a paucity of research in the long-term follow up of treatment effects.[54–56]

EVALUATION OF STUDIES

Several approaches to evaluating the confused literature help to clarify the state of the art. Perhaps the most direct approach is to give examples of good studies which used the two most commonly applied strategies (described below) for ameliorating back pain. Another valuable approach is to tabulate all of the studies we find in the literature which have enough information to permit adequate evaluation. This provides a semi-quantitative idea of how many patients of various diagnostic categories have been helped to various degrees, through various strategies.

General Awareness and Relaxation Strategy

Studies using the "general awareness and relaxation strategy" include those by Keefe et al.[57,58] and Johnson and Hockersmith.[59] The latter reported their experience with 510 consecutive chronic low back pain patients with undifferentiated diagnoses treated over a 7-year period. Ninety-four percent had prior "extensive" medical treatment. Many had a record of surgical interventions, and 97% carried a medical diagnosis of organic involvement. Their biofeedback strategy was oriented toward developing the ability to control and relax the body's muscles and to understand the pain-tension-anxiety cycle as related to their reactions to environmental stressors. Feedback was from a signal generated from electrodes placed on the flexors of each forearm. Johnson and Hockersmith feel that this gives an approximation of tension in the upper body. Microvolt levels were carefully recorded, and patients worked toward a variety of success criteria. Average pain among all patients decreased by about half from beginning to end of treatment (change from 4.3–2.3 on a scale of 0–7). We cannot tell from the report how many people improved to what extent or how long individual follow-ups were. We can estimate that the treatment was unevenly effective as the variance in average pain intensity changed from 1.9 before treatment to 3.4 after treatment, while the range

remained about the same (6.8 and 7.0 respectively).

This study is rather typical in that readers can tell that some of the patients must have been helped significantly, but insufficient data are provided to determine: *a*) what was probably wrong with those most and least helped (if, indeed, there was any etiology-based difference); *b*) how long individual follow-ups were; and *c*) which patients helped most needed further intervention. It is also difficult to determine what types of concurrent "home" practice (e.g., relaxation training) was given.

The study by Keefe et al.[58] is very different in its method of data presentation. Although their strategy also centered on general tension awareness and control, they were concerned with individual differences in pain relief. Feedback was from the forehead or upper back areas of 111 chronic low back pain patients. This intervention was part of a multifactor treatment which included relaxation training. They compared the 28 most successful subjects with those having the least success and found that the successful patients had been in pain for fewer years but had higher initial pain intensity ratings. They reported the diagnostic breakdown of their group but did not relate individual diagnoses to treatment success. The study also did not report a follow-up success rate or indicate that subjects were being followed-up. The subjects showed an overall decrease in reported pain intensity of about 29%, as well as a decrease in use of pain medications, but, again, individual improvement was not reported.

Specific Muscle Groups Strategy

The other major strategy is oriented toward training specific muscle groups either while subjects are still or, more rarely, in motion. In this approach, attempts are frequently made to identify abnormal patterns which are corrected through use of the feedback signal. Typical studies include those by Wolf et al.,[60] Stuckey and Jacobs,[61] Nouwen,[62] and Flor et al.[63] An early example is found in a study by Freeman et al.[64] who trained eight patients (no diagnoses reported) to work toward preset criteria—to reduce tension in the paraspinal muscles 50% by attending to feedback from those muscles. After 10 sessions, half of the subjects met the criteria, one came close, and three did not. Of those who reached criteria, all progressed toward reaching goals of increased work- and school-related activities. They also reported less pain at a 3-month follow-up. Two of the subjects not meeting the criteria showed some improvement, and two did not.

Flor et al.[63] limited their study to rheumatic patients, so there can be little doubt about the relationship between diagnosis and outcome. Biofeedback was given from the paraspinal or trapezius muscles, depending on where most of the pain was reported. They were careful not to give an attendant relaxation training along with the biofeedback, to avoid mixing the effects of the two procedures. The data showed significant decreases in both EMG activity and pain which were sustained through follow-up.

Reports of Studies Analyzed

We have tabulated all of the reports of studies we could locate which provide even minimal information about the back pain patients, biofeedback methods, and results. Table 8.1 contains the results of the 15 published studies that deal with the biofeedback treatment of low back pain that have less than 10 subjects in the biofeedback group. It also contains the results of our criteria outlined above. As can be seen from the table, most of the studies are single-subject case designs, anecdotal reports, or single group studies. Only two studies, both by Flor and her colleagues,[63,65] stand out in this group.

In Flor's first study,[63] 24 patients who suffered from rheumatic back pain were given either paraspinal EMG biofeedback, a credible pseudotherapy treatment, (presumed to be psychophysiologically inert), or conventional medical treatment. Results indicated that at 4-month follow-up the biofeedback group patients "showed significant improvement in the duration, intensity, and quality of their back pain as well as their EMG levels, negative self-statements, and utilization of the health care system. In contrast, the pseudotherapy group showed minimal, but non-significant improvements, and the medically treated group remained unchanged" (p. 21). Unfortunately, there was a 25% drop-out rate from each group—a significant rate. Moreover, an unspecified number of the subjects suffered from shoulder pain, instead of back pain, and were given feedback from that area.

Flor's second study[65] was a 2.5 year follow-up of the subjects in the original 1983 study. The findings indicated that treatment effects remained the same. In summary, with the exception of the studies by Flor and her colleagues, and sophisticated single-subject experimental designs by Wolf and his colleagues,[60,66] demonstrating the possible efficacy of using EMG biofeedback during dynamic movement with low back pain subjects, all that other studies add to the literature are confusion and a great deal of methodologically-flawed research.

Table 8.2 contains the results of the twelve published studies that deal with the biofeedback treatment of low back pain that have at least 10 subjects in the biofeedback group. It also details how well the study fit our study criteria outlined above. As can be seen from this table, most of the large scale studies are as methodologically limited as are the smaller scale ones. Three studies, however, do stand out as being more methodologically sophisticated than the others.

Bush, Ditto, and Feuerstein[67] published the most methodologically "tight" study to date. Low back pain subjects were randomly assigned to one of three groups: biofeedback, placebo, or wait-list control. Regardless of treatment, all groups showed significant reductions in pain, anxiety, depression, and paraspinal EMG following treatment and at follow-up. No group differences were found on any variable. With the exception of a lack of clearly defined diagnostic groups and a failure to measure subjects in different positions, this study appears to fit our criteria the best.

Clearly, its results suggest grave problems for those who believe biofeedback for back pain sufferers works through a straight "psychophysiological" mechanism. (Interestingly, these results mirror those of the pain literature in general—see Holroyd et al.[68] for the most sophisticated study to date, done with tension headache subjects.)

Two other reports deserve note, both by Arie Nouwen. In the first study,[69] 18 low back pain subjects of musculoskeletal origin were given EMG biofeedback training and 7 subjects were placed on a wait list. At follow-up there were significantly lower pain levels in the treatment group. However, the treated group suffered from a large drop-out rate (13 subjects—42%). In a second study,[62] 20 chronic low back pain subjects with high standing paraspinal EMG levels on pretreatment assessment were evenly divided into two groups: EMG biofeedback and wait-list control. No significant decreases in pain between the two groups were found at post-treatment assessment.

There are a number of observations that can be made on the basis of Tables 8.1&2. First, all of the studies on the biofeedback treatment of chronic low back pain suffer from serious methodological problems. Second, the majority of the studies do not specify the diagnosis of the subjects, do not assess medication usage, and only three studies had adequate follow-ups. More importantly, two of the three studies from Table 8.2 (which contains the studies with sample sizes of at least 10) that "best fit" our criteria for a low back pain study to have internal and external validity, had negative results. Thus, the available research is seriously methodologically flawed, and the best of the current research does not support the efficacy of biofeedback, as a modality by itself, in the treatment of chronic low back pain.

THE PRACTICAL VIEW

The Field Today

Two outstanding conclusions can be reached from our review of the literature. First, bio-feedback of many types can be an effective adjunct to standard therapeutic interventions for low back pain. It can help some people a great deal and many people significantly. However, it has not been shown to help most people reduce their back pain sufficiently so that no further intervention is requested. Thus, a trial of biofeedback is worth attempting with most patients having low back pain which does not require immediate surgery, because many of them will experience significantly less discomfort while other therapies are being tried. And some will achieve a sufficient reduction in pain so that no further intervention is necessary. At least theoretically, biofeedback should be most effective among subjects whose pain has a muscle tension related etiology. For those patients who have failed virtually every standard treatment, biofeedback may play an important role in helping them disrupt pain tension cycles which intensify pain not otherwise controllable. This can result in a reduced need for medications and increased socialization.

The second conclusion is that (a) the evaluative studies reviewed here do not permit us to know which etiologic categories of low back pain patients are most likely to respond to biofeedback, and (b) we cannot recommend one training strategy over another. There is no evidence that use of biofeedback from muscle groups (to correct demonstrated muscle tension pattern abnormalities) is more effective than use of biofeedback from the frontal or general upper trunk regions (as part of general muscle tension awareness and relaxation training).

Future Directions

Before biofeedback can be truly accepted as a valuable part of the low back pain treatment armamentarium, very large, well-controlled studies must be performed, and they must clearly demonstrate long-term effectiveness upon 1-year follow-up with specific etiologic groups of patients. Comparative studies will have to be performed which relate different biofeedback strategies (e.g., generalized muscle tension awareness and control vs. correc-

Table 8.1
Studies of Biofeedback in the Treatment of Low Back Pain with Less than 10 Subjects

Criteria	Studies						
	Belar and Cohen[78]	Biedermann et al.[79]	Biedermann et al.[80]	Flor et al.[63]	Flor et al.[65]	Freeman et al.[64]	Gentry and Bernal[76]
1. Diagnosis Specified	No	No	No	Yes	Yes	No	No
2. Inclusion Criteria	No	No	No	Yes	Yes	No	No
Exclusion Criteria	No	No	No	Yes	Yes	No	No
3. Acute/Chronic	Chronic	Chronic	Chronic	Chronic	Chronic	Chronic	Chronic
4. Number of Subjects[1]	1	6	24 (8 "high success" BF)	24 (8 BF)	24 (8 BF)	8	1
5. Control Groups[2]	None	No	Yes (see #20, below)	Yes (PsT and CMT)	Yes (PsT and CMT)	No	None
6. Adaptation Period	None	No	No	No	No	No	Yes
7. Preassessment	No	No	No	Yes	Yes	No	No
8. Instrumentation/ Procedural Issues	Adequate	No	No	No	No	No	No
9. Learning Demonstrated	Yes	Yes	Yes	Yes	Yes	Yes	Yes
10. Biofeedback Described	No	No	No	Yes	Yes	No	Yes
11. Generalization Attempted	Yes	No	No	Yes	Yes	No	Yes
12. Practice Defined	Yes	No	No	Yes	Yes	Yes	Yes
13. Positions Measured	No	No	No	Yes	Yes	No	No
14. Paraspinals Measured[3]	No (TR)	Yes	Yes	Yes	Yes	Yes	No (FR)
15. Pain Diary Kept	Yes	No	Yes	Yes	Yes	No	No
16. Multiple Outcome Measures	Yes	No	Yes	Yes	Yes	Yes	No
17. Medications Measured	No	No	Yes	No	No	No	No
18. Statistical/Clinical Sig.	Both	Statistical	Both	Both	Both	Neither	Neither
19. Length of Follow-Up	8 weeks	None	3 months	4 months	2.5 years	3 months	6 weeks
20. Description of Study Results and Design	Systematic, single-case study. BF and R_x decreased EMG levels and frequency of pain but did not affect medication usage.	Confusing study. Average improvement 62%. It is unclear as to how and when pain was measured.	Confusing study. Average improvement rate was 63%. No group effect ("high success," "low success," or "linear" BF.	Sophisticated study. BF > PsT > CMT in terms of pain intensity, duration and quality, as well as EMG levels, negative self-statements and health care utilization.	Follow-up of 1983 study. All Ss in BF group stated they were improved; 68.3% improvement in BF group compared to only 13.8 in others.	Uncontrolled study. Authors concluded, "all patients showed improvement," no pain measure other than pre-post pain questionnaire.	Anecdotal report. Results are not clear; some increase in time able to work and decrease in pain intensity.

NOTES: BF = biofeedback
CMT = conventional medical therapy
PL = placebo
PsT = credible pseudotherapy
FR = frontalis
TR = trapezius
R_x = standard treatment

Table 8.1 (continued)
Studies of Biofeedback in the Treatment of Low Back Pain with Less than 10 Subjects

				Studies				
Jones and Wolf[66]	Large and Lamb[77]	Nigl[73]	Nigl and Fisher-Williams[74]	Peck and Kraft[75]	Stuckey et al.[70]	Todd and Belar[71]	Tung et al.[72]	Wolf et al.[60]
No	Yes	No	No	No	No	Yes	No	No
No	Yes	No	No	No	No	No	No	No
No	Yes	No	No	No	Yes	No	No	No
Chronic	Chronic	Chronic	Chronic	Both	Chronic	Chronic	Chronic	Acute
1	2	7	4	8	24 (8 BF)	1	7	1
No	No	No	No	No	Yes (8 R_x, 8 PL)	No	No	No
No	No	No	No	No	No	No	No	No
Yes	No	No	Yes	Yes	No	Yes	No	Yes
Yes	No	No	No	No	No	No	No	Yes
Yes	No	Yes	Yes	Yes	Yes	Yes	No	Yes
Yes	No	No	No	No	No	No	No	Yes
Yes	No	No	No	Yes	No	No	No	Yes
Yes	No	Yes	No	Yes	No	No	Yes	No
Yes	No	No	No	No	No	No	No	Yes
Yes	No (FR)	Yes	Yes	Yes (TR also)	Yes (TR also)	Yes	No (FR)	Yes
No	No	Yes	No	Yes	No	Yes	Yes	No
Yes	No	No	No	No	Yes	No	No	No
Yes	No	No	No	Yes	No	No	No	No
Clinical	Statistical	Statistical	Both	Both	Statistical	Clinical	Clinical	Clinical
10 weeks	None	None	1 month	3 months	None	None	6 weeks	None
Sophisticated case report, using EMG BF to reeducate muscles during move- ment; about 80% relief.	Confusing study; 18 Ss; only 2 had LBP. Results were that both EMG BF and a within- Ss control condition were useful in reducing pain.	BF and R_x > R_x in a within Ss design; (2 other ex- periments in article previously published).	Four case reports with varying so- phistication and diag- noses; all significantly reduced pain and EMG levels.	Simple outcome study—no changes in pain or medi- cation—con- founded by some Ss having shoul- der pain, others LBP.	Three group design, con- founded by no pain diary recording and no clinical significance given. Results were R_x > BF > PL.	Anecdotal case report; a combination of BF, R_x, and stress innoc- ulation; BF had no effect on pain levels.	Uncontrolled, unsystematic outcome study; 43% were "some- what im- proved" (no definition of this categor- ization was given).	Well-designed single case study that suffers from lack of pain diary— dynamic move- ment BF decreased EMG and questionnaire pain.

Table 8.2
Studies of Biofeedback in the Treatment of Low Back Pain with More than 10 Subjects

Criteria	Studies					
	Adams et al.[84]	Asfour et al.[85]	Biedermann et al.[86]	Bush et al.[67]	Hendler et al.[82]	Johnson and Hockersmith[59]
1. Diagnosis Specified	No	Yes	Yes	No	No	No
2. Inclusion Criteria	No	Yes	Yes	Yes	No	No
Exclusion Criteria	No	Yes	Yes	Yes	No	No
3. Acute/Chronic	Unspecified	Chronic	Chronic	Chronic	Chronic	Chronic
4. Number of Subjects[1]	30	30 (15 BF)	14	66 (23 BF)	13	510
5. Control Groups[2]	None	Yes (No BF)	None	Yes (PL and WLC)	None	None
6. Adaptation Period	None	No	No	Yes	No	None
7. Preassessment	No	No	No	Yes	No	No
8. Instrumentation/ Procedural Issues	Adequate	Inadequate	Inadequate	Adequate	Inadequate	Inadequate
9. Learning Demonstrated	Yes	Yes	Yes	Yes	Yes	Yes
10. Biofeedback Described	Yes	Yes	No	Yes	Yes	Yes
11. Generalization Attempted	Yes	No	No	Yes	No	Yes
12. Practice Defined	No	No	No	Yes	No	Yes
13. Positions Measured	No	No	Yes	No	No	Yes
14. Paraspinals Measured[3]	No (FR)	Yes	Yes	Yes	No (FR)	No (FR & FA)
15. Pain Diary Kept	No	No	Yes	Yes	No	Yes
16. Multiple Outcome Measures	No	Yes	Yes	Yes	Yes	Yes
17. Medications Measured	No	No	Yes	Yes	No	No
18. Statistical/Clinical Sig.	Statistical	Statistical	Both	Statistical	Neither	Neither
19. Length of Follow-Up	None	None	4–12 weeks	3 months	1 month	30 days
20. Description of Study Results and Design	Uncontrolled experimental study—a decrease in pain levels from pre- to post-BF sessions.	Simple 2-group design; EMG BF added to a comprehensive pain treatment program did not affect pain levels.	Uncontrolled outcome study; BF led to 50% of Ss with at least a 67% decrease in pain, 21% with 33–67% reductions.	Sophisticated, well-controlled study; results indicated no differences between groups on any measure.	Uncontrolled study; 6 of the 13 subjects "felt they were getting some relief" (p. 506).	Uncontrolled outcome study; inpatients seen 2 × day for 6 weeks; 47.5% overall pain improvement.

NOTES: BF = biofeedback
CMT =conventional medical therapy
FA = forearm
FR = frontalis
NP =non pain
PL = placebo
PsT = credible pseudotherapy
R_x = relaxation

Table 8.2 (continued)
Studies of Biofeedback in the Treatment of Low Back Pain with More than 10 Subjects

			Studies			
Keefe et al.[57]	Keefe et al.[58]	Nigl[73]	Middaugh and Kee[20]	Nouwen[62]	Nouwen and Sollinger[69]	Strong et al.[81]
No	No	No	Only for 8 Ss	Yes	Yes	No
No	No	No	No	Yes	Yes	No
No	No	No	No	Yes	Yes	Yes
Chronic	Chronic	Chronic	Chronic	Chronic	Chronic	Chronic
111	18	20 (10 LBP)	23	20 (10 BF)	26 (19 BF)	40 (20 R_x and BF)
None	None	Yes (10 NP)	No	Yes (WLC)	Yes (WLC)	Yes (R_x)
No	No	Yes	No	No	Yes	None
No	No	Yes	Yes	Yes	Yes	No
Inadequate	Adequate	Inadequate	Adequate	Adequate	Inadequate	Adequate
Yes	Yes	Yes	No	Yes	Yes	No
No	Yes	No	No	No	Yes	Inadequate
Yes	Yes	No	No	Yes	Yes	No
Yes	Yes	No	No	No	Yes	No
Yes	No	No	Yes	No	Yes	No
Yes	No (FR)	Yes	Yes	Yes	Yes	No (TR)
Yes	Yes	No	No	Yes	Yes	No
Yes	Yes	No	No	No	No	No
Yes	Yes	No	No	No	No	No
Statistical	Statistical	Statistical	Neither	Statistical	Statistical	Statistical
None	Mean = 1.3 yrs.	None	1 year	None	3 months	X = 8 months (3–15 months)
Uncontrolled outcome study; BF-assisted R_x led to significant decreases in EMG, subjective tension, and pain levels.	Uncontrolled single group design. 69% of BF-assisted R_x Ss at follow-up reported decreases in subjective tension and pain.	2 × 2 within Ss design; compared binary and analog feedback within sessions; binary was better at reducing pain levels within session than analog.	"Overall two-thirds success rate at 1 year follow-up" (p. 164); success not defined; effect on EMG.	Controlled study; BF and WLC had no effect on pain levels; BF had a significant effect on EMG.	Controlled study; BF had sig. decreases in pain levels at 3 months; however, EMG returned to pretreatment levels.	Controlled study which lacks good outcome measures; no diff. R_x and BF vs. R_x; at 3 months R_x and BF better on pain rating index.

tion of specific pattern abnormalities) to clearly defined groups of patients. Although it would be scientifically valuable and of considerable interest to know just how a technique is affecting the pain, that is not as important as determining whether the technique works. When that determination has been made, more effort can be applied to determining mechanisms.

Biofeedback from recordings of the paraspinal and other muscles has certainly not been thoroughly proven to be an effective treatment for any and all low back pain problems. Large studies incorporating careful differential diagnostic categories of patients, and long-term follow-ups of clearly defined interventions, will have to be performed before definitive decisions about the technique's usefulness for particular problem groupings can be made. These studies will have to incorporate outcome data which relate changes in pain to the extent goals are met (for making sustained changes in physiological systems shown to function abnormally during initial assessment).

Such studies are far more difficult to do than to recommend because of the idiosyncratic nature of each individual's low back pain. Finding an acceptable basis for making relevant differential diagnoses for grouping patients will be exceedingly difficult, and it will count on using techniques, such as ambulatory recording, which are still in their infancy. Definitive evaluation of each patient's precursors to changes in pain will have to be accomplished so that treatments can be individualized for each participant. This can be accomplished through a combination of careful clinical and environmental evaluations. Patients in a clinic can be recorded from multiple sites simultaneously as they move, so abnormal patterns of muscle function can be defined. During the recording, musculoskeletal responses to physical stresses, such as pulling against a dynamometer, and to psychological stresses, such as discussing the pain and other problems, can be evaluated. Longitudinal recordings can be made over several days (while the patient functions in the normal

work and home environment) to assess relationships between types of activities and interactions, muscle tension, and many types and forces of movement.

The specific signals to feed back will have to be developed and tested. There is little reason to feed back tension in the paraspinal muscles if it has little to do with the pain. Tension patterns from combinations of other muscle groups may have to be related to types, amounts, and forces of a variety of movements and, perhaps, other factors as well, before a useful composite feedback signal can be generated. Subjects will have to receive feedback as they recreate the conditions that lead to increased pain, so they can learn to avoid or correct the situation.

The individual elements of equipment already exist in a variety of forms. They are capable of performing the required types of in-laboratory and environmental recordings and of combining multiple signals into useable feedback, while patients reproduce dynamic situations which lead to their pain. Figure 8.3 illustrates a subject receiving feedback under these circumstances. Beneath is a photograph of a device currently in use which can perform the required environmental evaluations, while the figure beneath that pictures a standard ambulatory biofeedback device which can provide feedback to subjects while they are in their normal environments. These devices will have to be combined with computer-based systems already available, to provide a useable feedback signal to moving subjects, before biofeedback for low back pain can really be a success.

Biofeedback is likely to continue as an important part of the armamentarium of pain treatment centers.[87] However, its growth is dependent upon use of component analysis techniques to demonstrate how much of the change in pain is likely to be related to use of biofeedback.

ACKNOWLEDGMENTS

This work was entirely supported by the U.S. Army Health Services Command's Department of Clinical Investigation and by the U.S. Department of Veterans Affairs. The illustrations were finalized by Karen Wyatt, medical illustrator at Fitzsimons Army Medical Center.

REFERENCES

1. Schwartz M. Biofeedback: a practitioner's guide. New York: Guilford Press, 1987.
2. Revised applications standards and guidelines for practitioners of biofeedback. Denver: Association for Applied Psychophysiology, 1991.
3. Basmajian J. Biofeedback: principles and practice for clinicians. 3rd ed. Baltimore: Williams & Wilkins, 1989.
4. Hatch J, Fisher J, Rugh J. Biofeedback: studies in clinical efficacy. New York: Plenum Press, 1987.
5. Bonica J. The management of pain. Philadelphia: Lea & Febiger, 1990:1395–1514.
6. Horenstein S. Chronic low back pain and the failed low back syndrome. Neurol Clin 1989; 7:361–385.
7. Sherman R. Relationships between strength of low back muscle contraction and intensity of chronic low back pain. Am J Phys Med 1985; 64:190–200.
8. Arena J, Sherman R, Bruno G, Young T. Electromyographic recordings of five types of low back pain subjects and non-pain controls in different positions. Pain 1989; 37:57–65.
9. Arena J, Sherman R, Bruno G, Young T. Temporal stability of paraspinal electromyographic recordings in low back pain and non-pain subjects. Int J Psychophysiol 1990; 9:32–37.
10. Arena J, Sherman R, Bruno G, Young T. Electromyographic recordings of low back pain subjects and non-pain controls in six different positions: effect of different pain levels. Pain. In press, 1992.
11. Sherman R, Arena J, Searle J, Ginther J. Development of an ambulatory recorder for evaluation of muscle tension related low back pain and fatigue in soldier's normal environments. Milit Med In press, 1992.
12. Sherman R, Sherman C. Relationships between continuous environmental recordings of posterior trunk muscle tension and patterns of low back pain and tension headaches. Biofeedback Self Regul 1989; 14:168.
13. Sherman R, Varnado S, Caminer S. Ambulatory recordings of relationships between paraspinal muscle tension and low back pain in the normal environment. In preparation for submission for publication.
14. Weisenberg M. Pain. St. Louis: C.V. Mosby, 1975.
15. Nouwen A, Bush C. The relationship between paraspinal EMG and chronic low back pain. Pain 1984; 20:109–123.
16. Wolf S, Wolf L, Segal R. The relationship of extraneous movements to lumbar paraspinal muscle activity. Biofeedback Self Regul 1989; 14:63–74.
17. Headley B. Muscle scanning: interpreting EMG scans. St. Paul: Pain Resources, 1990.
18. Cram J. Clinical EMG: muscle scanning and diagnostic manual for surface recordings. Seattle: Clinical Resources, 1986.
19. Headley B. Dynamic EMG evaluation: interpreting postural dysfunction. St. Paul: Pain Resources, 1990.
20. Middaugh S, Kee W. Advances in electromyographic monitoring and biofeedback in the treatment of chronic cervical and low back pain. Adv Clin Rehabil 1987; 1:137–172.
21. Campbell D, Stanley J. Experimental and quasi-experimental designs for research. Skokie: Rand McNally, 1963.
22. Arena J, Blanchard E, Andrasik F. The role of affect in the etiology of chronic headache. J Psychosom Res 1984; 28:79–86.
23. Arena J, Blanchard E, Andrasik F, Dudek B. The headache symptom questionnaire: discriminant classificatory ability and headache syndromes suggested by a factor analysis. J Behav Ass 1982; 4:55–69.
24. Sherman R, Ernst J, Barja R, Bruno G. Invited editorial: phantom pain: a lesson in the necessity for careful clinical research on chronic pain problems. J Rehabil Res Dev 1988; 25:vii–x.
25. Common orthopedic procedures and codes: a reference guide. New York: American Academy of Orthopedic Surgery, AAOC, 1986.
26. Garfield S. Research problems in clinical diagnosis. J Consult Clin Psychol 1978; 46:596–607.
27. Arena J, Blanchard E, Andrasik F, Cotch P, Myers P. Reliability of psychophysiological assessment. Behav Res Ther 1983; 21:447–460.
28. Arena J, Goldberg S, Saul D, Hobbs S. Temporal consistency of psychophysiological stress profiles: analysis of individual response stereotypy and stimulus response specificity. Behav Ther 1989; 20:609–618.
29. Barlow D, Blanchard E, Haynes S, Epstein L. Single case experimental designs and clinical biofeedback experimentation. Biofeedback Self Regul 1977; 2:221–239.
30. Biederman H. Comments on the reliability of muscle activity comparisons in EMG biofeedback research with back pain patients. Biofeedback Self Regul 1984; 9:451–458.
31. Arena J, Sherman R, Bruno G, Young T. Electromyographic recordings of five types of low back pain subjects and non-pain controls in different positions. Pain 1989; 37:57–65.
32. Arena J, Sherman R, Bruno G, Young T. Temporal stability of paraspinal electromyographic recordings in low back and non-pain subjects. Int J Psychophysiol 1990; 9:31–37.
33. Sturgis E, Arena J. Psychophysiological assessment. In: Hersen M, Eisler R, Miller P, eds. Progress in behavior modification (Vol. 17). New York: Academic Press, 1984:1–30.

34. Beck J, Andrasik F, Arena J. Group comparison designs. In: Bellack A, Hersen M, eds. Research methods in clinical psychology. New York: Pergamon Press, 1984:100–138.

35. Arena J. Inter- and intra-reliability of psychophysiological post-stress adaptation periods. J Behav Assess 1984; 6:247–260.

36. Lichstein K, Sallis J, Hill D, Young M. Psychophysiological adaptation: an investigation of multiple parameters. J Behav Assess 1981; 3:111–121.

37. Myers A, Craighead W. Adaptation periods in clinical psychophysiological research: a recommendation. Behav Ther 1978; 9:355–362.

38. Sallis J, Lichstein K. The frontal electromyographic adaptation response: a potential source of confounding. Biofeedback Self Regul 1979; 4:337–339.

39. Lippold D. Electromyography. In: Venables P, Martin I, eds. Manual of psychophysiological methods. New York: John Wiley, 1967:245–299.

40. Hillenberg J, Collins F. The importance of home practice for progressive relaxation training. Behav Res Ther 1983; 21:633–642.

41. Blanchard E, Nicholson N, Taylor A, Steffek B, Radnitz C, Applebaum K. The role of regular home practice in the relaxation treatment of tension headache. J Consult Clin Psychol In press, 1991.

42. Blanchard E, Andrasik F, Neff D, Jurish S, O'Keefe D. Social validation of the headache diary. Behav Ther 1981; 12:711–715.

43. Bergner M, Bobbitt R, Carter W, Gilson B. The sickness impact profile: development and final revision of a health status measure. Med Care 1981; 29:787–805.

44. Turk D, Wack J, Kerns R. An empirical examination of the "pain-behavior" construct. J Behav Med 1985; 8:119–130.

45. Keefe K, Block A. Development of an observation method for assessing pain behavior in chronic low back pain patients. Behav Ther 1982; 13:363–375.

46. Blanchard E, Applebaum K, Radnitz C, Jaccard J, Dentinger M. The refractory headache patient: I. Chronic, daily, high intensity headache. Behav Res Ther 1989; 27:403–410.

47. Michultka D, Blanchard E, Applebaum K, Jaccard J, Dentinger M. The refractory headache patient: II. High medication consumption (analgesic rebound) headache. Behav Res Ther 1989; 27:411–420.

48. Coyne L, Sargent J, Sergerson J, Olbourn R. Relative potency scale for analgesic drugs: use of psychophysical procedures with clinical judgments. Headache 1976; 16:70–71.

49. Hugdahl K, Ost L. On the difference between statistical and clinical significance. Behav Assess 1981; 3:289–296.

50. Arena J, Hightower N, Chang G. Relaxation therapy for tension headache in the elderly: a prospective study. Psychol Aging 1988; 3:96–98.

51. Arena J, Hannah S, Bruno G, Meador K. Electro-myographic biofeedback training for tension headache in the elderly: a prospective study. Biofeedback Self Regul In press, 1991.

52. Blanchard E, Andrasik F, Neff D, Arena J. Biofeedback and relaxation training with three kinds of headache: treatment effects and their prediction. J Consult Clin Psychol 1982; 50:562–575.

53. Sherman R, Gall N, Gormly J. Treatment of phantom limb pain with muscular relaxation training to disrupt the pain-anxiety-tension cycle. Pain 1979; 6:47–55.

54. Holroyd K, Holm J, Penzien D, Cordingley G, Hursey K, Martin N, Theofanous A. Long-term maintenance of improvements achieved with (abortive) pharmacological and nonpharmacological treatments for migraine: preliminary findings. Biofeedback Self Regul 1989; 14:301–308.

55. Blanchard E, Andrasik F, Guarnieri P, Neff D, Rodichok L. Two, three, and four year follow-up on the self-regulatory treatment of chronic headache. J Consult Clin Psychol 1987; 55:257–259.

56. Radnitz C, Blanchard E. A 1- and 2-year follow-up study of bowel sound biofeedback as a treatment for irritable bowel syndrome. Biofeedback Self Regul 1989; 14:333–338.

57. Keefe F, Block A, Williams R, Surwit R. Behavior treatment of chronic low back pain: clinical outcome and individual differences in pain relief. Pain 1981; 11:221–231.

58. Keefe F, Schapira B, Williams R, Brown C, Surwit R. EMG assisted relaxation training in the management of chronic low back pain. Am J Clin Biofeedback 1981; 4:93–103.

59. Johnson H, Hockersmith V. Therapeutic EMG in chronic back pain. In: Basmajian J, ed. Biofeedback: principles and practice for clinicians. 3rd ed. Baltimore: Williams & Wilkins, 1989:311–315.

60. Wolf S, Nacht M, Kelley J. EMG feedback training during dynamic movement for low back pain patients. Behav Ther 1982; 13:395–406.

61. Stuckey S, Jacobs A, Goldfarb J. EMG biofeedback training, relaxation, training, and placebo for the relief of chronic back pain. Percept Mot Skills 1986; 63:1023–1036.

62. Nouwen A. EMG biofeedback used to reduce standing levels of paraspinal muscle tension in chronic low back pain. Pain 1983; 17:353–360.

63. Flor H, Haag G, Turk D, Koehler H. Efficacy of EMG biofeedback, pseudotherapy, and conventional medical treatment for chronic rheumatic back pain. Pain 1983; 17:21–31.

64. Freeman C, Calsyn D, Paige A, Halar E. Biofeedback with low back pain patients. Am J Clin Biofeedback 1980; 3:118–122.

65. Flor H, Haag G, Turk D. Long-term efficacy of EMG biofeedback for chronic rheumatic back pain. Pain 1986; 3:195–202.

66. Jones A, Wolf S. Treating chronic low back pain:

EMG biofeedback training during movement. Phys Ther 1980; 60:58–63.

67. Bush C, Ditto B, Feuerstein M. A controlled evaluation of paraspinal EMG biofeedback in the treatment of chronic low back pain. Health Psychol 1985; 4:307–321.

68. Holroyd K, Penzien D, Hursey K, Tobin D, Rogers L, Holm J, Marcille P, Hall J, Chila A. Change mechanisms in EMG biofeedback training: cognitive changes underlying improvements in tension headache. J Consult Clin Psychol 1984; 52:1039–1053.

69. Nouwen A, Solinger J. The effectiveness of EMG biofeedback training in low back pain. Biofeedback Self Regul 1979; 4:103–111.

70. Stuckey S, Jacobs A, Goldfarb J. EMG biofeedback training, relaxation training, and placebo for the relief of chronic back pain. Percept Motor Skills 1986; 63:1023–1036.

71. Todd J, Belar C. EMG biofeedback and chronic low back pain: implications of treatment failure. Am J Clin Biofeedback 1980; 3:114–117.

72. Tung A, DeGood D, Tenicela R. Clinical evaluation of biofeedback relaxation training. Penn Med 1979; 46:18–19.

73. Nigl A. A comparison of binary and analog EMG feedback techniques in the treatment of low back pain. Am J Clin Biofeedback 1980; 4:25–31.

74. Nigl A, Fischer-Williams M. Treatment of low back strain with electromyographic biofeedback and relaxation training. Psychosomatics 1980; 21:495–499.

75. Peck C, Kraft G. Electromyographic biofeedback for pain related to muscle tension: a study of tension headache, back, and jaw pain. Arch Surg 1977; 112:889–895.

76. Gentry W, Bernal G. Chronic pain. In: Williams R, Gentry W, eds. Behavioral approaches to medical treatment. Cambridge: Ballinger Publishing Company, 1977:173–181.

77. Large R, Lamb A. Electromyographic (EMG) feedback in chronic musculoskeletal pain: a controlled trial. Pain 1983; 17:167–177.

78. Belar C, Cohen J. The use of EMG feedback and progressive relaxation in the treatment of a woman with chronic back pain. Biofeedback Self Regul 1979; 4:345–353.

79. Biederman H, Monga T. Relaxation oriented EMG biofeedback with back pain patients: evaluation of paraspinal muscle activity. Clin Biofeedback Health 1985; 8:119–123.

80. Biedermann H, McGhie A, Monga T, Shanks G. Perceived and actual control in EMG treatment of back pain. Behav Res Ther 1987; 25:137–147.

81. Strong J, Cramond T, Maas F. The effectiveness of relaxation techniques with patients who have chronic low back pain. Occup Ther J Res 1989; 9:184–192.

82. Hendler N, Derogatis L, Avella J, Long D. EMG biofeedback in patients with chronic pain. J Clin Psychiatry 1977; 38:505–509.

83. Johnson H, Hockersmith V. Therapeutic electromyography in chronic pain. In: Basmajian J, ed. Biofeedback principles and practice for clinicians. Baltimore: Williams & Wilkins, 1989:311–315.

84. Adams J, Pearson S, Olson N. Innovative crossmodal technique of pain intensity assessment with lower back pain patients given biofeedback training. Am J Clin Biofeedback 1982; 5:25–30.

85. Asfour S, Khalil T, Waly S, Goldberg M, Rosomoff R, Rosomoff H. Biofeedback in back muscle strengthening. Spine 1990; 15:510–513.

86. Biderman H, Monga T, Shanks G, McGhie A. EMG biofeedback in the treatment of back pain patients: treatment protocol. Clin Biofeedback Health 1986; 9:139–145.

87. Loeser J, Egan K. Managing the chronic pain patient. New York: Raven Press, 1989.

9

Soft Tissue Mobilization

ALAN J. GRODIN and ROBERT I. CANTU

The broad concept of soft tissue mobilization incorporates many schools of thought: myofascial release, muscle energy, traditional massage, rolfing, and movement approaches including: Feldenkrais, Traegering, and Proprioceptive Neuromuscular Facilitation. While other chapters in this book address myofascial release, PNF, and muscle energy, this chapter will concern itself with the "direct" manipulation of soft tissue structures which include muscle and its associated fascia, tendon, and ligament.

A rationale for soft tissue mobilization will be based upon the structure and function of soft tissue from a histologic, biomechanical, and gross morphological standpoint. The effects of immobilization and remobilization after it upon the soft tissue structures will also be analyzed to explain the basis of soft tissue mobilization. A review of the literature will explore the effects of soft tissue mobilization upon the blood, blood flow, metabolism, reflexive behavior, and mechanical factors. In order to understand the effects of soft tissue mobilization, one must first understand the structures being affected from a histological standpoint.

HISTOLOGY OF CONNECTIVE TISSUE

Connective tissue is subdivided into five principal groups: ordinary connective tissue, blood cells, cartilage, adipose, and bone.[1] From a direct soft tissue mobilization ap-

proach we are concerned primarily with ordinary connective tissue which includes superficial and deep fascial sheaths, nerve and muscle sheaths, supporting framework of internal organs, aponeuroses, ligaments, joint capsules, periosteum, and tendons.

Connective tissue is composed of cells and extracellular matrix. The most abundant cell is the fibroblast. The fibroblast produces the extracellular components, including collagen, elastin, reticulin, and ground substance. The fibroblast differentiates and matures into the fibrocyte.[1–2]

Macrophages and histiocytes are found in the connective tissue primarily in pathological and posttraumatic states. These cells are part of the reticuloendothelial system, being responsible for phagocytosing foreign matter and bacteria, and thereby playing a significant role in the inflammatory process.[1–2]

Mast cells are found primarily in loose connective tissue and secrete histamine, a vasodilator, and in some mammalian species, heparin, an anticoagulant. An appreciation for the function of the mast cell is important in order to understand the histamine response common in application of soft tissue technique.

Plasma cells found in connective tissue are also associated with the reticuloendothelial system and are responsible for synthesizing antibodies. Because of this specialized function, plasma cells are found primarily in pathological conditions.

Extracellular Matrix

Extracellular matrix includes all components of connective tissue except cells (i.e., ground substance and the various fibers). The fibers include collagen, elastin, and reticulin.

Collagen is subdivided into four types: *Type I collagen* is found in ordinary connective tissue, both loose and dense. *Type II collagen* is found in hyaline cartilage. *Type III collagen* lines arteries and is in the fetal dermis, and *Type IV* is in the basement membranes (Table 9.1).

Elastin is a great deal less tensile than collagen and has more elastic features. Elastin is found lining blood vessels in abundance.

Some ligaments also have a high density of elastin, such as the ligamentum flavum.

Reticulin is responsible for providing a meshwork supporting the glands and lymph nodes.[3] Connective tissue response to immobility and the effects of immobilization upon fascial mobility will be discussed in detail in later sections.

The extracellular matrix also consists of ground substance, a viscous gel-like substance in which the cells and connective tissue fibers lie. The *ground substance* serves as a mechanical barrier for foreign matter and acts as a medium for the diffusion of nutrients and waste products. A prime function of the

---

Table 9.1
Histological Makeup and Classification of Connective Tissue

I. Components

  A. Cells (fibroblasts): Synthesize collagen and ground substance
    (Cousins are the chondroblast and osteoblast)

  B. Extracellular matrix

    1. Fibers

      a. Collagen
        i. Type I: Ordinary connective tissue (loose and dense) and bone
        ii. Type II: Hyaline cartilage
        iii. Type III: Fetal dermis, arteries
        iv. Type IV: Basement membranes

      b. Elastin: Lines the arteries

      c. Reticulin: Supports glands and lymph nodes

    2. Ground substance: Viscous gel with much water content. Substance in which collagen lies.

      a. Purpose
        i. Diffusion of nutrients and waste products
        ii. Determines to some extent the histological characteristics of the tissue
        iii. Maintains "critical interfiber distance"
        iv. More abundant in early life—decreased with age
        v. Mechanical barrier against bacteria

      b. Components
        i. GAG's lubricating effect, maintain critical interfiber distance, minimize collagen crosslinking
        ii. Proteoglycans: primarily bind water

II. Types of connective tissue

  A. Dense regular: Forms ligaments and tendons. Sinusoidal and parallel configuration. Dense parallel arrangement of collagen fibers

  B. Dense irregular: aponeuroses, joint capsules, periosteum, dermis of skin, and fascial sheaths (in areas of considerable mechanical stress

  C. Loose irregular: Superficial fascial sheaths, muscle, and nerve sheaths (support sheaths of internal organs); thin meshwork of collagen

---

From Grodin A, Cantu R. Myofascial manipulation: theory and clinical management. Berryville, VA: Forum Medicum Publishers, 1989. Reprinted with permission.

ground substance is the role it plays in providing a lubrication system in addition to maintaining distance between adjacent collagen fibers.

Ground substance consists of *glycosaminoglycans* (GAGs) and water. In early literature GAGs are referred to as *mucopolysaccarides*. GAGs consist of two primary groups: sulfated and nonsulfated. The sulfated group is responsible for the cohesiveness of the tissue and the nonsulfated group for its water-retaining capability. The ratio between the ground substance and the connective tissue fibers may possibly contribute to the overall pliability or "tension" of the tissue.

Classification of Connective Tissue

Connective tissue is classified by arrangement and density of fibers. Ordinary connective tissue is divided into *dense* and *loose* types,[1–2] and is also subdivided into regular and irregular.

Dense Regular Connective Tissue. This includes tendons and ligaments. It is characterized by a dense, mostly parallel arrangement of collagen fibers. The high proportion of collagen fibers to ground substance and the parallel arrangement of the fibers, allow for little extensibility of the tissue but high tensile characteristics. The high density of the fibers and the low density of ground substance relate directly to the limited vascular supply and account for decreased metabolic activity and a slow rate of healing.

Dense Irregular Connective Tissue. Aponeuroses, joint capsules, periosteum, and dermis of skin and fascial sheaths are included. It is characterized by a dense multidirectional arrangement of collagen fibers. This multidirectional arrangement provides the ability to resist forces in a three-dimensional manner. A high proportion of the connective tissue is collagen. There is a slightly greater degree of ground substance, and, therefore, the vascularity is greater than that of dense regular connective tissue.

Loose Irregular Connective Tissue. It includes, but is not limited to, the superficial and deep fascia, nerve and muscle sheaths, and the endomysium, which binds together individual muscle fibers. Also included is the supportive framework of the lymphatic system and the internal organs. Loose irregular connective tissue is characterized by a sparse, multidirectional framework of collagen and elastin. There is more ground substance per unit area in loose irregular connective tissue, and the vascularity is greater than in other types of connective tissue.

EFFECTS OF IMMOBILIZATION AND REMOBILIZATION ON MYOFASCIAL TISSUE

Connective Tissue Immobilization

Many studies have been performed to identify the results of immobilization on soft tissue structures of animals. Caution must be shown when extrapolating to human tissues. Much of the work has been by Akeson et al. and Woo et al.[4–9] In these studies various animals with previously nontraumatized knee joints were immobilized for at least 9 weeks. The periarticular connective tissues were analyzed biomechanically and histologically. The authors also described a fibrofatty infiltrate in the joint space, especially in the capsular recesses. With prolonged immobilization, the infiltrates developed a more fibrotic appearance, creating adhesion in these recesses.

Histological and histochemical analysis of the connective tissues showed significant changes in the water content and ground substance, with no significant loss of collagen, in connective tissues immobilized less than 9 weeks. There was a 30–40% loss in GAGs (both sulfated and nonsulfated). The primary change was in the loss of hyaluronic acid. Since the primary purpose of GAGs is to provide pliability and serve as a lubricant between adjacent collagen fibers as well as to maintain interfiber distance, Akeson et al. postulated that the loss of GAGs results in an approximation of adjacent collagen (fibers) and/or an increase in abnormal cross-linking of the fibers. They hypothesized that when the distance between existing collagen fibers is too great for cross-linking, the cross-linking takes place by the aggregation and cross-linking of new fibers with the preexisting fibers.[5–9]

Consistent with the half-lives of collagen and ground substance, no significant amounts of collagen were lost in contrast to the significant amounts of ground substance lost. (Normal collagen has a half-life of 300–500 days, while GAGs have a half-life of 1.7–7 days.[10–12] Akeson's group[7] demonstrated that an actual increase in abnormal cross-link formation occurs after 9 weeks of immobilization (See Fig. 9.1.). This cross-linking results in decreasing pliability of the tissue.

Biomechanical analyses in these studies indicate that 10 times the torque of a normal joint is required to mobilize the immobilized joint. After several repetitions of mobilization, the amount of torque required to move the joint is reduced to three times that of a normal. Akeson's group implicated both the macroadhesions (fatty infiltrate) and the increase in microscopic crosslinks as the cause of the decreased pliability of the connective tissue.

Ligaments and periarticular connective tissue also showed histologic, biomechanical, and biochemical changes to immobilization. "Histologically, there is a pattern of increased

randomness and loss of parallelism of collagen fibers in cruciate ligaments, which has been observed in an animal model after 9 weeks of immobilization."[7]

After several weeks of stress deprivation a ligament becomes more compliant. The decrease in tensile characteristics are due to changes in the tissue substance, rather than tissue atrophy.[12] *The period of immobilization is critical to the degree of degradation of the ligament.* After 12 weeks of immobilization, collagen degradation exceeds synthesis by 28%, and after 9 weeks, collagen degradation exceeds synthesis by 14%. Before 9 weeks of immobilization there is a balance between collagen synthesis and degradation. After 9 weeks of immobilization collagen degradation exceeds synthesis, resulting in a net loss of collagen.

Effects of Immobilization on Insertion Sites

There are also significant changes that take place at the bone-ligament-bone complex or junctional zone. Noyes et al.[13] demonstrated the result of avulsion of the anterior cruciate in a primate model was in part a result of cortical atrophy at the insertion sites, with a 39% decrease in maximum load to failure.

Soft tissue insertions (ligament, tendon, joint capsule) to bone are major stress points, since there is a transition from a flexible tension-bearing structure to a noncompliant rigid tissue. To help accommodate for this stress area, ligament and tendon insert through fibrocartilage to bone. Different insertion site mechanics are due to differences in macrostructure near attachments. Irrespective of these differences all the structures insert by superficial and deep fibers. The superficial fibers become continuous with the adjacent periosteum, and the deep fibers insert into bone directly or through fibrocartilage.[7]

Although ligament, tendon, and joint capsules are vascularized and have rich nerve supply, the insertion site has no nerve endings and relatively no vascular supply. Stress and

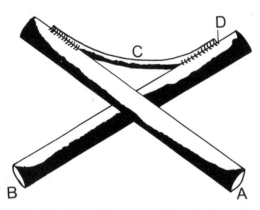

Figure 9.1. Schematic representation of collagen fibers and abnormal crosslink formation. **A** and **B** represent preexisting fibers, **C** represents a newly synthesized collagen fiber, and **D** represents abnormal crosslink formation which decreases the mobility of the two fibers. (From Donatelli R, Owens-Burkhart H. Effects of immobilization on the extensibility of periarticular connective tissue. JOSPT 1981; 3:67–72. Reprinted with permission.)

joint motion are critical in maintaining the tissue integrity of insertion sites.[13] Few if any studies reveal the effects of immobilization on insertion sites. Twenty years ago Barfred[14] noted a decline of soft tissue bone junctional strength with joint immobilization. Soon after Woo's group[4] demonstrated a softening effect on ligament substance with immobilization, and Noyes et al.[15] concluded that the loss of cortex immediately below the ligament insertion reduced the strength of the entire ligament-bone unit. The strength loss of the cortex immediately below the ligament may be at least two times that of the midsubstance of the structure, making this region susceptible to injury.

Crimp. One possible reason for the increased incidence of strain at insertion sites is the difference in collagen fiber *crimp* period. Crimp in connective tissue fibers results in a particular amount of elasticity, so that the ligament acts like a spring when a load is applied (the "slack" taken out of the tissue that results in elastic elongation).[16] Crimp periods are smaller and crimp angles larger near attachment sites. As load is sustained, larger strains are required to remove the end region crimp than the midsubstance crimp, resulting in higher stress concentrations at insertion sites.

Effects on Muscle Tissue

Muscle shows profound changes due to immobilization as well.[17–20] In normal muscle, the number of sarcomeres in series is important in determining the distance through which the muscle can shorten during normal limb movement. The tension of the tendon determines how the individual sarcomeres are stretched, which in turn determines tension development. When muscle is immobilized in the shortened position, sarcomeres are lost, and when immobilized in the lengthened position sarcomeres are added.[21] While in a shortened position a sarcomere's functional length is decreased. Actin/myosin filament overlap is increased beyond the optimal range;

therefore, maximum contracture strength cannot be developed.

After immobilization, muscle weighs approximately half as much as nonimmobilized control muscles. The muscle also shows a decrease in total protein, mitochondria, and soluble enzymes as well as decrease in extensibility. This results in atrophy of the muscle. Fast as well as slow twitch muscle fibers atrophy during immobilization.

The muscle adapts to shortened length by losing sarcomeres, while remaining sarcomeres lengthen somewhat. Optimal sarcomere length is reestablished with maximum filament overlap over a period of approximately 3 weeks. The muscle is adaptively shortened and contains fewer sarcomeres in series, even though the sarcomeres are at optimal length.[21] Length tension curves show a shift to decreased extensibility in the slow twitch muscle. Tabary et al.[21] suggests that this is due to an increase in connective tissue in the belly of the muscle.

In muscle immobilized in a lengthened position (over-stretch), the sarcomere is pulled to a length where overlap of myofilaments decreases, also causing reduction in a maximum tension. Normal muscle develops maximum tension when muscle length is 90% of its maximum. The tension in the muscle is translated to the tendon through the musculotendinous junction, which is a highly specialized area histologically. Biomechanically the junctional zone is the weakest link during muscle strain. The site of failure appears to be within the terminal muscle fibers near the myotendinous junction. Healing occurs by an inflammatory reaction followed by a proliferation of fibroblasts. The net result is increased fibrosis at the site of injury.

The most frequent type of muscle contraction that leads to strain is the eccentric (lengthening) contraction since it is able to generate greatest force.[22] This is an indirect type of injury as compared to a direct laceration or contusion. The direct injury occurs at the site of trauma, but the indirect occurs as a result of stretching or overactivation (excessive force). The most common site of an indirect strain is at the weakest part—the musculotendinous junction. As stated earlier, length changes in muscle are associated with changes in sarcomere number and length.

When new sarcomeres are added they are incorporated in the region of the myotendinous junction. Maintaining mobility and a proper length tension relationship is therefore critical at the myotendinous junction. Muscle immobilized in the shortened position compared with controls develop less force and stretch to a shorter length before tearing.

Lacerations. Another type of muscle pathology that results in immobilization is muscle laceration from a direct trauma of a sharp object. Following complete laceration and suture repair, muscle fragments heal primarily by dense connective tissue.[23] Garrett et al.[23] found that muscles lacerated near the midbelly recovered approximately 50% of their ability to produce tension and could shorten about 80% of normal amount.

Contusions. Muscle contusions result from nonpenetrating blunt injuries. An inflammatory reaction and hematoma may occur. Healing consists of the formation of scar tissue consisting of dense connective tissue with variable amounts of muscle regeneration.[24] More inflammatory reaction was seen in mobilized muscle as compared to immobilized muscle, but it disappeared more rapidly with more scar formation than immobilized muscle.[25] Biomechanical testing showed faster recovery of tensile strength in mobilized muscles.[26]

Mobilization

Movement is a primary factor in maintaining homeostasis between collagen synthesis and degradation.[27] Since collagen is a nonliving tissue, synthesis depends upon the ability of cells to transduce mechanical force into biochemical action. Mechanical force upon the tissue provides the biological activation for alignment of fibroblasts and/or myofibroblasts in the direction of stress. Movement also inhibits contracture by facilitation of proteoglycan synthesis, thus maintaining interfiber distance and lubrication between collagen fibers.[28]

Evans et al.[29] took experimentally weak, immobilized, rat knees and remobilized them by high velocity manipulation, passive range of motion or by both methods. The group receiving manipulation showed that the macroadhesions were ruptured and partial joint mobility restored. If joint motion was allowed subsequent to the manipulation, functional range was regained. Range of motion of the joint, along with freedom of movement, produced the same effect although more gradually, and after 35 days of remobilizations the joints were histologically indistinguishable. Rat knee joints immobilized for more than 30 days did not regain full functional range. The hypothesis is that movement restores normal histologic collagen balance. However, the longer the period of immobilization, the lower the potential for achieving optimal rehabilitative results.

The probable explanation for this phenomenon lies with the maturation of collagen fibers and collagen fiber crosslink. In immobilized connective tissue, collagen is laid down in haphazard arrangement and is crosslinked to adjacent collagen fibers. With time, these crosslinks increase in number and in strength. The early bonding of these crosslinks consists primarily of hydrogen bonding (weak electrostatic bonds). The hydrogen bonds are eventually replaced by stronger covalent bonds, which require more energy to be broken. The connective tissue changes become more comprehensive with longer periods of immobilization, eventually involving the entire tissue and resulting in a more permanent state of inextensibility.[30]

To further understand the effects of mobilization on connective tissue, the *viscoelastic properties of the connective tissue* must be considered. In the viscoelastic model, two components of extensibility (viscous and elastic) combine to give connective tissue its unique deformation quality. The first is the elastic component, which represents the temporary change in the lengthening of connective tissue subjected to mobilization or stretch. The elastic component has a postmobilization recoil or memory, in which extensibility gained during a mobilization session is lost over a short period of time (Fig. 9.2).

The elastic component is not well understood, but it is believed to be the "slack" taken out of the collagen fibers during a stretch. For example, the dense regular connective tissue of a tendon has a very small elastic component because of the parallel, less wavy, arrangement of the collagen fibers. The loose irregular connective tissue of a muscle sheath has a greater elastic component, presumably because of the random orientation of the collagen fibers, i.e., more slack in a nonparallel arrangement of fibers.

The viscous component (plastic component) represents the permanent change in connective tissue when subjected to mobilization or stretch and is sometimes referred to as the hydraulic cylinder model. The plastic component does not have a postmobilization recoil. Any change in the plastic component of connective tissue results in permanent change in the length of extensibility of connective tissue. Presumably, the permanent changes result from breaking intermolecular and intramolecular bonds between collagen molecules, fibers, and crosslinks (Fig. 9.3).

The viscoelastic model is simply the viscous and elastic components together, arranged in series. After stretch or mobilization, the elastic component of the connective tissue returns to normal length, while the plastic portion remains elongated (Fig. 9.4).

The *stress-strain curve* (Fig. 9.5) further illustrates the viscoelastic nature of connective tissue.[31-36] By definition, *stress* is force applied per unit area, and *strain* is change in length divided by original length (percent change in length).[37] Initially, very little force is required to elongate the tissue; however, as more force is applied, the percent elongation is decreased. The early part of the curve, sometimes called the toe region, represents the easily stretched, elastic portion of the tissue. The latter portion of the curve represents the plastic or viscous portion of the tissue.

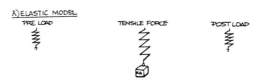

Figure 9.2. Schematic representation of the elastic portion of the viscoelastic model of elongation. No permanent elongation occurs after the application of tensile force. (From Grodin A, Cantu R. Myofascial manipulation: theory and clinical management. Berryville, Va: Forum Medicum Publishers, 1989. Reprinted with permission.)

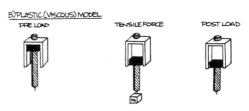

Figure 9.3. Schematic representation of the plastic or viscous portion of the viscoelastic model of elongation. Permanent elongation occurs after the application of tensile force. (From Grodin A. Cantu R. Myofascial manipulation: theory and clinical management. Berryville, Va: Forum Medicum Publishers, 1989. Reprinted with permission.)

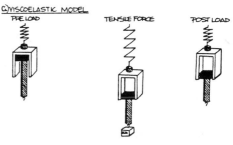

Figure 9.4. Schematic representation of the viscoelastic model of elongation. Some elongation is lost and some is retained after application of tensile force. (From Grodin A. Cantu R. Myofascial manipulation: theory and clinical management. Berryville, Va: Forum Medicum Publishers, 1989. Reprinted with permission.)

The roles of the elastic and plastic components of connective tissue become more evident when plotted against time (Fig. 9.6). The initial elongation, which requires little force, takes place in a short period of time. The plastic portion, requiring more force

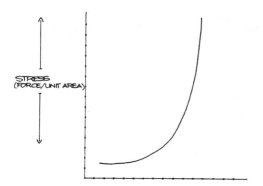

Figure 9.5. Graphic representation of viscoelastic deformation—force applied (stress) is plotted against percent deformation (strain). (From Grodin A, Cantu R. Myofascial manipulation: theory and clinical management. Berryville, Va: Forum Medicum Publishers, 1989. Reprinted with permission.)

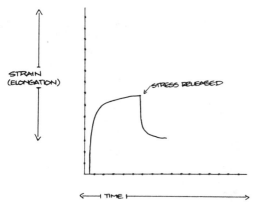

Figure 9.6. Elongation of connective tissue (strain) plotted against time. (From Grodin A, Cantu R. Myofascial manipulation: theory and clinical management. Berryville, Va: Forum Medicum Publishers, 1989. Reprinted with permission.)

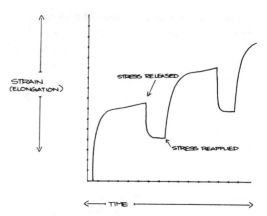

Figure 9.7. Repeated elongations of connective tissue (strain) plotted against time. (From Grodin A, Cantu R. Myofascial manipulation: theory and clinical management. Berryville, Va: Forum Medicum Publishers, 1989. Reprinted with permission.)

Scar Tissue

Scar tissue mechanics differ from nontraumatized, connective tissue mechanics. The primary differences lie in the biomechanics and histology of the different stages of healing of traumatized tissue—scar formation. There are four major phases of scar tissue formations: the inflammatory phase, the granulation phase, the fibroplastic phase, and the maturation phase.[30]

Inflammatory Phase. This begins immediately after insult or trauma to the tissue. Clotting begins almost instantly and is followed by an influx of macrophages and histiocytes to start debriding the area. Debridement facilitates healing in a clean environment and helps prevent infection. The inflammatory phase last approximately 24–48 hours. At this time immobility is important because of the potential for further damage with movement.

Granulation Phase. The second phase of scar formation is the granulation phase. It is characterized by increased vascularity of the tissue, necessary for the transport of debris away from the area and of nutrients into the area. The time required for the granulation phase varies greatly, depending on the nature of the tissue and the extent of the damage.

Fibroblastic Phase. The third phase of

than the elastic portion, also requires more time. When the stress is released, a portion of the gained length is lost almost instantly, while a portion remains permanently.

When this process is repeated, the tissue continues to gain length progressively (Fig. 9.7). Clinically, this is evident in the stretching of a restricted joint capsule. After a mobilization session, a certain amount of range of motion is gained. On a subsequent visit, some range of motion previously gained is lost, while some is retained.

scar formation includes proliferation of fibroblasts and an increase in fibroblastic activity. The rate of collagen and ground substance formation is increased, but the collagen is being laid down in haphazard arrangement and is very weak, since the new collagen is bound by weak hydrogen bonds. The fibroplastic phase lasts 3–8 weeks, depending on the histological makeup of the damaged tissue.

Maturation Phase. The last phase in scar formation is when the collagen is maturing, solidifying, and shrinking. During this phase, the collagen is strong enough to endure some stress without incurring further damage. Since collagen synthesis is still accelerated, significant remodeling can be performed on the tissue if appropriate mobilization and therapeutic techniques are used to stress the tissue.

If left unchecked and untreated, the haphazard arrangement of the collagen fiber and contracture of the tissue will solidify, and some extensibility will be permanently lost. If long periods of immobilization are required, the effect of immobilization on traumatized connective tissues is compounded. Not only is there a loss of ground substance and an increase in intermolecular and intramolecular cross-linking, but there are also macroadhesions formed from scar tissue that adheres to adjacent nontraumatized connective tissues. Scar then limits the extensibility of healthy surrounding tissues.

Although there is a good deal more information regarding remobilization effects on muscle, their effects upon junctional sites of ligament, tendon, and joint capsule with bone is inconclusive. Changes in the number and size of collagen fibrils and ground substance may change insertion strength. The use of many different animal models and different experimental procedures have made the correlation of information difficult. The following conclusions nevertheless can be drawn.

It appears that junctional zones become stronger with exercise. However, maximum force and energy to failure returned to only 80% of control values. Histologically the insertion site showed evidence of bone formation at sites of previous reabsorption. Laros et al.[38] demonstrated that the effects of immobilization are relatively reversible in dogs after 4–12 months of exercise in large open pens. Tipton et al.[39] studied endurance exercise and its effect upon ligament insertion in rats. They reported that ligaments show larger diameter collagen fiber bundles and higher collagen content in trained animals compared with untrained controls. The ligament bone complex showed a higher separation force per body weight.

MYOFASCIAL MANIPULATION AND PHYSIOLOGIC EFFECTS OF MASSAGE

Massage may be defined as systematic, therapeutic, and functional stroking and kneading of the body. Since "massage" and "soft tissue mobilization" are interchangeable in concept, the available research as to the effect of massage upon the body should be explored. In particular, known effects upon circulation, blood flow, capillary dilation, cutaneous temperature, and upon the morphology of blood vessels require documentation. Most of the studies performed in this area were done prior to 1950.

Effect of Massage on Blood Flow and Temperature

In an early study, the effects on blood flow in the extremities of 17 adult men and women were analyzed by Wakim.[40] Groups were subdivided into those with no medical problems, those with rheumatoid arthritis, those with flaccid paralysis, and those with spasmatic paralysis. The subjects received moderate depth stroking and kneading massage described as a modified Hoffa-type massage, and deeper vigorous stimulating, kneading, and percussion massage for 15 minutes (as practiced in some European schools of physical therapy). The massaged areas were the upper and lower extremities. Plethysmography was used to evaluate venous occlusion. This system incorporated a compensating spirometer recorder as described by Berry and associates.[41]

Wakim concluded that there was a consistent or clinically significant increase in total blood flow and cutaneous temperature after deep stroking and kneading massage of the extremities in normal subjects, patients with rheumatoid arthritis, and subjects with spasmatic paralysis. A much milder effect was noted with the more superficial Hoffa-type massage and primarily in the paralyzed group. The greatest increase in circulation after deep stroking and kneading massage to the extremities occurred in subjects with flaccid paralysis. Significant increases in blood flow and temperature were still apparent in all groups receiving the deep massage when remeasured at 30 minutes. Blood flow increases diminished markedly after 30 minutes. Neither deep stroking, kneading, or vigorous stimulating massage of the extremities resulted in consistent, significant changes in blood flow of the contralateral unmassaged extremity.

Wakim's primary significant finding of temperature change in the extremities resulting from increased blood flow to the part may well depend upon the manner in which the massage is administered. He found that modified Hoffa massage increased the blood flow only of subjects with flaccid paralysis, while stimulating massage (non-Hoffa) had the effect of increasing the blood flow of all subjects treated.

In another early study by Wolfson, the effects of deep kneading massage on venous blood flow were also examined.[42] He used an animal model (anesthetized dogs) and measured blood flow by cannulation of the femoral vein. Massage was applied to the limbs above and below the knee. The blood draining out was measured and reinjected into the opposite limb at the same rate the blood was being removed. The kneading massage was described as a "deep kneading type." The massage initially caused a fairly rapid increase in blood flow followed by a decrease in blood flow to a rate less than normal. This decrease in blood flow continued throughout the administration of the massage. Immediately following cessation of the massage, blood flow slowly returned to normal. Thus, Wolfson

concluded that massage causes an increase in the rate of blood flow by mechanically emptying the blood vessels and allowing them to refill with fresh blood.

The studies of Wakim and Wolfson are in substantial agreement: deep kneading massage, performed on normal subjects, increases the blood flow to the area being treated, even though the massage applied by Wolfson was of the nonstimulating type. However, generalizations cannot be made because Wakim studied human subjects while Wolfson worked with anesthetized animals that had just undergone surgery to expose the femoral vein for cannulization.

The morphology of normal blood vessels and their reaction to stimuli were microscopically examined even earlier by Carrier.[43] Gross visual observation of skin reaction was made following mechanical stimulation of the skin by a blunt instrument. The following reactions were noted. Light stroke: the area in the path of the stroke blanched after a latent period of 15–20 second; the blanching lasted for several minutes. A harder stimulus resulted in a hyperemic line in the immediate path of the stimulus. With microscopic investigation, light pressure resulted in instantaneous opening of all capillaries in the microscopic field. A heavier pressure opened the underlying capillaries for a longer duration, which was not specified.

The observations of Carrier may correlate with the results of the studies by Wakim and Wolfson. If the Hoffa-type massage (nonstimulating) is similar to the light stroke produced by a blunt instrument in Carrier's study, an immediate capillary reaction is probable with massage. The light stroke or Hoffa massage creates capillary dilation but for too short a duration to affect blood volume, blood flow, or temperature in the underlying area stroked. With the vigorous stimulating massage as administered by Wakim and heavy pressure administered by Carrier, the result is a longer lasting dilation of the underlying capillaries, creating both a change in blood flow and skin temperature. Indeed, a vigorous stimulating massage and heavy pressure are used in connective tissue massage or myofascial release. In connective tissue massage the strokes are three in succession, and the skin response is an immediate hyperemia, lasting a few minutes. The hyperemia may be followed by an increase in blood flow and cutaneous temperature and can be measured by a thermocouple.

A review of the literature before 1950 pertaining to the physiologic effects of massage was reported by Pemberton[44] in that year. He described the work of Clark and Swanson who studied the capillary circulation in the ear of a rabbit following massage, using a permanent window surgically created in the rabbit's ear to observe the capillaries.

Following massage an increase in rate of blood flow as well as actual changes in the vessel walls occurred. The change in the vessel wall was evidenced by the "sticking" and emigration of leukocytes. Clark and Swenson concluded that massage is accompanied or followed by an increase interchange of substances between the blood stream and the tissue cells. The change in vessel wall promotes a heightened tissue metabolism.

Although massage is not defined in Clark and Swenson's study, the findings of increase in blood flow and change in vessel-wall support the notion that massage or soft tissue mobilization has an effect on the vascularization of the region underlying the massage. The conclusion by Clark and Swenson supports Carrier[43] who reported an immediate capillary reaction underlying the stimulus of light and heavy pressure.

Cutaneous temperature of an extremity following 5–10 minutes of modified Hoffa massage was studied by Martin et al.[45] Normal adults and those with rheumatoid arthritis were studied, and cutaneous temperature of the digits was measured with thermocouples. Martin et al. found (in every instance) superficial cutaneous temperature increases in the extremity lasting 15–90 minutes. In a related investigation of three subjects, the peripheral cutaneous temperature of extremities was examined after back massage. There was no change in the cutaneous temperature of the extremities.

Whereas some studies addressed the effects of massage on the volume of blood flow,[40,42] others addressed the effects of massage on capillaries,[43] and Martin et al.[45] examined cutaneous temperature. All these studies are in agreement on one point: massage causes capillaries to dilate in the region underlying the massage. If capillary dilation occurs, the increased blood volume brought to the skin surface results in an increase in cutaneous temperature.

Effect of Massage upon Blood

The effects of massage upon blood cell type, specifically red blood cells, and blood platelet count has been studied. An indirect physiologic effect of massage is believed to influence blood. Pemberton's 1950 review of the literature[44] quoted Mitchell: "in health and anemia the red cell count is increased after massage." In Pemberton's own work (unpublished) the red cell count increased after massage, but details were not provided.

In a study of the blood in six human subjects at high altitude (initial exposure and extended exposure), Schneider and Havens[46] showed an increase of red corpuscles in the peripheral capillaries after abdominal massage. Kneading administered to the abdomen for 5 minutes or longer elicited the red corpuscle increase; however, further details were not presented. The significance of this early study is the effect of a peripheral increase in the red cell count. The increase in red cell count suggests that massage is effective in temporarily increasing red cell counts in localized areas of the body, albeit by diversion from other areas of the body.

The thrombocyte or blood platelet count after massage was studied by Lucia and Rickard.[47] The massage was performed by stroking the ear of five rabbits in a "gentle but firm manner," at a rate of 25 strokes per minutes for 1 minute at 5-minute intervals. The ear was then punctured and the first drop of blood studied. They found an increase in the blood platelet count of the massaged ear, but no change on the opposite untreated ear.

In summary, there is some reasonable evidence that increased cutaneous temperature and increased blood flow result from massage with a local elevation of the cellular components. These may have a positive therapeutic effect upon parts of the body with compromised circulation. Dysfunctional areas are by definition in need of increased nutrition that increased blood is capable of supplying.

Effect of Massage upon Metabolism

The effect of massage on metabolic processes includes the effect upon vital signs and waste products of the body. An early review of the literature on the effect of massage on metabolism in humans was performed by Cuthbertson.[48] He concluded that there was an increase in the output of urine after massage, especially following abdominal massage. The excretion of acid was not consistently altered nor was there a change in nitrogen content, inorganic phosphorus, and sodium chloride. The increased output of urine occurred within 3 hours of the massage, but the total net output of urine in a 24-hour period was unchanged. In normal subjects there was no increase in basal consumption of oxygen, pulse rate, or blood pressure. All the above metabolic effects apply to a systemic process. Although localized increase in basal consumption may also occur, none has been studied directly.

Because the basal metabolism is not influenced by massage, a likely explanation for the increase in urine output is that it is secondary to the effect of massage on the circulation of the part concerned. Another possibility is related to the increase in blood volume assumed to occur following an increase in cellular components of the blood. The body rids itself of excess fluids during the recovery time following the effects of massage, thereby increasing urine output.

If the finding of a temporary increase in metabolism under the area massaged is correct, as reported in Pemberton's review, the metabolic effects carry strong implication. An increase in the circulation to the area[40,43,44] may be required to deal with the increased metabolic processes. Both the increase in metabolic processes, which produce heat as a byproduct and the increase in blood flow would increase cutaneous temperature. To accommodate for the increase in metabolic processes in the part treated with massage, an increase in red blood cells is required to bring the needed oxygen to the tissues being influenced.[46] Hence there is some support for the traditional notion that massage is strongly applicable in areas where increased circulation and nutrition to the tissue are desired.

Physiological Reflexive (Autonomic) Effects of Massage

The literature on the effects of massage on a reflexive base consists of limited studies of the effects of connective tissue massage distal to the area being treated. In support of connective tissue massage, Dicke and Ebner[49,50] reported that viscera, blood vessels, supporting tissue, and muscle cannot function as separate entities. Connective tissue massage stimulates the circulation to an area of the body that in turn, reflexively opens up increased circulatory pathways to other regions of the body. The cause for the initial increase in circulation is secondary to the mechanical tension by the connective tissue massage strokes, thereby stimulating the tissue.

Investigation of the skin temperature of three patients after connective tissue massage was reported by Ebner,[50] who found an increase in skin temperature (1–2°C) of the foot following 20 minutes of connective tissue massage carried out on the sacral and lumbar segments of the back. Volker and Rostovsky (as reported by Ebner[50]) also carried out experiments using connective tissue massage and found a maximum increase in temperature approximately 30 minutes after its termination.

The mechanical friction of the massage stroke stimulates structures within the connective tissue, including mast cells. When stimulated, mast cells produce histamine, a vasodilator. Vasodilation creates increased blood flow to the local area treated and to other areas receiving histamine through the blood stream. The increased permeability of the capillaries and small venules allows for quicker and more complete diffusion of waste products from the tissues to the blood. The blood components when filtered by the kidney and excreted as urine, show increased nitrogen content, inorganic phosphorus and sodium chloride, as reported by Cuthbertson.[48]

SCHOOLS OF THOUGHT IN MYOFASCIAL MANIPULATION

There are various other treatment approaches that also deal with the autonomic and/or mechanical nature of soft tissue work. At best, these are poorly documented, but they appear through testimonials to have profound effects upon the body. The following descriptions are systems that are popular today, although the list is by no means comprehensive.

Soft Tissue Mobilization

The approaches being utilized by practitioners are too numerous to detail all in this chapter. The term soft tissue mobilization encompasses all the systems into a common language. A few of the systems of soft tissue manipulation are briefly outlined below.

Connective Tissue Massage. Under the heading soft tissue mobilization falls connective tissue massage or *Bindegewebsmassage*,[49] a system originated by Elisabeth Dicke of Germany in the 1920's and 1930's.[49] It was further developed by Maria Ebner.[50] In her book Dicke wrote that she was suffering from endarteritis obliterans of the right leg secondary to a tooth infection. The leg gave the appearance of incipient gangrene. She was also experiencing acute pain of the low back. She was able to relieve her pain by stroking over the sacrum and iliac crest. When stroked, these areas were hypersensitive, but this gradually subsided as did the low back pain. The affected leg gradually felt warm, and superficial venous circulation reappeared. Over time

her other problems (gastritis, enlarged liver, and angina) also were relieved. She described a phenomenon corresponding to what we now call a visceral somatic response. Her work was investigated further by Dr. Veil of Jena, Professor Kohlrausch of Freiburg, and Dr. Leube of Breisgau. They incorporated the work of Dr. Head (who had described the changes in skin areas) and Mackenzie[53] who had noted changes in muscle tone and sensitivity in areas that share the same nerve root supply with pathologic organs. In essence the system became focused on normalization of the *autonomic reflex pathways*, with strong influences on the circulation of various types of tissues.

Hoffa Massage. Hoffa massage is a system approach employing traditional effleurage and petrissage.[51] Effleurage is described by Hoffa as follows: "The hand is applied as closely as possible to the part. The hand ... glides on it (the body), distally to proximally ... with the broad part of the hand. Use the ball of the thumb and little fingers to stroke the muscle masses, and at the same time glide along at the edge of the muscle with the fingertips to take care of the larger vessels; stroke upward." Petrissage is described by Tappan[51] as part of the Hoffa technique as follows: "Apply both hands obliquely to the direction of the muscle fibers. The thumbs are opposed to the rest of the fingers. This manipulation starts peripherally and proceeds centripetally, following the direction of the muscle fibers. The hand goes first and tries to pick the muscle from the bone, moving back and forth in a zigzag path." The primary purpose of the Hoffa massage is to increase circulation and decrease muscle tone.

Rolfing. Rolfing (structural integration)[52] is a system used to correct inefficient posture or integrate structure. The technique involves manual manipulation of the soft tissue (myofascia) with the goal of balancing the body in the gravitational field. Rolfing is a standardized, nonsymptomatic approach to soft tissue manipulation, with a set number of treatment sessions in basic and advanced sequences. The basic sequence usually involves 10 sessions, each focusing upon a different aspect of postural integration. The advanced sequence is usually 2 or 3 sessions, with "tune up" sessions done as needed following the advanced sequence.

Other Approaches. Connective tissue massage, Hoffa massage, and rolfing collectively incorporate manual intervention that deals either with the autonomic nervous system or mechanical motion limitation in the connective tissue. Another category of soft tissue work includes the movement approaches, where the main goal is to break up abnormal movement patterns so that more efficient patterns can be initiated. This category includes approaches such as proprioceptive neuromuscular facilitation (PNF), Feldenkrais, Alexander technique, and Aston patterning, etc. These approaches will be discussed separately in another chapter.

Choice of Approach

Autonomic techniques include connective tissue massage and Hoffa massage. Mechanical limitation can be treated with myofascial release, cross friction, and rolfing, and movement techniques such as Alexander, Feldenkrais, and proprioceptive neuromuscular facilitation. Any stimulus to the human body may have autonomic effects, since the skin is a sensory organ that contains many proprioceptors. The skin proprioceptors respond positively to appropriate touch or negatively to inappropriate touch.

The choice of approaches depends upon the condition being treated. Soft tissue problems occur for various reasons which include:

—Metabolic-hormonal, collagen vascular disease,
—Posttraumatic response,
—Postural imbalance, poor body language,
—Mechanical stress from underuse and overuse, and
—Combination of the above.

In any of these conditions the patient may present with either hypomobility or hypermobility. Hypermobility is best treated by stabilization and an autonomic approach. Hypomobility is best treated by soft tissue

mobilization. A direct approach utilizing an appropriate force of passive movement of the musculofascial elements through its restrictive directions is recommended.

These are but a few of the most prominent approaches that work with the soft tissues to achieve bodily harmony. Each of the systems offers specific strengths. A clinician is limited only when one school of thought is utilized to the exclusion of the others. In dealing with human pathology, it is essential to draw upon all of the resources and be in touch with the capabilities in each. An appropriate treatment approach is one that integrates all of these systems.

TARGETS AND GOALS OF MYOFASCIAL MANIPULATION

In 1945, Mennell[53] stated, there were two and only two possible effects of any movement of massage—reflexive and mechanical. Some of the mechanical effects of soft-tissue mobilization from a histological standpoint have already been discussed. Movement or mobilization rehydrates the connective tissue, stimulates the production of ground substance, assists in the orienting of collagen fibers, and breaks fibrofatty macroadhesions.

Mobilization results in plastic deformation of the connective tissue, thereby increasing extensibility, length, and mobility. The tissues clinicians attempt to affect—muscle sheaths, ligaments, tendons, aponeuroses, joint capsules, superficial fascia, and deep fascia—can be classified as connective tissue. All of these tissues can be affected by soft tissue mobilization.

Autonomic Effects

As previously stated, the reflexive, or autonomic, component is primarily affected through the skin and superficial connective tissues.[49] MacKenzie[54] defined the reflexive, or autonomic, component as "that vital process which is concerned in the reception of a stimulus by one organ or tissue and its conduction to another organ, which on receiving a stimulus produces the effect." When soft tissue mobilization is performed for autonomic effect, sensory receptors in the skin and superficial fascia are stimulated. The stimuli pass through afferent pathways to the spinal cord and may be channeled through autonomic pathways, producing effects in areas corresponding to dermatomal zones being mobilized.[51]

Dicke[49] refers to certain aspects of this phenomenon as the cutivisceral reflex. Dicke uses the example of the application of a mother's warm hand to alleviate a child's stomach ache. Obviously, the intestine would not be affected from the surface of the skin and the reaction must be "a reflex which affects the intestines from the skin." The skin is the primary organ for the reception of outside tactile stimuli and is densely innervated.

The idea of affecting areas of the body by stimulation of the skin and superficial connective tissue has been utilized in areas apart from soft tissue mobilization. For example, part of the theory of transcutaneous electrical nerve stimulation (TENS) is direct stimulation of large myelinated nerve fibers which modulate noxious stimuli through small unmyelinated fibers at various mediating points of the nervous system. Aside from its application for pain control, TENS has been used to control postsurgical nausea and menstrual cramping.

Though it is only conjecture at this point, it is possible that an autonomic component factors into the therapeutic response from stimulation. In acute patients, affecting the autonomic system is an important stepping stone to more "aggressive" mechanical work. In subacute patients, autonomic techniques are most often used at the beginning of treatment to provide an entry (to bring about relaxation), and at the end of treatment to provide an exit from mechanical technique.

The effects of autonomic technique should not be overemphasized. Some practitioners use this autonomic phenomenon to justify treatment of disorders unrelated to the neuromusculosketetal system. While the autonomic effect cannot be denied, judgment should be exercised by the clinician in evaluating the extent of autonomic effect.

Mechanical Effects

The mechanical effects of myofascial manipulation were discussed in detail in earlier sections. The histologic changes caused by myofascial manipulation have the overall effect of decreasing myofascial tone and increasing extensibility. The patient is then prepared for postural reeducation and therapeutic exercise. When myofascial imbalances exist, the patient has difficulty in postural self-correction. For example, in the forward head posture, tight subcranial myofascial elements may not allow the patient to assume a more axially extended position. After releasing the subcranial myofascia, proper posturing is facilitated. The patient is no longer struggling against his or her myofascial limitations. As the subcranial myofascia releases, axial elongation is possible, and a positive feedback loop is established.

When the subcranial myofascia is not released before correct posturing is attempted, fatigue and increased symptoms often ensue, establishing a negative feedback loop. As a result, the patient assumes old posturing patterns. Therefore, soft tissue mobilization is often needed prior to any instruction on posture. The clinician must be confident that soft tissue changes have occurred before attempting postural reeducation.

CLASSIFICATION OF MYOFASCIAL PAIN

In recent years, a multitude of techniques associated with osteopathic and physical therapy concepts have become popular. These include myofascial release, myofascial mobilization, unwinding, muscle energy, and soft tissue mobilization.

The techniques can be learned by a skilled clinician. The criteria for usage of myofascial technique must be established. Pathologies can be categorized into 3 distinct areas: (*a*) fibromyalgia, (*b*) myofascial pain syndromes, and (*c*) soft tissue lesion—mechanical dysfunction.

Fibromyalgia

First described by Stockman in 1904 fibromyalgia was defined as a pathology based on "inflamed circumscribed parts which are tender, painful on pressure and if large, can be easily felt."[55] Over the years the lack of diagnostic laboratory and radiographic findings associated with fibrositis (fibromyalgia in more recent literature) had placed this pathology in the area of psychologic disorders.[56]

Over the past 10 years, the pathology has been reexamined and specific findings have been associated with fibrositis.[56] The patient presents with diffuse aches and pains not associated with a specific joint or structure, disturbed sleep with morning stiffness and fatigue, and 11 of 18 multiple characteristic tender points, a few of which are:

- midpoint, upper trapezius muscle
- medial fat pad of knee
- just distal to lateral epicondyle of elbow
- middle to upper quadrant of buttock at iliac crest
- midpoint of sternocleidomastoid muscle
- just distal to medial epicondyle of elbow
- second costochondral junction

"Hypersensitivity to cold or to heat; frequent bouts of abdominal pain, constipation, and diarrhea; recurrent fronto-occipital headaches, sensations of numbness or swelling in the hands and feet; and anxiety or depression"[57] are other clinical signs.

Seventy to ninety percent of cases are female and fall into the age bracket of 20–50 years. The patient usually presents with chronic pain, headaches, and fatigue over many years, but the process is nondegenerative and nondeforming in nature. X-ray, CAT scan, MRI testing, and blood studies are normal. The above symptoms are frequently associated with hypermobility and occasionally with mitral valve prolapse.[57]

Myofascial Pain Syndrome

Myofascial pain syndrome follows a sequence of events usually associated with hypermobility or hypomobility, postural imbalance, trau-matic insult to the tissue—such as an automobile accident—and stress and strain from under- or overuse. As with fibrositis, this syndrome has no clear diagnostic criteria based on x-ray findings or blood studies. One of the main differences distinguishing myofascial pain syndrome from fibromyalgia is that the symptoms are more regional, rather than global. The head, neck, and upper thoracic areas, for example, may be diffusely tender and painful, while other areas generally associated with fibromyalgia may not.

Postural imbalance is usually the most common denominator in myofascial pain syndrome. The imbalance leads to areas of hypomobility, resulting in abnormal force levers and stresses to other tissues which may result in hypermobility.

A Prime Example. The forward-head posture is a common occurrence in a sedentary population. The patient presents with forward bending of the midcervical facet joints (decreased cervical lordosis). The resulting compensation by the occiput-atlas joints creates a backward-bending position to maintain the eyes level. Shortening of the suboccipital muscles may lead to impingement of the greater or lesser occipital nerves and result in occipital to frontal headaches. The supportive musculature of the cervical spine develops poor length tension relationships—specifically the sternocleidomastoid, levator scapulae, upper trapezius, and infrahyoid/suprahyoid muscles. The forward-head posture also results in shoulder girdle protraction and potential shortening of the glenohumeral joint internal rotators—subscapularis, teres major, latissimus dorsi, and the pectoralis minor. The shortening of the internal rotators and the loss of external rotation result in a potential rotator-cuff impingement condition. The scapula also loses range of motion in the direction of posterior depression.

The patient often presents with an increased thoracic kyphosis as well. Secondary to a decreased lumbar lordosis, or to the anterior forces of the increased thoracic kyphosis, the patient will bring in a posterior force from backward bending at L5/S1.

Respiration. Increased activity in the accessory muscles with poor diaphragmatic breathing is apparent. The ability of the lower rib cage to expand decreases, as does the respiratory diaphragm's ability to descend. This leads to increased activity on the part of the upper respiratory muscles. The scalenes being accessory muscles of respiration, exhibit increased activity, elevating the first rib. First rib elevation, increased scalene activity, and pectoralis minor activity increase the potential for impingement of the neurovascular bundle, resulting in thoracic outlet symptomatology.

Muscular Imbalance. When one motion is impaired to a joint, other directions will also be limited. Since the cervical facet joints are in forward bending in the forward head posture, there is loss of rotation. Since rotation must take place somewhere, the cervical/thoracic junction as well as the atlanto-axial articulation become overused, overstressed areas, leading to early joint changes.

The muscular imbalance causes some muscles to become facilitated (decreased threshold to firing) resulting in increased excitation to stimulation. The formation of trigger points is likely. A trigger point is defined by Travell[58] as a "focus of hyper-irritability in a tissue that, when compressed, is locally tender and, if sufficiently hypersensitive, gives rise to referred pain and tenderness, and sometimes to referred autonomic phenomenon and distortion of proprioception." Maintaining joints in the short range results in associated soft tissue tightness (Table 9.2).

The typical symptoms will be:

- intermittent cervical, thoracic, or lumbar pain
- bilateral headaches and facial pain
- trigger points in multiple muscle sites
- upper extremity pain and/or tingling in the absence of neurological findings (typically early in the process)
- difficulty sitting for a long period of time, especially in deep, soft chairs or bucket seats that accentuate forward-head posture
- ache on prolonged standing
- pain decreased by rest or gentle movements.

Table 9.2
Postural Sequence for the Forward Head Posture

Forward bending of the midcervical facet joints

Backward bending (extension) of the occiput atlas

Shortening of suboccipital muscles, resulting in potential impingement of the greater or lesser occipital nerves

Imbalance between the sternocleidomastoid, the levator scapulae, and the trapezius

Imbalance between the anterior cervical musculature (including the suprahyoid and infrahyoid muscles) and posterior cervical extensors

Shoulder girdle protraction with internal rotation, (the latissimus, subscapularis, pectoralis, and teres major being involved)

Increased thoracic kyphosis with decreased lumbar lordosis

Increased activity of the accessory respiratory muscles due to poor diaphragmatic breathing and expansion of the lower rib cage

Elevation of the first rib by increased scalene activity

Anterior and posterior restriction of the first rib articulations

Tendency toward thoracic outlet symptomatology

Cervical imbalance with a tendency toward degenerative joint disease from C5 through C7

Muscular imbalance leading to abnormal muscle-firing (some muscles become facilitated with trigger points)

Joints and soft tissues maintained in shortened range lead to restriction of joint capsules and loss of proprioception.

From Grodin A., Cantu R. Myofascial manipulation: theory and clinical management. Berryville, VA: Forum Medicum Publishers, 1989. Reprinted with permission.

Soft-Tissue Lesion/Mechanical Dysfunction

Soft tissue lesion/mechanical dysfunction is the most easily diagnosed, and its treatment is more specific. There is usually overuse or direct trauma to the tissue which leads to inflammation. Sometimes a partial or full tear—as in a hamstring tear or "pull," gastrocnemius group tear, tennis elbow, are a few examples. Reproduction of pain through palpation, contraction of muscle, or stretch to the tissue helps localize the lesion to a specific tissue.

PRINCIPLES OF MYOFASCIAL EVALUATION

The evaluation for fibromyalgia and myofascial pain syndromes emphasizes palpatory examination. The purpose is to identify and define areas of somatic dysfunction and to attempt to categorize the findings into one of the previously mentioned categories (fibromyalgia, myofascial pain syndrome, soft tissue lesion mechanical dysfunction).

Observation

Somatic dysfunction can be defined as impaired or altered function of related components of the somatic (body framework) system, skeletal, arthrodial, and myofascial structures. The first part of any evaluation for somatic dysfunction consists of the observational examination. The primary purpose of observation is to help direct the clinician to the areas or regions where the palpatory examination should be directed. The structure of the body dictates the location of movement disturbance and where stress by overuse or trauma will take place.

Body Asymmetry. Its observation is important. However, the clinician must remember that the human body is by nature's design asymmetrical. We have hand and leg dominance as well as eye dominance, all of which cause us to function asymmetrically.

Gross Imbalance. This observation yields more important clinical information. For instance, some individuals have significant hypertrophy of one of the paraspinals. This is common with serious golfers. The pattern creates a situation in which there is an asymmetrical force of transmission through left and right paraspinals, causing abnormal and uneven forces at the lumbosacral spine. Paraspinal hypertrophy on one side frequently causes hypomobility on one side and hypermobility on the other side of the lumbosacral spine. In addition, the increase in muscle activity of the hypertrophied musculature results in development of trigger points within muscle or facilitated spinal motion segments, especially at the lumbosacral and thoracolum-

bar junctions. The observation of unilateral muscle hypertrophy should focus the clinician on active and passive motion of the trunk as well as direct palpation of the thoracolumbar junction and lumbosacral junction. The stress/strain or lever arm-fulcrum forces are greater at transitional areas of the spine.

Myofascial treatment in this scenario would focus on mobilizing the restricted myofascia unilaterally to facilitate harmony of motion. The transitional areas of the spine would be emphasized even if pain is not present in these areas. Once the myofascial tissues become more extensible, the joints may be mobilized to create further movement balance. Postural reeducation techniques may then be emphasized in order to reduce the stresses on the transitional areas.

Another example of imbalance is seen when there is lack of development of musculature in the mid thoracic spine. This nearly always is accompanied by a reversal of the thoracic kyphosis in the mid thoracic area. This can occur with postural dysfunctions or as a structural problem with an underlying genetic basis.

Because the trunk has a reversal of the kyphosis, normal movement through the thoracic spine becomes abnormal and unbalanced. The reversal of the kyphosis creates a straightening of the mid thoracic spine. The line of gravity consequently does not fall as anteriorly as it normally does in the mid thoracic spine. The erector spinae muscles are underused because of the decreased vector forces, and weakness eventually results. The ligamentous and capsular structures subsequently become more involved in checking motion (especially forward bending), and hypermobility eventually occurs. Compensatory activities take place above and below the mid thoracic spine (cervicothoracic and thoracolumbar junctions), which are also undergoing the stresses associated with transitional zones. Hypertrophy of the upper thoracic musculature occurs, specifically the upper trapezius and levator scapulae. Frequently, there may be an overuse pattern in which these muscles become the focal area of a myofascial pain pattern. Joint stiffness can occur in this area due to the consistently increased myofascial tone and hypertrophy, which restrict normal movement. The cause of the pain in the cervicothoracic junction is myofascial, and can be considered a product of overuse. The cause of the pain in the mid thoracic area is also a product of overuse, but with hypermobility occurring and the pain coming from overused ligamentous and capsular structures.

The focus of treatment in this scenario would be myofascial and joint mobilization and manipulation to the cervicothoracic junction to decrease myofascial and joint restrictions. Stabilization exercises are directed to the mid thoracic spine to promote healthy myofascial tone and decrease the strain on the ligamentous and capsular structures. Again, postural education is necessary to maintain changes made with therapy.

After visual observation the clinician knows where the focus of attention needs to be for the active range of motion, passive range of motion, and palpation examinations. An important Rolfing concept comes into play here: when dealing with an area of pain, always look elsewhere for the cause.

Range of Motion

During range of motion testing the examiner is observing for lever arms (hypomobility) and fulcrums (hypermobility). As previously mentioned, soft tissue overuse (in the form of connective tissue and muscular restrictions and/or hypertrophy) usually takes place over the lever arm. Soft tissue overuse in the form of mechanical breakdown (stress/strain) takes place over the area of hypermobility. Myofascial pain can be associated with both the overused hypomobile area, and the overused hypermobile or unstable area.

Even more important than range of motion quantity is the quality of movement. Ideally, the movement should be brisk without hesitation or compensation (deviation to avoid pain). There should be fluidity of movement without any cogwheel-type pattern. Cogwheel movement occurs where there is a hesitation of movement and then when the body accelerates to overtake the dysfunction. This pattern may repeat itself during the entire movement. Often this is seen in areas of hypermobility where the body is trying to protect itself.

During this test both range of motion and quality can vary with many factors including age, which makes motion all the more important. Quality of movement can be influenced by myofascial or joint involvement as well as the degree of pain present. It is also determined by the recruitment of tissue. Movement should ideally be brisk and purposeful without compensations. Other factors identified are smoothness, sequence of tissue recruitment, deviation of movement from the norm, guarding such as nonreversal of the lumbar lordosis during spinal flexion.

Passive Range of Motion

This is most important for identification of hyper and hypomobility as well as the recruitment of the tissues. It is imperative that the patient be relaxed during this part of the examination so an accurate assessment can be made. The spine must be in a neutral position with proper trunk support, as with cushions.

Layer Palpation

Layer palpation allows for systematic identification of soft tissue pathology: for didactic purposes this can be broken down into minute proportions, but for practical clinical purposes superficial and deep palpation should suffice. The superficial palpatory examination includes:

Light touch—superficial connective tissue
Tissue temperature and moisture
Mobility of superficial fascia
Skin rolling

Superficial Palpation. Targeted are:

Epidermis—keratinized stratified epithelium
Dermis—mechanical strength and elasticity secondary to fibrous content. Contains the vascular supply of the skin.
Papillal layer—superficial layer
Reticular layer—deep layer interlacing bands

of white fibrous tissue with some elastic fibers. The fibers run parallel giving cleavage lines.

Loose connective tissue layer—superficial fascia

Deep Palpatory Exam. This includes:

Deep fascia—parallel layers of collagen fibers
Ligament
Joint capsule
Myofascial unit
Tendon
Periosteum

Deep palpation. The clinician can employ the following palpatory techniques:

Compression: palpation through layers of tissue perpendicular to the tissue.
Shear: Movement of tissues between layers parallel to tissues.

Findings. The descriptions used for palpatory findings are:

superficial—deep   acute—chronic
compressible—rigid   painful—nonpainful
moist—dry   circumscribed—diffuse
soft—hard   rough—smooth
hypermobile—hypo-   thick—thin
          mobile

PRINCIPLES OF TREATMENT APPLICATION

Once the pathology has been identified by examination, appropriate goals are set and a soft tissue approach used as necessary. When dealing with hypermobility, stabilization is utilized, and when dealing with hypomobility, mobilization is stressed. The proper sequence of the patient should ideally consist of:

1. Soft tissue mobilization to the area of hypomobility,
2. Joint mobilization following normalization of the soft tissue,
3. Soft tissue elongation based on the new range of motion,
4. Neuromuscular reeducation to restore normal movement to the area of aberrant motion,
5. Home program to maintain the increase in range of motion, quality of movement, and

to remove lever arms and fulcruming on the area of aberrant motion.

Important Factors

When considering a manual soft tissue approach the following factors must be considered:

Position of the Patient. The patient must be comfortable and supported. A neutral spinal position is necessary during most soft tissue techniques, but there are times when full length of the tissue is required for elongation techniques. Tissue tone is inhibited best when the myofascial unit is in a shortened range.

Position of the Therapist. The therapist must be comfortable. There must be minimal expenditure of energy by the therapist. Proper posturing and body mechanics are essential. A patient cannot relax when confronted with tension and imbalance on the therapist's part. Ergonomic chairs and high-low tables are helpful for achieving therapist comfort and increasing the efficiency of the treatment delivery.

Depth of Penetration. If during the palpatory examination the findings reveal superficial involvement, then the treatment techniques must be superficial in nature. For example, if the therapist penetrates the tissues too quickly, the posttreatment reactivity can be excessive. If it produces soreness for greater than 24 hours, then treatment was too vigorous or inappropriate techniques were chosen. Once the superficial connective tissue reacts normally to pressure stimuli, then deeper structures can be approached. It is imperative to follow the findings of the layer palpation examination.

If the patient's pain is acute, then the superficial techniques must also be considered. The primary goals would be more autonomic in nature rather than mechanical. The main goals here are the reduction of muscle tone, patient relaxation, restoration of normal diaphragmatic breathing, and desensitization of hyper-reactive tissue as in a "reflexive sympathetic dystrophy" type of behavior. After superficial tissues are successfully penetrated, techniques become more mechanical by design.

Amplitude of the Technique. The amplitude should be enough to produce a deformation of the desired myofascial structure. An example is the bending of a metal hanger, which results in a convex/concave relationship and a change in the metal surface tension. The net effect often results in a release of heat. The myofascial structure likewise, must be deformed to create changes in the collagen and the GAGs. In superficial techniques the frictioning creates an angular deformation of the connective tissue by shearing one layer upon another. The hard resistance found in the tissue is then broken down.

Direction of Technique

Soft tissue mobilization takes place into the direction of restriction. The direction is determined by the palpatory examination. The restriction may be in oblique, perpendicular, or parallel planes. Stretching will usually take care of parallel restrictions, but many tissue restrictions are in oblique planes. For example, an individual who does a great deal of sitting is subjected to a force from the edge of the chair perpendicular to the hamstrings. This may cause a "milking" out of the ground substance in the immediate contact area causing an approximation of collagen fibers and a restriction of the myofascial unit. During the palpation examination, the restriction is often found to be perpendicular to oblique: the direction of force during mobilization is perpendicular or oblique to the muscle.

Another example is the laying down of scar tissue, which is multi-directional. In an attempt to mobilize the tissue in the direction of function, all planes of restriction must be released.

Contraindication

Soft tissue mobilization should not be employed over tissues that are in a state of active inflammation. It should also be avoided over hypermobile or unstable segments of the spine such as in spondylolisthesis. However, soft tissue techniques would be quite appropriate above the displaced segment to remove any lever arms that may be influencing the positional fault.

REFERENCES

1. Ham AW, Cormack DH. Histology. Philadelphia PA: JB Lippencott, 1979.
2. Copenhaver WM, Bunge RP, et al. Bailey's textbook of histology. Baltimore: Williams & Wilkins, 1975.
3. Warwick R, Williams PL. Gray's anatomy, Vol 35. Philadelphia: WB Saunders Co, 1973.
4. Woo S, et al. Connective tissue response to immobility. Arthritis Rheum 1975; 18:257–264.
5. Akeson WH, Woo S, et al. The connective tissue response to immobilization: biochemical changes in periarticular connective tissue of the rabbit knee. Clin Orthop 1973; 93:356–362.
6. Akeson WH, Amiel D, et al. The connective tissue response to immobility: an accelerated aging response. Exp Gerontol 1968; 3:289–301.
7. Akeson WH, Amiel D, et al. Collagen cross linking alterations in joint contractures: changes in the reducible crosslinks in periarticular connective tissue after nine weeks of immobilization. Connect Tissue Res 1977; 5:15–19.
8. Akeson WH, Amiel D, et al. The connective tissue response to immobility: a study of the chondroitin 4 and 6 sulfate and dermatan sulfate changes in periarticular connective tissue of control and immobilized knees of dogs. Clin Orthop 1967; 5:190–197.
9. Akeson WH, Amiel D. Immobility effects of synovial joints: the pathomechanics of joint contracture. Biorheology 1980; 17:95–110.
10. Schiller S, Matthew M, et al. The metabolism of mucopolysaccharides in animals: further studies on skin utilizing C^{14} glucose, C^{14} acetate, and S^{35} sodium sulfate. J Biol Chem 1956; 218:139–145.
11. Schiller S, Matthew M, et al. The metabolism of mucopolysaccharides in animals: studies in skin using labeled acetate. J Biol Chem 1955; 212:434–531.
12. Newberger A, Slock H. The metabolism of collagen from liver, bones, skin, and tendon in normal rat. Biochem J 1953; 53:47–52.
13. Noyes F, Torvik PM, et al. Biomechanics of ligament failure: an analysis of immobilization, exercise and reconditioning effects on primates. J Bone Joint Surg 1974; 56A:1406.
14. Barfred T. Experimental rupture of the achilles tendon: comparison of various types of experimental rupture in rats. Acta Orthop Scand 1971; 42:528–543.
15. Noyes FR, DeLucas JI, et al. Biomechanics of anterior criciate ligament failure: an analysis of strain

rate sensitivity and mechanism of failure in primates. J Bone Joint Surg 1974; 56A:236–253.

16. Stouffer DC, Butler D. The relationship between crimp pattern and mechanical response of human patellar tendon-bone units. J Biomech Eng 1985; 197:158–165.

17. Williams PE, Goldspink G. Changes in sarcomere length and physiological properties in immobilized muscle. J Anat 1978; 127:459–468.

18. Fishback GD, Robbins N. Changes in contractile properties of disused soleus muscles. J Physiol 1969; 201:305–320.

19. Williams PE, Goldspink G. Connective tissue changes in immobilized muscle. J Anat 1984; 138:343–350.

20. Jones VT, Garrett WE, et al. Biomechanical changes in muscle after immobilization at different lengths. Trans Orthop Res Soc 1985; 10:6.

21. Tabery JC, Tabery C, et al. Physiological and structural changes in the cat's soleus muscle due to immobilization at different lengths by plaster casts. J Physiol 1972; 224:231–244.

22. McCully KK, Faulkner JA. Injury of skeletal muscle fibers of mice following lengthening contractions. J Appl Physiol 1985, 59:119–126.

23. Garrett WE, Seaber AV, et al. Recovery of skeletal muscle after laceration and repair. J Hand Surg 1984; 9A:682–692.

24. Jarvinen M. Healing of a crush injury in striated muscle. Acta Pathol Microbiol Scand 1976; 142:147–56.

25. Jarvinen M, Sorvari T. Healing of a crush injury in rat striated muscle: 1) description and testing of a new method of inducing a standard injury to the calf muscles. Acta Pathol Microbiol Scand 1975; 83:259–265.

26. Jarvinen M. Healing of a crush injury in rat striated muscle: 2) a histological study of the effect of early mobilization and immobilization on repair process. Acta Pathol Microbiol Scand 1975; 83:269–282.

27. Amiel D, Woo S, et al. The effect of immobilization on collagen turnover in connective tissue. Trans Orthop Res Soc 1981; 6:85.

28. Gillard GC, Reilly HC. The influence of mechanical forces on the glucosaminoglycan content of the rabbit flexor digitorum profundus tendon. Connect Tissue Res 1979; 7:37–46.

29. Evans E, Eggers G, et al. Experimental immobilization and mobilization of rat knee joints. J Bone Joint Surg 1960; 42-A:737–758.

30. Cummings G, et al. Soft tissue changes in contracture. Atlanta, GA: Stokesville Publishing Co., 1985; 9–45.

31. Frankel VH, Nordin M. Basic biomechanics of the skeletal system. Philadelphia, PA: Lea and Febiger, 1980: 90–99.

32. Warren CG, Lehmann JF, et al. Heat and stretch procedures: an evaluation using rat tail tendon. Arch Phys Med Rehabil 1976; 57:122–236.

33. Woo, SC, Ritter D, et al. The biomechanical and biochemical properties of swing tendons: long-term effects of exercise on the digital extensors. Connect Tissue Res 1980; 7:177–183.

34. Fung YCB. Elasticity of soft tissues in simple elongation. Am J Physiol 1967; 213:1532–1544.

35. Stromberg DD, Weiderhielm DA. Viscoelastic description of a collagenous tissue in simple elongation. J Appl Physiol 1969; 26:857–862.

36. Hooley CJ, McCrum NG, et al. The viscoelastic deformation of tendon. J Biomech 1980; 13:521–528.

37. LeBan MM. Collagen tissue: implications of it's response to stress in vitro. Arch Phys Med Rehabil 1962; 43:461–466.

38. Laros GS, Tipton CM, et al. Influence of physical activity on ligament insertions in the knees of dogs. J Bone Joint Surg 1971; 53A:275–286.

39. Tipton CM, Scheld RJ, et al. Influence of physical activity on the strength of knee ligaments in rats. Am J Physiol 1967; 212:783–787.

40. Wakim KG. The effects of massage on the circulation in normal and paralyzed extremities. Arch Phys Med 1949; 30:135.

41. Beard G, Wood E. Massage principles and techniques. Philadelphia; WB Saunders Co, 1965.

42. Wolfson H. Studies on effect of physical therapeutic procedures on function and structures. JAMA 1931; 96:2020.

43. Carrier EB. Studies on physiology of capillaries: reaction of human skin capillaries to drugs and other stimuli. Am J Physiol 1922; 61:528–547.

44. Pemberton R. Physiology of massage. In: AMA handbook of physical medicine and rehabilitation. Philadelphia: Blakinston Co, 1950:133.

45. Martin GM, Roth GM, et al. Cutaneous temperature of the extremities of normal subjects and patients with rheumatoid arthritis. Arch Phys Med Rehab 1946; 27:665.

46. Schneider EC, Havens LC. Changes in the content of haemoglobin and red corpuscles in the blood of men at high altitudes. Am J Physiol 1915; 36:360.

47. Lucia SP, Rickard JF. Effects of massage on blood platelet production. Proc Soc Exp Biol Med 1933; 31:87.

48. Cuthbertson DP. Effect of massage on metabolism: a survey. Glasgow Med J 1933; 2:200–213.

49. Dicke E, Schliack H. A manual of reflexive therapy of the connective tissue (connective tissue massage) (bindegwebbsmassage). Scarsdale, NY: Sidney S. Simon Publishers, 1978.

50. Ebner M. Connective tissue massage and therapeutic application. Huntington, NY; Kreiger, 1975.

51. Tappan F. Healing massage techniques: a study of

eastern and western methods. Reston, VA: Prentice Hall, 1975.

52. Rolf, I. Rolfing: the integration of human structures. Santa Monica, CA: Dennis-Landman Publishers, 1977.

53. Mennell JB. Physical treatment by movement, manipulation and massage. Philadelphia: Blakeston, 1945.

54. MacKenzie J. Angina pectoris. London, England: Henry Frowde and Hodder and Stroughton, 1923: 47.

55. Stockman, R. The courses, pathology and treatment of chronic rheumatism. Edinb Med J 1904; 15:107–116.

56. Hudson JI, Hudson MS, et al. Fibromyalgia and major affective disorder: a controlled phenomenology and family history study. Am J Psychiatry 1985; 142:441–446.

57. Goldenberg D. Fibromyalgia syndrome: an emerging but controversial condition. JAMA 257:2782–2803.

58. Travell J, Simons D. Myofascial pain and dysfunction: the trigger point manual. Baltimore: Williams & Wilkins, 1983.

10

Myofascial Release Concepts

ROBERT C. WARD

This chapter discusses the evolution, principles, and examples of correlative research underlying myofascial release concepts.

MANUAL MEDICINE: CONCEPTS

Seven core concepts highlight American osteopathic principles and manual medicine education. They are discussed according to current teaching and clinical practices rather than in historical order. I have been privileged to see virtually every manual therapy system practiced in both western and oriental cultures, including China and Japan. With the exceptions of high-velocity/low-amplitude and articulatory techniques, the techniques described below have evolved, by and large, through American osteopathy.

Manual Medicine and the Locomotor System

Manual medicine's evolution has focused primarily on the locomotor system, emphasizing neurological, orthopedic and pain-related concepts. The resulting models overlap and coincide in many ways, with explanations often differing.

Biologic Functions

What seems increasingly clear is the notion that in varying measure, manual treatments directly access not only neuromusculoskeletal and orthopedic functions, but also more basic biologic processes. How changes occur remains unclear, but clues are gradually appearing from different disciplines, mainly the neurosciences. A few synthesis papers have tried to bridge gaps, but many mysteries and opportunities for research remain.[1,2]

Muscle Energy Technique[3]

Muscle energy concepts and treatments were first presented in the 1950s by Fred L. Mitchell, Sr. They were synthesized from a pool of information passed on as oral history reflecting the views and experience of T.J. Ruddy, an early osteopathic eye, ears, nose, and throat specialist, and William Neidner. With the aid of Paul Kimberly, an expert functional anatomist, Dr. Mitchell developed and taught his first tutorials in the 1960s and 70s. The concepts which Fred L. Mitchell, Jr. and colleagues helped to clarify in a widely used book are now widely quoted and taught. Karel Lewit, MD, a professor of neurology at Charles University in Prague has used similar principles in describing postisometric relaxation (PR) techniques.[4]

Flexion, extension, sidebending, and rotation movements are used to identify pathophysiologic vertebral and joint positions. Operator-directed maneuvers are precisely applied against "abnormal" vertebral motion barriers as the patient isometrically resists. The goal is to restore physiologic joint motions.

Strain and Counterstrain Technique[5]

Strain and counterstrain concepts were developed by Lawrence Jones, DO. He observed that the body has multiple anterior and posterior "trigger points," not to be confused with trigger points described by Travell and Simons.[6] The goal is to identify offending triggers and "turn them off" by moving the offending joint or limb away from pain to a maximum position of comfort and holding the position for 90 seconds.

Craniosacral Concepts[7]

Craniosacral concepts were developed by a student of Dr. Still, William Garner Sutherland. Initially thought highly implausible, his system now receives considerable international attention, including basic, advanced and research-related texts by Kimberly, Magoun, Upledger, Greenman, and Retzlaff.[8–16] Some dentists and rehabilitation specialists dealing with craniocervical trauma and closed head injuries have begun to learn the system while many physicians and scientists remain puzzled and skeptical.

Sutherland suggested the possibility of subtle, identifiable, patterned cranial bone movements. He postulated that these movements are at least partially controlled by cerebrospinal fluid (CSF) mechanics inside the closed dural tube stretching from cranial to sacral attachments—hence the name craniosacral. Cranial bone movements have been documented by osteopathic physicians in a number of papers and presentations.[7–16] Using specially trained and highly developed palpatory skills, they assert that bony positions and movement patterns can be identified as readily as elsewhere in the body. However, their correlation with CSF dynamics, as suggested by Sutherland and others, has not been scientifically documented. A series of low-amplitude whole body wave-like pulses which ebb and flow averaging 8–10 cycles per minute appear to be a factor. They were discovered by Sutherland and his colleagues and documented by Adams,[16] and by myself and others at Michigan State University in the late 1980s in a series of unfunded pilot projects.

Cranial bone movements, amplitudes, and frequencies are highly variable in both normal and pathologic situations, varying from as low as 1–3/min in profoundly depressed patients to over 100/min in those with hypermetabolic or agitated psychiatric states.

The Treatment Goal. The objective is to restore functional symmetry to distorted cranial bone positioning and movements with the use of the palpating hands. Profound relaxation commonly occurs. Occasionally psychological responses become prominent. Whenever that phenomenon occurs, one assumes that a biofeedback-like series of autonomic responses are taking over. At this point treatment becomes infinitely more complex, esoteric, difficult and, to some extent, risky. The mind-body connection becomes real. The therapist should be ready and competent to handle the situation before venturing into this area.

Functional Concepts[17]

Functional concepts were developed by two groups of osteopathic physicians—a western group led by Lon Hoover, Sr., and an eastern group in the New England Academy of Osteopathy, led by William Johnston, Chester Bowles, and John Goodridge, along with Esther Smoot and George Andrew Laughlin.

Using subtle, highly sensitive, small, operator-induced maneuvers through a "motive" hand, the free hand monitors shifting areas of "ease" and "bind" in the spinal complex. The goal is to establish symmetrical joint movements, by monitoring small muscle changes and shifting vertebral joint activities.

High-Velocity/Low-Amplitude and Articulatory Concepts

These techniques, recipients of the most notoriety, have been used in varying ways for hundreds, perhaps thousands, of years. In essence, both high-velocity and articulatory maneuvers work to reestablish joint movements.

If done carefully and within ranges of joint

capability, articulatory maneuvers are by and large quite safe. High-velocity maneuvers, on the other hand, carry some risk and should be approached with caution. I know of and have served as an expert witness in several cases where manipulative disasters have occurred; these ranged from fractures to bilateral deafness, quadriparesis, quadriplegia, and four deaths. Two recent incidents, reported to me in August and September, 1990, included an undiagnosed prostatic carcinoma with metastasis to the vertebral column, including the neck, and a young man rendered bilaterally deaf following maneuvers to the upper neck, including backward bending thrusting force. In every reported fatal instance, the high-velocity maneuvers were followed by brainstem rupture and/or hemorrhage.[18]

Soft Tissue Release Concepts

Although used for many decades, little has been documented or written about myofascial release (fascial release) concepts. The system is as a complex form of soft tissue manipulation based on the operator's ability to monitor functional anatomic and neurologic influences.

Myofascial Release or Fascial Release (MFR)

Developed by American osteopathic practitioners, MFR led, with important exceptions, to clinically pertinent, fascially-based discussions almost exclusively in the osteopathic literature, but only after 1950.[19–26] Earlier practitioners often had learned varieties of these techniques from mentors and the oral tradition, and from concepts originated by Dr. Still.[27]

The concepts stand independently, but in practice are generally more effective when integrated with functional and craniosacral principles (described above). Even with only a little experience, it is apparent that powerful but poorly understood release mechanisms can be invoked to modify musculoskeletal relationships at many levels.

When substantial central, autonomic, and behavioral pathology exists, there are bound to be problems.[28] Under these circumstances, manual methods of any kind, including myofascial release can be either helpful or potentially aversive and counterproductive. Surprising help occurs in some situations with significant lack of success in seemingly similar cases. Many mysteries remain. Given these realities, the conclusion must be that disrupted neurohumoral, autonomic, and behavioral factors link soft tissue, arthrodial joints, and biomechanical changes in ambiguous ways.

MODELS AND MECHANISMS: FOUR MAJOR THEMES AT WORK

Four major themes highlight myofascial considerations: (a) genetics, conformation, and behavior; (b) impulse-based and nonimpulse-based factors;[29] (c) mechanical mechanisms; and (d) the *tight-loose* concept, a synthesis of the first three.

Genetics, Conformation, and Behavior

We often note how individuals reflect their genetic potential and this is true for responses to myofascial release. Each of us is configured in both obscure and obvious ways, e.g., children often look, move, and behave as their parents and grandparents; some are fearful, others fearless. There is a vast body of literature dealing with these issues, both concrete and esoteric.

Impulse-Based and Nonimpulse-Based Mechanisms

Impulse-Based Mechanisms. These highlight neural and electrical factors. For example, piezoelectric effects arising from shifting Na^+, K^+, Ca^{++}, and Mg^{++} pumps control complex cellular functions, synaptic transmissions, muscle contractions, and generalized skeletal forces. Reflexes are activated, chemical and electrical relationships change, muscles contract, and locomotor activities are carried out.

Muscle and joint receptors, including Golgi tendon organs, Ruffini endings, and Pacinian corpuscles, link up with annulospiral units, dense connective tissue, tendons, apo-neuroses, and fascial planes to provide joint movements and locomotion.[30]

Nonimpulse Based Mechanisms. These are marked by nutritional and biochemically mediated functions. Metabolic functions associated with axoplasmic flow, general neurotrophic functions, collagen, and elastin effects make up this category. Examples are: variable rates of rostral to caudal axoplasmic flow which are functions of neuronal size and volume; and proteoglycan-fibroblast-collagen turnover as influenced by myriad mechanical and neuroendocrine functions.[31] Excellent discussions of these concepts can be found in five texts: Basmajian's: *Muscles Alive*; Bonica's: *The Management of Pain*, Korr's edited work: *The Neurobiologic Mechanisms in Manipulative Therapy*, and White and Panjabi's: *Clinical Biomechanics of the Spine*.[32–36] Research delving into soft tissue and muscle pain factors is now common.[37–39] Multiple theories are appearing. Some are research-based like those in Bonica, Melzack, and Wall's texts noted above, while others are more speculative.[40–42]

Mechanical Mechanisms

Mechanical mechanisms highlight force, movement, acceleration, deceleration, i.e., rate of change, strain, and deformation—i.e., rheologic events and their effects. Mechanical events, based on Newtonian laws, deform vascular, neural, and cellular networks. Each exerts independent mechanical effects.[43–45] Movements of cytoskeletons and their contents, soft tissues, arthrodial joints, and complex kinesiologic and skeletal mechanics fall in this category.[46] For example, both local and general soft tissue and vertebral mechanics are commonly disrupted. Such alterations suggest mechanically-based changes, as well as reflex and neurovascular factors with broader biologic effects.

Vertebral motions: concepts, research, and teaching. Early in the 20th century, Harrison Fryette, DO, after studying the 1903 work of Robert Lovett, MD, reported on vertebral motions and their properties in a 1918 paper.[47] Later, his concepts were refined by Beal and Beckwith.[48,49] Citations of this early work are virtually absent in world literature. Subsequent work by Aho[50] and Moll,[51] along with more recent studies by Pearcy[52] and many others continue in this important area.

The Tight-Loose Concept—a Synthesis of Other Factors

Looseness and tightness are coexisting asymmetrical three-dimensional phenomena that can be traced systematically anywhere in the body.[53] They are natural, but complicated, responses to seemingly chaotic asymmetrical loads and forces imposed on an already asymmetrical biological system of soft and hard tissues. The phenomenon reflects complex physiologic and behavioral factors interacting mechanically with passive support systems. Responses are nonlinear and asymmetrical.

Nonlinear Mechanics Characterize All Biologic Systems. Both symmetrical and asymmetrical forces deform a heterogeneous soft tissue matrix. Bending, twisting, shearing, compression, and extension forces create predictably unpredictable responses—particularly if sudden and/or repetitive forces load the system excessively. Varying amounts of intrinsic elasticity, i.e., stiffness, permit either slow or rapid deformations. Return to pre-stress configurations depends on the loads and forces involved and whether damage occurs. Some areas unload and become looser, while others simultaneously load and become tighter. This phenomenon is independent of all other effects and results from both small and large accommodations to every imaginable biologic and behavioral activity.

Loosening and tightening arise from mechanical, thermal, neural, endocrinologic and behavioral events:

- **Mechanical forces** bend, twist, compress, shear, and extend, i.e., distract.
- **Thermal activities** heat and loosen or cool and tighten.
- **Neural events** create central, peripheral, and autonomic effects.
- **Endocrinologic events** increase and de-

crease all other activities, e.g., enhancing and inhibiting neural activities or changing fluid volume and mechanics as a function of renin-angiotensin activity.

- **Behavior is the net result**, contributing to the others through both conscious and unconscious mechanical efforts. Feedback loops are closed. Structure and function are inseparable.

If forces and movements are benign and there is no injury, tissues and joints gradually return to previous shapes, usually within minutes to hours. However, if there is even a small breakdown in the passive support system, accommodative tightening and loosening occur both in the immediate vicinity and elsewhere. A cycle has begun.

For reasons not entirely clear, the loosened site is frequently accompanied by inhibited muscle activity.[54] Muscles fire, and they fatigue sooner. The area is proprioceptively and kinesthetically more active, with patients commonly reporting heightened sensations of "tightness" or pain when actual loosening is present.

An example: Inhibited, loose soft tissues such as the left quadratus lumborum often are accompanied by accommodative tightening of right quadratus lumborum. Deeper ipsilateral rotatores and intertransversarii are also tight with inhibited facet joint movements. If the examiner's focus is limited to vertebral mechanics, discs and facets—as commonly occurs—much will be missed.

Available technology cannot regularly and accurately differentiate the important from the unimportant. Given this clinical reality, it becomes realistic to use sensitively trained palpation for exploration and clarification. (See Table 10.1.)

Tethering. Tethering inhibits any and all movements away from tightness and compression almost always permits further compression. The rule holds true for small and large areas alike. Mechanical lines of force alter the system as much or more than anatomical groupings.

Patterns. Forces come in many forms. Long-lasting gravitational effects change pos-

tural patterns over a lifetime. When sudden uncontrolled bending and twisting injuries superimpose new and often irreversible effects, new patterns are created. Whether and to what extent old patterns can adapt to new demands often defines subsequent disability.

For example, normal thoracic and lumbar sidebending create vertebral rotations toward the formed convexity. With aging comes progressive loss of joint movement capabilities—some earlier, others later. General soft tissue responses tighten concavities while convexities loosen. The system becomes stiffer. Gravitational and weight-bearing loads are superimposed on the failing skeleton. Muscles weaken, particularly extensor groups. Stiffening fascia, ligament, and bone, the passive supports, carry increasing loads. Kyphotic, lordotic and scoliotic curves progress, further inhibiting "normal" mechanics. Sudden twisting trauma, regardless of type, forces an already weakened system to accommodate. Disability, seemingly greater than the injury might cause, commonly follows.

The only way of assessing these effects is through skilled palpation, because, perversely, both concavities and convexities often feel superficially tight due to passive support stiffening.

Table 10.1
A Good Rule to Remember[a]

TIGHTNESS IS AN AREA OF COMPRESSION. INDUCTION OF EITHER ACTIVE OR PASSIVE MOTIONS GENERALLY CREATES GREATER MOVEMENT TOWARD TIGHTNESS

AND

TIGHTNESS HAS A TETHERING EFFECT. INDUCTION OF EITHER ACTIVE OR PASSIVE MOTIONS PERMITS LESS MOVEMENT AWAY FROM TIGHTNESS.

COROLLARY 1

TIGHTNESS CREATES AND LOOSENESS (WEAKNESS) PERMITS POSITIONS OF DEFORMITY

COROLLARY 2

ISOLATED MUSCLE WEAKENING COMMONLY ACCOMPANIES BOTH TIGHTNESS AND LOOSENESS

[a]A good way to remember the rule: tightness reflects shortening. The area in question has become either relatively or absolutely compressed and tethered down.

FUNCTIONAL ANATOMICAL CONSIDERATIONS

This section discusses general anatomical factors influencing the hard and soft tissues of the myofascial system from a clinical perspective.

Definitions

Hard Tissues. For purposes of this discussion, hard tissue is mainly bone. Movement capability is inhibited by stiffness imposed by the proteoglycan matrix and calcium salts. Bones are anchors for soft tissues, i.e., the myofascial complex. Bony and joint configurations directly influence available motion.

Soft Tissues. Soft tissues are here defined as anything other than bone. Included are skin, subcutaneous tissues, fascias, muscles, ligaments, viscera, nerves, blood vessels, lymphatics, groups of cells, as well as individual cells and their contents. They are a physically diverse, multifunctional, biologic amalgam of reflex, vascular, endocrine, and nutritional factors. To coin a metaphor, "we live in our soft tissues." They are where most biologic functions occur. As life progresses, both normal and abnormal movement patterns are established in response to myriad loads and forces.

Injuries

Clear diagnoses of soft tissue and somatically-based pain are blurred by complex primary and secondary mechanical responses. Obviously neural, vascular, and mechanical factors play large roles. Characterizing such changes is another question entirely.

Neurally-based currents of injury come from many sources. For example, in the early 1970s, Fernandez and Ramirez demonstrated increased muscle fibrillation by blocking axoplasmic transport.[55] Constant aversive autonomic stimuli have been shown to create vague burning responses, even though causalgia and reflex sympathetic dystrophy are not classically present.[56]

Some Soft Tissues Function as Hard Tissues

Because of high stiffness factors, tendons, some ligaments, thicker fascias, and scars demonstrate some hard tissue functions. After submaximal deformations these relatively immobile and avascular tissues return to their original shapes rather quickly, usually within minutes to a few hours. Importantly, they often anchor other soft tissues—muscles, nerves, and blood vessels.

Wolff's Law Applies to Hard and Soft Tissues Alike

Wolff's law implies that deformations occur along directions of force. A corollary might suggest that new loads impose new movement patterns forcing further adaptations.

In an unpublished 1983 study, Reynolds, White, and I studied a series of 15 skeletons in the Hamann-Todd Collection at Case Western Reserve University. Consistent deformation patterns were identified among series of vertebrae, ilia, and sacra, suggesting that Wolff's Law can be applied throughout the skeletal complex (Fig. 10.1). The August 1990 Gordon Conference on Biomechanics in New Hampshire was devoted exclusively to this phenomenon.

Overlapping Mechanical Properties of Active and Passive Tissues

All active tissues have passive functions and vice-versa. Each has distinct characteristics that can be systematically explored.

Active Tissues. Nerves, muscles, blood vessels, lymphatics, and active components of cells carry out active physiologic functions. While carrying on functions they deform elastically and plastically. Therefore, all active tissues have passive functions and vice-versa.

Passive Tissues. By supporting and separating, they give form while permitting and constraining movement. Collagen and elastin predominate. They are: bone, cartilage, fascia, tendon, aponeuroses, ligaments, vascular and neural support tissues, and cell membranes.

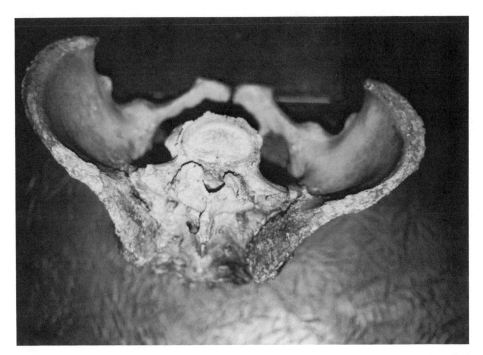

Figure 10.1. L5 and pelvis from above: Wolff's Law in action. Note major bony asymmetries, including pubic ramus, brim of the pelvis, and facets. Bridging is extensive, and effects of long-term asymmetrical loading are evident.

Examples

Neural tissues, usually defined as active, have varying amounts of collagen and elastin. Dorsal roots contain more collagen, are thicker and less elastic, while longer peripheral nerves and autonomic plexuses are more elastic and flexible.

Sudden, unhindered mechanical deformations often disrupt stiffer collagenized tissues with resulting pathologic disruption and fibroblastic healing. Both mechanical and neural connections have been permanently altered, some areas tighter, others looser.

Two common clinical examples are:

1. *Congestive heart failure* with pathologically altered neurohumoral feedback mechanisms creating generalized edema, including changes in skeletal, lymphatic[57] and myofascial mechanics.
2. *Inversion ankle sprain* with both local and generalized mechanical accommodations to injury, with hemorrhage, swelling, and pain-related postural accommodations for plantar surfaces upward.

Cadaveric Research

In a 1988 study, George and the author demonstrated that fascias and aponeuroses at multiple levels demonstrate long-term effects of both loading and age-related changes in a cadaver of an elderly person. Loss of structural and neurovascular coherence in fascial sheaths was particularly striking in this ninth decade cadaver (Figs. 10.2–10.4). This observation links well with others, noting that Golgi tendon organs are found not only in myotendinous junctions, but also in fascial sheaths as well as fine and dense connective tissues everywhere in the body.[58]

Inferences

From the foregoing we make three inferences:

1. There is little functional separation between muscle and fascia.
2. Normal and pathophysiologic form and function are intimate inseparable parts of the whole.
3. Altered myofascial relationships signal both

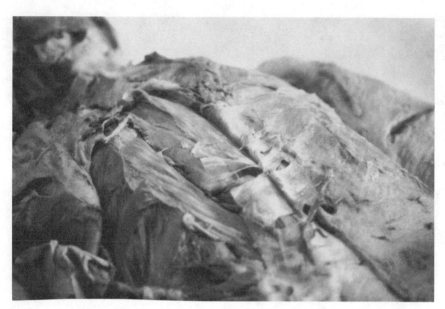

Figure 10.2. Fascia in gross dissection. Fat is minimal. Fascial layers are variably dense. Some are thin, others thicker and heterogeneous. Note differences in myotendinous attachments of the erector spinae. Observe also, the fine layering and integration of muscles in relation to fascias. The latter are simultaneously continuous with some muscles while covering and separating others.

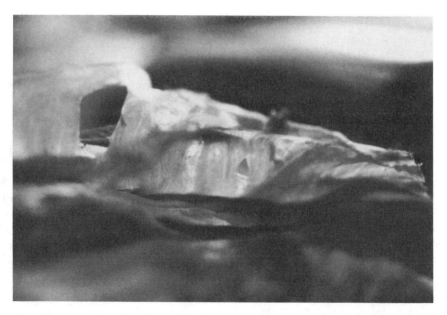

Figure 10.3. Avascular fascia and deformation effects. This is a closer, backlit view, of a portion of fascia from Figure 10.2. Note its avascularity and heterogeneity. Collagen predominates. The holes are artifact from preparation. Note the heterogeneity suggesting that a lifetime of variable stresses and loads strained fibers in multiple directions. Some are still strong, but many have disappeared, leaving a filmy collagenous covering where stronger supports predominated earlier in life. Wolff's Law applies to bones and soft tissues alike. A second finding was rather startling. It was virtually impossible to separate muscle from fascia in many areas. Sharp dissection was needed and myofascial attachments were often damaged in the process. (See Fig. 10.4)

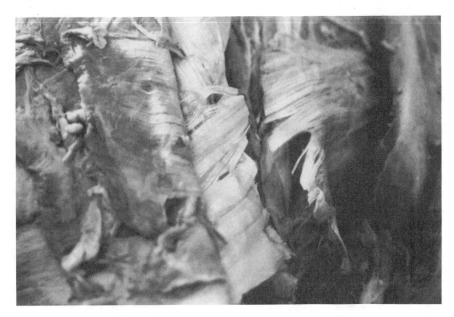

Figure 10.4. Sharp dissection difficulties. This is the cut edge of a rhomboid muscle. Note directional differences in myotendinous and muscle fiber attachments. The reflected portion was impossible to sep-arate from heavier collagenous myotendinous attachments. Based on this finding, it appears that tendon, muscle, and fascia (myofascias) are functionally inseparable.

local and distant mechanical, neural, and vascular effects.[59,60]

Clinical Inferences. What does this mean clinically? Altered movement patterns imposed by aging, injuries, disease, and lifestyle create pathomechanical adaptations. Stress-induced deformations occur at interfaces between hard and soft tissues. Often, not surprisingly, this is problematic.

For example, sudden twist of the craniocervical spine in a motor vehicle accident commonly creates permanent soft tissue and arthrodial joint changes with accompanying central autonomic and peripheral neurologic effects. Similar effects occur with varieties of low back injuries.[58]

Active and Passive Tissues Create and Respond to Movements

The ability to create and respond to movements are functions of: 1) skeletal and soft tissue conformation; 2) neurologic status including pain-related factors; 3) thermoregulatory states; 4) constantly shifting locomotor demands, 5) physical conditioning, and 6) body positions.

Skeletal and Soft Tissue Conformation. We are all accustomed to identifying those we know from long distances. They may stand tall, slump, hold their head in a special way, or swing the arms asymmetrically. Whether they are moving, sitting, standing, or lying down, makes little difference; we know who they are. Their conformations are readily identifiable to an intimate—the body as "fingerprint." Conformation patterns enhance and constrain all movements from the cell to the whole body.

Neural Factors

These play important roles. Neurologic status includes behavioral, cognitive and pain-related factors. Locating purely neural disability in long-term problems is a real challenge because they are both common and difficult to sort out. Deficits are hard to change when central, autonomic, and peripheral processing is fundamentally altered. Assistance is often temporary and relapse common.

Variables. Bonica suggests analyzing variables in four ways: 1) the peripheral nervous system; 2) the spinal dorsal horn, and medullary dorsal horn (trigeminal caudal nucleus); 3) the ascending systems, including substrates of head pain; and 4) the supraspinal systems.[61]

Tightness, Looseness and the Sensory Experience. These are affected by neural factors. Altered peripheral transmission arises from many sources. Soft tissue injuries and their painful sensations occur through electrical, thermal, chemical, and mechanical processes.[62] The information network is centrally controlled and behaviorally driven.

The clinician must decide: Is tightness and looseness a mainly neurologic phenomenon? How many of the phenomena are impulse or nonimpulse based? How important are they?

For example does looseness result from direct injury with inhibited muscle function[63] or is it associated with secondary degenerative factors such as diabetes or hypothyroidism? OR: is generalized tightening in an isolated site a combination of normal response to agonist-antagonist loosening in the immediate area as well as at points distant and also a reflection of accommodations to an old sports injury?

Other examples: Paresis associated with isolated nerve injuries and mild to severe postpolio paresis.

Neural Networks Have Memory. With only a little experience, one soon learns that neural networks have memories that are asymmetrical. Patient complaints and motor problems recur in the same sites even after healing, particularly when under stress. Some of these changes occur at the cord level.[60]

Identifying Sensory Asymmetries. In oneself this is fairly easy. Locate areas of previous injury. Notice how quickly sensory feedback is available from allegedly recovered sites. Our bodies literally encode and remember.[64] *Patients relay this information to health care providers in their own words.*

Immediately, problems of communication arise. Responses aggregate into many or few ambiguously defined aversive, hyperalgesic sensations that may or may not be identifiable using current technology. Given the complexities, there should be little wonder such information is commonly misinterpreted.

Shifting Locomotor Demands

At different ages we perform different tasks. As the nervous system learns, the myofascial and skeletal systems respond. As general tasks involving the whole body take over, such as standing, sitting, walking, and running, genetically determined response patterns are built in and reinforced. Each skill places special demands that alter myofascial and skeletal response patterns. Each movement pattern creates variable tight-loose demands at different sites.

New learnings are superimposed on preexisting skills and patterns. Some adapt and work well and others not at all. Playing basketball does not imply one can play the piano, although it neither includes nor excludes the possibility. Working and playing with injuries add further complications.

Pathologic learning creates accommodative loosening and tightening. Linking with effects of previous injury, conditioning, and advancing age, *the myofascial complex usually weakens.* The process is always asymmetrical, and vulnerability to further injury is common.

Thermoregulatory State

Both local and distant normal and pathophysiologic processes generate thermal effects. Skin and other soft tissue temperatures change periodically and dramatically. Thermal factors affect circadian, nutritional, central, autonomic, peripheral neural, and hormonal states, and vice-versa. Mechanical factors are influenced.

Acute, subacute, and long-term thermoregulatory alterations often work aversively in an otherwise normal system. Some areas have increased temperatures, others cooler. Energy is consumed in the process. Acute and subacute sites are warmer, chronic sites generally cooler. Such changes are often palpable.

Technologies, such as thermography, readily identify differences. With some exceptions, however, they have not proved generally practical. Unfortunately, correlations with other diagnostic methods is not high.[65] Whether or not magnetic resonance imaging will assist diagnosis in a cost-effective manner has yet to be determined.

Physical Conditioning

Usually thought of in terms of general cardiovascular-cardiopulmonary and neuromusculoskeletal terms, physical conditioning should be broadened to understand effects of asymmetrical tightening and loosening in the myofascial system. Loose joints, for example, the knee, often trigger asymmetrical tightening and loosening from plantar fascias to the head and neck.

Athletes and Others. Well-conditioned athletes, such as runners, basketball players, gymnasts, and dancers frequently are disabled because of a failure to appreciate the tight-loose phenomenon. News media regularly report these effects among high profile athletes. On the other hand, repetitive daily activities in the general public create the same problems. Deconditioning follows disuse and is followed by asymmetric combinations of loosening and weakness. Disability has begun or is made worse.

Body Positions

Body positions are obviously affected by gravity, but neurologic and conformational accommodations create major and minor weight-bearing shifts. Both general musculoskeletal and less apparent myofascial forces behave differently at the same site.

An example is the thoracolumbar junction which acts as a major mechanical transitional zone. It anchors the costal cage, diaphragm, and iliopsoas complex, as well as thoracolumbar fascias, trunk rotators, quadratus lumborum, latissimus dorsi, and trapezius. Proximal craniocervical and shoulder girdle factors directly relate to lumbopelvic and lower extremity mechanics across this area. Careful static and dynamic observation and palpation are essential, as will be described below.

DIAGNOSIS
Broad Approach Essential

Myofascial diagnosis requires a broad approach. Somatically-based diagnoses should always include multiple hypotheses from many possible sources. It is not the task here to cover all diagnostic possibilities, but an adequate and detailed history is essential.

Most manual medicine systems are taught narrowly from a vertebral and joint mechanics perspective. Strong emphasis on one or two such areas to the exclusion of other possibilities, while common, is fraught with problems, particularly for the patient.

Patient Characteristics and History

At a minimum, inferences should be made based on knowledge of the individual's:

● *Genetics and Sex-Linked Factors.* For example a tall, slender woman with Marfan-like features is more vulnerable mechanically than a short, stocky, muscular male office worker.

● *Symptoms.* Those associated with loose skeletal tissues, or life-threatening vascular problems must be thoroughly explored. I have encountered many cases of previously undiagnosed diabetic neuropathy, coronary heart disease, metastatic disease, and aorto-femoral disease with associated muscle weakening and claudication symptoms.

● *Chronological Age.* For example, if a 36-year-old sedentary male office worker persistently exercises for more than 30 minutes once a week and experiences neck and left shoulder pain, is the complaint heart, vascular, neurological, postural, mechanical—or some of each?

● *Work and Sports History.* For example, repetitive combined bending and twisting movements for either short or long periods should be explored. Does persistent strain and load aggravate preexisting problems?

● *Socioeconomic Status and Educational Level.* These are important. For example, an inability to financially cope often accompanies difficulty with abstract reasoning. Often this leads to additional stress, frustration, social paralysis, and depression signaled by somatic complaints.

• *Expectations of Patient, Family, and Examiner.* These include context and payment mechanisms for the evaluation. Perception and context are crucial. Stress and somatic complaints are common when third parties and litigators are in the picture. Problems arise, for example, around how disability is defined by each party. One person's disability, no matter how severe, can be a mere annoyance to another.

• *History Should Include—*

—directions of externally imposed forces; for example in auto accidents and sport injuries often help map superimposed soft tissue alterations.
—general health status
—general medical issues such as endocrine status or osteoporosis
—general neurological status
—central and peripheral neurologic insults such as closed head injuries, loss of consciousness, herpes zoster, cerebrovascular accidents, and Parkinsonism.
—mechanical traumas of all types over a lifetime including, birth trauma, physical abuse, and head trauma
—diseases affecting soft tissues, such as polio, the arthritides, diabetes, gout, endocrinopathies in general.

• *Psychological Influences Include—*

—*Understanding the role of both depression and somatization* in sustaining soft tissue pains is an essential ingredient in the process. Central and operant learning, as well as autonomically mediated pain and hyperactivity often aggravate the picture. Sleep disturbance is common. One should remember that affective/behavioral disabilities are more often a disability's consequences rather than causes.
—behavioral and psychological factors, associated psychological and sexual abuse, helplessness, poor ego, strength and low self esteem
—psychopathology independent of abuse

When the foregoing are clarified, palpatory diagnosis and design of a treatment plan can begin.

• *Injury History.*

—All the usual factors plus relationship of biomechanical forces imposed by those injuries

Palpation

Joint movements are affected by soft tissues, and vice-versa. Skilled palpation identifies both gross and subtle abnormalities when other methods, such as electophysiologic testing, imaging, blood chemistries, and even surgical explorations yield ambiguous information. The process can assess discrete small sites or whole body effects for asymmetry, tissue texture abnormalities, and motion changes or whole body changes. With some practice, three-dimensionally-related tight-loose effects become apparent.

Palpation: The Sensory Experience. The goal is to locate subtle and even gross, otherwise hidden dysfunctional sites. Careful, knowledgeable exploration frequently uncovers changes that correlate perfectly with the reported sensory experience. Sites can be either loose or tight, exhibiting either tissue laxity or muscle spasm as well as joint looseness or tightness. Sites are often asymptomatic unless mechanically stressed.

Observation and Palpation Clarify Myofascial Factors—Myofascial Assessment

• Static palpatory analysis identifies tight-loose changes without inducing active or passive movement.

• Dynamic palpatory analysis identifies changes using varieties of actively and passively induced forces.

• Both general and local assessments examine the same sites in multiple positions.

• Symptomatic and dysfunctional sites are repetitively examined using the four primary positions: standing, seated, prone, and supine and the four primary movements: forward bending, backward bending, rotation, and sidebending.

With experience, it becomes apparent that more is going on than classic orthopedic and neurologic assessments suggest.

Functional Analysis: Static and Dynamic Posture and the Tight-Loose Concept

Local and distant patterns are compared and correlated. Sometimes myofascial structures are loose, sometimes they are tight. Learning to think three-dimensionally helps.

Because shifting from one mode to the other creates different loading demands, static findings often hide dynamic effects and vice-versa. Tightness and looseness factors shift.

After palpating for static tightness and looseness patterns, have the patient move about. Motions are either greater in the direction of tight concavities or lesser as convexities are straightened. Myofascial findings may or may not correlate with skeletal and vertebral motions in the immediate vicinity. Most of the time they do, but they fail this criterion often enough that one must be alert and remember to go beyond mere skeletal and joint analysis. With practice, both large contractions and subtle, smaller movements can be appreciated. The eye can lead the hand and vice-versa.

Patterns

Systematically assess local sites in a context of the whole, because patterns come from many sources. Remember that body conformation has a lot to do with tightness and looseness. A finely tuned athlete is as apt to demonstrate clinically important asymmetry as a stroke patient. The dimensions are simply different.

Standing, walking, bending, and twisting create total body responses from plantar fascias to cranial vault. For example, lower extremity and lumbopelvic mechanics interact intimately and directly with diaphragm, costal cage, shoulder girdle, and craniocervical systems.

You must consider:

- total body configuration remembering that everyone is asymmetrical;
- individual and group muscle configurations;
- shifts in three-dimensional static and movement-related tightness and looseness of bilaterally similar muscle groups.

Examples. These include—

1. Right versus left gluteus maximus and medius relationships to hamstrings, quadriceps, and pelvic mechanics.
2. Standing hip extension quickly identifies widespread, three-dimensionally-related, asymmetrical, tightening and loosening effects.
3. Lower extremities frequently flex or extend reciprocally; thus lumbopelvic mechanics become more or less oblique, or the thoracolumbar junction and sacral base often flatten or become lordotic.
4. Costal cage and trunk rotators commonly shift in a variety of directions both individually and together according to which hip is extended.
5. The "hip drop test," flexing one knee while keeping the other leg straight with both heels on the floor, often identifies startlingly different hip, sacroiliac joint, sacral base, and general lumbopelvic shifts.
6. Seated postures, both slumped and erect, give further information, as do prone and supine assessments.

Gait and the Tight-Loose Concept

After findings are documented, walk the patient back and forth a few times. Correlate lower extremity movements with lumbopelvic, costothoracic, shoulder girdle, and craniocervical mechanics. Frontal, posterior, and side views are essential.

Focus on the low back, noting changes in hamstring and knee relationships, sacroiliac joint, sacral base, lumbar muscles, trunk rotaters, and diaphragm. Link them to costothoracic, shoulder girdle, and craniocervical spine. Always explore tightness and looseness, because tightness and looseness often vary according to the layer of tissue palpated.

A Common Craniocervical Pattern

One common pattern demonstrates tight left cervical tissue from basiocciput to thoracic inlet. The cervical spine is sidebent toward the tightness. Its curve is concave on the left.

Right sidebending is inhibited because of tethering effects.

One or two vertebrae may be partially immobile or tend to rotate toward the formed convexity (so-called Type I mechanics), while individual soft tissues behave idiosyncratically and unpredictably. Tightness or looseness can occur on either the inside or outside of the formed curve.

Example. Induction of left cervical sidebending should create a smooth firm feeling on the inside of the curve as vertebrae rotate toward the formed concavity. Commonly, C3, 4, and/or C5 coupled movements fail to move smoothly as the concavity forms. Locally the area becomes even tighter near and around synovia on the inside of the curve. Overlying soft tissues are tight. Facets either open or close with the net effect that already tight areas become tighter. Not surprisingly, both unilateral and bilateral neurologic complaints are common with this phenomenon. Knowledgeable palpation helps clarify.

Sacral, Sacroiliac, and Iliosacral Mechanics

These are subtle and two definitions are required—

Sacroiliac responses refer to activities associated with spinal and proximal body factors.

Iliosacral responses refer to activities associated with lower extremity factors.

Pure sacroiliac movements are alleged to be similar to cervical movements,[66] but one cannot be sure. Some even continue the argument that the sacroiliac joints fail to move, although such movements have been documented many times.[67–71]

Lumbopelvic Functions and the Tight-Loose Concept

Although many texts separate sacral and innominate movements, sacroiliac and iliosacral mechanics, the concepts are more theoretical than practical. The lower lumbar spine, sacrum, pelvis, lower extremities, and shoulders often operate as an integrated unit. For example, prone hip extensions by patients with chronic low back pain complaints commonly engage contralateral trapezius, latissimus dorsi, and glenohumeral external rotaters. This may or may not be the case in other primary positions, i.e., standing, seated, or supine.

For all intents and purposes, lower lumbar motion is inseparably linked with sacral and innominate mechanics through:

- sacroiliac, sacrotuberous, and sacrospinous ligaments from below,
- lumbodorsal fascia and iliolumbar ligaments above, and
- anterior ilioinguinal, hip, and trunk rotator attachments, which include but are not limited to myofascial attachments across the pubic rami and rectus fascias.

Example. Anterior rotation of the right innominate is frequently associated with:

—loosening of antagonists, both ipsilateral and contralateral

—tight ipsilateral anterior thigh groups (quadriceps and adductors) with associated ipsilateral loosening of the right hip joint along with inhibited (loose) hip extensors and thigh abductors.

—tight close-packing of the left sacroiliac joint and left L5-iliolumbar ligament system. These involve the posterior left innominate, a tight left sacrotuberous ligament, a tight left hamstring, and apparently L5 rotates left. Statically, the left transverse process feels posterior. Dynamically, the system moves more easily left and less easily right. Sometimes findings are the opposite, so one must be alert.

Form and Function Are Inseparable

Now that we are aware that form and function interact together, varieties of tightness and looseness should become evident.

Example. The patient is neurologically intact. The lumbar curve is convex left at L4–5, then right at L1–2. Accompanying myofascial asymmetry involves tightness of the right lumbodorsal fascias near the sacral base with relative loosening on the opposite side. Quadratus lumborum is tight beneath the right lumbodorsal fascias and relatively loose on the left. Right trunk rotators are loose left and tight right. There is a *three-dimensional corkscrew effect*. Charting the findings might look like Table 10.2.

What Does It All Mean

Even with all these "positive" findings, one cannot be sure. Because identifiable neuromusculoskeletal dysfunction does not imply an accurate and appropriate diagnosis, avoidance of under- and overtreatment is essential. Failure to respond to treatment always calls for appropriate referral and consultation.

Ultimately and empirically, all we can know is that soft tissues work against hard tissues in myriad ways. Hard tissue movements force soft tissues to asymmetrically accommodate, and vice-versa. Wolff's law is always at work: bones, and by extension myofascial tissues, deform according to loads placed upon them. Tightness and looseness result.

If loading is excessive, tissues accommodate by forming new patterns. Mechanical, anatomical, neurologic, and neurovascular adjustments occur. Muscles and their investments, the myofascial system, become asymmetrically tight or loose.

PRINCIPLES OF MYOFASCIAL RELEASE TREATMENT

Goal of Treatment

The goal is to establish functional three-dimensional whole body symmetry within the ability of the patient to adapt. There are thirteen principles on the following pages.

Principle 1. The palpating hands should become as sensitive as a blind persons's.

Principle 2. Functional assessments three-dimensionally integrate, both local and whole body findings.

Principle 3. Because of different load and force demands, assessments work best by separating out effects of the four primary positions and the four primary motions.

The *four primary positions* are: standing, seated, prone, and supine.

The *four primary motions* are: flexion, extension, sidebending, and rotation.

Principle 4. Palpatory evaluations should test the same sites passively, because passive testing gives more accurate information.

Principle 5. Static and dynamic assessments continuously evaluate tightness, looseness, and asymmetry from skin to deepest spinal structures.

Principle 6. Releases are more efficient when the patient is completely relaxed.

Principle 7. Releases use both direct and indirect approaches.

Principle 8. Tightness is the focus for all releases. Sometimes pain and tightness correlate, often they do not. Palpation is the only way of knowing.

Principle 9. Barriers, both direct and indirect, are released using combinations of direct and indirect maneuvers.

Direct maneuvers traverse relatively short motion ranges to end-points. Joints and soft tissues feel tight and compressed; the end-feel is quite firm.

Indirect maneuvers seek end-points by traversing longer ranges of motion reciprocal to the direct. The end-feel is usually, but not always, much softer.

How Releases Occur

Releases occur by applying carefully directed forces against barriers, i.e., tightness. They occur in at least four ways:

Forcible Separation or Compression of Joints. As external loading either separates or

Table 10.2
Sample Chart of Findings

Tight	Loose
1. Left L 4–5 convexity	1. Right L4–5 concavity
2. Right lumbodorsal fascias near sacral base	2. Right lumbodorsal fascias opposite side
3. Right quadratus lumborum	3. Left quadratus lumborum
4. Right trunk rotators proximally	4. Left trunk rotators distally

compresses, everything from skin surfaces to deepest components of the spinal complex is forced to respond. Examples are direct release of barriers at the sacral base in relation to inferior aspects of L5 and release of the thoracolumbar junction.

Forcible Loading of Asymmetrically Tightened Myofascial Tissues. For example, the left thoracolumbar junction is commonly tighter than the right (the tight-loose concept). Usually this involves both a reflex tightening on the left and reciprocal loosening on the right. Lumbar spine, lower costal cage, diaphragm, and skeletal mechanics are usually asymmetrically involved.

General, Myotatically Controlled, Mechanoreceptor Responses. Altered proprioception highlights many asymmetries. The Golgi tendon organ (GTO) is centrally involved in the process. Golgi tendon organs pervade all soft tissues including joints, fascial sheaths and aponeuroses. Since Golgi tendon organs are either "on or off" and do not exhibit neural plasticity, they readily respond to outside forces, such as manual maneuvers. They can easily assume new behaviors either normal or pathologic. Using manual forces, release maneuvers permit GTO's to return to more normal firing patterns, at least for a time.

Muscle Tightening and Asymmetries. Muscle tightness and asymmetry is maintained through Ia afferents acting at the segmental levels interacting closely with descending central mechanisms. Gamma efferent effects are particularly important. Emotional and stress-related mechanisms often are major contributors.

Traumatic accleration-deceleration forces massively stimulate Ia afferents at the segmental level of the spinal cord. Descending central inhibitory factors suddenly become insufficient to control the overwhelming, uncontrolled input. Modulation breaks down with accompanying neurosensory and sensorimotor changes.

Often these "asymmetries" are dramatic such as cord injuries, fractures, and plexus-related disruptions. Sprains, strains, and myofascial disruptions with pain syndromes,

however, are more frequent. Asymmetrical muscle spasms, pains, paresthesias, dysesthesias, and autonomic changes follow.

Centrally Controlled Relaxation. Effects occur as myofascial tightness and muscle spasm releases. Assertive, slow, carefully directed soft tissue loading can overcome many of these effects assuming massive neural and other soft tissue damage has not occurred. Although there is no direct evidence at present, we assume that such loading invokes inverse myotatic (clasp-knife) reflexes.

Principle 10. Using an interactive process of treatment and constant reevaluation tight-loose analysis is integrated with changes in myofascial tone, so-called inherent tissue motion. (See Principle 11, below.)

Tight-loose myofascial comparisons and contrasts are made among:

—loading asymmetries
—movement asymmetries
—reflex-related asymmetries
—muscle strength asymmetries
—force tension relationships, including immediate strength versus endurance
—joint-related changes, including joint play.

Continuing reassessments of the same area, e.g., thoracolumbar junction, is essential. The four primary positions of load and the four primary movements are always integrated.

Principle 11. Monitoring inherent tissue motions increases the probability that myofascial release will be both efficient and long lasting.

Inherent Tissue Motion. This is noted as asymmetrical waves of tightening and loosening, both locally and throughout the body. Little research has occurred regarding the phenomenon. Current technology and fast Fourier transform analysis has difficulty dealing with pulsatile waves below 20 Hz. Some empirical evidence suggests the phenomenon is related to ebbing and flowing tonic and phasic changes in muscle tone, but has not been published to my knowledge.

Whatever the source, inherent tissue motion tightens and loosens the myofascial complex. Expert clinician-technicians are able to enter this system, monitor shifting asymmetries and invoke specific loads that change the patterns, at least temporarily, if not permanently.

Principle 12. Release enhancing maneuvers increase both speed and efficiency of treatment.

Examples are:

—Eye movements activate brainstem feedback loops that alter craniocervical and shoulder girdle mechanics.
—Deep and shallow breath holding as tethered asymmetries are systematically stressed.
—Directed movements of the limbs while monitoring tightness and looseness.

Principle 13. Exercise and lifestyle changes are essential for continuing and maintaining change.

GENERAL SUMMATION

Manual therapies in general have been an ongoing source of controversy for most of the twentieth century. Unfailingly popular and used by a variety of practitioners, clinically trained and lay alike, there continues to be little hard scientific data supporting their use.

At the time of this writing, over 50 outcome and efficacy studies have been published. Most suggest that for a subset of patients with acute low back problems, manual treatments shorten morbidity and functional disability.[72,73] Problems most studies encounter are the significant variability of manipulations used and the assumptions made by the researchers.[74-76]

Outcome measures are difficult to study, at best. When and if multivariate protocols can be made consistently reliable and valid and if excessive sensitivity[77] can be linked with reliable specificity, then perhaps alleged versus real efficacy will be clarified. Reliance on single approaches, for example, ambiguously defined single manual therapies, such as just rotational manipulation, while scientifically correct, is methodologically flawed. They not only weaken the research, but also beg the issue of clinical complexity.

The more approaches employed, the better the outcome.[78,79] That ambiguity surrounds the specifics should not be surprising. However, this must not be a cause for discontinuing searching for clarity and new knowledge.

REFERENCES

1. Farfan H. The scientific basis of manipulative procedures. Clin Rheumat Dis, 1980; 6:159–177.
2. Zusman M. Spinal manipulative therapy: review of some proposed mechanisms, and a new hypothesis. Aust J Physiother 1986; 32:89–99.
3. Mitchell FL, Moran PS, Pruzzo N. An evaluation of osteopathic muscle energy procedures. Valley Park, Kansas City: Pruzzo, 1979.
4. Lewit K. Manipulative therapy in rehabilitation of the motor system. London: Butterworths, 1985; 214.
5. Jones L. Strain and counterstrain. Newark, OH: American Academy of Osteopathy, 1981.
6. Travell J, Simons D. Myofascial pain and dysfunction: the trigger point manual. Baltimore: Williams and Wilkins, 1983.
7. Magoun HI. Osteopathy in the cranial field. Newark, OH: American Academy of Osteopathy, 1966.
8. Kimberly P. An introduction to cranial technique: a course outline. Des Moines: Des Moines Still College of Osteopathy, 1948.
9. Neumann H-D. Introduction to manual medicine. New York: Springer Verlag, 1989.
10. Goodridge JP. Muscle energy technique: definition, explanation, methods of procedure. J Am Osteopath Assoc 1981; 81:249–253.
11. Heilig D. The thrust technique. J Am Osteopath Assoc 1981; 81:244–248.
12. Upledger JE. Craniosacral therapy I. Seattle: Eastland Press, 1985.
13. Upledger JE. Craniosacral therapy II. Seattle: Eastland Press, 1987.
14. Greenman PE. Principles of manual medicine. Baltimore: Williams and Wilkins, 1989.
15. Retzlaff EW, Mitchell FL Jr. The cranium and its sutures. New York: Springer-Verlag, 1987.
16. Adams T. Documentation of rhythmic parietal suture separation in the anesthetized cat. Seminar presentation, Dept of Physiology, East Lansing, Michigan State University, June 1990.
17. Bowles CH. Functional technique: a modern perspective. J Am Osteopath Assoc 1980:326–331.
18. Schmidt H. Brain stem injury and death associated with manual medicine maneuvers. Workshop on Complications of Manipulation of the Cervical Spine. Denmark: Aarhus, 1990.
19. Snyder G. Fasciae: applied anatomy and physiology. Newark, OH: American Academy of Osteopathy Yearbook, 1956; 65–75.
20. Cooper GJ. Clinical considerations on fascia in di-

agnosis and treatment. Newark, OH: American Academy of Osteopathy Yearbook, 1977; 73–84.

21. Page LE. The role of fasciae in the maintenance of structural integrity. Newark, OH: American Academy of Osteopathy Yearbook, 1952; 70–73.

22. Travell J, Rinzler SH. The myofascial genesis of pain. Postgrad Med 1952; 11:425–34.

23. Becker RF. The meaning of fascia and fascial continuity. Osteopath Ann 1975; 35–47.

24. Cathie AG, England RW, eds. The clinical importance of fascia. Newark, OH: Academy of Applied Osteopathy Yearbook, 1968; 87–103.

25. Sucher BM. Thoracic outlet syndrome—a myofascial variant: Part 1. Pathology and diagnosis. J Am Osteopath Assoc 1990; 90:686–704.

26. Sucher BM. Thoracic outlet syndrome—a myofascial variant: Part 2. Treatment. J Am Osteopath Assoc 1990; 90:810–823.

27. Still AT. The philosophy and mechanical principles of osteopathy. Kirksville: Osteopathic Enterprise 1892, Re-published 1986; 76–86.

28. Bonica JJ. The Management of pain, 2nd ed. Malvern: Lea and Febiger, 1990; 211–243.

29. Korr IM. The neurobiologic mechanisms in manipulative therapy. New York: Plenum, 1978.

30. Bonica JJ. The management of pain, 2nd ed. Malvern: Lea and Febiger, 1990; 32.

31. Uitto J, and Perejda AJ. Structure and biology of the components of the extracellular matrix. In: Connective tissue diseases: the molecular pathology of the extracellular matrix. New York: Marcel Dekker; 1987; 12:3–100.

32. Basmajian, J. Muscle alive. 4th ed. Baltimore: Williams & Wilkins, 1978.

33. White AA, Panjabi M. Clinical biomechanics of the spine. Philadelphia: Lippincott, 1978.

34. Bonica JJ. The management of pain, 2nd ed. Malvern: Lea and Febiger, 1990; 28–94.

35. Korr IM, ed. The neurobiologic mechanisms in manipulative therapy. New York: Plenum, 1978.

36. White AA, Panjabi M. Clinical biomechanics of the spine. Philadelphia: Lippincott, 1978.

37. Cobb CR, et al. Electrical activity in muscle pain. Am J Phys Med 1975;54:80–87.

38. Elliott FA. Tender muscles in sciatica: electromyographic studies. Lancet 1944; 1:47–49.

39. Fricton, JR. Myofascial pain syndrome: electromyographic changes associated with local twitch response. Arch Phys Med Rehabil 1985; 66:314–317.

40. Korr IM. Sustained sympathicotonia as a factor in disease. In: The neurobiologic mechanisms of manipulative therapy. New York: Plenum Press, 1978; 229–268.

41. Thompson JM. Tension myalgia as a diagnosis at the Mayo Clinic and its relationship to fibrositis, fibromyalgia and myofascial pain syndrome. Mayo Clin Proc 1990; 65:1237–1248.

42. VanBuskirk RL. Nociceptive reflexes and somatic dysfunction: a model. J Am Osteopath Assoc 1990; 90:792–809.

43. Dunn MG, Silver FH. Viscoelastic behavior of human connective tissues: relative contribution of viscous and elastic components. Connect Tissue Res 1983;12:59–70.

44. Sunderland S. Traumatized nerves, roots, and ganglia. In: The neurobiologic mechanisms in manipulative therapy. Korr, IM, ed. New York: Plenum, 1978; 137–166.

45. Viidik A. Interdependence between structure and function in collagenous tissues. In: Biology of collagen. Viidik A, Vuust J, eds. New York: Academic Press, Harcourt, Brace, Jovanovich, 1985; 256–279.

46. Viidik A. Adaptability of connective tissue. In: Biochemistry of exercise VI. Saltin B, ed. Champaign: Human Kinetics Publishers, 1986; 545–562.

47. Fryette HH. Principles of osteopathic technic. Newark, OH: American Academy of Osteopathy, 1966; 15.

48. Beckwith CG. The vertebral joint lesion, etiology and diagnosis. J Am Osteopath Assoc 1944; 43:263.

49. Patriquin D. Letter to the editor. J Am Osteopath Assoc 1990; 90:759, 766, 768.

50. Aho A, Vartianinen O, Salo O. Segmentary mobility of the lumbar spine in antero-posterior flexion. Ann Med Fenniae 1955; 44:275.

51. Moll JMH, Wright V. Normal range of spinal mobility: an objective clinical study. Ann Rheum Dis. 1971; 30:381–386.

52. Pearcy M, Portek I, Shepherd J. The effect of low back pain on lumbar spinal movements measured by three-dimensional x-ray analysis. Spine 1985; 10:150–153.

53. Bagnall KM, et al. The histochemical composition of vertebral muscle. Spine 1984; 9:470–473.

54. Janda V. Muscles, central nervous motor regulation and back problems. In: The neurobiologic mechanisms in manipulative therapy. Korr IM, ed. New York: Plenum Press, 1978; 27–41.

55. Fernandez HF, Ramirez B. Muscle fibrillation induced by blockage of axoplasmic transport. Brain Res 1974; 49:385–389.

56. Bonica JJ. The management of pain, 2nd ed. Malvern: Lea and Febiger, 1990; 220–230.

57. Roddie IC. Lymph transport mechanisms in peripheral lymphatics. N Physiol Sci 1990; 5:85–89.

58. Bonica JJ. The management of pain, 2nd ed. Malvern; Lea and Febiger, 1990; 32.

59. Wells MR et al. Phasic morphological changes in rat dorsal root ganglion neurons after sciatic nerve section. J Am Osteopath Assoc 1990; 90:721.

60. Sugimoto T, Bennett G, Kajander K. Transsynaptic degeneration in the superficial dorsal horn after sciatic nerve injury: effects of a chronic constriction injury, transection, and strychnine. Pain 1990; 42:205–213.

61. Bonica JJ. The management of pain, 2nd ed. Malvern. Lea and Febiger, 1990; 28.

62. Wall PD, Melzack R. Physiologic responses associated with tissue injury and acute pain. In: Textbook of pain, 2nd ed. Edinburgh: Churchill Livingstone, 1989; 285–305.

63. Janda V. Muscles, central nervous motor regulation and back problems. In: The neurobiologic mechanisms in manipulative therapy. Korr IM, ed, New York: Plenum Press, 1978; 27–41.

64. Wall PD, Melzack R. Peripheral neural mechanisms of nociception. In: Textbook of pain, 2nd ed. Edinburgh: Churchill Livingstone, 1989; 22–45.

65. Wall PD, Melzack R. Textbook of pain, 2nd ed. Edinburgh: Churchill Livingstone, 1989; 312.

66. Fryette HH. Principles of osteopathic technic. Newark, OH: American Academy of Osteopathy, 1966; 67–77.

67. Egund N, et al. Movements in the sacroiliac joints demonstrated with roentgen stereophotogrammetry. Acta Radiol Diag 1978; 19:833–835.

68. Lavignolle B, et al. An approach to the functional anatomy of the sacroiliac joints in vivo. Anatomia Clinica, 1983; 5:169–176.

69. Sturesson B, Selvik G, Uden A. Movements of the sacroiliac joints: a roentgen stereophotogrammetric analysis. Spine 1989; 14:162–165.

70. Vleeming A, et al. Relation between form and function in the sacroiliac joint: Part I: clinical anatomical aspects. Spine 1990; 15:130–132.

71. Vleeming A, et al. Relations between form and function in the sacroiliac joint: Part II: biomechanical aspects. Spine 1990; 15:133–136.

72. MacDonald RS, Bell CMJ. An open controlled assessment of manipulation in non-specific low back pain. Spine 1990; 15:364;370.

73. Schmidt KE, et al. Correlation of palpatory and electromyographic findings in patients with low back pain. J Am Osteopath Assoc 1990; 90:639.

74. Seffinger MA, Johnston WJ. Relationship between musculoskeletal findings and somatic dysfunction. J Am Osteopath Assoc 1990; 90:636.

75. Roberts GF, Ikner CL, Hassen JB. Audition brainstem response variability in subjects with tinnitus over time (effects of manipulative treatment). J Am Osteopath Assoc 1990; 90:638.

76. Greene CH, et al. The effect of helium-neon laser and osteopathic manipulation on soft-tissue trigger points. J Am Osteopath Assoc 1990; 90:638.

77. Beatty DR. Incidence of cervical somatic dysfunction in ambulatory subjects. J Am Osteopath Assoc 1990; 90:637.

78. Bergquist-Ullman M, Larsson U. Acute low back pain in industry: a controlled prospective study with special reference to therapy and confounding factors. Acta Orthop Scand Suppl 1977; 170:1–117.

79. Meade TW, et al. Low back pain of mechanical origin: randomised comparison of chiropractic and hospital outpatient treatment. Br Med J 1990; 300:6737.

11

Proprioceptive Neuromuscular Facilitation

VICKY L. SALIBA, GREGORY S. JOHNSON, and CHERYL WARDLAW

Proprioceptive Neuromuscular Facilitation (PNF) is a dynamic approach to the evaluation and treatment of neuromusculoskeletal dysfunction with particular emphasis on the trunk. Over the past couple of decades substantial progress has been made in the conservative care of spinal problems.[1–5] The shift towards evaluating and treating them from a functional or neuromuscular perspective enhances and complements the symptomatic and structural approaches.[6–14] A functional or neuromuscular approach looks beyond the classical diagnosis, identifying their habitual patterns of posture and movement; their dynamic strength, flexibility, and coordination; and the specific muscle recruitment and motor control of the symptomatic region, as well as contributing factors in the patients' environment.

PNF applies neurophysiological principles of the sensory/motor system to manual evaluation and treatment of neuromuscular skeletal dysfunctions. PNF provides the therapist with an efficient means for evaluating and treating neuromuscular and structural dysfunctions.[15–19]

Structural dysfunctions (myofascial and articular hyper- and hypomobilities) affect the body's capacity to assume and perform optimal postures and motions and often are associated with symptoms.[2,5,15,20–22]

Neuromuscular dysfunctions (inability to coordinate and efficiently perform purposeful movements) cause repetitive, abnormal, and stressful usage of the articular and myofascial system, often precipitating structural dysfunctions and symptoms.[3,6,12,19,23,24]

The goal of the PNF approach is to facilitate an optimal structural and neuromuscular state. This helps to reduce symptoms, to improve the distribution of forces through the symptomatic region, and to reduce the inherent functional stresses caused by poor neuromuscular control.[15,19,23,24]

The principles and procedures of PNF are especially effective when integrated with appropriate use of joint and soft tissue mobilization techniques. The basic philosophy and principles of PNF can be universally integrated into any treatment approach, since the foundation is the evaluation and treatment of posture and movement. The utilization of PNF for spinal dysfunction is enhanced by a working knowledge of arthrokinematics, neurophysiology, and possible pathomechanics of the spine.

THE EVOLUTION OF PNF

The PNF approach was developed by Herman Kabat, MD, and Margaret Knott, PT, (Fig. 11.1), during the 1940s and early 1950s, primarily as a method to treat patients with neurological dysfunctions.[16,25,26] Dr. Kabat desired to offer more to the neurologically involved patient population than walkers and passive range of motion exercises. He

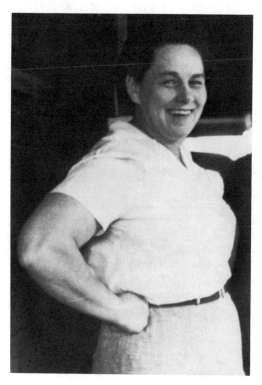

Figure 11.1. Margaret Knott, PT (December 18, 1978)—Devoted to her patients, dedicated to her students, and a pioneer in her profession.

searched the literature to uncover basic neurophysiological principles which could serve as the foundation for a more dynamic and functional approach. His studies led him to the works of Sherrington, Gellhorn, Coghill, Gesell, Hellebrandt, and others.[15,17] These researchers identified that a muscle response could be influenced by resistance, stretch reflex, irradiation, and other proprioceptive input. Stimulated by his studies, Dr. Kabat searched for clinicians whose treatment approach could serve as a foundation for the clinical application of these neurophysiological principles. His search then led him to Sister Elizabeth Kenny, who was successfully using manual resistance and neurophysiological principles to facilitate active functional movement in polio patients.

Dr. Kabat, a physician who liked to physically work with his patients, began to put into action the knowledge he had acquired

through his research, along with the clinical knowledge he gained from watching Sister Kenny. His goal was to meet the needs of the neurological population by focusing on the reeducation of the patient's developmental postures and movements. He believed this approach facilitated the patient toward more efficient function and independence during ADL.[16]

The effectiveness of PNF evolved with its specificity. When Margaret Knott began to work with Dr. Kabat in the mid-40s, they focused their attention toward utilizing the concepts of resistance, stretch reflex, approximation, traction, and manual contact to the facilitation of efficient motor recruitment patterns. Their goal was to facilitate efficient responses in specific muscles and muscle groups. This commitment towards developing specificity laid the groundwork for the effectiveness of PNF as a broadly applicable manual therapy approach.

Regardless of the underlying pathology, evaluation and treatment of structural and neuromuscular dysfunctions depend upon an assessment of specific motor recruitment and control. The PNF approach offers the trained clinician tools to quickly and effectively evaluate these motor components. It builds on the concept that motor recruitment can be enhanced through appropriately utilized reflex and proprioceptive input. From this initial foundation, PNF continues to evolve to new levels of proficiency through clinical experience and scientific advances, but the initial concepts and principles developed by Kabat and Knott have withstood the test of time.

PHILOSOPHY

The philosophy of the PNF approach is based upon the premise that *all human beings have untapped existing potential*. Therefore, the role of the physical therapist is to identify dysfunctions and facilitate the patient's optimal physical capacity.[10,15,17,27]

To facilitate the patient's optimal functional level and insure total involvement in the rehabilitation program the therapist must develop effective rapport. An important aspect of developing rapport is to capitalize and place emphasis upon the individual's physical, mental, and emotional strengths, rather than his or her deficits. A person's strengths become the foundation from which reeducation and learning take place. Working from one's strengths, rather than one's deficits, tends to achieve success, not frustration—physically, mentally, emotionally, and spiritually.

Strengths are best utilized by mutually agreeing upon clear and attainable short- and long-term goals. These goals should be developed both from a thorough evaluation and the needs and desires of the patient. Based upon established goals, the treatment program is specifically designed to address the identified functional limitations.

When treating neuromuscular dysfunctions, complex motor patterns are reduced to their basic movement and developmental components. The emphasis is placed upon selective reeducation of individual motor elements, through developing the fundamental skills of trunk control, stability, and coordinated mobility. These basic motor skills are built upon by progressing to less stable postures and more complex functional activities. Each movement and posture learned is reinforced through repetition in an appropriately demanding and intense training program. This program may consist of manual treatment, a home program, an exercise class, and or a gym program. The intensity of the physical program is graded to meet the patient's specific strength and endurance needs for performing efficient postures and movements during daily activities.

PRINCIPLES

The principles of PNF are based upon sound neurophysiological and kinesiological principles and clinical experience.[10,15] Each is an essential component of the approach and provides the basis for developing consistency throughout the evaluation and treatment process. Through applying these basic principles, the patient's postural responses, movement patterns, strengths, and endurance can be assessed and enhanced.

Manual Contacts

The psychological effect of manual contact is well known.[15,28,29] The comment "You are the first one to really touch me where it hurts" is frequently made after the initial evaluation by a manual medicine or therapy practitioner. The inherent responsibility of a manual therapist is to maximize the psychological benefit by establishing trust and cooperation without facilitating dependency.

The quality of touch influences the patient's confidence and the appropriateness of the motor response and relaxation. Therefore sensitivity and specificity should be utilized when applying a manual contact. The therapist should be consistent and specific with all manual contacts to allow for accurate evaluation, effective treatment, and continuous reassessment.

On a physical level, manual contacts to the skin and deeper receptors influence neuromuscular responses.[30,31] Through the use of appropriate and specific manual contacts, the therapist can influence and enhance the direction, strength, and coordination of a motor response. *Appropriate manual contacts are applied to the skin surface on the side to which the movement or stabilizing contraction is desired.*[10,15] If inappropriate contacts are applied, the sensory input is confusing and affects the motor response. One testing for shoulder flexion strength to access the effectiveness of the applied manual techniques can distort the findings if consistent manual contact is not maintained during the pre and post treatment testing. Use of a lumbrical grip is the most effective means of applying appropriate manual contacts. This allows for a less compressive grip, while still facilitating specific unidirectional contact (Fig. 11.2).

Therapist Position and Body Mechanics

An essential aspect in applying appropriate manual contacts is the use of proper body position and mechanics.[13] *The therapist needs*

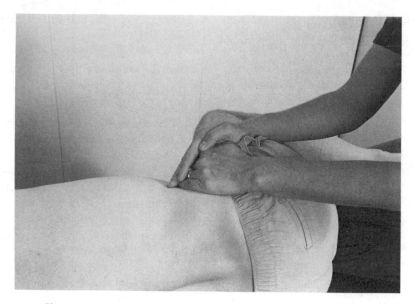

Figure 11.2. Appropriate manual contact—utilizing a lumbrical grip.

to position his center of gravity and base of support in line with the direction of motion being resisted. This position allows the movement to occur either towards or away from the therapist, so that weight transference and acceptance can be coordinated and smooth. The therapist's total body and arm movement should equal the same excursion and reflect the same arc of motion as the body part being treated. The therapist's spine should remain in a neutral alignment with motion occurring primarily in the hips, legs, and arms (Fig. 11.3).

Appropriate manual contacts and body position provide resistance from the therapist's trunk rather than the upper extremities. Therefore, the arms can relax and better translate the resistance and evaluate the motor response. The slightest deviation from the use of appropriate position and body mechanics can alter the desired response and distort the therapist evaluation.[10,13,15]

Appropriate Resistance

Appropriate resistance[10] is the amount of resistance which facilitates the desired motor response through a smooth, coordinated, and optimal muscle contraction.[15] Appropriate and variable resistance is applied to an active contraction for two purposes.

- Initially, the resistance allows the therapist to evaluate the patient's motor response. Characteristics such as control, strength, initiation, stabilization, endurance, relaxation, and quality of contraction are effectively assessed when manual resistance is applied to the patient's contraction.[10,15,19]
- If a dysfunction is identified in any of these characteristics, appropriate resistance applied in conjunction with various PNF techniques, facilitates the relearning and rehabilitation process.[10,15,18]

During normal activity the neuromuscular system utilizes a variety of muscle contractions to meet the normal demands of efficient motor control.[32] The patient's capacity to stabilize (isometric), as well as move (isotonic), can be specifically evaluated through manual resistance. The use of resistance allows the therapist to determine the patient's ability to selectively and efficiently perform and integrate each of these contractions. Identified dysfunctions are specifically treated to facilitate optimal function.

The kinesiological definitions of isometric and isotonic contractions vary within the lit-

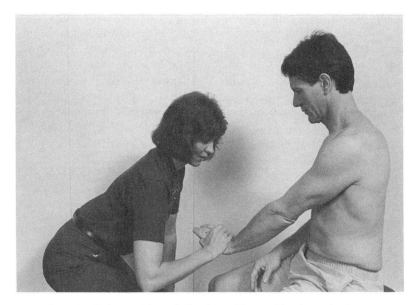

Figure 11.3. Proper therapist body position and body mechanics—promotes smooth and coordinated movements.

erature. We have chosen to define these terms to correspond with "functional evaluation and treatment" represented by the approach of PNF.

Isometric Contractions. The traditional definition of an isometric contraction is one in which "the external force is equal to the internal force developed by the muscle and no external movement occurs."[32,33] The functional definition of PNF builds on this definition to include the intention of the contractions. According to the authors, this contraction is a stabilizing contraction "in which the patient's intention is to maintain a consistent position in space."[10]

Isotonic Contractions. The traditional definition of an isotonic contraction is, "a contraction in which the external force is constant and motion occurs."[32,33] An isotonic contraction as defined in the PNF approach is one "in which the patient's *intention* is to create movement."[10]

These are subdivided into *concentric* (a dynamic shortening of the muscle), *eccentric* (a dynamic controlled lengthening), and *maintained contractions.* A maintained contraction is a dynamic contraction in which the patient's

intention to produce movement is limited by a greater external force. This contraction differs from an isometric contraction in that the intention of an isometric contraction is to maintain a stabile position.[10]

> An **example** of the interaction of these various contractions occurs during the removal of a bowl from a high shelf. When reaching, the arm must concentrically raise, perform a maintained contraction to stabilize the weight of the bowl as it leaves the shelf, and eccentrically lower the bowl and arm to the counter. During this motion components of the trunk perform isometric contractions to maintain a stable position in space.

Each of these functional types of contractions needs to be specifically evaluated and facilitated. Nonvarying mechanical resistance cannot create the variables needed to stimulate these differentiated contractions. The PNF principle of manually applied appropriate resistance allows for this selective differentiation to occur. The therapist varies the type and degree of resistance to facilitate the appropriate response. The resistance must vary in application, power, and endurance to evaluate and treat the patient's dysfunctions of selective motor control, coordination, range of motion, strength, initiation, stabilization, and/or relaxation.

Irradiation. Resistance can also be used to produce appropriate irradiation.[10] Irradiation is defined as the overflow of excitation from stronger components to weaker or inhibited components.[15,34,35,36] This is accomplished through the application of graded resistance to stronger components to facilitate irradiation and produce an appropriate and enhanced contraction in weaker ones.

There are many variables which the therapist must consider while utilizing appropriate resistance to facilitate an efficient motor response such as: the patient's position, gravity, existing normal and abnormal reflexes, therapist's manual contacts, and body mechanics. The encouragement of controlled breathing further reinforces efficient movement.

> **Example.** Various forms of resistance can be applied to the shoulder girdle as an effective treatment of cervical dysfunction.
>
> - In cases of acute pain, gentle, slowly built isometrics can often decrease tone, mobilize articulations, improve circulation, and decrease pain through indirect means.
> - In many individuals with cervical dysfunction, abnormalities in neuromuscular control of shoulder girdle motions are identified. This alteration of neuromuscular control is effectively treated using the various forms of isotonic contractions combined with isometric contractions. The isometric contraction allows the therapist to monitor the slowly building contraction to assure proper muscle recruitment, followed by the retraining of the isolated group with various isotonic contractions. In these cases appropriate resistance is utilized in conjunction with the appropriate technique for training control.
> - In patients where more trunk or neck facilitation is desired maximal resistance is given to the shoulder girdle to facilitate appropriate irradiation.

Traction and Approximation

Traction and approximation utilize force vectors to assist the resistance and in facilitating the desired motor response.[15,36] They supply a reflex enhancement to the volitional response to resistance. Therefore, the therapist must be aware of blending traction or approximation with resistance to ensure smooth and appropriate resistance (Fig. 11.4).

Traction. This is the elongation of a segment and separation of joint surfaces which facilitates an enhanced muscular response to promote movement or enhance stability.[10,15] The direction of traction is always applied away from the apex of the arc of motion (Fig. 11.4).

> **Example.** Use of general traction when treating a patient with an acute cervical spine can assist the patient in his/her ability to perform controlled contractions without pain. The PNF approach utilizes traction differently than distraction which is designed to specifically separate joint surfaces.[20]

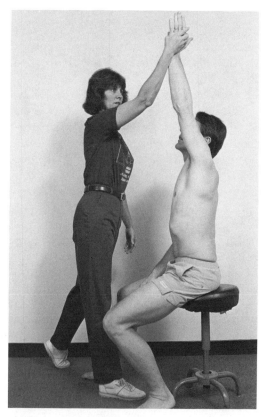

Figure 11.4. The force vectors of resistance and traction or approximation—combine to provide appropriate resistance and facilitation.

Approximation. A compression force towards the axis of motion resulting in an approximation of joint surfaces is Approximation. It facilitates an increased muscular response and promotes stability, and is often used when facilitating stability in weight bearing postures or positions.[15,19,37,38] The desired response can be initiated or reinforced by a reflex—producing quick approximation, followed immediately by a maintained approximation and resistance.

Example. Use of approximation can be used to retrain postural awareness in sitting by facilitating a more stable and improved response of the trunk musculature and improve trunk stability (Fig. 11.5).

Even though reflex responses can be facilitated through use of traction and approximation, these responses are not therapeutic un-less coupled with a volitional contraction and appropriate resistance.

Cautions. When applying traction or approximation care must be taken to avoid increasing pain, and consideration must be given to the underlying pathology. In many cases where the joint is the source of pain, such as arthritis, judicious use of traction or approximation may decrease symptoms and allow for a more intensive rehabilitation program. Pain which is secondary to articular instability may be reduced with a combination of resistance and traction or approximation, allowing for greater facilitation of neuromuscular stabilization.

Quick Stretch

In the presence of weakness, incoordination, poor initiation, or poor endurance a volitional contraction can be heightened and reinforced through the use of spinal reflexes. PNF uses a facilitating cue termed quick stretch to offer a stretch stimulus and produce a desired stretch reflex.[15,18]

Gelhorn defined stretch stimulus as the "increased state of responsiveness to cortical stimulation that exists when a muscle is placed in an elongated position."[39] The stretch reflex is a spinal reflex that is facilitated by a quick elongation of a muscle on stretch. This stretch stimulates the extrafusal and intrafusal muscle spindles fibers to fire and produce a reflex contraction.[18,40] This reflex response, if isolated, produces a quick, short-lived contraction. However, if resistance is applied immediately to the contraction in conjunction with an appropriate verbal command, the result is a facilitated muscular response.

The use of these neurophysiological principles, such as the stretch reflex, allows the therapist to facilitate the initiation, force, direction, or endurance of a specific motor response through quick stretch. While these principles can affect the response of individual muscles, the tool is most effective when applied to a synergistic group of muscles or a PNF pattern of facilitation. Quick stretch can be applied at the beginning of a contraction

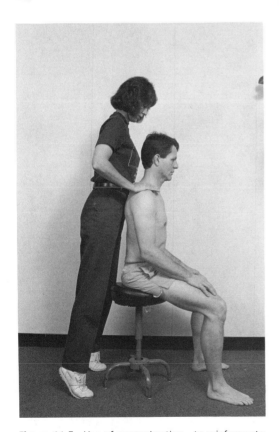

Figure 11.5. Use of approximation—to reinforce stability and reeducation.

when the muscle group is lengthened or throughout an active contraction. When utilized throughout an active contraction, the stretch reflex is facilitated from existing tension within the contracting muscle. A contraindication to the application of quick stretch is increased pain.[15]

> **Example.** Consider the posterior elevation pelvic pattern which is functionally utilized in stepping backwards and scooting. To perform this pattern the latissimus dorsi, erector spinae, and quadratus lumborum must function together to achieve an efficient movement. If the patient has difficulty in initiating the contraction, just placing the muscles on stretch often will facilitate a stronger more effective pattern. If that is not sufficient, a stretch reflex can be applied to initiate the contraction and repeated either at the beginning or through the range.

Verbal Stimuli

The therapist's verbal command is a primary link between reflex responses and the patient's volitional response.[15] Without the use of verbal commands, there is no cognitive reeducation taking place, only reflex responses to proprioceptive input. This is a primary functional consideration with all patients because a reflex response must become volitional to facilitate the patient's independence in motion activities.

Verbal commands, coupled with manual contacts, provide the therapist with the primary tools for establishing communication and cooperation. Verbal commands should be simple, concise, and unidirectional. In addition, the quality of the verbal command should vary depending upon the type of motor response desired from the patient.[15]

> **Example.** In a sports rehabilitation setting, when a patient is stable with minimally irritable symptoms, the goal of treatment is a heightened motor response and strength. The therapist's energetic and enthusiastic verbal commands can facilitate the patient's excitement and participation in the treatment. However, with a patient who has acute, highly irritable cervical dysfunction, the commands are most effective when given in a quiet and assuring manner. This is to promote relaxation and to not trigger

heightened or easily aroused neuromuscular responses.

Summary. Verbal commands are used to:

- coordinate volitional effort with reflex response,
- define the type of muscular contraction,
- define the direction of motion,
- signal timing of relaxation of contraction,
- facilitate increased involvement and arousal,
- stimulate generalized relaxation.

Visual Stimuli

The visual system is important in normal development and coordinated use of the body (Fig. 11.6). The therapeutic utilization of visual stimuli goes beyond the use of vision to teach an activity. Developmentally, the neuromuscular system gains its control in a ce-

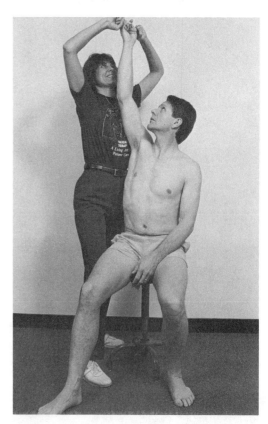

Figure 11.6. Visual stimuli—reinforces the other principles of facilitation and enhances the patient's response.

phalic-caudal direction. Movement of the trunk and extremities can be facilitated by the incorporation of the visual system, which requires integration of the head and neck. Failure to evaluate and include the visual system in a rehabilitation program can inhibit or retard the development of complete and coordinated trunk and extremity control. In addition, balance and equilibrium responses rely heavily on visual input for accurate interpretation of spatial relationships.[15,30,41,42]

Patterns of Facilitation

The patterns of facilitation were discovered by Kabat in the final stages of his development of PNF.[15,27] Through the utilization of all the previously identified principles, he began to understand and recognize the inherent movement patterns which humans utilize to perform normal functional and athletic activities. He observed that normal coordinated activities are accomplished by the moving of the extremities and trunk in diagonal and spiral motions in relationship to each other. He observed that muscular responses were strong and coordinated when resisted within specific diagonal patterns. In addition, the use of reflex facilitation, such as the stretch reflex, was most effective when the part was elongated in its specific diagonal. This observation made Kabat question the validity of using cardinal plane motions in the rehabilitation of functional activities, because normal motion is performed in diagonal and spiral patterns. Through trial and error, Kabat and Knott developed the specific trunk and extremity patterns.

Patterns of facilitation provide the therapist with tools to evaluate and treat dysfunctions of neuromuscular control and mobility of selective spinal articulations, as well as the ability to integrate synergistic muscle groups within the patterns. As control is developed, synergistic muscle activity is integrated into functional whole body movements. Through use of patterns of facilitation, the patient is provided the opportunity to correctly perform and learn the desired motor response and in-

tegrate that response into daily functional activities.

The patterns exist in narrow diagonals in relationship to the central axis of motion of the extremity and trunk. Each pattern is as wide as the part being treated and moves within a smooth arc of motion. Three components of motion are blended within each diagonal movement pattern.

In the Trunk. The components are: flexion/extension, lateral movement, and rotation (Figs. 11.7A,B,C).

In the Extremities. The components are: flexion/extension, abduction/adduction, and rotation (Figs. 11.8A,B).

Parameters. Each pattern can be identified by the following parameters.[10,23,24]

1. When in the elongated position all synergistic muscles are equally on stretch. In this manner the patient's functional range can be evaluated.
2. The stretch reflex is optimally facilitated within a synergistic group of muscles at one time.
3. Clinically, it can be shown that a muscle contraction is stronger when performed within a facilitation pattern than outside of the pattern. It is theorized that muscles work together more efficiently when placed within these patterns and the contraction is more readily enhanced by irradiation. An example is the function of thumb and little finger opposition, which is easily demonstrated to be not only stronger, but more easily recruited when the upper extremity is placed within the extension-abduction pattern.
4. Resistance to an extremity pattern will facilitate a contraction within the related trunk patterns.
5. Increased tone and clonus are generally reduced when the part is specifically placed within a component of the diagonal. This is often dramatically illustrated in a patient with increased abnormal tone of the upper extremity or an immediate reduction in tone when the scapula of that same extremity is placed into posterior depression.[10]

By using the PNF patterns of facilitation, the therapist can more quickly and effectively

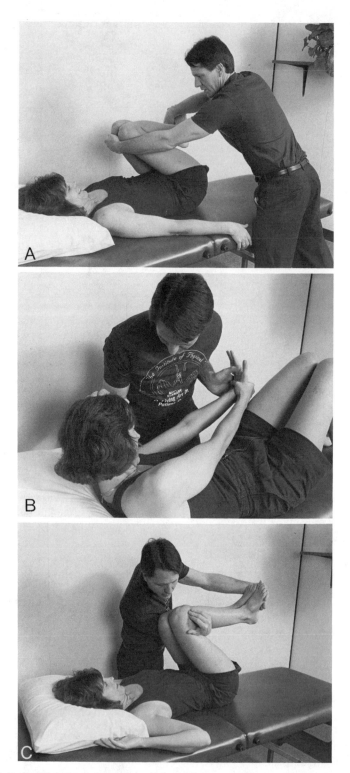

Figure 11.7. Available trunk patterns include: **A**) lower trunk flexion; **B**) upper trunk flexion with chopping; **C**) lower trunk lateral flexion with rotation.

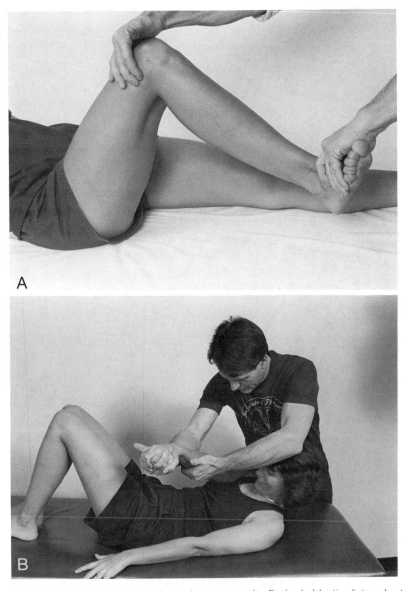

Figure 11.8. Extremity patterns include: **A)** lower extremity flexion/adduction/internal rotation, **B)** upper extremity flexion/adduction/internal rotation.

evaluate neuromuscular control and range of motion within synergistic muscle groups. When dysfunctions are identified, specific PNF techniques are applied to enhance the desired movement.

    Example. The lower trunk extensor pattern can be utilized to selectively evaluate for hypo- and hypermobilities of the spine, and then treat the identified dysfunction through specific

treatment procedures described later in the chapter.

Timing

Normal timing refers to the *efficient sequencing* of dynamic muscle contractions to achieve a desired functional result.[10,15,43] This includes the sequence in which the muscle fires and the controlled interaction between mobility and stability of the selected components of a movement. In the orthopedic and sports injured population there is often a deficit in normal timing of motions during the performance of a pattern within symptomatic regions. These deficits are identified through manual and observational assessment.

Example. Orthopedic patients frequently demonstrate an inability to brace, or to stabilize the lumbar spine during normal or stressful activities.[21,44] The contraction of the trunk muscles should occur reflexively in response to any external demand which could potentially stress the spinal structures. Often the trunk muscles will test strong with conventional muscle testing, but when tested within a mass movement pattern or during a functional activity (such as push/pull activities) the contraction will be delayed or nonexistent. Through appropriate use of reeducation techniques abnormal timing can be improved and integrated into normal functional activities. (See Fig. 11.9)

Appropriate Techniques. Treatment of dysfunctions of normal timing can occur through multiple avenues.

- Reduce the motion or activity to the simplest components and facilitate an optimal

contraction of each individual component. Then combine these individual components together into the desired functional motion or activity.
- Appropriate use of resistance, quick stretch, and verbal command are used to reinforce normal timing.
- If abnormal timing is evaluated in a complex skill such as walking, less complex motions such as rolling and crawling can be used initially to train timing and kinesthetic awareness.

Example. One of the most valuable activities to observe for the assessment of a patient's inherent patterns of motions is rolling. To roll efficiently all components of the neuromuscular skeletal system must function in integrated and coordinated patterns. Each person should have the capacity to perform rolling from supine to sidelying in flexion, and roll from prone to supine with extension (Fig. 11.10). The initiation and performance should be executed with minimal effort. If the patient rolls with any other pattern, attempt to see if the efficient pattern is an option by providing verbal clues. All identified dysfunctions are selectively treated by beginning with the most basic motion and progressing to the

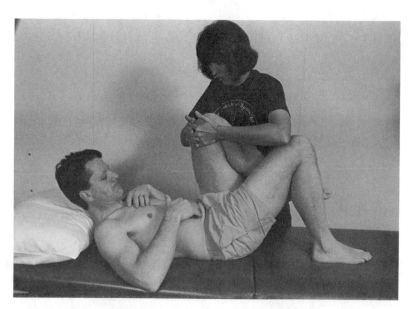

Figure 11.9. Utilization of resistance to the lower extremity flexion/adduction pattern to facilitate irradiation to the abdominals for functional bracing.

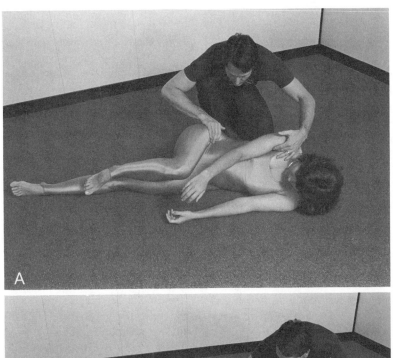

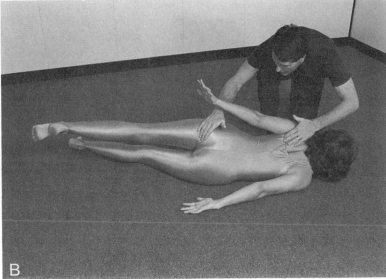

Figure 11.10. Rolling is facilitated through the principles of PNF to reeducate both flexion and extension.

complete roll. This motion should be a part of the patient's home program, through the use of tubing, pulleys, or sports cords.

FUNCTIONAL EVALUATION

The integration of PNF treatment techniques into a comprehensive rehabilitation program is dependent upon a thorough and continuous evaluation system. Initially this should include

an in-depth subjective and objective evaluation.[2,3,5,20]

Initial Evaluation

The subjective evaluation provides insight into the patient's symptoms, and his/her history, irritability, and normal course. Clear and concise subjective data can assist both the patient and therapist in gauging the effectiveness of treatment.

The orthopedic objective evaluation and standard neurological testing provide objective parameters by which the therapist and patient can assess progress. These parameters include specific measurements and documentation of the patient's posture, range of motion, symptom-producing motions, joint and soft tissue mobility functional capacities, and neurological involvement.

The neuromuscular assessment [10,13,15] generally begins with observing activities which can reveal the functional capacity of the symptomatic region. One assesses the interaction of the symptomatic region with related segments of the kinematic chain for activities performed both efficiently and inefficiently. Are the movements smooth and coordinated, and is there an effective interaction between stability and mobility?

Characteristics of Neuromuscular Control

In conjunction with the results of the subjective and objective evaluations, specific movement patterns are selected for manual neuromuscular assessment. Utilizing the principles of PNF, this manual assessment reveals the functional status of the neuromuscular system or characteristics of neuromuscular control. The patient is evaluated in various postures and movements to identify and assess the following characteristics of neuromuscular control and their effect on pain and symptoms:[10,23,24]

—Ability to relax and allow the part to be moved passively.
—Quality of initiation of movement.
—Coordination and control of contraction.
—Speed of contraction.
—Power of contraction.
—Ability to adjust power to meet functional demands.
—Ability to actively and with resistance to achieve a desired ROM.
—Ability to effectively produce an isometric contraction.
—Ability to perform a combination of isotonics

(concentric, eccentric, and maintained contraction).
—Ability to coordinate and smoothly reverse direction of motion.
—Neuromuscular balance between antagonists and agonists.
—Ability to coordinate contraction with synergistic muscle groups.
—Ability to produce appropriate irradiation to synergistic parts of the body

The PNF approach is organized upon the foundation of identifying dysfunctions of neuromuscular control through feeling the motion, palpation, and observation. Each of the above characteristics is an essential component for optimal function of the system as a whole. A dysfunction of one characteristic may indicate not only the necessity for neuromuscular reeducation, but can also require the utilization of other manual techniques, such as joint and soft tissue mobilization.[23,24] Therefore, it is necessary to fully understand how to manually assess each characteristic in order to integrate the findings into a total subjective and objective evaluation.

IDENTIFYING DYSFUNCTIONS

Passive Mobility

Passive movement of a segment through the arc of a PNF diagonal assists in the identification of the accessible passive range of motion, the patient's ability to relax, and the presence of neuromuscular holding patterns.[10,15] *Neuromuscular holding patterns* are unconscious states of unnecessary increased tone, which restrict passive and active mobility. To assist in selecting the appropriate treatment techniques, a differentiation needs to be made between neuromuscular dysfunctions and those stemming from soft tissue or articular restrictions.

Example. In patients with a forward head posture and/or anteriorly displaced shoulders, passive limitations will often be identified into the scapula pattern of posterior depression. This limitation can be a result of increased tone in the pectoral, cervical, or upper thoracic muscle groups. On the contrary, the patient may demonstrate the ability to totally relax the segment being moved, but still have motion interference which clearly indicates possible soft-tissue or joint involvement.

Active Mobility

The source of an identified limitation can be further clarified by active performing of the PNF diagonal previously assessed passively. If there is more range actively than passively it is an indication that the patient has difficulty relaxing. When less active than passive range exists, this is an indication of neuromuscular dysfunction. Observing a pattern performed actively provides information about the initiation, quality, control, range, and directional capabilities.[10,41]

Initiation

To evaluate the quality of initiation, the part is taken to the elongated portion of a pattern. The therapist couples verbal commands with resistance to determine the patient's ability to initiate the motion. The response is evaluated for sluggishness, delayed response, hyperactive responsive, or inappropriate recruitment.

The inappropriate recruitment would allow for movement, but not in the appropriate direction.

Example. Patients with lumbar pain often demonstrate a poor responsiveness of the abdominal musculature. This is often revealed through sluggish initiation of the pelvic anterior elevation pattern (Fig. 11.11). This assessment supplies critical information about the patient's ability to effectively recruit the trunk muscles at the demand of environmental stresses. Once this dysfunction is identified, a specific treatment program is designed to improve neuromuscular responsiveness.[6,12,22,44]

Coordination and Control

Through the use of resistance, coordination and control can be evaluated. From initiation, the contraction should be smooth and coordinated throughout the available range of motion. If the pattern of movement is dysfunctional, the patient often demonstrates muscle substitution to accomplish the movement. This is evident if the pattern is jerky, incoordinated, and deviates from the appropriate direction of movement.

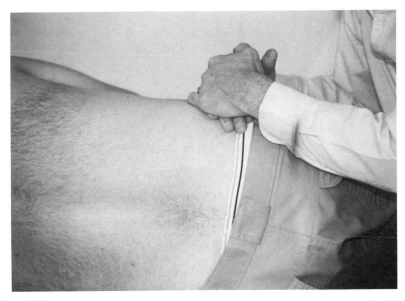

Figure 11.11. Evaluation of the anterior elevation pelvic pattern reveals the quality of responsiveness of the abdominal muscles and coordination with lateral flexors and extensors.

Example. In patients with fixed kyphotic thoracic curves, there exist anterior to posterior structural and muscular imbalances, which can diminish neuromuscular control and directional capabilities. In this example, the scapular stabilizers are often overstretched, while the pectoralis major and minor are shortened or over-developed. As a result, resistance to posterior depression of the scapula (which requires contraction of the scapula stabilizers) often results in pure depression, retraction, or anterior depression. The posterior depression motion may be altered by the dominance of the anterior musculature, the fixed structural thoracic position, and the loss of efficient recruitment and contraction of the posterior depressors and stabilizers.[6,10] This imbalance and necessary compensation places added strain on the lumbar and cervical spine.

The demand of manual resistance produces a functional response which clarifies the patient's ability to efficiently recruit the scapular stabilizers, inhibit the pectoral musculature, and move the shoulder girdle on the underlying rib cage. Treatment should emphasize initial lengthening of the anterior and superior structures and reeducation of the scapular depressors.

Strength and Speed

Through the application of resistance the therapist can assess the patient's strength and speed capacity. Traditional strength testing through manual muscle testing procedures may not be a complete or accurate predictor of functional capabilities. Efficient function is not solely dependent upon an individual muscle's strength, but also the appropriate motor response of synergistic muscle groups.[6,15,32,45] Therefore, functional strength testing must incorporate an analysis of each muscle group's ability to respond to the functional requirements as a primary mover, secondary mover, antagonist, neutralizer, stabilizer, and its synergistic capacities.

Patients often demonstrate a diminished ability to vary the speed of a contraction in response to the demands of activity. This characteristic is assessed by applying resistance and varying the verbal control to determine the patient's ability to recruit and execute a specific speed of motor response.

The patterns and techniques of PNF provide a comprehensive system for the assessment and retraining of strength and speed. The PNF diagonals requires functional combinations of muscles' actions, which allows each one to function in various capacities (i.e., primary mover, stabilizer, etc). A quick assessment of all the diagonals in the region being tested gives a more accurate functional strength analysis than individual muscle testing.

By varying the resistance, the therapist also determines the patient's ability to adjust the strength and speed of the contraction to meet the diversified functional demands placed on the segment during daily activities. This will identify segmental weaknesses which can cause altered arthrokinematics, postural deviation, and increased soft tissue strain.

Combination of Isotonics

In addition to the evaluation of general strength, there needs to be an assessment of performance and transition between the three type of isotonic contractions (concentric, eccentric, and maintained). Each isotonic contraction must be specifically evaluated and retrained, since the control and strength developed while performing one type does not necessarily directly translate to the others. We have termed this evaluation and treatment tool: combination of isotonics.[10]

Concentric Contractions. To evaluate and treat the ability to perform concentric contractions, the patient is given the command, "Push" or "Pull," while the therapist applies appropriate and variable resistance throughout the desired or available range.

Eccentric Contractions. These are evaluated and treated by giving the command, "Slowly let go" while the therapist applies appropriate lengthening resistance.

Maintained Contraction. To perform

them the patient is given the command, "Keep it there, don't let me move you," while the therapist quickly applies matching resistance to prevent motion. If a dynamic contraction is not facilitated, the therapist may use the command "Push" or "Pull" while applying a stronger resistance that allows only minimal motion.

Isometric Contraction

The patient's ability to produce an isometric contraction is evaluated in addition to the combinations of isotonics. For assessing and retraining the ability to perform this contraction, the patient is given the command, "Hold, don't let me move you, don't push into me." The therapist *gradually* applies and releases the resistance, attempting to *match* forces with the patient. The verbal command is important to reinforce to the patient that he is not to push or pull, only maintain his position. In cases where the patient is unable to perform an isometric contraction, low level maintained isotonic contractions may have to be initially utilized. The goal is to progressively facilitate the patient's capacity to perform true stabilizing contractions on demand, or to facilitate a selective motor recruitment where substitution is prevalent.

Reversals

The ability to reverse direction is a primary control feature of the neuromuscular system.[32,47-49] Inadequate control, speed, or strength of a reciprocal motion can result in altered arthrokinematics[6,23,24] and the development of compensatory movement patterns.

Example. By resisting flexion/adduction/external rotation of the lower extremity, followed by extension/abduction/internal rotation of the lower extremity, the therapist evaluates the patient's ability to perform reciprocal motions. The change in directions is critiqued for smoothness, direction, proper speed, and synergistic control of the prime movers versus the stabilizers. At the same time, while the extremity is performing the reciprocal motion, the trunk is assessed for its capabilities to stabilize.

Agonist/Antagonistic Balance

Secondary to structural dysfunctions, herniated nucleus proposus, or overuse syndromes, a functional imbalance may occur between the use of the antagonistic muscle groups. This manifests itself as many of the dysfunctions previously discussed, such as poor coordination, inefficiency at reversals,[6,12,44] or neuromuscular holding patterns such as backward bending of the lumbar spine.

Trunk Control

Trunk control depends upon the integration of stability and mobility. It is essential for efficient function and the health of associated structures.[41,50] Dysfunctions of trunk motor control lead to aberrant movement patterns, and places abnormal stress on the soft tissues and articular structures. This stress, if repetitive or excessive, often precipitates symptoms and degeneration. Motor dysfunctions are often overlooked in the normal course of evaluation and treatment, as emphasis is placed on the structural components. Therefore, a basic tenant of PNF is to evaluate trunk motor control with any musculoskeletal problem in an extremity or the trunk.

For efficient trunk or extremity function to occur these interconnecting segments of pelvis and scapula must have the capacity to function independently and in coordinated manner with the extremity and trunk. In an efficient state the trunk provides appropriate proximal stability or controlled mobility to support optimal task or postural performance.

A functional trunk assessment is conducted by first evaluating the pelvic and shoulder girdles for appropriate characteristics of neuromuscular control and the pelvis and shoulder integration with the axial skeleton.

SYMPTOMS AND SELECTION OF TREATMENT TECHNIQUES

During the performance of passive, active, or resisted PNF diagonals, the therapist is always alert to the reproduction of the symptoms. The combinations of functional demands placed upon articular and soft tissue structures during any given pattern may identify restrictions or reproduce symptoms in a dynamic way that isolated structural assessment may not.

Assessment

A skilled practitioner can accomplish a full neuromuscular assessment in a few minutes and integrate the treatment of identified dysfunctions within the treatment program.

Example. In cases of recurrent inversion sprains of the ankle, the lower extremity patterns are assessed. Each aspect of the lower kinetic chain, including trunk, is evaluated for the multiple components of efficient neuromuscular control. A frequently identified dysfunctional component is poor control of dorsiflexion with eversion and hip internal rotation in the flexion-abduction pattern. When identified, a specific facilitory technique is chosen and applied during the performance of the pattern, a more responsive contraction of dorsiflexion with eversion. As the technique is being applied, the status of the dysfunction continues to be evaluated.

If an improvement is noted during the treatment process the facilitation techniques used are gradually eliminated until the pattern can be performed with minimal facilitation. The improved pattern is integrated into more complex patterns of movement and functional activities, specifically those movements and activities that have been previously assessed as symptomatic or dysfunctional. As coordination, muscle recruitment, strength, and control improves normal activities become less stressful upon the symptomatic structures and the potential of reinjury is reduced.

THE TECHNIQUES OF PNF

Because proprioceptive neuromuscular facilitation is defined as the utilization of the proprioceptors to hasten or make easier the learning of a neuromuscular task,[27] application of ideal technique is essential. The success achieved through PNF is derived from the therapist's ability to appropriately identify faulty characteristics of neuromuscular control and analyze and select the appropriate PNF technique. These techniques focus upon the functional attribute of the patient's motor response, utilizing facilitory tools such as resistance, stretch reflex, approximation, and traction.

Once a technique is selected and applied, the therapist evaluates the results and proceeds by choosing from the list of options (Table 11.1).

The following techniques were developed in response to clinically identified dysfunctions. Each techniques evolved through a trial and error application of the principles of PNF and subsequent observation of variations in the patients functional needs.

Rhythmic Initiation (RI)[15]

Purpose. RI is used to evaluate and treat the patient's ability:

Table 11.1
Options during PNF Procedures

1. If there is no improvement in the motor response—
    a. Evaluate whether the technique was effectively applied, and if not, correct the technique and apply again, or
    b. Select and apply another technique, or
    c. Utilize irradiation from a stronger synergistic component, or
    d. Address an associated dysfunction in conjunction with applied technique.

2. If a partial resolution has occurred in the motor response—
    a. Continue to utilize the technique to gain further improvement, or
    b. Integrate improvement into functional activity, or
    c. Teach patient self exercise program to maintain and enhance gains between treatments, or
    d. Wait until next treatment to address dysfunction again.
    e. Address an associated dysfunction in conjunction with applied technique.

3. If dysfunction is resolving or has resolved—
    a. Judiciously reduce use of facilitory technique and train patient to move efficiently against resistance without facilitation, or
    b. Integrate improvement into mass movement patterns and functional activities.

- to allow passive motion,
- to actively contract in a smooth, rhythmical fashion
- to perform movement at a consistent rhythm against resistance.

Indications. RI is utilized for the treatment of dysfunctions which affect the initiation, speed, direction, or quality of the contraction.

Application. In preparation to apply the technique, the patient is positioned in a posture conducive to relaxation. The technique is divided into three distinct components; passive, active, and resisted.

Passive. The technique is initiated by requesting the patient to relax and allow the therapist to perform the desired motion passively. An appropriate rhythm of movement is established as the patient relaxes. Manual contacts can be nonspecific.

Active. When a smooth and rhythmical passive motion is achieved, the therapist asks the patient to minimally assist with the motion. With each successful repetition, the patient increases the force of contraction. If the patient's participation interrupts the smooth rhythmical motion, the therapist resumes passive motion and tries again to have the patient participate at a lesser degree. Manual contact must be specific to direction of movement.

Resistive. Appropriate resistance is applied as the patient increases active participation. The goal is to slowly increase resistance with each repetition while maintaining the same rhythm and excursion of motion. Resistance is pivotal to the reinforcement of volitional control.

Example. The rhythmic initiation technique can be helpful to progressively facilitate active and resistive contractions in patients with acute pain. For acute lumbar symptoms, passive pelvic motion in pain-free range can provide oscillatory inhibition. As the patients relax and allow the motion, they are requested to provide a minimal active contraction. This active contraction can begin to inhibit pain and spasm, and provide a muscular pumping action for the region. If the active contraction is built to a point where resistance can be added, it is added minimally at first and, if possible, with traction.

Often reversals of these small motions are helpful.

Combination of Isotonics (COI)[10]

Purpose. COI is used to evaluate and develop the ability to perform controlled purposeful movements. This is accomplished through assessment of the patient's capacity to alternate between the three types of isotonic contractions (concentric, eccentric, and maintained).

Indications. COI is indicated for the treatment of deficiencies in strength, the ability to appropriately perform these three isotonic contractions, ROM, and decreased neuromuscular coordination and awareness.

Application. This technique is coupled with the evaluation process. The therapist begins by assessing the patient's capacity to perform and transition between the three types of isotonic contractions within the normal range of a selected agonistic contraction. The exact timing and speed of the transitions will depend upon the individual patient and the goals of treatment. When a dysfunction is identified the technique is initiated by utilizing the type of contraction the patient performs best.

Identified Dysfunction. Included are—

Poor Concentric Control: Problems with initiation, power of concentric contraction, coordination, and direction of motion are treated through use of maintained and eccentric contractions.

Example. If the patient is unable to easily move a body part to a specific target position, the body part is placed at that point. A maintained contraction is built followed by a short-range eccentric contraction with an immediate concentric contraction to return to the target position. This procedure is repeated until the concentric contraction can be performed to the target point.

Poor Eccentric Control: Difficulty in controlled eccentric contractions with appropriate strength is treated through utilization of maintained and concentric contractions.

Example. A ratchety quality of an eccentric contraction performed against appropriate resistance. Once the ratchety type of contraction begins, a maintained contraction is initiated, then a short-range concentric followed by an eccentric. This procedure is repeated until optimal control is gained, which is determined by reassessing motion quality.

Inefficient Maintained Isotonic: The inability to perform a maintained contraction, with optimal strength and endurance is treated through utilization of concentric and eccentric contraction.

Example. The inability to hold a position would be treated by slowly switching between short-range concentric and eccentric contractions until a maintained one can be established.

Inefficient Neuromuscular Control: The goal is to be able to functionally combine these three contractions in a smooth and coordinated manner.

Example. Combination of isotonics can be utilized to train ADL activities such as training push/pull activities. Initial training begins with resisted gait to facilitate the proper pelvic and lower extremity mechanics. Once developed, resistance is applied to the upper extremities through direct or indirect (use of a dowel) to train through combination of isotonics appropriate weight shift, weight acceptance, balance, force production, and shoulder girdle stability. (See Figs. 11.12, a, b, c).

Decreased Range of Motion: COI is used to treat decreased ROM and offers an alternative to traditional hold or contract relax. The repetition of the internal shortening and lengthening of the muscle fibers against resistance yields a lasting increase in ROM of the soft tissues and subsequently affects associated joint motion. This is effectively demonstrated by applying COI to the scapula patterns when decreased cervical-thoracic translation is observed during active cervical rotation.

Repeated Quick Stretch (RQS)[15,16]

Purpose. RQS is the repeated use of the stretch reflex to assist with initiation of a muscular response or to enhance strength and endurance of a preexisting contraction. This is based upon the principle that repeated excitation of a pathway in the central nervous system promotes ease of transmission of impulses through that pathway.[16]

Indications. RQS is a valuable tool for enhancing initiation and force of a weak contraction, for reducing fatigue, improving endurance, and increasing the patient's awareness of the motion.

Application. There are two basic forms of RQS. It can be performed from elongation or it can be superimposed upon an existing contraction.

Repeated Quick Stretch from Elongation (RQS-E)[10]

Purpose. RQS-E is utilized to treat the following dysfunctions: sluggish or delayed initiation, inability to pull through complete range, fatigue, and poor coordination of the motion.

Application. RQS-E is applied by placing each of the muscle components in their lengthened range. In most cases this will be the beginning position of a PNF pattern of facilitation. A contraction is initiated by a stretch stimulus and coordinated with a timed verbal command. The reflex contraction is reinforced through the immediate application of appropriate resistance. The contraction is resisted through the active range of motion or to fatigue. The part is then passively or actively returned to the elongated position and process repeated. Because the stretch reflex is facilitory, the motion can be repeated multiple times to enhance the learning, strengthening, and conditioning process, with minimal fatigue.

Repeated Quick Stretch Superimposed upon an Existing Contraction (RQS–SEC)[10]

Purpose. RQS-SEC is utilized to treat the following dysfunctions: a weakening contraction, fatigue, poor control in a specific portion of the range, inability to actively complete the desired range, diminished control of selected

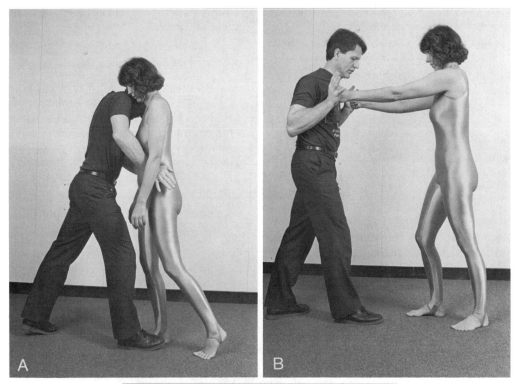

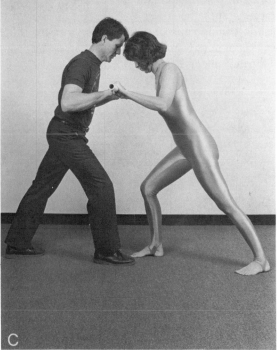

Figure 11.12. Push-pull activities broken down into: **A**) resisted gait; **B**) direct resistance through the extremities; **C**) indirect resistance through a dowel.

components of the motion, and inability to move in desired direction.

Application. RQS-SEC is a quick stretch applied to the tension of the existing contraction at the desired point in the range. This is possible because resistance maintains tension on the contracting muscles, to which a stretch reflex is superimposed, followed by immediate resistance applied to the subsequent reflex contraction. The number and frequency of repeated quick stretches varies according to the dysfunction and the goal of treatment. Multiple repetitions of the motion can be performed while applying repeated quick stretches through the range. As with any facilitory technique the therapist should begin to reduce the use of RQS to train the patient to function efficiently without the facilitation.

Example. Resisted crawling is an important developmental activity which influences and retains the trunk's ability to maintain stability while the extremities support and move the trunk. The goal of treatment is to train the patient to maintain a stable neutral lumbar spine, while the therapist resists the lower extremities. Often specific components of a lower extremity pattern do not initiate and/or fire during the range of the movement. RQS-E

and -SEC are both valuable tools to facilitate these movements.

Reversal of Antagonists (ROA)[10,15]

Purpose. Most activities depend upon coordinated control of antagonistic muscle groups. This control is essential to produce efficient interaction between the demands for mobility and stability. When an antagonist fails to work in accordance with the demand of the activity, function is immediately impaired. The techniques are based upon Sherrington's principle of successive induction.[49]

Indications. The ROA techniques are designed to:

—Facilitate coordinated transitions between reciprocal contractions,
—Facilitate a weaker antagonist,
—Reduce fatigue,
—Improve coordination,
—Increase active ROM,
—Enhance carry-over of reciprocal function into functional activities (Fig. 11.13), and
—Produce a reduction in antagonistic activity.

Application. There are two techniques involved in ROA: isotonic reversals and stabilizing reversals.[10]

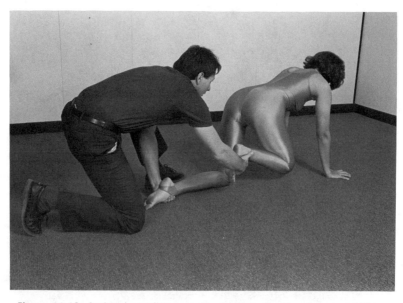

Figure 11.13. Resisted crawling—used to facilitate functional trunk stability.

Isotonic Reversal (IR)

IR is applied by resisting alternating concentric contractions. The speed and the range of motion utilized is dependent upon the individual's needs and abilities. Techniques such as RI, COI, and RQS can be combined with IR to enhance the motor response.

Application. The technique is begun by initiating a concentric contraction, either through a verbal command alone or one that is timed with a stretch reflex. At the point in the range, if a reversal of directions is desired the therapist smoothly shifts from applying resistance with both hands to one (usually freeing the proximal hand). The free hand then applies manual contact to the antagonistic surface, and for a brief time the hands are contacting both surfaces. A reversal of direction is elicited through a verbal command and if necessary a quick stretch. The goal is to train the patient to shift smoothly and effectively from one pattern to the other.

A weaker agonist group can be facilitated by applying manual resistance to the antagonist pattern before the reversal or by combining the repeated quick stretch techniques within the IR.

When there is difficulty in reversing direction smoothly, the therapist may use a maintained isotonic to the agonistic motion. This maintained isotonic contraction will facilitate the antagonists motion and allow the therapist time to change manual contacts.

If the patient fatigues easily in one direction while applying RQS-E, an IR can be combined to reduce fatigue.

As the patient learns to reverse directions smoothly with simple nonweight-bearing patterns the skills are advanced to more complex functional activities.

Stabilizing Reversal (SR)[10]

SR, also called *Rhythmic Stabilization*,[15] is applied by resisting alternating isometric contractions. The goals of the technique are to improve stability around a segment, to increase positional neuromuscular awareness, to improve posture and balance, and to enhance strength or stretch sensitivity of extensors in the shortened range. The technique can also be applied to reduce pain, facilitate relaxation, and increase ROM. This technique also offers the therapist a significant amount of information about the patient's ability to reinforce the contractions through appropriate irradiation.

Application. Manual contacts can be placed either on one side of the trunk or extremity, or on both sides. The therapist begins by gradually increasing resistance through both hands coupled with a verbal command, "Keep it there; don't let me move you." The therapist slowly increases the resistance in direct proportion to the patient's response. This matching or isometric contraction is built to a maximal level without promoting a concentric response. Once the contraction has plateaued, the therapist can slowly change the manual contacts to place a varying demand on the stabilizing muscles. To shift a manual contact, one hand must adjust resistance to maintain the contraction while the other hand slowly releases its resistance. The free hand is then shifted to another appropriate surface. The transition must be smooth, not allowing for any relaxation or initiation of attempted motion. If the patient is not able to perform an isometric contraction a maintained isotonic contraction is used.

Example. A good illustration is the application of resistance to the shoulder girdle region to promote trunk stability in sitting. As the patient is instructed to maintain a balanced position, the therapist slowly begins to apply resistance to the trunk through manual contacts at the shoulder region. If the resistance is applied too quickly, the patient may respond with an active isotonic contraction of the shoulder girdle muscles. By applying the resistance slowly, the therapist not only encourages an isometric contraction of the shoulder girdle region, but facilitates irradiation to the trunk muscles in an isometric mode. As the therapist increases the resistance, the patient's response builds to the level at which the trunk is holding a maximum isometric contraction. At this time, the therapist slowly changes the manual contacts in a smooth and coordinated manner, so as to maintain the isometric nature of the trunk contraction (Fig. 11.14).

Contract Relax (CR)[15]

Purpose. Contract relax utilizes the development of muscle tension through an concentric or maintained contraction to facilitate relaxation and stretching of the intrinsic connective tissue elements of that muscle.

Indication. To increase range of motion of the myofascial unit, by facilitating relaxation and improving extensibility of the myofascial tissues. Relaxation of unnecessary muscle tension may also serve to improve local circulation.

Application. To perform a *CR technique*, the therapist first places the segment at the point of limitation within the movement pattern. Resistance is given to a concentric contraction of either the restricted agonist (direct contraction), or to the antagonist (reciprocal relaxation). All components of the pattern should be resisted and a few degrees of motion allowed to occur. Special emphasis should be placed on the rotatory component of the pattern, as it will facilitate a more complete contraction and relaxation. The duration and intensity of the contraction should be sufficient to generate a strong contraction within the target muscles. Following the contraction, the patient is asked to completely relax, and upon full relaxation the segment is passively or actively taken into the new available range. Resisted motion into the new range can be used for reinforcement, strengthening, or further reciprocal inhibition.[5,15,18,52–55]

Hold Relax (HR)[10]

Purpose. Like contract relax, HR is used to facilitate relaxation and increased range,

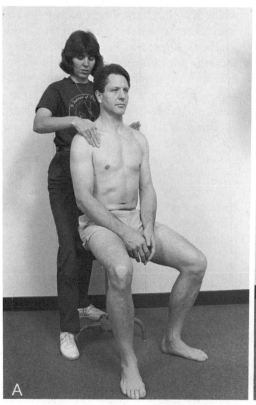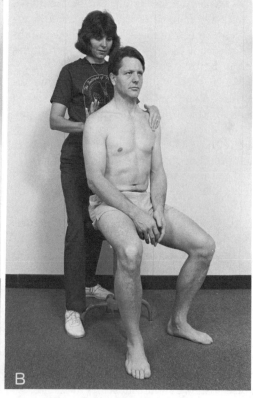

Figure 11.14. The technique of Isometric Reversals (IR)—applied to the shoulder girdle region in sitting to facilitate a better stabilizing response and postural awareness.

utilizing an isometric rather than an isotonic contraction.

Indication. In the presence of pain or when the concentric contraction is overpowering, an isometric contraction provides greater control of the procedure.

Application. The part is placed in a pain-free portion of the range and the isometric contraction is slowly built. The verbal command, "Hold, don't let me move you" is given. In cases with highly irritable symptoms the facilitated contraction may be minimal. In some cases, the technique is most effectively applied to a pain-free portion of the body to create indirect relaxation through irradiation. The segment may then be moved actively or passively to the new range, or the technique may be repeated without motion to gain further relaxation or pain reduction.[10,15]

SPECIFIC DYSFUNCTIONS

Pain

Determining the level of irritability is the first consideration in the treatment of pain.[2] If the symptoms are highly irritable the goal of treatment is the reduction of symptoms, with extra caution taken not to exacerbate those symptoms.

The first aspect of treatment is to identify positions which reduce symptoms and provide appropriate supports. In addition, an important adjunct to treatment is the use of ice, which is most effective if utilized while treatment techniques are being applied. The authors personally prefer the icing system developed by Kabat and Knott, which uses towels soaked in a bucket of shaved ice and water. These towels are wrung out and placed over the painful and surrounding regions, and changed every few minutes.[15,56]

The techniques of choice for *irritable symptoms* are stabilizing reversals and hold relax. These techniques are applied to components which facilitate appropriate irradiation. As relaxation occurs and if symptoms reduce, controlled use of combinations of isotonics can begin to assist in improving mobility, circulation, and relaxation of the symptomatic region. Also mid-range active short-arc motions can provide oscillatory inhabition and relaxation. If pain increases, the techniques are discontinued.

If symptoms are *minimally irritable* the primary goal of treatment is to assess for dysfunctions (characteristics of neuromuscular control) and to provide appropriate manual therapy (soft tissue and joint mobilization and neuromuscular reeducation).[23,24]

Throughout the evaluation process, care must be taken to differentiate between the primary symptoms and those which are secondary to compensations, inflammation, and inactivity. Pain is rarely localized to the primary dysfunctional structure, partially due to the compensatory movement patterns and altered postures. These compensations, if chronic, precipitate muscular imbalances and strength loss. Secondary dysfunctions serve to reinforce the primary dysfunction and ultimately need to be addressed.

Example. Patients suffering from cervical pain and demonstrating restricted cervical movements, often have restriction of scapula patterns as well. Since the cervical spine and shoulder girdles share many of the same muscles, treatments of shoulder girdle dysfunction often have dramatic effects on cervical dysfunctions and symptoms. In addition, in highly irritable patients in which the cervical spine cannot be treated, the shoulder girdle may often be successfully utilized. As limitations in the scapular patterns are identified, HR, CR, or COI techniques can be applied to enhance relaxation. Muscle tension reduction may produce immediate changes in arthrokinematics, extensibility, and proprioceptive input of the shoulder girdle and cervical spine.[6,57] Improved movement patterns often result in pain reduction. As compensations are resolved, the therapist can work directly into the primary dysfunction, much like peeling the layers of an onion.

Limited Functional Excursion and Muscular Imbalance

Dysfunctional effects occur secondary to limited myofascial excursion, muscle play, and muscular imbalance.[6,21,22,58] Such effects are:

1) Greater susceptibility for muscle pulls or tears.[9,59]

2) Altered primary fulcrum of motion—*an example* is seen when there is restricted extensibility of lower extremity muscles. This limits hip and pelvic mobility and places the primary fulcrum of motion in the lumbar spine. With moderate hamstring restriction the lumbar spine becomes the improper primary axis of motion during most forward-oriented tasks. In addition, with psoas restriction, efficient vertical alignment and weight attenuation is impossible and the hips are limited from contributing to backward bending activities.

3) Altered posture and normal mobility—this is observed in patients with limited functional excursion of the muscles of the cervical and upper thoracic spine. The following muscles are often the most frequently involved and most dramatically contribute to cervical pathomechanics: suboccipitals, scaleni, longus coli, levator scapulae, SCM, multifidus, pectoralis minor, posterior superior serratus, etc.

4) Joint dysfunction and pathomechanics—alterations in the excursion and mobility of either the myofascial unit or the articulation serve to facilitate or reinforce dysfunctions in the other.[6,12,19]

5) Agonistic tightness inhibits antagonistic function.[6,56]

6) Unilateral restriction increases emphasis for motion on opposite side.[20]

Clinical Example. The utilization of PNF strategies can be effective for improving these types of conditions:

Many patients with lumbar symptomatology have marked anterior to posterior muscle imbalances (Figs. 11.15, 11.16). The trunk extensor and hip flexors have limited functional excursion, while the trunk flexors and hip extensors are weak, with sluggish or absent responsiveness. These patients often stand with the thoracic cage posterior to the pelvis, increasing the lumbar lordosis. During forward oriented functional activities, most of the motion occurs in the lumbar spine. This compares with the efficient state where the primary axis of motion occurs in the pelvis

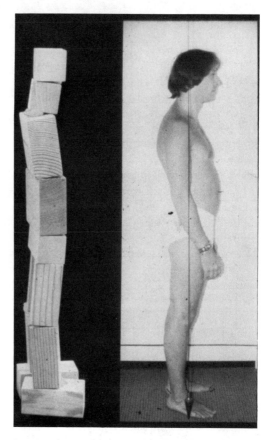

Figure 11.15. The frequently observed dysfunctional standing posture of thoracic cage posterior and backward bent in relationship to the pelvis often precludes inefficient movement patterns.

and hips, and minimal motion occurs in the lumbar spine (Fig. 11.17).

The initial focus of neuromuscular treatment is facilitating efficient pelvic girdle patterns. Both structural and neuromuscular components are evaluated and treated using the diagonal of anterior elevation and posterior depression. During the resisted motion of anterior elevation, the pelvis should move in a straight line in relationship to the body, while the lumbar spine remains in a stable anteroposterior position. To accommodate the motion occurring in the plane of the facet joint, the lumbar spine will sidebend to allow the pelvic motion. (See Figs. 11.18, 11.19).

For the anterior elevation pattern to occur

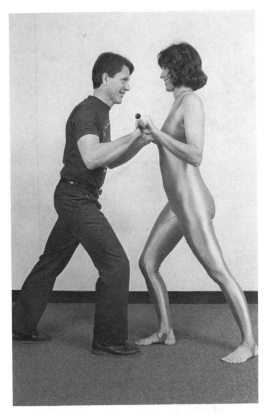

Figure 11.16. Existence of muscular imbalance of the trunk muscles leads to trunk instability, inefficient fulcruming within the spine, and inability to stabilize spine against external forces.

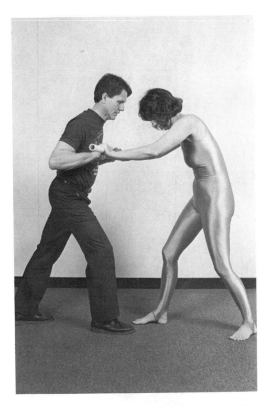

Figure 11.17. Muscular balancing allows the trunk to stabilize and the base of support to generate and translate the force.

efficiently, the lower abdominals, trunk extensors, body of psoas, and quadratus lumborum must perform in a coordinated sequence of contractions and elongations. The primary tools for treating dysfunctions in the pattern are *contract* or *hold relax* to increase mobility and *combination of isotonics* to improve the proper sequencing of muscle recruitment and dissociation of the pelvic girdle from the lumbar spine. As the motion becomes integrated, lower extremity flexion can be resisted to develop synergistic lumbopelvic/lower extremity control. This is an important motion for the initiation and progression of swing through in the gait cycle.

The *posterior depression pattern* occurs along the same track of motion but requires efficient

antagonistic muscles function to develop coordination of pelvic/hip motions and dissociation of pelvic/lumbar motions. This is an important pattern for push-off during the gait cycle.

As indicated in the example, there is a correlation between soft tissue dysfunctions and the identified muscular imbalance. In many traditional manual therapy approaches, soft tissue changes have been treated as secondary dysfunctions and believed to be treated indirectly by joint mobilization. Often the soft tissues feel improved following joint mobilization. Therefore, it has been theorized that they do not need to be addressed separately. However, through a more dynamic palpatory assessment, the experienced therapist can often identify structural dysfunctions of muscle play,[21] accessory mobility, and ex-

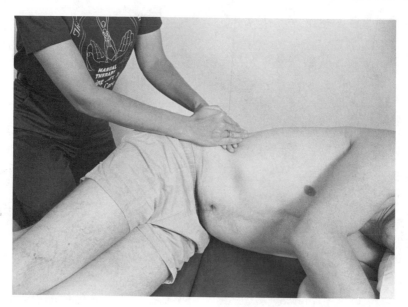

Figure 11.18. Pelvic anterior elevation.

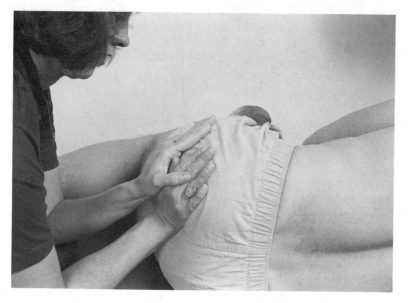

Figure 11.19. Pelvic posterior depression.

tensibility, which the conventional evaluation will not reveal. Throughout the procedures of PNF these dysfunctions can be identified and normalized.

Motor Control

Assessment and treatment of inefficiencies in motor control should consider: elements of recruitment, sequencing, coordination, balance, and fine motor control.[10,15,32] Inefficiencies in these elements may be secondary to: altered arthrokinematics, soft tissue trauma, muscular tension, pain, CNS irritability, posture, or receptor damage.

Efficient muscle recruitment is the ability to initiate and grade a muscle contraction to the appropriate internal and external demands of the environment. The neuromuscular system, in most cases, is trying to identify the most efficient and coordinated manner to perform tasks, but in dysfunctional states is unable to make the appropriate corrections. Through the use of techniques of neuromuscular reeducation, the system experiences the more efficient and coordinated recruitment, and through the use of repetition and resistance the system learns this as a new option for movement. Recruitment can be assessed by varying the type, direction, and amount of resistance given, such as combination of isotonics or stabilizing reversals. If the patient's *recruitment is in excess* of demand, rhythmic initiation can be used, starting with passive and slowly progressing to the desired amount of recruitment. Inversely, when *recruitment is deficient* in meeting demand, the contraction can be augmented by reflex facilitation (repeated quick stretch, traction, or approximation). If the patient's selective recruitment is inappropriate and more responsive, overactive muscles substitute for the movement. Then the PNF patterns and COI (combination of isotonics) or hold relax techniques can be emphasized to ensure appropriate recruitment.

Sometimes the muscles are not recruited in an efficient order and there is an *altered pattern of motor sequencing.* In this case a repeated quick stretch can be applied to the latent muscle at the appropriate point in the range to facilitate more efficient recruitment patterns. Also, a combination of isotonics can be utilized, beginning with a maintained contraction in a range where all the components of the pattern can be recruited, and then through the use of eccentric and controlled concentric contractions, one can retrain the efficient pattern.

Inefficiencies in coordination, balance, and fine motor control can be addressed by reducing the task to its simplest and easiest component. These components are generally learned most efficiently in the least demanding positions and postures. As skill develops, they are progressed to the more complex functional postures, motions, and tasks.

Example. During lifting activities, patients often demonstrate inefficiency of mechanics, recruitment, balance, and motor control. Dysfunctions of these components can be effectively retrained by reducing the more complex activity into simpler components.[10,13,15]

Initially, retraining of smooth and coordinated *weight shift* is accomplished through appropriate resistance to the pelvis. If the bipedal position is too premature, weight shift can be first trained in quadruped, half kneeling, or sitting (Fig. 11.20).

Proper *sequencing* of the hips and trunk, should occur with the primary motion occurring at the hips with trunk providing controlled stability. The proper coordination of the motion is often trained more effectively in sitting, then progressing to standing.

To train the proper use of the *base of support,* balance and control can be emphasized through the use of resistance. Once the

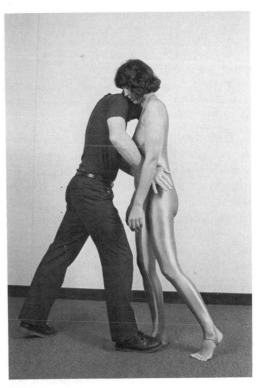

Figure 11.20. Resisted gait—used to retrain efficient weight shift.

smaller components are developed they are integrated back into the larger activity of lifting; the technique of combination of isotonics is used to effectively retrain the components into the whole throughout various portions of the task.

Segmental Limited Mobility

Treatment of limited mobility has been covered previously in this chapter. This section is designed to provide examples in the cervical, thoracic, and lumbo-pelvic regions.[23,24] Segments with restricted mobility can be identified through:

- Restriction in range of a pattern,
- A section of the range in which the motion "jumps" past a region,
- A deviation in the performance of the pattern at a specific segment,
- Palpation of the spinal structures while the pattern is being performed.

The general principle for utilizing PNF to restore segmental mobility is to:

- Localize the restricted motion,
- Lock the segments above and below to provide specificity,
- Place manual contact upon the restricted region to provide a fulcrum and kinesthetic feedback.

If the localization is done well, many times substantial mobility can be gained through the use of selective breathing. The patient is instructed to breath into the manual fulcrum and build up to the point of comfort; then, on exhalation, to relax and allow a new range to be gained. Once the segment is moved into the new range, the technique is performed again until progress plateaus or normal mobility is reinstated. Facilitation techniques are then applied to reeducate the new range. If breathing does not provide adequate force, a hold or contract relax can be performed when the symptoms are not too irritable.

Cervical Spine. Each segment is evaluated for its ability to move both into flexion and extension within the patterns. In the flexion motion, the anterior aspect of the facet joints are palpated for limited mobility. This is the region to which the treatment fulcrum is placed. In the same manner the posterior articular pillars are palpated into extension to that side. The options for facilitating a contraction are: breathing, use of shoulder girdle, jaw opening and closing, eyes movement, side-bending of the trunk specificity, or contractions within the pattern (Fig. 11.21).

Thoracic Spine. A frequently restricted motion in the thoracic spine is backward bending. The following procedure is adapted from a thoracic spine mobilization technique. The restricted segment is localized through a hand placed posterior at the level of restriction, and the resisted force is placed through the patient's elbows. The treatment technique is applied by having the patient lift the elbows up or down (Fig. 11.22). This will localize the force to the restricted movement segment. As the range increases, neuromuscular reeducation is performed in the new range. If a manipulative thrust is used, neuromuscular reeducation can help to retrain the surrounding muscles to functionally maintain the gains.

Lumbar. Through the use of standard localization techniques (see Fig. 11.23) instead of passive mobilization techniques, the more dynamic PNF approach can add a more functional option. *Hold relax* is often the technique of choice to assure the proper recruitment and avoid substitution or too forceful of a response.

Pelvic Girdle. Figure 11.24 illustrates the use of a position to dynamically mobilize and reeducate an innominate bone that is restricted into posterior torsion.

Instability

Spinal stabilization is the capacity of the intrinsic and extrinsic trunk musculature to provide both segmental and general stability to the spine in response to movement demands and external forces.[13,32] This protective stability or lumbar protective mechanism[36,44] requires adequate strength and responsiveness of the trunk musculature. Adequate strength includes both sufficient force production and

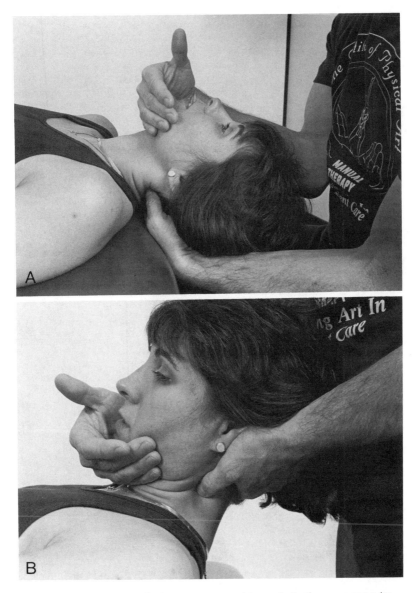

Figure 11.21. Cervical flexion pattern—used to evaluate the neuromuscular control and arthrokinematics of the cervical spine.

endurance, while responsiveness is the speed and appropriateness of the reflex reaction to external demands.

Segmental Stability. This is the capacity of primarily the one joint intrinsic muscles (i.e., in the lumbar spine the multifidi, rotatores, interspinales, intertransversarii, and the one-joint fibers of the quadratus lumborum and psoas) to provide controlled sta-

bility and mobility at each movement segment.

General Stability. This is the capacity of the multijoint extrinsic muscles (rectus abdominis, obliques, erector spinae, multi-joint fibers of the quadratus lumborum and psoas) to provide controlled stability and mobility of the lumbar spine in relationship to the pelvis and thoracic cage.

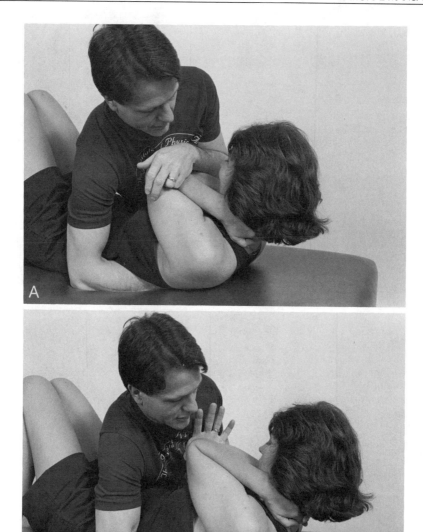

Figure 11.22. Resisted trunk flexion and extension patterns are combined with thoracic joint mobilization.

Integration. These two components must work together in a coordinated pattern to provide adequate stabilization. The neurophysiological principle that normal timing occurs from proximal to distal applies to the spinal musculature. The intrinsic muscles should provide the initial contraction to stabilize the segment to prepare for the extrinsic demands of stability or mobility.

If there is inadequate spinal stabilization of a region or individual segment, those structures are more vulnerable to sustaining injury during stressful activities or trauma. They also will receive repetitive microtrauma during normal activities, particularly those performed with rotation or end-range positions. These segments often develop degenerative changes and become hypermobile from the

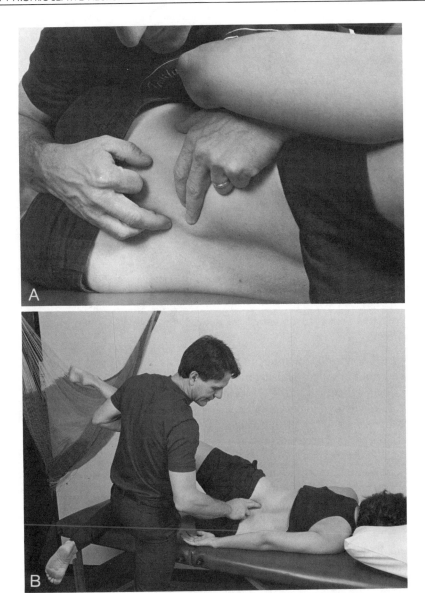

Figure 11.23. Hold Relax and Contract Relax techniques—used to facilitate lumbar mobilization; this treatment tool was later used in the development of "Muscle Energy Techniques." **A)** lumbar rotation; **B)** lumbar side bending while in extension and right rotation.

overstretching and demands to the discs, ligaments, and articular structures.[6,20,60]

Posture

Another mechanism which precipitates instability is posture. In efficient posture the individual spinal structures are positioned so that weight is distributed to the base of support and force is attenuated through the structure. However, many individuals have habitually developed postures which abnormally converge the weight distribution, force attenuation, and motion to individual regions and segments.

Example. A common postural dysfunction is the thoracic cage positioned in backwardbending in relationship to the lumbo/pelvic region. This posture creates an abnor-

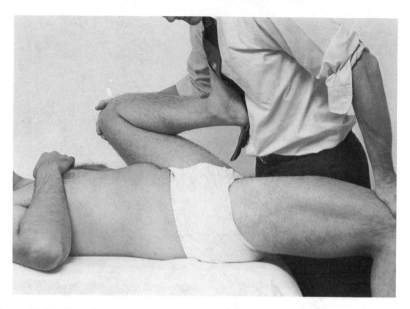

Figure 11.24. Use of contract relax to improve the mobility of a restricted innominate.

mal sharp angle (fulcrum) in the mid-lumbar spine, with the center of gravity shifting more to the posterior elements. During vertical loading this region will tend to buckle or bend backward, further stressing the posterior elements. In addition, the posture places the posterior myofascial structures in a shortened position and the abdominal muscles on stretch, altering the normal agonistic/antagonistic balance.[6] The abdominals tend to become weak, over-stretched, and delayed in their responsiveness, while the extensors general become shortened, with increased tone, and delayed responsiveness. The underlying movement segment progresses through the degenerative cascade.[4] In addition, due to reduced motion demands the regions above and below usually develop some degree of hypomobility.

Tests

Efficient alignment can be assessed through the *vertical compression test*, where a vertical pressure (approximation) is placed to the shoulders and the stability of the spine assessed (Fig. 11.25).[21,44] Regions where buckling is felt or seen are considered dysfunctional.

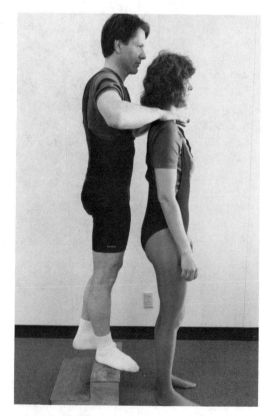

Figure 11.25. Vertical Compression Test (Johnson, 1984).

Responsiveness is tested through the *lumbar protective mechanism test* (Fig. 11.26). The test is administered with the patient in standing or sitting, while the therapist applies unidirectional pressure to the shoulders in posterior, anterior, and diagonal directions. The patient is instructed to hold, and the responsiveness and strength of the resulting contraction is graded. In the efficient state there is minimal lumbar motion.

Therefore, the treatment strategy for instability must address the structural, postural, and neuromuscular components.

Components

Structural. The soft tissue and myofascial dysfunctions need to be addressed through appropriate manual therapy techniques so the region has improved mobility and postural potential (Fig. 11.27).

Postural. Through graded and guided resistance and repetition the individual can be trained to attain an improved posture and to efficiently move in and from that posture. To assist their ability to maintain and their kinesthetic awareness of the posture, possibly through re-biasing of the muscle spindles, stabilizing reversals are applied in the optimal posture.

Neuromuscular. Education and training are required to prepare a patient to efficiently respond to the external forces which necessitate a stabilization response. The neuromuscular element of the structural and postural dysfunctions is evaluated and treated for the integral role this system plays in posture and movement retraining. The philosophy and principles of PNF give the therapist the tools to retrain the neuromuscular elements to support the stabilization response.

The process of stabilization training or functional rehabilitation is an integrated process, which includes the gamut of manual therapy techniques. The interrelated use of PNF with soft tissue and joint mobilization allows the therapist to progress the patient rapidly through the rehabilitation. Because the effects of structure and function are interdependent PNF may be used to address both aspects during the course of treatment, balancing one system as the other is altered through techniques.

Such utilization of PNF during the stabilization or functional rehabilitation program may include:

1. The use of contract or hold relax techniques as an adjunct to soft tissue mobilization to facilitate elongation in shortened muscles.

2. The use of trunk, shoulder girdle, and pelvic PNF patterns to localize the unstable segment and facilitate contractions of the intrinsic muscles. This is generally accomplished through the application of prolonged isometric and stabilizing reversals. The manual approach of PNF gives direct feedback to the therapist which is needed to assure proper recruitment is occurring. Otherwise, new movement patterns using old, habitual recruitment motor patterns are being retrained.

3. The use of combination of isotonics to manually reinforce and train controlled movement. This trains the extrinsic muscles to coordinate with the intrinsic muscles.

4. The next progression is to use the extremities in activities such as resisted rolling and crawling, while stability and control are maintained in the dysfunctional segment (Figs. 11.28, 11.29). This is coupled with an independent exercise program.

5. Progression to resisted functional activities such as lifting, walking, pushing, pulling, etc. is evaluated first through the manual principles of PNF, then trained and progressed to an independent exercise program (Fig. 11.30). Once again, the emphasis of PNF at this stage is to assure the patient does not substitute previous movement patterns during the more complex activities.

6. Balancing reactions through treatment adjuncts such as the Swiss ball (Fig. 11.31). Feldenkrais foam roll, balance boards, etc. offer the advanced training necessary to facilitate functional and spontaneous carry-over of stabilization to activities of daily living.

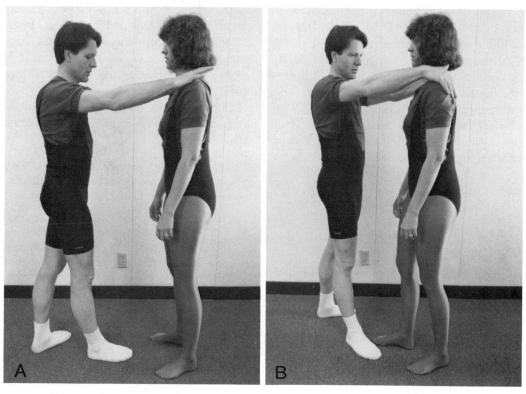

Figure 11.26. Lumbar protective Mechanism (Johnson, 1984). **A)** Flexors; **B)** Extensors.

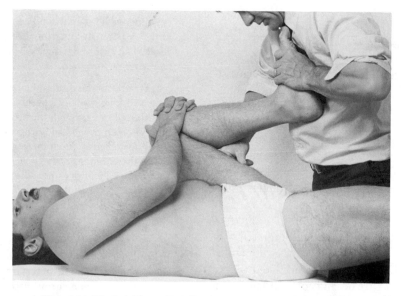

Figure 11.27. Soft Tissue Mobilization technique (Johnson, 1978).

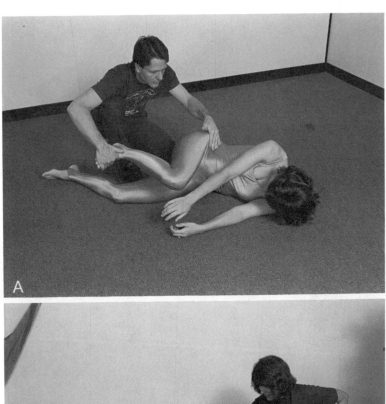

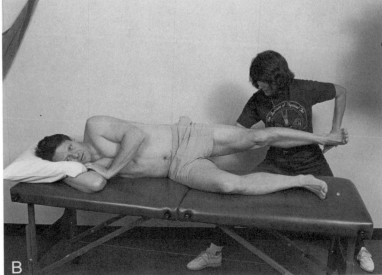

Figure 11.28. Use of lower extremities to facilitate rolling.

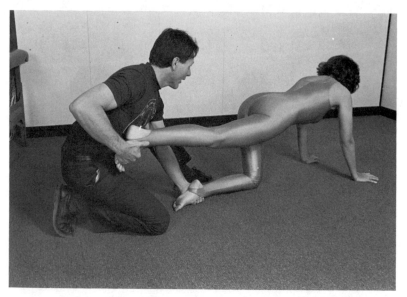

Figure 11.29. Facilitation of crawling—through resistance and facilitation to the extremities.

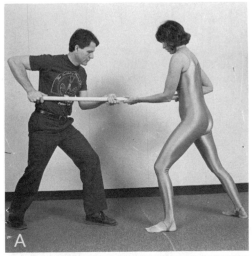

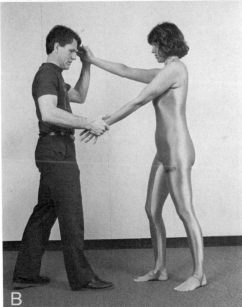

Figure 11.30. Resisted functional activities to ensure appropriate motor recruitment.

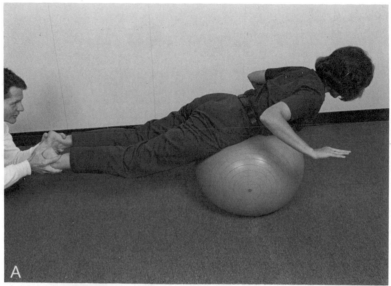

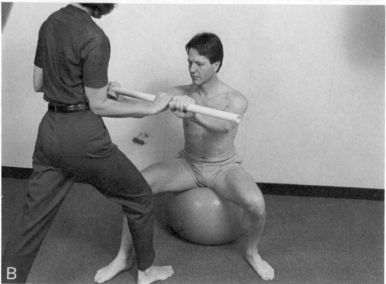

Figure 11.31A & B. Use of PNF facilitory techniques to enhance responsiveness training while working on the Swiss Ball.

CONCLUSION

The ability of a therapist to clearly assess the underlying structural and/or neuromuscular dysfunctions which perpetuate an identifiable alteration in a person's functional activities of daily living is the foundation of physical therapy. This ability is enhanced by the understanding and utilization of the manual therapy approach of Proprioceptive Neuromuscular Facilitation. Through the principles, procedures, and techniques of PNF the therapist can identify and treat many of these structural and functional aberrations. In addition, the approach of PNF allows the therapist to fully integrate the treatment of structure and function by continuously integrating structural changes into functional improvements. The results achieved through structural techniques such as soft tissue mobilization and joint mobilization are enhanced when incorporated into the neuromuscular system.

REFERENCES

1. White A, Anderson R. The conservative care of low back pain. Baltimore: Williams & Wilkins, 1990.
2. Maitland GD. Vertebral manipulation, 5th ed. London, England: Butterworths, 1986.
3. Grieve GP. Common vertebral joint problems. London, England: Churchill-Livingstone, 1981.
4. Kirkaldy-Willis WH. Managing low back pain. 2nd ed. New York: Churchill-Livingstone, 1988.
5. Greenman PE. Principles of manual medicine. Baltimore: Williams & Wilkins, 1989.
6. Janda V. Muscle weakness and inhibition (pseudoparesis) in back pain syndromes. Chapter 19 in: Grieve, Gregory, ed. Modern manual therapy of the vertebral column. London, England: Churchill-Livingstone, 1986.
7. Mayer TG, Gatchell RJ, Mayer H, Kishino N, Keeley J. A prospective two-year study of functional restoration in industrial low back injury: An objective assessment procedure. JAMA, 1987;258:1763–1767.
8. Saal JA. Rehabilitation of sports-related lumbar spine injuries. Phys Med Rehab: State of the Art Reviews 1987; 1:613–638.
9. Saal JS. Flexibility training. Phys Med Rehab 1987; 1:537–554.
10. Johnson GS, Saliba VI. PNFI: the functional approach to movement reeducation. San Anselmo, CA: The Institute of Physical Art, 1978:90.
11. Kendall HO, Kendall FP, Boynton DA. Posture and pain. Huntington, NY: Robert E. Krieger Pub. Co., 1977.
12. Lewit K. The contribution of clinical observation to neurological mechanisms in manipulative therapy. In: Korr, I, ed. The neurobiologic mechanisms in manipulative therapy. London, England: Plenum Press, 1978.
13. Johnson GS, Saliba VL. Back education and training, course outline. San Anselmo, CA: The Institute of Physical Art, 1988.
14. Morgan D. Concepts in functional training and postural stabilization for the low-back-injured. Top Acute Care Trauma Rehabil 1988; 2:8–17.
15. Knott M, Voss B. Proprioceptive neuromuscular facilitation. 2nd ed. London, England: Balleire, Daintily & Cogs, 1968.
16. Kabat H. Proprioceptive facilitation in therapeutic exercise. In: Licht E, ed. Therapeutic exercise. 2nd ed. New Haven: E Licht, 1961.
17. Voss DE. Proprioceptive neuromuscular facilitation. Am J Phys Ther 1967; 46:838–899.
18. Sullivan PE, Markos PD, Minor MAD. An integrated approach to therapeutic exercise: theory and clinical application. Reston, VA: Reston Publishing Company, Inc., 1982.
19. Guyner AJ. Proprioceptive Neuromuscular Facilitation for Vertebral Joint Conditions. In: Grieve GP, ed. Modern manual therapy of the vertebral column. London: Churchill Livingstone, 1986.
20. Paris S. S-1 Course notes. Institute for Graduate Health Sciences, 1401 West Paces Ferry Road, Suite A-210, Atlanta, GA 30327, 1977:3.
21. Johnson GS, Saliba VL. Functional orthopedics I, course outline. San Anselmo, CA: The Institute of Physical Art, 1988.
22. Johnson GS, Saliba VL. Soft tissue mobilization. In: White A, Anderson R, eds. The conservative care of low back pain. Baltimore: Williams & Wilkins, 1991:112–119.
23. Johnson GS. Functional orthopedics III: upper quadrant, course outline. San Anselmo, CA: The Institute of Physical Art, 1990.
24. Johnson GS. Functional orthopedics III: lower quadrant, course outline. San Anselmo, CA: The Institute of Physical Art, 1990.
25. Kabat H. Studies on neuromuscular dysfunction. I. Neostigmine therapy of neuromuscular dysfunction resulting from trauma. II. Neostigmine therapy of hemiplegia. Facial paralysis and cerebral palsy. III. Neostigmine therapy of chronic rheumatoid arthritis and subacromial bursitis. Public Health Rep 1944; 59:1635.
26. Knott M. In the groove. Phys Ther 1973; 53:365.
27. Knott M. Course notes. Vallejo, CA: Kaiser Rehabilitation Center, 1972:77.
28. Montagu A. Touching: the human significance of skin. 2nd ed, New York: Harper & Row Publishers, 1978.

29. Miller B. Learning the touch. Phys Ther Forum, Western ed. King of Prussia, PA: Forum Publishing, Inc., 1987.

30. Hagbarth KE. Excitatory and inhibitory skin areas for flexor and extensor motorneurons. Acta Physiol Scand 1952; 26:1.

31. Nicholas JA, Melvin M, Saraniti AJ. Neurophysiologic inhibition of strength following tactile stimulation of the skin. Am J Sports Med 1980; 8:181.

32. Gowitzke BA, Milner M. Scientific basis of human movement. Baltimore: Williams & Wilkins, 1988.

33. Basmajian, JV. Muscles alive: their functions revealed by electromyography. Baltimore: Williams & Wilkins, 1978.

34. Sherrington CS. Selected writing. D. Denny-Brown, ed. New York: Paul B. Hoeber 1940:1–2.

35. Moore JC. Excitation overflow: an electromyographic investigation. Arch Phys Med Rehabil 1975; 56:115.

36. Buchwald JS. Exteroceptive reflexes and movement. Am J Phys Med 1967; 46:121.

37. Ratliffe KT, Alba BM, Hallum A, Jewell MJ. Effects of approximation on postural sway in healthy subjects. Phys Ther 1987; 67:502–506.

38. Adler S. Effects of "approximation" on normal walking. Master's Thesis. Downey, CA: University of Southern California, 1982.

39. Simonds HC. The inside story: Kabat-Kaiser Institute. Vallejo, CA: Kabat-Kaiser Institute Publishers, 1951.

40. Peele TL. The neuroanatomical basis for clinical neurology. New York: McGraw-Hill, 1954.

41. Feldenkrais M. Awareness through movement. New York, Harper & Row, 1977.

42. Shahani M. Visual input and its influence on motor and sensory systems in man. In: Shahani M, ed. The motor system: neurophysiology and muscle mechanisms. New York: Elsevier, Publisher, 1976.

43. Harrison VF. A review of the neuromuscular bases for motor learning. Res Quart 1962; 33:59.

44. Johnson GS, Saliba VL. Lumbar protective mechanism. In: White AH, Anderson R, eds. The conservative care of low back pain. Baltimore: Williams and Wilkins, 1991:112–119.

45. Aston J. Aston Patterning. Selected writings. Mill Valley, CA: The Aston Training Center, (undated).

46. Smidt GL. Trunk muscle strength and endurance in context of low back pain. Chapter 15 in: Grieve G, ed. Modern manual therapy of the vertebral column. London, England: Churchill-Livingstone, 1986:151–164.

47. Angel RW. Antagonistic muscle activity during rapid arm movements: central versus proprioceptive influences. J Neurol Neurosurg Psychiatry 1977; 40:683–686.

48. Wannstedt G, Mayer N, Rosenholtz H. Electromyographic features of an antagonistic muscle. Read at the 4th Congress of the International Society of Electrophysiological Kinesiology, Boston, 1979.

49. Sherrington C. The integrative action of the nervous system. New Haven: Yale University Press, 1961:340.

50. Bobath B. Adult hemiplegia: evaluation and treatment. London: William Heinemann Medical Books Limited, 1978.

51. Frankle VH, Nordin M. Basic biomechanics of the skeletal system. Philadelphia, PA: Lea & Febiger, 1980.

52. Smith JL, Hutton RS, Eldred E. Postcontraction changes in sensitivity of muscle afferents to static and dynamic stretch. Brain Res 1974; 78:193–202.

53. Medieros JM, Smidt GL, Burmeister LF, Soderberg GL. The influence of isometric exercise and passive stretch on hip joint motion. Phys Ther 1977; 57:518–523.

54. Sady SP, Wortman M, Blanke D. Flexibility training: ballistic, static or proprioceptive neuromuscular facilitation? Arch Phys Med Rehabil 1982; 63:261–263.

55. Tanigawa MC. Comparison of the hold relax procedure and passive mobilization on increasing muscle length. Phy Ther 1972; 52:725–735.

56. Knight KL. Cryotherapy: theory, technique and physiology. Chattanooga, TN: Chattanooga Corporation, 1985.

57. Shahani M. Visual input and its influence on motor and sensory systems in man. In: Shahani M, ed. The motor system: neurophysiology and muscle mechanisms. New York: Elsevier, 1976.

58. Gossmand MR, Sahrmann SA, Rose SJ. Review of length-associated changes in muscle. Phys Ther 1982; 62:1799–1808.

59. Zachezewski JE. Flexibility for the runner: specific program considerations. Top Acute Care Trauma Rehabil 1986; 10:9.

60. Paris SV. Physical signs of instability. Spine 1985; 10:277–279.

12

Elements of Muscle Energy Technique

FRED L. MITCHELL, JR.

Muscle Energy (ME) is a system of manual therapy that combines the precision of passive mobilization with the effectiveness, safety, and specificity of reeducation therapies and therapeutic exercise. The precision, localization, and control of the procedures are provided by the therapist, while the patient provides the corrective forces and energies as instructed by the therapist.

The concepts of ME are so interrelated that linear exposition of principles is difficult. Discussion of treatment principles is predicated upon an understanding of diagnosis, which cannot be understood without knowing the concepts and techniques of physical examination, which, in turn, requires a grasp of the psychophysics of observation and palpation. By comparing and contrasting ME with alternative approaches to clinical problem solving, decision making, and therapy, one may enhance comprehension of its concepts and principles. Three brief glossaries are included to define terms related to the barrier concept, motion descriptors, and muscle contractions. Inasmuch as striated muscles will be considered both as potential restrictors of articular motion, and as potential agents for the restoration of articular motion, the reader may need to review the section on neuromuscular physiology.

HISTORY AND ORIGINS

The ME technique was originally developed into a systematic clinical skill and art by Fred L. Mitchell, Sr. (1909–1974). It continues to evolve and expand, first in the hands and minds of his first generation of students, and now, as the second and third generation of students apply it in their practices and develop its teaching methodology.

Fred Mitchell's first application was in the manipulative treatment of the joints of the pelvis, which are passive joints, i.e., not moved by direct muscle action. Viewed from the present perspective, this seems a strange beginning. Currently, a central ME concept considers the function of muscles as flexors, extenders, rotators, and side-benders of joints *as well as restrictors of joint movements*. Mitchell began by developing techniques which used the patient's muscles to restore physiologic movement to the joints of the pelvis. His basic principles are the same for all passive joints: *voluntary muscle contractions are exerted against a precisely executed counterforce to loosen the specifically localized joints for passive articulation during postcontraction relaxation.*

The sacroiliac joints were considered immovable by most physicians and anatomists. However, a number of osteopathic physicians[1,2] were convinced that not only was mobility detectable by physical examination, but also that manual treatment of impairments of sacroiliac mobility was an important contribution to the practice of medicine.

Beginning with the pelvis Mitchell went on to develop ME techniques for the treatment of all the joints except cranial sutures.

Initially he developed techniques for the spine employing concentric isotonic contractions of the patient's muscles to pull the vertebra through restrictions. The concept behind these techniques was based on Sherrington's observation that contracting the antagonist of muscle A caused reduction of muscle A's tonus in proportion to the force of contraction developed against a strong counterforce. Assuming that muscle A's hypertonus or spasm is the cause of vertebral motion restriction, decreasing its tonus would help remove the restriction. By allowing the contracting antagonist to produce motion (concentric isotonic) the actual movement is restored as muscle A relaxes. This concept is particularly useful when applied to the ME treatment of acute torticollis, where it is especially effective.

Postisometric stretch techniques are now the principal ME procedure for treating somatic dysfunctions of the spine. The forceful isotonic procedures are usually reserved for the treatment of (antagonist) muscle spasm, e.g., acute torticollis. When polyarticular muscles of the extremities, or the spine, especially in scoliotic patients, need to be elongated, forceful isometric contractions or sustained contractions against an oscillating counterforce (allasotonic, or sometimes called "isolytic" contraction) are indicated. However, the post-contraction stretch actually accomplishes the therapeutic change.

The Pelvic Paradigm and Chapman's Reflexes

In the late 1940s, Mitchell was challenged by Paul Kimberly, DO to write an explanation [3] of what Charles Owens (author of *An Endocrine Interpretation of Chapman's Reflexes*) had meant by "balanced pelvis" in relation to Chapman's Reflexes.[1] Mitchell's interest in Chapman's reflexes grew from observing Charles Owens, DO, use them in 1934 to treat his only child, the author, who was comatose and moribund from severe third degree burns over 50+% of the body surface. In 1934 such a condition was regarded as uniformly fatal,

yet Owens' applications of Chapman's reflexes miraculously restored renal function and, in effect, saved the patient's life.

This paper generated so much controversy that Mitchell was driven to research and develop a unified kinematic model of the pelvis (explained later in this chapter). A paper explaining this paradigm was published in 1958 under the title "Structural Pelvic Function" and was slightly revised and reprinted in 1965.[4] This model of the pelvis remains a central concept in ME, and its consistency and predictability have been demonstrated for over 30 years.

Two germinal ideas were presented to Mitchell at a meeting in the 1950s. Thomas J. Ruddy, DO, an ophthalmologist, demonstrated his "Rapid Rhythmic Resistive Duction Technique" for exercising the extraocular muscle by moving the eyes against a resisting finger on the eyelid, in order to reduce orbital edema. Karl Kettler, DO, demonstrated a manipulative procedure which required the patient to press a leg against "*a precisely executed counterforce.*" According to Mitchell's 1948 paper,[3] the techniques he had used previously to treat the pelvis were passive, mainly thrust (high velocity, low amplitude) procedures—the style of osteopathic manipulation learned in medical school for the treatment of vertebral, costovertebral, and extremity joints. Soon after his exposure to Ruddy and Kettler, Mitchell's pelvic thrust techniques were replaced by techniques requiring the active participation of the patient.

After appropriate positioning, the patient now was told to push a designated part of the body in a specific direction against a *precisely executed counterforce* provided by the operator. Mitchell reasoned that the anatomically unique joint structures in the patient's own pelvis were more precisely and intimately known to the patient's muscles than they could be to any examiner. And so he chose to use the energy of the patient's muscles instead of his own for the corrective forces of treatment, hence the name, "Muscle Energy Technique."

DIAGNOSTIC CONCEPTS

A New Perspective on the Musculoskeletal System

A central postulate in osteopathic physical diagnosis is the assumption that the musculoskeletal system contains important information (data base) about the patient's health history: evidence of the physical, toxic, immunologic, and psycho-emotional stresses to which the patient's body has made inadequate responses. The assumption is that all information necessary for diagnosis is present if we know how to read the record. In this remarkable medical record system there are three functioning components, (*a*) the nervous system, which perceives and learns; (*b*) the striated muscles, which react; and (*c*) the fascia, which "remembers"; they comprise the neuro-musculo-skeletal system.

How the neuro-musculo-skeletal system adapts to the stresses of injury, illness, impairment, and disability may not only leave a "scar" in the system (the data base function) but may play a role in expressing (manifesting) the symptoms (e.g., pain) of injury, disease, impairment, and disability. The experience of pain involves the musculoskeletal system, regardless of whether the pathology exists in the muscles, joints, or fascia, or in a viscus, nerve, or vessel. Striated muscles react reflexively to noxious stimuli, and such reactions serve to identify and amplify the conscious experience of pain. Striated muscles are also involved in generalized conditions where symptoms such as chills, fever, and malaise exist. In the words of Korr,[5] "Striated muscles are the primary machinery of life." Striated muscle is involved in everything the human body does, somatically, viscerally, and mentally.

Symmetry of structure and function is a basic physiologic concept in need of elaboration and clarification. Diagnostic judgments related to the musculoskeletal system are customarily based on the assumption that the normal structures and functions of the body are bilaterally symmetrical and that a state of harmony, rhythm, and periodicity should exist in the body. True anatomic symmetry, however, is a fiction, especially in the arrangement of the internal organs. We shall assume that the musculoskeletal system is supposed to be *approximately* symmetrical, taking into account the slight variance due to cerebral hemispheric dominance, the altered contour of the central tendon of the diaphragm due to embryonic visceral rotation, occupation and life style, etc.

Departures from approximate symmetry lead to the diagnosis of abnormal structure and/or function in the musculoskeletal system, and to the manipulable diagnosis, *somatic dysfunction* (discussed later in this chapter). But suppose that abnormal alteration of structure or function occurs in a bilaterally symmetrical fashion. How can it be detected? Just as left/right asymmetry produces an imbalance, anterior/posterior imbalances are also possible. Judging such anterior/posterior imbalances requires a more holistic, global, or *Gestalt* view of the distribution of body masses in the context of the whole body posture. Such a perception of the whole body is equally important in evaluating the relative importance of left/right asymmetries. Naturally, successful treatment of *one side* of a symmetrical somatic dysfunction would result in asymmetry, and, incidentally, prove the diagnosis as the signs of unilateral somatic dysfunction may be observed.

SOMATIC DYSFUNCTION

Identifying Somatic Dysfunction

The diagnosis of somatic dysfunction in the context of the ME paradigm is *not* based on the presence or absence of pain, or the location of pain. Instead, the diagnosis is based on objective physical findings, which will be described under the heading, *Principles of Physical Diagnosis*. A detailed understanding of the adaptations evoked by the somatic dysfunction may lead one to an explanation of the mechanism of the pain. For example, a causal relationship exists between the adaptation to somatic dysfunction and the presence of Travell's myofascial trigger points, in the sense that the trigger point seems to be a part of the adaptive mechanism. In the case of somatic dysfunctions of the third or fourth thoracic intervertebral joints, unilateral Travell points are commonly found in the iliocostalis muscles of the fourth or fifth ribs and in the center of the infraspinatous muscle of one scapula. These exquisitely tender points appear to generate and maintain spasm in their respective muscles, presumably as a protective function.

Terminology and Natural History

For various reasons, the musculoskeletal system may acquire somatic dysfunctions, which may be acute or chronic, primary or secondary. In terms of acuteness or chronicity, the inflammatory changes of associated tissues may be at any stage of resolution. Greenman's triad of Asymmetry, Range-of-motion Restriction, and Tissue Texture abnormality (ART)[6] describes, in general, the characteristics of somatic dysfunction regardless of its etiology, history, or stage of resolution. Primary somatic dysfunctions are acquired by physical trauma. When acute, primary somatic dysfunctions manifest soft tissue trauma characteristics, many are reversible using conservative physical therapy treatment, such as ice. When chronic, the range of motion restriction tends to be greater, and the motion barriers (q.v.) have distinctive qualities, indicating degrees of fibrosis, edema, and tonic muscle hypertonus. Both acute and chronic somatic dysfunctions are typically correctable almost immediately with light isometric ME treatment.

Ira Rumney[7] DO, persuaded the publishers of the 1973 edition of the *International Classification of Diseases—Hospital Adaptation*[8] to include the classification of "osteopathic lesion," and coined the term "somatic dysfunction" defined as: "Impaired or altered function of related components of the somatic (body framework) system; skeletal, arthrodial, and myofascial structures; and related vascular, lymphatic, and neural elements." But its inclusion in that publication, and in the current ICD-9-CM[9] under the heading: "739 Non-allopathic lesions" has done little to clarify the concept. As global and general as the definition is, it fails to mention one crucial aspect which distinguishes somatic dysfunction from some orthopedic conditions, i.e., somatic dysfunction is *correctable* by manipulative treatment.

Implied in the global definition is the concept that the somatic dysfunctions are related to other body structures, including the internal organs. Secondary somatic dysfunctions are produced by neural reflex reactions to pathology in some other part of the body, either through viscerosomatic reflexes or somatosomatic reflexes, and thus are part of the signs and symptoms of disease, acute or chronic.

Secondary somatic dysfunctions may be acquired either through pathologic viscerosomatic reflexes from irritated viscera, or from stresses imposed on somatic structures by the necessity to adapt their function to compensate for primary somatic dysfunctions, or other acquired or congenital impairments.[10] Secondary somatic dysfunctions may stay in the acute phase for a long time, yet remain readily, or even spontaneously, reversible as soon as the primary stressor is removed. Secondary somatic dysfunctions are compensatory in nature, and are the consequences of the body's efforts to adapt.

As adaptation leads to compensation which leads to readaptation, somatic dysfunctions may become layered in ever increasing complexity. Older somatic dysfunctions may become obscured by ones more recently acquired through adaptation stress or superimposed trauma. Treating such complex problems of layered compensations and dysfunctions has been compared to peeling an onion. Decisions regarding the sequence of areas treated influence the efficiency of the treatment process.

Characteristics of Somatic Dysfunction in Different System

Many different paradigms related to the concept of somatic dysfunction, as well as to the clinical applications of manipulative therapy, are currently in use. Each paradigm has its own definition(s) of somatic dysfunction, based primarily on the *methods* used to diagnose and treat them.

Treatment methods such as Mobilization, High Velocity Low Amplitude Thrust, and ME share the same objective—an increase in range of motion—and are classed as *direct* techniques, i.e., treatment is localized by moving the affected bone to a position just short of the restricted movement barrier. Of the three characteristics described by Greenman[6] (asymmetry, restricted motion, and tissue texture abnormality) the central feature is restricted motion. Asymmetry—the appearance of a "bone out of place"—is variable depending on whether body movements are attempted which require the bone to move in the direction of its restriction. Tissue texture abnormality is also variable, depending on acuteness or chronicity, and the manner in which the body's adaptations and compensations are constituted.

Range of motion restriction is not to be confused with reluctance to move in certain directions, a behavioral characteristic of compensating joints and tissues. Reluctant movement behavior in response to the demand for motion is referred to as "bind" by manual therapists utilizing the *indirect* treatment method known as *Functional Technique* (see Barrier Concept Definitions). It is beyond the scope of this chapter to elucidate Functional Technique (the topic of Chapter 14) other than to point out the important difference between "bind" and range of motion restriction.

"Bind" and its opposite, "ease," refer to *subtle* responses of tissues to passive movement *anywhere* within the range of motion of a dysfunctional body region. Somatic dysfunctions defined this way are not the same as somatic dysfunctions defined as having restricted range of motion. "Normal" joints do not exhibit either "ease" or "bind," but they are essential information in the application of Functional Technique.

It follows, then, that practitioners of Func-tional Technique define somatic dysfunction in terms of a "trinary" system of physical examination in which the three variables are "normal," "ease," and "bind." The variables are elicited by passive challenge movements called "motion demand," and the variables are termed "responses to motion demand," which are determined by the examiner's light surface palpation of the region being examined. True adherents of the Functional method studiously avoid conceptualizations beyond the confines of this basic paradigm, such as "what causes the 'bind'?" or "what anatomic structures are involved?".

THE BARRIER CONCEPT

In somatic dysfunctions treatable by *direct* techniques the motion barrier is encountered before the physiologic barrier is reached (Fig. 12.1). Such a dysfunctional barrier has distinctive qualities due to the mechanism of motion restriction. If restriction is due to increased myotonus (neuromuscular barrier), e.g., hypertonus of a tonic muscle, the barrier will have a consistent elastic quality. If the mechanism is fibrosis (fascial barrier), the barrier will be relatively inelastic. If edema is involved (passive congestion barrier), the barrier will also be quite abrupt but will fade slightly to sustained pressure. Intra-articular joint locks[11] are also quite abrupt, but do not yield to sustained pressure. Hypermobile joints have lost some of the end-field resiliency characteristic of the physiologic barrier; thus one reaches the anatomic barrier abruptly without warning after traversing an increased range of passive motion.

Barrier Concept Definitions

Active Technique.—manipulative procedure in which the patient actively participates through voluntary muscle contractions on request, to provide corrective force. Opposite of PASSIVE, q.v.

Anatomic Barrier.—requires operator assistance to reach. Hard, rigid end-field. Movement past Anatomic Barrier results in tissue damage.

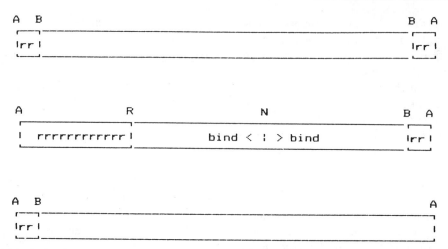

Figure 12.1. Barrier Concepts.

Top: Normal Range of Motion. A—Anatomic Barrier, B—Physiologic Barrier, B—B: Active range of motion, A—A: Passive range of motion. Mid-range center, N, or "neutral," may be mathematically defined, but is difficult to identify by physical examination in normal joint range of motion. rr—rapidly increasing resistance.

Middle: Somatic dysfunction with minor (<50%) motion restriction. A—Anatomic Barrier, B—Physiologic Barrier, R—Restrictive Barrier (if the restriction occupies more than half the normal range of motion, dysfunction is major), N—Mid-point of ease, more easily detected in these circumstances due to "bind" (mild resistance) when attempting to passively move in either direction from N. R—B: active range of motion; may be painful.

Bottom: Hypermobile joint. A—Anatomic Barrier, B—Physiologic Barrier. With no physiologic barrier on the right end of the range, the anatomic barrier is met abruptly with no warning. Active or passive movement in this direction may be painful.

Barrier.—A point within the range of active or passive motion where resistance to farther movement (hysteresis) *suddenly* increases. It does not refer to the phenomenon of "BIND" used in the application of functional technique.

Bind.—a term used in Functional Technique to describe a lesioned area's response to passive motion demand. It specifies a subtle reluctance to allow the passive movement, whereas passive movement in the opposite direction is characterized by an equally subtle "ease." Normal areas do not exhibit these reactions. NOT A BARRIER!

Direct Technique.—classification of manipulative techniques based on how the elements of the joint are positioned in relation to the point of restriction (the barrier) for treatment. If the barrier is engaged (met) the technique is *Direct.* All ME techniques[12] are classed as *Direct.* However, ME isometric procedures should be classed as *Direct Passive,* since the corrective motion is provided by the operator during patient relaxation. On the other hand, ME isotonic procedures are classed as *Direct Active,* since the patient's muscles provide the corrective motion. Other examples are: muscle stretching, thrust techniques, "joint play" articulation, and reduction of luxations and subluxations.

Indirect Technique.—class of manipulative techniques in which the point of restriction (barrier) is avoided in a search for a position of least tension, maximum comfort or lesion exaggeration. Examples are: Functional[13,14,15,16] (Hoover-Bowles-Johnston technique), *Cranial*[17] ("balance and hold"), *Counterstrain*[18] (Lawrence Jones' "Release by Positioning"), *Robert Maigne's*[19] *technique* (thrust in the direction of freer permitted motion), *unwinding* (as taught by Viola Fryman[20] and adapted by John Upledger[21]), inherent force technique (*Sutherland technique* according to Howard Lippincott[22]).

Myotatic Unit.—a group of muscles which share a common spinal reflex system. The simplest myotactic unit is a single motor unit plus its sensory and gamma efferent nerve supply and the associated spinal cord synapses. More complex myotatic units may include agonist and antagonist muscle groups and their shared spinal cord reflex systems.[23]

Passive Technique.—manipulative procedures in which the patient remains relaxed. Corrective forces are supplied by the operator.

Physiologic Barrier.—the limits of active movement. Feeling of resilience and elasticity.

Pathologic Barrier.—various qualities denoting the specific nature of the abnormal tissue change causing the restriction. Can distinguish edema, fibrosis, hypertonus, and spasm by the quality of the end-field. Fibrosis and hypermobility have an abrupt, hard, sudden end-feel. Edema also has a hard stop, but it fades with persistent testing force. Hypertonus has increased elasticity. Spasm reacts erratically to testing movements. In Europe the term BLOCKAGE is used with the same connotation.

Cautions

As important as the distinction between "barrier" and "bind" is, the distinction has not been identified in the literature. Lewit[13] (p. 14) reports that Stoddard[24,25] uses the term "binding" to mean what has been defined as "barrier" in this chapter.

It is important to distinguish between subluxation and somatic dysfunction. A subluxation is a bone out of place (from "luxation": a dislocation). In subluxation (minor dislocation) there is no discernible hemorrhage or tissue avulsion, but there is impaired and altered function secondary to the dislocation. Subluxation typically occurs in the pelvic joints or costovertebral joints, not in intervertebral joints. Somatic dysfunction, in contrast, is impaired or altered function WITHIN the physiologic range of motion of any joint, including intervertebral joints.

Diagnostic Labels

Labeling of somatic dysfunctions has been the source of frequent confusion and misunder-

standing. Some of the confusion has resulted from careless use of the English language, as well as from vague conceptualizations of the nature of the lesions. Beginning students of musculoskeletal structural diagnosis often use expressions like, "The lesion is on the left," to indicate that they have found the left transverse process of a vertebra to be abnormally posterior. The problem may actually be due to the inability of the vertebra to backward bend on the right side. The preposition, "on" is used by the student inappropriately.

Some practitioners like to describe somatic dysfunctions by observable positions, since it is not difficult to understand that a vertebra with its left transverse process more posterior than the one on the right is in a *left rotated* position when compared with the bone *inferior* to it (a generally agreed upon convention). The functional understanding of this observation is that the vertebra is free to turn to the left but is not free to turn as far to the right in relation to the bone inferior to it. Table 12.1 summarizes.

Positional descriptors require the past tense ending (actually the past participle serving as an adjective). For example, describing the L5/S1 motion segment, "Lumbar 5 Flex*ed*, Rotat*ed* left, Sidebent left" not only means that the fifth lumbar can freely flex (forward bend), rotate left and sidebend left on the sacrum, but also implies that the muscles which cause those movements may be too short. Movement of the body into the direction of free movement conceals the dysfunction. Therefore, *some* of the bone's position is observable whenever the region of the body containing the somatic dysfunction is posi-

Table 12.1
Labeling of Somatic Dysfunctions

Positional
Names the free movements
Indicates which muscles of the joint may be too short.

Motion Restriction
Names the restricted movements.
Identifies the movements to be restored by treatment.

Left rotated = (means the same as) Restricted right rotating

tioned far enough in one of the restricted directions.

The alternative to positional descriptors is motion restriction descriptors, which define the directions of movement to be restored by the treatment. Expressing the same example in motion restriction terms requires nouns (verbals with -ion endings or gerund -ing endings), e.g., "Lumbar 5 has restricted Extension, restricted right Rotation, and restricted right sidebending." To save writing the word "restricted" (meaning "reduced range of motion") repeatedly, some practitioners prefer to use the Greek omega sign (for "ohms"). However, omega is also used to denote the Functional term "bind."

Adding to the confusion is the practice of mixing motion restriction and positional terms, along with the preposition "in," as in the expression, "Restricted in extension, rotation to the left." Here it is not clear whether flexion or extension is the restricted motion. Is the left rotation a restriction or a position? Did the examiner mean to say "rotated to the left"?

Ways to avoid confusion in communication include not mixing position and restriction descriptors in the same expression, not using prepositions, and using correct word endings. Some colloquial expressions are quite clear in their meanings. Thus, if one describes a vertebral dysfunction as "anterior on the right," it is clear that the right zygapophyseal joint has restricted extension motion, resulting in the vertebra rotating and sidebending to the left whenever full extension of the joint is attempted. Its positional description, therefore, is "Flexed, Rotated and sidebent left." Note that "posterior on the left" does not mean the same thing. It means that the left zygapophyseal joint is not free to flex fully, and the vertebra is Extended, Rotated and sidebent left."

LEXICON OF MOTION DESCRIPTORS

Definitions

Apex.—point of maximum rotation of a neutral (q.v.) sidebent vertebral group. Each vertebra in the group contributes a small amount to the rotation (below the apex) or derotation (above the apex) of the group, which may be a functioning adaptation or a compensatory scoliotic lesion (see SCOLIOSIS).

Crossover.—in an "S" curve scoliosis, the vertebral joint where the sidebending changes direction. See SCOLIOSIS.

Extension.—to bend backward from the anatomic position, or, more precisely, ROTATION OF A VERTEBRA AROUND A TRANSVERSE AXIS SO THAT ITS SUPERIOR SURFACE MOVES POSTERIORLY RELATIVE TO THE BONE INFERIOR TO IT. Vertebral extension is bending backward on the inferior vertebra. Occipital extension is bending backward on the atlas by sliding the condyles forward. Moving the base of the sacrum posteriorly is sacral extension (postural), but it is craniosacral flexion. Opposite of FLEXION (q.v.).

Flexion.—to bend (forward) around a transverse axis in a sagittal plane, where the term applies segmentally to the superior part in relation to the inferior part when speaking of vertebral flexion. See EXTENSION.

The Physics definition of flexion is "approximation of two ends of an arc." Harrison Fryette applied this definition to spinal joint movement and confused some of his students. Because of the kypholordotic curves of the spine, he said the posture of the normal spine is already flexed. The cervical and lumbar arcs are concave posteriorly. Approximating their ends (backward bending) he called "flexion." Forward bending the thoracic kyphosis would also be "flexion" in Fryette's definition. The secondary (lumbar and cervical) arcs (curves), usually meet the primary (thoracic) curve at the tenth and third thoracic vertebrae, respectively, but not always. The Physics definition, therefore, leads to some ambiguity in describing spinal joint movements. Hence, the preferred definition of vertebral "flexion" is anterior bending from the anatomic position, or, more precisely, ROTATION OF A VERTEBRA AROUND A TRANSVERSE AXIS

SO THAT ITS SUPERIOR SURFACE MOVES ANTERIOR RELATIVE TO BONE INFERIOR TO IT.

In human kinesiology, "flexion" means movement in a sagittal plane (as if the part were in the anatomic position—even if it isn't).

Forward Bending.—A deformation of a flexible body such that its anterior surface becomes more concave (or less convex). In the axial skeleton the superior portion rotates about a transverse axis. Regardless of what moves in relation to the external world, the inferior portion is always regarded as the stationary reference in the axial skeleton. In the extremities the proximal bone is the stationary reference. Synonymous with some senses of the term "flexion" (Q.V.)

Neutral.—in reference to vertebral joints, any position in which the facet joints are not engaged, i.e., sufficiently space, or gapped, that the facets do not guide or control the rotation or sidebending movements of the vertebrae. The neutral position permits group sidebending with secondary uncoupled (but obligatory) rotation toward the convexity up to the apex (q.v.) of the group. See TYPE I SOMATIC DYSFUNCTION.

Nonneutral.—in reference to vertebral joints, any position in which the facet joints are engaged, i.e., sufficiently flexed or extended to create a pivotal point in one or the other facet joint. Under these circumstances rotation and sidebending are coupled to the same side. See TYPE II SOMATIC DYSFUNCTION.

Rotation.—with a qualifier, "left" or "right," this term is used to describe movement of a midline or central structure around a vertical (superior-inferior) axis. The anterior surface of the superior part moves to the left or right. The rotating midline part is assumed to be moving in relationship to the structure immediately inferior to it. In extremities the moving bone is assumed to be in relationship to its proximal neighbor, and is designated "internal" or "external," depending on the direction the anterior surface moves. In the

pelvis rotations of the sacrum between the ilia are called "torsions"; rotations of the ilia on the sacrum are labeled "anterior" or "posterior" rotations, depending on the movement of the iliac crest (upon a transverse axis).

Rotoscoliosis.—see SCOLIOSIS

Scoliosis.—an abnormal (pathological) lateral curvature of the spine due to (*a*) structural deformity of some part of the spine, (*b*) adaptation to structural deformity or asymmetry of the lower limb, pelvis, or cranium, or (*c*) developmental asymmetries of the soft tissues (q.v.) related to the spine. Descriptive adjectives, "left" or "right" refer to the side of convexity. Generic configurations are designated "C-curve" (regardless of side of convexity), "S"-curve, and "multi-curve." Functional scoliosis is often seen as an adaptation to vertebral somatic dysfunction, which is manipulable and curable.

Sidebending.—with a qualifier, "left" or "right," this term is used to describe movement of a midline or central structure around an antero-posterior axis. The superior surface of the part moves to the left or right. The designated bone is assumed to be moving in relationship to the structure immediately inferior to it. In extremities the abducting or adducting bone is assumed to be moving in relationship to its proximal neighbor. The prefix "ab-" means "away from the sagittal plane; "ad-" means "toward the sagittal plane."

Soft Tissues. any tissue in the body which is not bone, blood, lymph, cerebrospinal fluid, an internal viscus, or a part of the central or peripheral nervous systems. Includes deep fascia, muscles, ligaments, skin, and superficial fascia. All such tissues are in constant motion due to the body's pulses and respiratory motions. The terms inhalation and exhalation may be used to describe some of these motions.

Translation or Translatory Movement.—is movement parallel to a plane, either in a straight line or in an arc. Arcuate translatory movements occur in the parts of bones which are not on the rotational axis. Thus, a flexing vertebra translates its anterior surface in an anterior-inferior arc and its posterior surface in a superior-anterior arc.

SPINAL KINEMATICS AS RELATED TO MUSCLE ENERGY CONCEPTS

Theories related to spinal joint movement have developed gradually, beginning with Hippocrates or earlier and are still developing. Particularly useful to the application of ME techniques are the theories developed by Harrison Fryette. Taking a reasoned approach to the analysis of spinal motion, he referred to the research of two contemporaries, Lovett[26] and Halladay,[27] who drew conclusions from cadaveric dissections of the spine and its ligaments.

Lovett sawed a coronal section through the spine separating the vertebral bodies and discs from the neural arches at the pedicles. He observed that the posterior part containing the zygapophyseal joints permitted sidebending only if it was preceded by rotation—much in the manner of a flexible plastic ruler, as Fryette analogized. While the anterior part sidebent like a flexible column of blocks under load, the middle portion "twisted out from under the load." Lovett's conclusions mystified Fryette[28] who wrote:

> Notwithstanding these facts, Dr. Lovett's conclusions in regard to rotation in the various areas of the spine were as follows:
> *1. The Lumbar*
> "The rotation accompanying sidebending in the lumbar is *always* with the bodies turning to the concavity of the lateral curve."
> *2. Thoracic Region*
> "The rotation of the vertebrae in sidebending in the thoracic region is *always* toward the convexity of the lateral curve."
> *3. Cervical Region*
> In the cervical region, "sidebending is accompanied by rotation of the bodies of the vertebrae to the concavity of the lateral curve, as in the lumbar."

Fryette guessed that Lovett's concern was with the structure and etiology of spinal cur-

vatures and that he had no idea of the existence of individual vertebral dysfunctions.

Fryette introduced the notions of "neutral" (q.v.) (facet joints *not* engaged) and "non-neutral" (q.v.) (facets in control of vertebral motion), based on the observations of Halladay, who had perfected a method of treating cadaver ligaments with phenol and glycerin which preserved the tissues but kept them flexible. According to Fryette, Lovett's rule for thoracic spine sidebending-rotation coupling applied to any part of the spine as long as the facets were "idling," i.e., not engaged (vertebral joint "neutral"). This is an easily observable phenomenon in the lumbar and especially the thoracic spine, in spite of the prevailing opinion of anatomists that lumbar rotation is prevented by the shape of the vertebral facets. Fryette identified this as the *First Law of Physiologic Movements of the Spine* and characterized it as the "neutral" or "easy normal" law.

Students learned this principle as "neutral sidebending is coupled with rotation to the opposite side." The sidebending curves of the scoliotic spine show where rotation and sidebending, respectively, reverse their direction at the apices and crossover areas. The apices and cross-overs do not correspond, but are, in fact, approximately 90° out of phase with each other, the apices (vertebrae showing maximum rotation in relation to the cardinal planes of the body) occurring about midway between the points of sidebending alternation. The vertebrae at, or inferior to, the apex rotate toward the convexity of the curve. Vertebrae forming the part of the curve above the apex rotate in small increments toward the concavity. Thus, there is no abrupt change in the the rotation increments through the cross-over.

Such configurations, more aptly described as "rotoscolioses" of the spine, occur with natural sidebending movements of the trunk (thoracic and lumbar spine), or as adaptations to inherent or acquired structural asymmetries of the posture, such as leg length inequality or dysgenesis of the pelvis. Rotoscolioses also occur as adaptations to the asymmetries caused by pelvic or vertebral somatic dysfunctions. While the rotational component of individual vertebral segments within the sidebending group is small and secondary to the sidebending component, the rotation is additive. As a result, rotation becomes the group's most observable feature at its apex.

In the thoracic region, the rotation effect is most visible because of the distortion of the rib cage. In the lumbar spine, rotation is more visibly prominent because the axis of lumbar rotation is posterior to the neural arch,[29] resulting in a small shift of spinous processes toward the concavity of the sidebend curve and a relatively large arc of movement of the tips of the transverse process. Lateral shearing of the intervertebral discs also occurs in the direction of the posterior transverse process.

As a result of tests performed on cadaveric dissections, Fryette concluded that maximal "flexing" (decreasing the radius of curvature) of the spinal A-P curves caused rotation-sidebending coupling to the same side, but of a single vertebra.

Fryette's Laws: Physiologic Motion of the Spine

Law I. Neutral (q.v.) sidebending produces rotation to the other side, or, in other words, the sidebending GROUP rotates itself toward the convexity of the sidebend, with the maximum rotation at the apex (q.v.).

Law II. Non-neutral (q.v.) (vertebra hyperflexed or hyperextended) rotation and sidebending go to the SAME side, individual vertebral joints acting one at a time.

Law III. Introducing motion to a vertebral joint in one plane automatically reduces its mobility in the other two planes.

The types (I and II) of vertebral somatic dysfunction are based on Laws I and II.

Unfortunately, it is quite difficult to demonstrate the validity of the first two "laws." Obscure radiographic "evidence" has cropped up from time to time, but the concepts have not been generally accepted. Nevertheless, as a model for analysis of vertebral joint *dysfunction* there is no other theory with

the predictive power of Fryette's formulation. See Table 12.2.

Restrictors—Mechanisms, Theories, Assumptions

Etiology of Restriction. In order to understand somatic dysfunction as movement restriction, some consideration must be given to the mechanisms responsible for restriction. Explanations have been proposed suggesting that intra-articular structural anomalies, such as meniscoids (Lewit[11] p. 18) and cartilage deformation could produce a joint lock or block. Meniscoid entrapment and cartilage interlocking sometimes occur, but do not account for more than a small percentage of motion blockages. Much has been said and written about the role of connective tissue in somatic dysfunction. Gelosis of the colloidal ground substance and scar tissue formation in the fascia have been proposed as mechanisms of range of motion restriction. How often this occurs in the absence of myotonus is a legitimate question.

In terms of the etiology of somatic dysfunction, there exists a misguided tendency to blame the victim for faulty lifting, bad posture, etc. Frequently, no such information is forthcoming from the patient, except when the somatic dysfunction is caused by recent trauma. Most somatic dysfunctions are the result of automatic processes, mediated by the central nervous system, and this activity rarely impinges upon consciousness. Neumann[30] (p. 13) characterizes the etiology of somatic dysfunction as abnormal *neuroreflexive* feedback mechanisms.

Once striated muscle comes under consideration as a mechanism for restricting motion, the theory comes closer to matching common experience. I propose that the most common event resulting in loss of range of motion is a neuromuscular one, a temporary loss of coordinated harmonious muscle actions. In order to develop this idea further we must study the gross and microscopic structure of striated muscles of the musculoskeletal system.

Table 12.2
Vertebral Somatic Dysfunction and Adaptation

	Somatic Dysfunctions			Adaptations
	Non-neutral Flexed	Non-neutral Extended	Neutral	Varies
Positional Names	FRSLt	ERSLt	NSRLt	Not a Lesion
Restricted Motions ("-ing" endings)	SRERt	SRFRt	SLRRt	None
Lesion Type	Type II	Type II	Type I	None
Number	Single	Single	Group	Group
Cause (Etiology)	Trauma	Trauma	Adaptation	
Facet Motion impairment	Right	Left	None	
Effect of hyperextension	Worse	Increases symmetry	Less Deform.	Depends on Lesion
Effect of hyperflexion	Increases symmetry	Worse	Less Deform.	Depends on Lesion
Coupled rotation— sidebending	Same Side (e.g., Lt, Lt)	Same Side (e.g., Lt, Lt)	Group Left rotated, Right sidebent	
Observed posterior transverse process(es)	Left	Left	Left	

F = Flexed
E = Extended
R = Rotated
S = Sidebent
Rt = Right
Lt = Left

MUSCLE CLASSIFICATIONS APPLICABLE TO ME TECHNIQUE

Accepting Korr's principle[5] that striated muscle is the "primary machinery of life" puts manipulative medicine in proper perspective. A functional (kinesiologic) classification of striated muscle presents a simple conceptual framework in which to discuss its role in somatic dysfunction. Three pairs of antagonist muscles exist in this classification system: sagittal plane muscles (flexors, extenders), coronal plane muscles (right and left sidebenders), and transverse plane muscles (right and left rotators).

All the *named* striated muscles of the body contain fibers which belong in at least two of the six classes (the anconeus seems to be an exception). For example, the *rotatoris* muscle on the right side of the spine both left rotates and extends the vertebral joint which it crosses (actually it stabilizes the joint in these dimensions). Myology and kinesiology are tremendously simplified by this functional classification, in which the Anatomic Position and the Cardinal Planes of the body are the bases for describing the actions of muscles and the movements of joints.

One anatomic classification of striated muscles is the monoarticular (crossing only one joint) and polyarticular (crossing more than one joint) classification. As simple as this classification is, it is important to separate these two types of muscles, since their roles in normal and pathologic movement are different. Polyarticular muscles fit the popular image of muscle—powerful, massive structures carrying out the will of the brain—"popular" because they correspond to most people's visual images of muscles. The visibility of polyarticular muscles is due to their external location in the body, where they enjoy the greatest mechanical advantage due to their attachments being some distance from the axes of rotation.

The polyarticular muscle role in normal movement is to contract in short, powerful bursts to produce motions in chains of bones and joints within fairly massive body parts. Once these parts of the body commence movement, the polyarticular muscles coast along as the ballistic inertia of the body part carries the motion in the same direction until the antagonist muscle act to slow the motion to a halt. Such muscle functions are called *phasic* functions.

Phasic muscles spend more time resting than working. The microscopic structure of phasic muscles is consistent with their lifestyle. Their sarcoplasmic reticulum is complex and designed for fast oxidation, glycogenolysis, and rapid calcium ion exchanges. A single polyarticular motor unit is composed of many muscle fibers (sometimes hundreds), distributed rather randomly throughout the entire muscle, all activated by a single motor nerve. Thus power and speed are provided at the expense of precision and stamina.

When phasic muscles are required to contract continuously, as in reflexive guarding and spasm, they become acidotic, congested, and sometimes very sore. An important question concerns how phasic muscles become involved in behavior for which they are so poorly designed. Barry Wyke[31] traced the Pacinian-like mechanoreceptors (nociceptors) found in facet joints to the cord where they synapse directly with efferents in the intermediolateral cell column. Activation of the nociceptors in facet joints may produce an immediate sympathetic response, which may be multiplied more than a hundred-fold at the divergent synapses in the paravertebral ganglion. The net result is a redirection or shunting of the blood supply to the overlying skin and large muscles. This suggests a mechanism whereby the norepinephrine released within the substance of the large polyarticular muscles overlying the irritated facet has an inotropic effect on motor endplate receptivity, as intimated by Basmajian.[32] The gamma system becomes more sensitive to stimuli causing a facilitation and guarding contraction of large muscles, which ultimately become a source of conscious pain. The palpable muscle guarding response from viscerosomatic reflexes probably works in a similar manner. Travell's myofascial trigger points also serve to maintain the guarding tension in the muscle via a feedback reflex system.

Nociceptors are more likely to be stimulated by joint movements, especially abnormal movements due to adaptation or hypermobility, than by restriction of joint movement. This would explain the frequent observation that, if symptoms occur at a dysfunctional vertebral segment, they are usually on the unrestricted side of the vertebral joint, or arise from vertebral segments above or below the dysfunction. Stating the principle more generally, pain is usually, if not always, generated by the parts of the body which are adapting, not by the parts with impaired function.

The role of polyarticular muscles in pathologic movement (faulty movement patterns resulting from somatic dysfunctions, stressful postural statics, and injuries) is an adaptive one. For example, a single spinal joint non-neutral (see definitions of "neutral" and "non-neutral") somatic dysfunction which causes the vertebra to be sidebent and rotated to the left will require adaptive sidebending to the right in a group of vertebrae superior to the misaligned bone. This adaptive group sidebending is a complex activity involving coordination of polyarticular and monoarticular muscles, and yet, is amazingly predictable.

Almost as predictable and surprising is the reaction of the polyarticular muscles on the convex side of the adapting group curve. Frequently, they develop myofascial trigger points[23] which serve to generate and perpetuate spasms and referred pain. The pain and spasm are not confined to the precise site of the primary dysfunction.

The polyarticular muscles are normally able to do their work efficiently and painlessly only by virtue of the activity of the monoarticular muscles, whose role in normal movement is to make fine adjustments of the relative positions of the two bones and to stabilize that relationship in preparation for the more powerful leverage forces exerted by the polyarticular muscles. And when they are not participating in conscious voluntary movements (in the firing sequence demonstrated by electro-myography their activity precedes that of the polyarticular muscles by several milliseconds)[33] they are continually reacting to a complex sensory system which receives postural data in relation to gravity, inertial forces, and static stresses. Because of the precision required, they are richly innervated, each motor unit having only a few muscle fibers.

Because they must work tirelessly, their metabolism is energy conservative, slow oxidizing, and not prone to lactic acidosis. Such muscles are classed as *tonic* in contrast to *phasic*.

The anatomic, histologic, functional, and biochemical comparisons of striated muscle types just discussed cannot be made as clearcut as we have implied. It is much harder to classify human striated muscle than it is to tell dark meat from white meat in a chicken. The tonic/phasic functions of muscles and the corresponding histologic and biochemical distinctions appear to permit a wide range of individual variations, and may be subject to morphologic alterations from trophic influences. Not all polyarticular muscles are phasic, nor are all monoarticular muscles tonic. Most muscles are composed of mixtures of the three fiber types. The simplistic classification presented here is retained for its heuristic value (Table 12.3).

Although ME theory appears to assume that abnormally shortened muscle is a part of the mechanism of somatic dysfunction, exceptions come readily to mind. Clearly, an abnormally short monoarticular muscle would

Table 12.3
Summary of the Anatomical, Histological, Neurological, and Functional Differences Between Long and Short Restrictors.

	Comparison Chart of Striated Muscle	
	Long	*Short*
Anatomy	Superficial	Deep
	Polyarticular	Monoarticular
Histology	Fast oxidizing fibers	Slow oxidizing fibers
	More defined sarcoplasmic reticulum for faster Ca^{++} influx and efflux.	Ill-defined sarcoplasmic reticulum
	Glycogenolytic	
	Fast twitch fibers	Slow twitch fibers
Neuro-Anatomy	Sparsely innervated	Richly innervated
	Large motor units (>200)	Small motor units (<30)
	Voluntary reflex control	Involuntary reflex control often the first to be recruited
Function	Phasic	Tonic
	Power, speed	Weak, slow
	Greater leverage	Stabilize joint
	Maintain Type I Somatic Dysfunction	Maintain Type II Somatic Dysfunction
	Prone to weakness	Prone to tightness
	Longer chronaxie	Shorter chronaxie

prevent a full range of motion of its joint in some plane. Similarly, a contractured polyarticular muscle would alter the range of motion of all the joints between its attachments. The works of Janda[34,35] Burke,[33,36] Edgerton,[33,37] MacConaill,[38] and Basmajian[32,39] support these concepts.

Several mechanisms explain the abnormally shortened muscle phenomenon: neuroreflexive (probably the predominant mechanism), fibrosis or gelosis (probably follows closely on the heels of neuroreflexive shortening), and active or passive congestion of muscle tissue (more likely to occur in polyarticular muscles with active myofascial trigger points). Congestion, gelosis, and fibrosis can also account for articular blockage in the absence of neuroreflexive muscular causes, e.g., in passive joints like the sacroiliacs, intertarsals, and carpals. As mentioned earlier, ME techniques have been developed to mobilize passive joints.

Other Mechanisms

Manual therapists from Hippocrates to Still have written about using manipulation to put bones back in place, as if, once returned to their proper position, the bones should remain forever in place. Such static thinking has largely been supplanted by a dynamic concept of using manipulation to restore function. However, the notion that subluxation is the condition treated by manipulation has not entirely been disposed of. Even though the vertebral "subluxation" theory, held principally by chiropractors, is not supported by either x-ray or other evidence (Lewit[11] p. 12), nevertheless, some body parts are vulnerable to subluxations (mild displacements without tissue avulsion). Subluxation of the costovertebral joints is occasionally detectable, and pubic symphysis subluxation is quite common. When it occurs one would assume that the joint involved would be relatively hypermobile, yet physiologic motion of the joint is usually found to be restricted.

Other non-muscular restrictive mechanisms have been proposed. The *Meniscoid* *Theory* (Emminger[40]) is popular in Europe, but has had limited acceptance in North America in spite of a body of evidence to support the notion. Cartilage is easily deformed by steady pressure, and it is easy to see how such deformation in a diarthrosis can interfere with normal physiologic joint motion. Active joints, as well as passive joints, may be restricted by altered tension in ligaments or fascia.

Mennell[41] points out that joint play is a requirement for painless normal joint mobility. Joint play motions are also treatable with ME techniques. Voluntary muscle contractions can be used to stress articular structures in a precisely localized way, allowing restoration of passive movements to joints.

CLINICAL APPLICATIONS

The Psychophysics of Physical Diagnosis

Range of Motion. Assessment of ROM is relevant to the application of ME or other direct manipulative techniques. Predominantly a *visual* process, it calls for a disciplined use of the eyes as diagnostic instruments. As left-right cortical specialization and dominance occurs, the use of the eyes becomes biased in special ways depending on the nature of the visual information being attended to. Quantitative observations—judgments about geometric symmetry, size, and length—are best made by providing visual advantage to the dominant eye as it functions with the whole body, i.e., putting the dominant eye in the best position with the least stress to the body.

Eye dominance varies between individuals and sometimes within the same individual. The examiner must be acquainted with eye dominance in order to use visual analysis reliably. Many physicians and physical therapists do not know how to determine which eye is dominant. The test is done by visually lining up a small space between the hands (plural, to avoid handedness bias) with a distant object while keeping both eyes open, and then closing one eye. If the dominant eye is open, the distant object will still be in the space between the hands. If closed, the object will not be.

The static asymmetries being looked for occur at right angles to a particular plane. If the line of sight is parallel to that plane the asymmetry will be more obvious and therefore more easily detected. In the visual estimating of angular degrees, it is important to know that the closer the unknown angle approaches either zero or 90° the more discriminating the visual sense becomes. In comparing the heights of standing iliac crests, for example, using shims under the foot of the low side until the crests appear to be perfectly horizontal decreases observational error to a level of ± 2mm.[42]

The peripheral visual fields are particularly sensitive to movements—many orders of magnitude more sensitive than the untrained palpatory senses. If one is comparing bilateral movements, such as the respiratory movements of the rib cage, the most reliable judgments are made by focusing the gaze at the midline of the body. By contrast, color comparisons are best made using the central visual field.

Palpation. Detection and precise location of bony landmarks must precede visual observation and judgment of symmetry, and requires palpatory search. For this purpose *stereognosis is the most important palpatory sense*. Stereognosis is the most highly integrated of the palpatory senses, combining the various senses of pressure mensuration, texture appreciation, and possibly radiesthesia as well.

Precise and reliable use of palpatory sense as a scientific diagnostic instrument requires special knowledge of neuroanatomy, neurophysiology, and perception psychology. Relaxation is a basic requirement for accurate physical diagnosis palpation. This is a significant hurdle for the neophyte, whose first attempts are extremely energy intensive and wasteful. The neophyte's extra effort overloads the sensory nervous system with proprioceptive static (the problem of the afferent signal to noise ratio). No wonder it is so hard for beginners to interpret what they feel.

The seemingly uncanny ability of expert diagnosticians to palpate anatomic structures through a complex medium of skin, fat, fascia, and muscle is due, in part, to the ability to visualize. Visualizing the anatomy enables one to pay closer attention to the anatomic structures being examined. The interplay between mental imagery and the palpatory sensory input is extremely complex, yet teaching and learning physical diagnosis is often seriously handicapped by the absence of conscious consideration of that process. All psychomotor skill learning is enhanced by imagery, a means of focusing attention on what is significant as well as a method of mentally rehearsing a performance by visualizing effortless integrated body movements. Performance anxiety and inhibitory self-consciousness are reduced. Many skilled athletes have discovered the importance of imagery.

The Musculoskeletal Screen

Physical examination of the musculoskeletal system usually begins with some regional tests which are done for the purpose of excluding some body regions from detailed analysis. Using pain or other symptoms for this purpose is rarely adequate. Physical tests are preferred. An adequate screen should be brief, and yet permit comparative evaluation of every body region. The number of test procedures per region may vary from patient to patient. A more satisfactory screen not only enables the examiner to prioritize body regions for specific detailed analysis, but also facilitates selection of treatment modalities or methods.

The choice of treatment method is too often dictated by the therapist's skills. Competence in several methods is desirable, but carries with it the necessity to choose the most appropriate method. A manual therapist's skills may include some, or all, of the following:

1. Soft tissue (massage) techniques
   a. Swedish massage
   b. Myofascial release
   c. Bindesgewebsmassage (Dicke)
   d. Peripheral stimulation therapies

(1) Acupressure
(2) Myotherapy (based on Travell's trigger points)
(3) Chapman's reflexes
(4) Polarity therapy
2. Direct positioning mobilization techniques
  a. Thrust techniques
  b. Muscle Energy techniques
    (1) Light isometric
    (2) Forceful isotonic
    (3) "Isolytic"
  c. Cranial decompression techniques[17]
3. Indirect positioning mobilization techniques
  a. Functional technique
  b. Counterstrain technique
  c. Maigne thrust technique
  d. Craniosacral "balance and hold" technique

While the above list, based on Kimberly's classification,[43] is by no means complete, its general outline will probably accommodate any other unlisted manual therapies. It is important that the appropriate treatment be selected early in the evaluation process, since each treatment method influences the examination parameters. For example, range of motion is not relevant to Functional Technique, nor is "ease"/"bind" information applicable to ME technique. Selection of treatment method should be based on indications and contraindications (Table 12.4).

The goals of soft tissue techniques are to stretch tissues, move fluids, and reflexly relax or tonify muscles. ME techniques accomplish these goals at times more efficiently than massage. Unlike thrust techniques, ME techniques rarely require preparatory massage.

Application of Physical Diagnosis Principles to Examination of Specific Anatomic Regions

Cervical Region. Range of motion diagnosis of the cervical vertebral joints, including the occipito-atlantal articulations, is done most easily by passive lateral translation of the superior member of the joint being tested. In cervicals 2 through 7 the vertebra is held by finger pads on the articular pillars, not on the tender transverse processes. To obtain appropriate relaxation the procedure is done with the subject lying supine, the head and neck supported comfortably and moved gently, keeping support underneath the center of gravity of the head-neck mass. Care is taken that the sagittal plane of the bone being translated remains parallel with the sagittal plane of the body. In this way the distance of translation is quantitatively related to the amount of sidebending permitted by the joint. Thus, 3 inches of right translation of the occiput is roughly equivalent to 6 angular degrees of occipito-altantal left sidebending. By varying the flexion-extension angle of the joint being tested one may determine if one or both facet joint(s) has/have diminished range of motion. Except for the atlanto-axial joint, sidebending and rotation are coupled motions in the cervical joints, allowing for deductive inferences. Here the qualitative palpatory experience of the end-feel is combined with the quantitative visual estimation of translatory distances in order to make a diagnosis specific to that joint. Such a diagnosis will quantitatively describe the ranges of motion in all planes, distinguish between various possible restricting mechanisms, and attempt to estimate acuteness or chronicity.

Thoracic Spine and Costovertebral Relationships. Diagnosing somatic dysfunction of the thoracic vertebral joints is done most easily and reliably by making sequential visual observations of static vertebral positions in varying degrees of trunk flexion and extension. Since thoracic spinous processes are not dependably straight, palpatory-visual identification and location of transverse processes is the more reliable indicator of vertebral rotated position. Because unequal paravertebral muscle tonus tends to obscure the precise location of transverse processes, observing changes in rib position is an alternative to transverse process evaluations. This is an acceptable alternative, provided there are no subluxations or deformations of the ribs. The stereognostic palpatory sense is utilized in combination with arranging the visual line of sight approximately at right angles to the plane of vertebral or rib asymmetry.

Asymmetry which is exaggerated by flexion and eliminated by extension clearly indicates dysfunction with some amount of flexion restriction of the facet joint toward which the vertebra has rotated. This, of course, does not imply that the restricting mechanism is within the facet joint. Exaggerated asymmetry with extension implicates the facet joint on the anterior side of the rotated vertebra. If asymmetry is not made worse either by flexion or extension, one must consider the possibilities of compensatory group dysfunctions or structural rotoscoliosis.

Thoracic vertebral dysfunctions have a strong tendency to cause secondary impairment of respiratory motions of the ribs, and are the most common cause of such impairment. Thus, assessing active rib respiratory motion to identify a specific pair of ribs with motion asymmetry can aid in the discovery of

Table 12.4
Selection of Treatment Methods

Indications	Contraindications
LIGHT FORCE (<500 gms, <3 sec) ISOMETRIC:	
a. To treat motion restriction of an individual joint (a Type II spinal lesion). Or,	a. Spasm, pain (relative contraindication)
b. An abnormally short monoarticular muscle.	
MODERATE FORCE (5–20 Kg, <3 sec) ISOMETRIC:	
a. To treat motion restriction of more than one adjacent joint (a Type I spinal lesion). Or,	a. Spasm, pain
b. An abnormally short polyarticular muscle.	b. Tissue fragility
MAXIMUM FORCE ISOMETRIC:	
a. Testing strength. Not treatment!	a. Tissue fragility
b. If you wish to hypertrophy a muscle.	b. corticosteroids
	c. anticoagulants
ANTAGONIST MUSCLE MAXIMUM FORCE ISOTONIC	
a. To treat motion restriction due to painful muscle spasm.	a. Tissue fragility
	b. corticosteroids
	c. anticoagulants
VIBRATORY ISOLYTIC (15 sec. ALLASOTONIC):	
a. To treat motion restriction due to fibrotic contracture.	a. Spasm
	b. Pain
CONCENTRIC ISOKINETIC (3 reps., <4 sec.):	
a. To treat articular hypermobility due to muscular weakness.	a. Tissue fragility
INDIRECT (FUNCTIONAL) TECHNIQUES	
a. When direct technique is contraindicated.	a. Fracture
b. Acute, painful dysfunctions.	b. Dislocation
THRUST TECHNIQUES (H.V.L.A.)	
a. Sub-acute or early chronic fibrosis.	a. Fracture
b. Intraarticular joint lock.	b. Dislocation
c. When ME Technique does not work.	c. Hypermobility
	d. Fragile tissue
	e. Some neoplasms
	f. Anticoagulants (relative)
	g. PATIENT NOT RELAXED
SOFT TISSUE TECHNIQUES	
a. For reflex stimulation.	a. Too painful
b. For reflex inhibition.	b. Inflammation
c. Fascial release.	c. Fragile tissue
d. Circulatory stasis.	d. Spasm

vertebral somatic dysfunction, as well as rule out dislocations and intraosseous strains which also impair respiratory motion. Collecting analytic data involves stereognosis combined with peripheral visual field observation. Rib positions and motions may be assessed with the patient erect, slumped in flexion, arched in extension, or recumbent prone or supine whenever such detailed analysis is called for; in cases of diagnostic ambiguity, for example.

Lumbar Region. Examining the lumbars is similar to thoracic spine examination, except that lumbars rarely have ribs. Fortunately, the lumbar transverse processes have a fairly wide wingspan—about 10 cm at the third lumbar—making rotated position of a vertebra very visible. Although they lie underneath large paravertebral muscles, palpating them is relatively easy, if one feels along the fascial plane separating the *iliocostalis* from the *quadratus lumborum* muscles. The lumbar muscles are most relaxed in the prone position, and remain so even in the prone extended position if the head is supported by the hands. The preferred way to flex the lumbars is seated bending to put the arms and shoulders between the legs. This position stretches the lumbar extensor muscles and makes them thin and taut, thus reducing thickness asymmetries, if any exist.

Pelvis. As previously discussed, identification of the pelvic landmarks requires stereognosis and visual parallax. Interpretation of the landmark observations leads to diagnoses of pelvic subluxations, sacroiliac dysfunctions, and iliosacral dysfunctions.

Vertebral Hypermobility. In extremity joints hypermobility is indicated by weakness of the joint muscles when manually tested. However, testing the muscles of individual vertebral joints for strength is obviously problematic. How, then, does one diagnose hypermobility of a vertebral segment? Often the diagnosis is a strongly suggested probability from a history of trauma or chronic adaptation to dysfunction. Janda's[34] concept of the alternating vertical arrangement of tonic and phasic muscles in the postural muscular chain can be helpful in making this determination. The diagnosis sometimes only becomes clear after a trial of ME treatment fails to restore symmetrical function.

The ME treatment for hypermobility is specific muscle strengthening with isokinetic technique. Isokinetics are easy to apply to specific extremity muscles, difficult for specific paravertebral muscles. The hypermobile vertebra must be protected from adaptive overuse, by removing the stressors, in order to heal. Treatment of neighboring somatic dysfunctions may provide the healing circumstances.

Manipulable Disorders of the Pelvis[12]

The theoretical model of pelvic kinematics, normal and abnormal, developed in the context of ME technique, has proven to be an effective tool in the analysis and manual treatment of pelvic joint somatic dysfunctions. The model assumes that movement functions are as important as stability in the sacroiliac joints and at the *symphysis pubis*. Impairment of movement functions significantly stress postural adaptive mechanisms, locomotor functions, and circulatory dynamics, as well as trophic and regulatory nervous system functions. Clinical and experimental evidence of sacroiliac mobility is abundant.[44,45]

Three types of manipulable disorders of the pelvic joints can be distinguished. There are, of course, other manipulable conditions involving pelvic muscles, fascias, vessels, and organs, which are of special interest to gynecologists and obstetricians. The three types of pelvic joint disorders are *subluxation*, *sacroiliac dysfunction*, and *iliosacral dysfunction*. The distinction between sacroiliac and iliosacral, which are anatomically the same joint, pertains to the difference between spinal movement functions of the sacrum between the ilia and lower limb movement functions of the ilium, both in relation to the sacrum and to the opposite ilium. Thus, sacroiliac movements are caused by spinal motion, whereas iliosacral movements are caused by movements of the lower limbs.

Subluxations of the Pelvis

Subluxations are fairly common in the pelvic joints, and, when present, may stress the whole body in the same way as somatic dysfunctions of the pelvis. In addition, subluxations impair the physiologic movement functions of the pelvic joints, sometimes bizarrely displacing the bony landmarks used in somatic dysfunction analysis. For this reason subluxations are looked for and treated, if necessary, before attempting to diagnose or treat somatic dysfunctions of the pelvis.

Pubic Shear. The most common subluxations of the pelvis are inferior or superior pubic shears. Without the aponeurotic extensions of the transversus, obliquus, and rectus abdominis and the adductor longus the pubic symphysis would permit 5–10 mm of vertical shear without avulsion. The symphysis has no intrinsic stabilizing structures to hold the pubic bones in place, symmetrically opposite each other (this statement is based on clinical observation). The diagnosis is made by precise palpatory location of the *pubic crests* while observing for superior/inferior asymmetry. When such asymmetry exists, one side is normal and the other side is subluxated. The subluxated side consistently has impaired (restricted) movement in the ipsilateral sacroiliac joint, which can be detected by a standing flexion mobility test.

Positional stability of the pubic symphysis is provided by the abdominal and thigh muscles whose motor nerves originate in the lower thoracic and upper lumbar segments. Thus, when the integrity of this myotonic stabilizing mechanism is compromised, it is no surprise that one frequently finds dysfunction and stress affecting the thoraco-lumbar region. The altered muscle tonus of pubic subluxation is sometimes palpable in the abdomen or thighs. ME treatment consistently restores integrity of the myotonic stabilizing system (at least temporarily) even when the spinal dysfunction is still present. ME treatment to the normal side will simply have no effect.

Sacroiliac Dislocation. The second most common pelvic subluxation is the "up-slipped innominate" (clinical observation). Originally describe by Fryette[46] in 1914 with several complicating variations, this lesion is essentially a vertical shear between the sacrum and ilium which shortens the distance between the sacrococcygeal attachment of the *sacrotuberous ligament* and its ischial tuberosity attachment. Fryette's variations tend to muddle the subluxation concept, mainly because in 1914 the distinctions between dysfunction and subluxation were not regarded as important. Thus, superior vertical shear was discussed in combination with anterior or posterior rotation of the iliac crest, without considering the possibility that the iliac rotations might be adaptive and not a part of the lesion mechanism *per se*. In the modern paradigm rotations of the ilium are not considered subluxations, but are actually restrictions of physiologic functions. The distinction is now considered to be important. Pratfalls (falls on a buttock) are probably the most frequent cause of ilial dislocations, which are diagnosed by observing the prone patient's superiorly displaced *ischial tuberosity* and palpating the comparative laxity of the corresponding *sacrotuberous ligament*. Clinical observations of 10 ± 5 mm superior displacements are typical. Reduction with longitudinal distraction of the involved hip is usually easy.[6] Reductions are stable to weight bearing about half the time.

Mobility Tests. Of particular interest is the effect of up-slipped innominate subluxations on mobility tests of the pelvis. A sacroiliac joint which has been subluxed can be expected to be hypermobile. Yet the standing and seated flexion tests of pelvic joint mobility manifest restricted mobility of the subluxed side most of the time (probably because of wedging of the weight bearing sacrum). Exceptions can usually be accounted for by concomitant dysfunctions on the opposite side of the pelvis. Non-weight bearing mobility tests, however, demonstrate hypermobility. These paradoxical mobility test findings may be the reason the standing flexion test is occasionally negative on the dislocated side, or positive on the opposite side.

From clinical experience, it appears to be

best to assume that the superior side is dislocated and treat is as such. Down-slipped innominate is a theoretical possibility (in a catcher in a trapeze act, for example), but rare enough to have eluded the author, possibly because of the therapeutic effect of gravity in the upright posture.

Pelvic Flare. The least common of the pelvic subluxations are the inflare and outflare lesions, labeled "dished in" and "dished out" by Fryette.[46] These are identified by measuring asymmetric distances of the *anterior superior iliac spines* (ASIS) from the midline of the abdomen. Fryette mentions a gapping of the pubic symphysis with these lesions, but I have more consistently noticed a slight anteroposterior shear of the symphysis. The rarity of flare lesions is probably due to an uncommon anatomic variation in which a convex sacral auricular surface causes instability in the transverse plane of motion.

With the patient's flexed femur as a lever, hip adductor and abductor muscles can be contracted to assist reduction of the flare isotonically.

When instability persists, as shown by recurring dislocations, either up-slipped or flare, a sacroiliac belt may be required for external stabilization following reduction of the dislocation.

Sacroiliac Dysfunctions

Once the subluxations have been ruled out or eliminated by appropriate treatment, the next consideration is sacroiliac dysfunctions. Here the application of physiological reasoning (as opposed to the "bone out of place" theory of pelvic dynamics) led Fred Mitchell, Sr., to formulate a unified theoretical model of sacroiliac motion physiology and dysfunctions. The model offers the clearest explanation of observable phenomena and the greatest power to predict outcomes of intervention.

According to Mitchell, there are two types of sacroiliac dysfunctions, flexions and torsions, both of which asymmetrically displace the sacral *inferior lateral angles* (ILA). Measuring pelvisacral angles radiographically,

Kottke[44] demonstrated a nutation mobility of the sacrum between the ilia associated with forward and backward trunk bending. The average pelvisacral angle change was 7.5 angular degrees, roughly equivalent to 12 mm of linear ILA movement. Even voluntary respiration[47,48] alters the pelvisacral angle 1–3°. In spite of accumulated research evidence it is still commonly believed that the articular movements of the sacrum are so small as to have eluded the attention of scientists. In my clinical observations, however, sacroiliac dysfunctions typically produce manipulable and correctable asymmetric displacement of the ILA of the sacrum in the magnitude of 6 ± 3 mm.

Inferior Lateral Angles (ILA). Descriptions of ILA have been incredibly vague both in the anatomy[49–61] and the manual medicine literature,[4,30] including my earlier publications. They[47] are well described recently by Greenman[6] (p. 236f). The ILA is best defined as the transverse process analog of the fifth sacral segment. As such, its left and right posterior surfaces can be palpated just lateral to the sacral cornua and observed for rotated positions of the sacrum. The ILA inferior surface can be palpated (avoiding the coccyx) and observed for sidebent positions of the sacrum. Physical examination and evaluation of the ten pelvic landmarks requires meticulous technique in order to reduce errors to a minimum. Landmarks previously mentioned are the *pubic crests, ischial tuberosities, sacrotuberous ligaments*, and *anterior superior iliac spines* (ASIS).

The special palpatory sense of palmar stereognosis (placing the whole hand on the surface of the body and sliding the skin around over the bone) is absolutely essential for accurate identification of these landmarks. The examiner's thumbs or fingers are then carefully placed on the specific landmark positions which have a high degree of inter-examiner reproducibility (based on my 27 years of conducting practical examinations in osteopathic colleges): the most superior points of the pubic crests, the most inferior points of the ischial tuberosities, the medial edges of the sacrotuberous ligaments just superior to the tuberosities, and the medial surfaces of the ASISs (for inflare-outflare diagnosis) or the inferior slopes of the ASISs (for iliac rotation diagnosis). The symmetry or asymmetry of these landmarks is not determined by palpation alone (unless the examiner is blind). The visual sense is much more reliable for making geometric judgments, especially if the examiner is trained in the disciplined use of eye dominance, visual fields, and visual parallax.[42]

Since S5 projects posteriorly more than any other part of the sacrum or the coccyx, it can be identified most easily on the prone patient by palmar stereognosis. Finger pad stereognosis may also be used to identify the *sacral cornua*, which are the bifid spinous processes on each side of the midline *sacral hiatus*, the inferior opening of the *sacral canal*, which normally opens at S5. If the hiatus is wide enough to accommodate one finger pad, the sacral cornua can be felt on each side of the finger. Since the coccyx also has cornua, care must be taken to detect the most superior opening of the sacral canal along the *median crest* of the sacrum. Occasionally the hiatus commences as high as S3, or more rarely is open the entire length of the sacrum. The two cornua are often of different sizes, and this may mislead one to believe a sacral positional fault exists.

Normal flexion and extension nutations of the sacrum appear to occur around more than one transverse axis. Weisl's ambiguity in locating these axes is probably due to his experimental method,[45] in which the hip bones were clamped in a vise. Kottke's method[44] eliminated this artifact. Voluntary deep breathing changes the pelvisacral angle (as defined by Kottke) an average of 1.8 angular degrees. The axis for this respiratory movement is thought to be a transverse axis located at the second sacral segment[47,48] Extreme forward bending of the trunk usually produces a posterior movement of the sacral base, called "counter-nutation" by Kapandji.[29] Under these circumstances the sacrum probably rotates around a transverse axis located in the region of the posterior sacroiliac ligaments as the taut erector spinae muscles apply cephalic traction to the sacrum, which moves superiorly on the auricular joint tracks.

Unilateral Sacral Flexion. Bilateral sacral restrictions are quite rare, but unilateral restriction is fairly common. Clinically, the most frequent of this species of dysfunctions is the left unilaterally flexed sacrum. Viewed from the posterior perspective, the sacrum is sidebent to the left, with the left ILA about a centimeter closer to the feet than the right. The left side of the sacral base also moves inferiorly along the auricular track and, therefore, moves anteriorly in relation to the left iliac crest (without movement on the right).

Assessing the position of the sacral base is done by palpation of the sacral sulci for depth: thumb pads are placed on the gluteal tubercles of the iliac crests and the thumb tips are curled mediad and anteriorly toward the base of the sacrum to determine which thumb sinks in deeper from the iliac crest. Differences in sulcus depths, however, are often too subtle to judge reliably. Supplemental landmark tests, such as prone leg length, the seated flexion test, or assessing ILA displacement against two planes (horizontal and coronal), may be necessary to confirm the diagnosis of *left sacral flexion*. For example, one would expect the seated flexion test to be positive (indicating restricted pelvic joint motion) on the left.

When the sacral base declines to the left, the normal lumbar adaptation is a neutral left convexity created by contraction of spinal right sidebender muscles. This usually has the effect of shortening the right leg in the prone position. In the straight prone position, leg length discrepancy is detected by observing the heel pads, preferably with the feet off the examining table. Anatomic differences must be taken into account. For example, if the standing left iliac crest height is one centimeter inferior to the right crest, indicating anatomic shortness of the left leg, and the prone position makes the heel pads symmetrical, one must assume the right leg to be functionally shortened one centimeter due to dysfunction and adaptation in the pelvis and lumbar regions.

The left ILA is prominent in both left sacral flexion and sacral torsions to the left. Left sacral flexion primarily sidebends the sacrum to the left, displacing the left ILA mostly inferior (6–10 mm) and only slightly posterior (3–5 mm). Left sacral torsions have less sidebending effect, and typically displace the left ILA more posterior (6–10 mm) then inferior (3–5 mm). When such comparisons are unambiguous, the differential diagnosis can be made with confidence.

Sacral Torsions. According to the ME model, sacral torsion motions occur normally during walking to accommodate the lateral shifts of the spine. During the right stance phase of walking the left lumbar sidebender muscles contract at midstride, elevating the left hip and shifting the center of gravity to the right. The right piriformis muscle stabilizes the sacrum against a pivot point on the lower right sacroiliac joint, creating an oblique axis between the pivot and the upper left sacroiliac area. As the right side of the sacral base is pushed inferiorly by the lumbar shift the sacrum rotates to the left on this axis, which is arbitrarily named the left oblique axis. The weight of the trunk is transmitted through the sacral pivot on the ilium to the stance leg.

Thus, sacral torsion to the left on the left oblique axis is maximum at midstride, during the right stance phase of the walking cycle. The theory presumes the sacrum is not rotated at heel strike, when contraction of the deep hip rotator-stabilizers commences. The term "torsion" describes the state of the lumbosacral joint, where the trunk and the sacrum are rotating, sidebending, and nutating in opposite directions.

When sacral torsion dysfunction occurs, the sacrum loses the use of one oblique axis. The sacrum can rotate in either direction on either axis. However, only the forward torsions (to the left on the left axis or to the right on the right axis) occur in natural movements. "Unnatural" movements of the body which result in ipsilateral co-contraction of lumbar sidebenders and hip external rotators force the sacrum to rotate its base backward on the oblique axis. These circumstances frequently produce acute low back pain and an antalgic position indistinguishable from that of psoas spasm. The typical clinical case gives a history of straightening his back from a right sidebent anteflexed position with a heavy burden in the right hand while simultaneously stepping off onto the left leg. This activity produces a co-contraction of left piriformis and left lumbar sidebenders, resulting in sacral torsion to the left on the right oblique axis.

ME treatment of unilateral sacral flexion dysfunction utilizes careful positioning of the prone patient to loose-pack the sacroiliac joint, focused sustained operator pressure against the S5 segment tangent to the arc of the joint (see Fig. 12.2), and deep inhaling efforts by the patient.

The treatment of torsions employs reciprocal inhibition of co-contracting antagonist muscles to relax the affected piriformis and lumbar muscles. Sacral torsion to the left on the left oblique axis is maintained by hypertonus of the lumbar left sidebenders and the right piriformis (an external rotator of the femur). By having the patient strongly contract (after appropriate positioning) the muscle groups which are their antagonists, the offending muscles are made to relax, and the sacrum is freed from its restraints.

Iliosacral Dysfunctions

Throughout the entire stance phase of the walking cycle the iliac crest rotates anteriorly, pivoting at the same point where the sacrum torsions.[4] The opposite iliac crest in swing phase rotates in the reverse direction, turning around a transverse axis through the symphysis pubis. A loss of anterior and/or posterior ilial rotation produces iliosacral dysfunction—right or left "rotated innominate" anterior or posterior.

Malalignment of the anterior superior iliac spines (ASIS) in the supine position, following successful treatment of pelvic subluxations and sacroiliac dysfunctions, is the best indica-

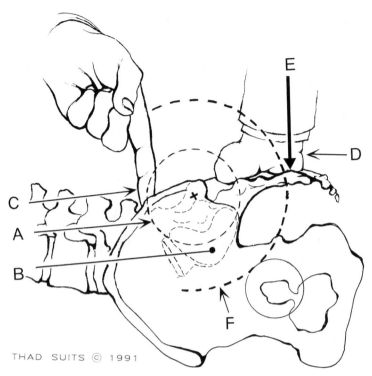

THAD SUITS © 1991

Figure 12.2. Geometric model for treatment of left unilateral sacral flexion. **A**, arc of circle with center **X**; **B**, sacroiliac joint surface track for sacral nutation; **C**, operator's index finger palpating for sacral base movement at sacral sulcus medial to gluteal tubercle, **D**, heel of operator's hand pressing on the left side of S5 in the direction of **Arrow E** which is tangent to circle arc **F** with the same center as arc **A**.

tor of iliosacral dysfunction. Inferior displacement of the ASIS on the side of a positive standing flexion test (relative to the contralateral ASIS) indicates an anterior innominate on that side, and not a posterior innominate on the other side, which has a relatively superior ASIS. Anterior rotation of the innominate also slightly displaces the posterior superior iliac spine (PSIS) superiorly, and moves the pubic crest very slightly anteriorly, *but not inferiorly.*

Leg length measured in the straight supine position by observing the inferior edges of the medial malleoli, against which the thumbs are placed firmly, is altered by innominate rotation because the acetabulum is in front of the iliosacral rotation axis. Thus, anterior rotation of the innominate lengthens the leg in the supine position. Innominate rotation influence on leg length is somewhat reduced in the prone position, since the two ASISs and

the pubic bones form a tripod support for the pelvis. With both iliosacral and sacroiliac dysfunctions present, moving the patient from prone to supine may at times reverse the side of the functional short leg!

Successful treatment is predicated on first treating subluxations and sacroiliac dysfunctions to restore alignment to the iliosacral axis. Muscle contractions produce transarticular forces which create compression or shear at the sacroiliac joint. With relaxation of the contraction the joint is looser packed than it was, and the rotation range may be increased by using the femur for leverage.

TREATMENT CONCEPTS

Balance, Relaxation, and Localization

In addition to diagnostic accuracy and good clinical judgment, there are three general principles—balance, relaxation, and localization. They are basic to all effective manual medicine treatment procedures, strongly influencing their precision and control. Relaxation of both the patient and the therapist requires balance, while localization requires relaxation.

Localization. This term refers to precision and specificity of the treatment effect. As Neumann[30] (p. 4) says, "The presence of a somatic dysfunction is the only indication for manual therapy!" Unless the treatment is applied precisely to the dysfunction, it will not be effective. Localization is achieved when the anatomic parts with the dysfunction are positioned so that the restrictive barrier is encountered. This means that the slack in the tissues has been taken up, and the very beginning (the "feather edge") of the restrictive barrier has been reached, or engaged. This precise positioning may be done by palpating the end-field quality, or by *passively* introducing motion in the direction of mobilization, stopping just before the next bone in the chain of bones moves. It must be emphasized that passive positioning requires that the patient be sufficiently relaxed so that he is neither assisting nor resisting the movement, either of which can defeat the localization.

Specificity. It is important to understand the relationship of localization to specificity. This is related to Greenman's term "Control"[6] (p.47), i.e., controlling the force, direction, and duration of muscle contraction, which has the effect of selecting which of the patient's muscles does the therapeutic work. Localization is passive positioning to the barrier; specificity is what you and the patient do after localization is achieved. Specificity is Kettler's "precisely executed counterforce."

Localization and specificity also apply to thrust techniques, as well as soft tissue or massage techniques. Localization is positioning the problem where you can do something about it. Specificity is doing the right thing to resolve the problem.

Relaxation. This means voluntary reduction of muscle tonus to a minimum level. Palpatory sensitivity is required for localization in treatment. The goal of rehearsing any psychomotor performance is to make it more efficient, i.e., reduce the effort expended. The therapist's conscious awareness of the amount of effort (muscle tension) being used to execute a particular procedure must be especially alert in order to overcome the initial inefficiency inherent in learning a new skill. Until performance inefficiency is overcome results will likely be disappointing.

Patient relaxation is equally important. The therapist must be alert to tension in the patient's body, so that appropriate steps can be taken to reduce it. Tension in the therapist is communicated non-verbally to the patient as soon as the therapist touches the patient. Other factors to be dealt with include patient comfort and security, both physical and psychological.

Balance. A part of physical security is balance, i.e., postural stability in relation to gravity. *Balance is essential for relaxation of both the therapist and the patient.* Balance is achieved through somatic proprioceptive awareness and by putting broad support underneath the center of gravity.

Reexamination. In addition to these three basic principles there is an important habit to acquire. *Always re-examine the area of dysfunction after it has been treated.* Re-examination should be the last step of every treatment procedure. Old hands at manipulation sometimes omit this step, confident that they "felt the release," but sometimes the release is only partial.

NEUROMUSCULAR PHYSIOLOGY UNDERLYING ME TECHNIQUE

An understanding of the anatomy and physiology of muscles is clearly relevant to a discussion of ME treatment.

Tonic and Phasic Muscles

Some classifications of muscles have already been discussed in the context of the etiology and the mechanisms of somatic dysfunctions. In addition to the publications of MacConaill[38] and Basmajian[39] on the classifications of muscle functions as tonic or phasic

agonists, synergists, stabilizers and antagonists, the works of Janda,[34] Burke[33,36] et al.,
Edgerton,[33,37] and Roy et al.[62] are relevant to
the following discussion. As we have already
indicated, the histological, biochemical, anatomical and functional classifications overlap
to a degree. Thus, stabilizer muscles tend to
be monoarticular, slow twitch, glycogen conservative, and tonic. There are many exceptions. The hamstring muscles, which have a
tonic, stabilizer function,[35,63] are histologically complex, and are polyarticular. In man
the stabilizer function of muscles has apparently become so efficient that continuous sustained contraction is rarely necessary to support posture (Basmajian[32] p. 178). Instead
intermittent contractions make fine adjustments in joint relationships.

The histology of phasic and tonic muscles
has been extensively researched in other ver-
tebrates, but human striated muscles are much
more complex and difficult to classify. Nevertheless, animal models provide very suggestive information on which to base a scientific
approach to ME technique. Cats with micro-
electrodes implanted in their soleus and gastrocnemeous muscles[33] were equipped with
tiny radio transmitters in order to study the
firing sequence of tonic (gastrocnemeous) and
phasic (soleus) muscles as the cats moved
about freely in their environment. For many
types of movement the tonic muscles fired
several milliseconds before the phasic muscles
(shorter chronaxie).

In humans there are striated muscles
which function and behave in a tonic-like way,
and there are others which are phasic-like.
When using isometric technique to treat somatic dysfunction involving tonic muscle,
such as somatic dysfunction of a single vertebral joint, it therefore makes sense to keep
the forces of contractions very light, whereas
the treatment of tightened and shortened
polyarticular phasic muscles with isometric
technique requires more forceful contractions.

The concept of the *motor unit* is important
to ME theory (see Chapter 4). Larger functional units, called myotatic units, are also

important, e.g., a unit composed of a motor
unit plus the intrinsic sensory systems arising
from the muscle fibers of the motor unit (including the spindle receptors) and their synaptic connections in the spinal cord, including
the gamma efferents. Still larger functioning
units are composed of the motor unit, the
intrinsic and extrinsic sensory systems and
central nervous system connections. These
latter units, or systems, have great clinical
importance, since they are the structural components of reflexes—somatosomatic,
viscerosomatic, somatovisceral, and "somato-
angiotaxic."

Intrinsic and Extrinsic Reflex Systems.
To understand the neurophysiologic mechanisms involved in isometric or isotonic ME
technique, let us examine the parts of the
nervous system concerned with the control of
muscle length. At the level of the spinal cord
effector mechanism there are two basic reflex
systems, intrinsic and extrinsic. The simplest
element of the intrinsic system is a myotatic
unit, in which the sensory nerves originate
from the bag or chain elements of the muscle
spindle, and from stimulatory synapses with
the alpha and gamma efferents to the same
muscle. Examples are the myotatic (stretch)
reflex and the hypertonic monoarticular muscle creating and maintaining a single vertebral
joint somatic dysfunction (see Type II Somatic Dysfunction, Table 12.2).

The spindle receptors in muscles are complex structures providing digital data to the
central nervous system which compiles the
data into information about the length of the
muscle as well as the rate of length change of
the muscle.[60] Spindle receptors are composed
of two types of intrafusal muscle fibers (nuclear bag and nuclear chain) which are bun-
dled together in a parallel fashion, and encap-
sulated. The larger nuclear bag fibers extend
beyond the capsule to attach to the endomysium of the surrounding extrafusal muscles.
Nuclear chain fibers attach to the inside of
the capsule. See Figure 12.3.

At least two kinds of sensory nerve endings
are found on the muscle fibers within the
spindle: annulospiral around the equatorial

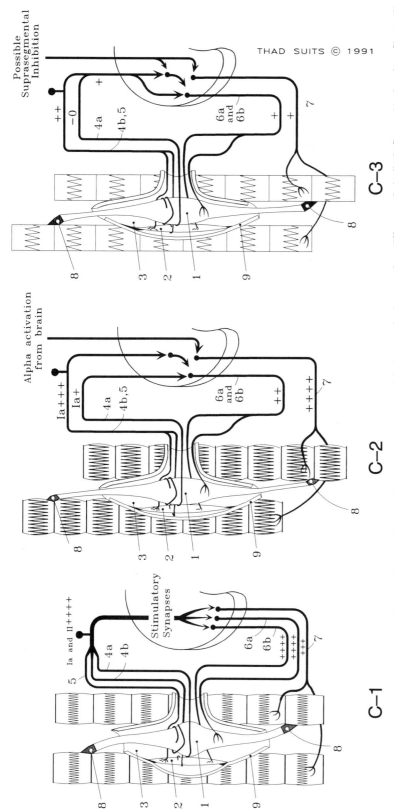

THAD SUITS © 1991

C-1

C-2

C-3

Figure 12.3. Effect of isometric contraction on hypertonic muscle.

C-1. Hypertonic Muscle. Gamma efferents (6a to bag, 6b to chain) keep nuclear bag fibers (1) and nuclear chain fibers (2) contracted, shortening and widening spindle capsule (9). Alpha motor (7) firing keeps extrafusal muscle contracted, stimulating the annulospiral proprioceptors (4a) of the bag fibers which extend beyond the ends of the spindle capsule (9) to attach to the endomysium (8) of the extrafusal muscles. Contraction of the nuclear chain fibers (2) slightly shortens the spindle capsule and stimulates the chain annulospiral (4b) and flowerspray (5) nerves. Cortical inhibition is absent, or decreased, allowing positive feedback reflex to continue operating.

C-2. Isometric Contraction. Effect on Spindle Reflexes. Nuclear bag fibers (1) are passively elongated by the contracting extrafusal muscle (8), the overall length of which does not change, even though muscle fibrils may shift in relation to each other. Extrafusal muscle pressure against capsule reduces subcapsular lymph space (3), slimming capsule (9) and slightly reducing nuclear chain flowerspray (5) stimulation. Bag annulospirals (4a) adapt more rapidly after initial response to stretch.

C-3. Postisometric Relaxation. Extrafusal muscle may now be stretched without farther elongating the bag fiber and stimulating spindle afferents. Repeating the isometric procedure further reduces the gamma gain.

regions of both bag and chain fibers, and flower spray endings toward the poles of the chain fibers.[64] The nuclear bag receptors are thought to be capable of rapidly adapting to changes in muscle length, velocity, and acceleration of contraction, whereas the nuclear chain fiber receptors are slow adapting tension transducers. In single segment somatic dysfunction of a vertebra, the alpha motor neuron activity of monoarticular muscle fibers has been abnormally re-set to a higher gain, keeping the muscle's resting length abnormally short, probably to reduce the tension on the nuclear chain fibers of the spindle. Re-setting the gamma bias of the spindle in order to reduce the alpha motor activity may occur by means of pre- and post-synaptic inhibition at the cord level. On the other hand, a precisely controlled isometric contraction may be sufficient to alter the spindle dynamics therapeutically in this manner (see Figure 12.3). At present, with much relevant basic laboratory research yet to be done, clinical empiricism is the principal basis of ME theory.

The intrinsic system may become autonomous when corticospinal inhibition is removed and not reinstituted. This may occur when muscular movement events are not as anticipated. A positive feedback reflex arc is established between the annulospiral spindle receptor and alpha and gamma motor nerves, resulting in maintained hypertonous of the muscle.

One ME hypothesis is that light, brief isometric voluntary contraction of the hypertonic muscle externally stretches the nuclear bag fibers of the spindles. The bag annulospirals, after brief excitation, promptly adapt to a lengthened muscle condition, even though the muscle length did not change. With post-isometric relaxation, the muscle may be actually lengthened without stimulating myotatic reflexes. The isometric contraction may also press fluid from the spindle lymph spaces, reducing the post-isometric tension in the capsule of the spindle. The slower adapting nuclear chain fibers which are attached to the capsule of the spindle may,

therefore, undergo a change in tension with a reduction of annulospiral stimulation.

The myotatic unit is a positive feedback reflex system which functions to keep a constant gain set in the gamma efferent-annulospiral loop, thereby keeping the muscle's resting length constant. In a tonic monoarticular muscle this constant must be exquisitely precise—to several digits beyond the decimal, so to speak—and is one of the determinants of the physiologic motion barrier, as well as the motion barrier of somatic dysfunction.

In the extrinsic system the anterior horn cells of the alpha and gamma efferents to the muscle receive synaptic impulses from sensory nerves originating in *other* muscles or organs. The elements of the extrinsic system are larger, more complex "neuromuscular units" which link together myotatic units from muscles which have some functional relationship to each other. Examples are reciprocal inhibition of antagonist muscles (Sherrington Law II), organized pain avoidance, conditioned reflexes involving learned firing sequences,[65] viscero-somatic muscle guarding reflexes, and polyarticular muscle spasm. Even though Basmajian[32] has shown by EMG apparent exceptions to the Sherrington reciprocal inhibition law, the principle has practical clinical application in ME technique, and works very predictably when applied correctly. Retzlaff[66] has demonstrated the role of the Mothner internuncial neuron in contralateral reflex inhibition. See Figure 12.4.

Clearly both intrinsic and extrinsic systems are almost constantly "supervised" by suprasegmental systems, which constitute such an inhibitory influence that is is often not possible to elicit a knee jerk reflex, for example, without first having the patient perform Jendrassik's maneuver. This is more common in trained athletes and dancers, suggesting that a significant component of these suprasegmental inhibitory influences is derived from sequential programs involving the cerebellum with its descending tracts in the lateral funiculus, from the *substantia gelatinosa*, and from cord interneurons involved in motor

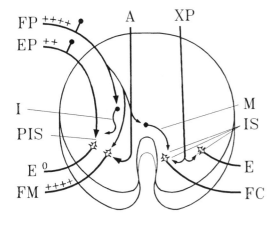

THAD SUITS © 1991

Figure 12.4. Two Kinds of Inhibitory Extrinsic Reflexes—Afferent reciprocal inhibition of antagonist muscles, and cross-pattern inhibition of muscle homologues. **A**—alpha activation from brain to flexor muscle (**FM**), **FP**—flexor proprioceptors, **EP**—extensor proprioceptors, **I**—interneuron, **PIS**—Presynaptic inhibitory synapse, **E**—Extensor alpha motor nerve, **M**—Mothner cell commissural interneuron to contralateral flexors (**FC**) by way of inhibitory synapse (**IS**). Extrapyramidal nerves (**XP**) from brain connect with anterior horn motor cells at inhibitory synapses.

coordination and spinal cord operant conditioning.[65]

It is thought that suprasegmental systems, as well as the muscle spindle receptors, are reprogrammed by ME technique procedures. Since voluntary actions are a part of ME technique, the cerebral cortex, extrapyramidal and limbic systems are probably involved in the treatment. They are also most likely involved in the adaptation to the somatic dysfunction. The muscles and spinal effector mechanisms involved directly in the dysfunction have temporarily or permanently, in some fashion, isolated themselves from suprasegmental control. The gamma loop to the monoarticular tonic muscle has become autonomous. Isometric ME technique is a means of coaxing the maverick muscle back into the system. It is assumed that during the isometric contraction there is a *re-setting of the "gain"* in the gamma loop, both at the level of the spindle

receptors as well as in the spinal cord through interneuron and suprasegmental inhibitory synapses. During the post-isometric contraction relaxation phase, an increase in the resting length of the muscle is permitted, as relaxation comes about from the resultant decrease in gamma efferent discharge to the spindles.

In the extrinsic systems the annulospiral and flower spray spindle receptor data are synapsed to spinal effector systems controlling other muscles: the synergists, stabilizers, and antagonists. These data are supplemented by input from many other sensory receptors—Golgi receptors, free unmyelinated nerve endings, and Pacinian-like receptors, such as the ones found in joint structures,[31] e.g., vertebral facet joints. Complex integration of somatic sensory proprioceptive postural and oculovestibular data results in immediate readaptation of the entire somatic system upon the occurrence of somatic dysfunction, or following its successful treatment.

Golgi tendon receptors are rarely stimulated in ME treatment, since most have a high stretch threshold. Their principal function is to protect muscle attachments from avulsion, utilizing a post-synaptic inhibitory synapse in the spinal effector mechanism. Recent theory implicates some types of Golgi receptors in alpha-motor excitation.[67] Their precise role is not clear. The free unmyelinated nerve endings in muscles are assumed to be C-fiber nociceptors. They may be the principal source of pain associated with visceral or joint inflammation and the neuroreflexive guarding response of the muscles which lie over the inflamed structures.

Classification of Muscle Contractions

Muscle contractions can be described with several quantitative variables:

1. Tension.—the amount of force applied by the lever to which the muscle attaches, or the amount of counterforce opposing the movement of the lever. This tension can be measured in Newtons, pounds, or ounces.

2. Time.—either the muscle firing sequence, in which intervals are measured in milliseconds, or the duration of the effort, usually measured in seconds.

3. Distance.—the amount of movement produced, usually measured in angular degrees, linear excursion, or a percentage of the potential range of motion. If movement is produced, it may be plus or minus (concentric or eccentric). Zero change = isometric contraction.

4. Rate. —with time and distance one can also express the variables of velocity (d/t), acceleration (d/t^2) and frequency (oscillatory movements).

Expanding the Definitions of Therapeutic Muscle Contractions

Isometric. —tensing a muscle with no resulting change in length.

Isotonic. —"constant force," literally. Actually means muscle tensing *with* a change in length.

Concentric (with shortening) or

Eccentric (with lengthening of the muscle).

Isolytic—a type of eccentric isotonic used to stretch fibrotic muscle. The speed of eccentric movement is very quick due to fast movement of the counterforce, or, preferably, a rapid vibratory oscillating counterforce (3–5 Hz.).

Isokinetic. —a concentric or eccentric isotonic contraction where the length change occurs at a constant velocity.

By precisely and specifically instructing the patient one may get voluntary contractions of muscles of sufficient variety to accomplish the goals of treatment. It is advisable to state what part of the patient's body is to be activated ("push your forehead against my resisting hand"), in what direction the effort is to be made ("toward your lap"), how hard ("with eight ounces of force"), and how long ("Stop now and relax"). Before and after, but not during, the patient's active participation, while the patient is sufficiently relaxed, the part being treated is precisely positioned passively for localization (q.v.). The counterforce

provided is an important communication to the patient. It precisely directs the patient's effort. If the effort is to be isometric, the counterforce does not yield. On the other hand, isotonic techniques require a moving counterforce. If constant velocity (isokinetic) contraction is desired, the counterforce must move at a uniform speed. Precise instructions to the patient are essential, and must be varied or elaborated for the patient to understand exactly what to do. In order to get a maximum force contraction, words of encouragement are sometimes appropriate.

Maximum force isometric contractions are used clinically to test the strength of muscles in their elongated state. During strenuous physical activities, when muscles perform an eccentric isotonic contraction in order to arrest the ballistic movement of a body part before the joint is damaged, or becomes hypermobile, the muscles are approaching their maximum resting length. Diminished performance strength at maximum resting length provides evidence consistent with a diagnosis of hypermobility. Sustaining the test contraction for 15 seconds will occasionally permit discovery of clinical weakness in a muscle which initially exhibits normal, or even increased, strength because of reflex guarding behavior.

By way of emphasizing the body building potential of isometric exercise, Spackman[68] at the University of Southern Illinois demonstrated that three repetitions of a maximum isometric contraction of an arm biceps muscle daily for two weeks would produce measurable enlargement of the arm. The clinical usefulness of this information is debatable. Muscle fiber splitting studies[62] seem to indicate that the gross hypertrophy of the muscle exercised in this way is due primarily to neovascularization, not to enlargement of the sarcoplasm, and that performance strength is not significantly increased.

Great force, but not necessarily maximum, is also required in the application of the Sherrington reciprocal inhibition of muscle antagonists (Law II) principle to relax a spastic muscle. The harder the force, up to a practical limit, the more the reciprocal inhibition. The same is true of the isokinetic treatment of pathologically weak muscles. The isokinetic treatment procedure is introduced to the patient by explaining and demonstrating what the patient is expected to do: "You will try to move your foot from here to here (manually demonstrating the full range of motion of the part) against my resistance in three seconds. I will tell you when to begin and will count the seconds for you aloud. You will have to work very hard to complete the movement in three seconds. Each repetition will require harder effort. We will do it only three times." Of course the isokinetic exercise can be done with an Orthotron or Cybex machine, but since nine seconds is usually sufficient to restore full strength, unless there is measurable atrophy of the muscle, the time and expense of automation may not seem justified.

For the treatment of abnormal muscle shortness or joint range of motion restriction, isometric contractions of the muscle opposing the restricted movement should be in the range of force to elicit action of the selected muscle with minimal activity of other muscles. Appropriate force for monoarticular muscles is less than a pound (<0.5 kg.). Polyarticular muscles are activated with moderate force. Too much force activates undesired muscles which may interfere with restoring range of motion.

The isometric techniques are the most widely applicable in ME treatment. They are used to treat vertebral somatic dysfunctions using the principle described in the previous paragraph. They are also used to treat the passive joints of the pelvis, foot, and wrist. When being used to treat passive joint movements, the treatment effect is localized by passive positioning to the restriction and holding. Isometric contractions which indirectly exert forces on the joint are performed to increase joint range of motion. Different muscle groups may be tried until the treatment objective is achieved. Even joint play motions, which, as Mennell[41] points out, are essential for full active range of motion function of extremity joints, may be treated by

articulatory localization and isometric contractions. See Figure 12.4 and Table 12.5.

The isolytic techniques are especially effective in the treatment of chronic muscle contractures. Originally they were performed with one quick stretch. In the updated techniques, the counterforce is oscillated in a rapid vibratory movement, in effect alternating concentric and eccentric isotonic contractions. It is postulated that the vibration has some effect on the myotatic units in addition to the mechanical and circulatory effects.

EXAMPLES OF CLINICAL APPLICATIONS OF ME TECHNIQUE

Initially, spinal somatic dysfunctions were treated utilizing the reciprocal inhibition of muscle antagonists. Thus, if right sidebending of the fourth lumbar (L-4) were restricted, the patient was positioned so that L-4 was at the "feather edge" of its restriction (precise localization was recognized as important from the beginning); then the patient was asked to forcefully contract the right sidebender muscles of the trunk by reaching the right hand down toward the floor. The operator resisted any movement of the patient's shoulders, so the action produced a left lateral translation of the first lumbar. As sidebending to the right was restored, the *left sidebender muscle was lengthened.* Even though the shoulders were not allowed to move, the contraction was expected to produce translatory vertebral movement, and, therefore, was concentric isotonic. (Example illustrated in Figure 12.6.) In retrospect, this also seems to be a reverse way to develop ME as a discipline.

Soon the forceful isotonic techniques were replaced by light force isometric procedures in which the abnormally shortened muscle was contracted against an unyielding counterforce for a few seconds and then relaxed (Example illustrated in Figure 12.5). During the post-isometric relaxation phase the muscle was passively stretched to its new resting length, and the procedure was repeated, if necessary. When using the isometric technique to treat a vertebral joint the force of

Table 12.5
Contractions: Light or Hard, Short or Long, Concentric, Eccentric, or Isometric; Summary of Clinical Applications

Isometric (6 variations)
Vary FORCE (ozs., lbs., maximum), Vary Duration (3, 8, 15+ seconds), Vary LENGTH

1. Maximum force, 8 second ISOMETRIC, any length—Stimulates neovascularization and muscle fiber splitting.
2. Maximum force, 15+ second ISOMETRIC with the muscle elongated—Tests joints for hypermobility and measures protecting/stabilizing power of the muscle.
3. Maximum force, 15+ second ISOMETRIC with the muscle shortened—Tests muscle holding power.
4. Moderate intensity (lbs) 2–3 second ISOMETRIC, muscle elongated to take out its slack to the feather edge of the motion barrier—Treats and lengthens abnormally shortened LONG RESTRICTORS.
5. Light intensity (ozs.) 2–3 second ISOMETRIC with the muscle's slack taken up to the motion barrier—Treats and lengthens an abnormally shortened SHORT RESTRICTOR, and mobilizes a restricted joint.
6. Light to moderate intensity intermittent rhythmic ISOMETRIC contractions (X9), called Ruddy's Rhythmic Resistive Duction—used to increase lymphatic flow from a region.

Isotonic (4 variations)
Vary LENGTH (concentric & eccentric) Vary SPEED (isokinetic and isolytic)

1. Moderate to maximum intensity, slow and controlled CONCENTRIC ISOTONIC—to relax a spastic antagonist muscle by reciprocal inhibition (Sherrington's 2nd Law), or to mobilize a restricted joint (e.g., costovertebral M. E. Technique).
2. Moderate to maximum intensity ISOLYTIC (either an ECCENTRIC ISOTONIC contraction with a quick stretch, OR a sustained contraction against a vibratory oscillating counterforce—ALLASOTONIC, or alternating eccentric and concentric isotonic)—used to stretch fibrotic muscle shortness.
3. ISOKINETIC (uniform velocity of movement—concentric or eccentric)—used to strengthen muscles for specific functions, and to increase muscle tonus.

contraction needed to be only a few ounces, just enough to activate the monoarticular muscles of the joint (e.g., *intertransversari, rotatores*).

In Figure 12.5, the isometric technique for treatment of restricted flexion-right side-bending/rotation (ERSLt, positionally) of the 4th Lumbar vertebra begins with L4 in neutral (facets not engaged). If restriction is major (>50%) lumbar lordosis may be increased extremely in order to position L4 at the flexion end of its neutral range. L4 is then sidebent to the right to its barrier by passively shifting the patient's weight to the left, maintaining the patient's postural balance. Fine adjustments are then made in the patient's trunk position, flexing by translating the vertebra posteriorly (to maintain postural balance) and rotating to the right until the restrictive bar-

rier in engaged in all 3 planes (being careful not to disturb the engagement of barriers in the other two planes). The operator must turn his/her whole body with the patient's shoulders in order to maintain flexion localization. The operator's position must also be balanced and stable. The patient is then instructed to pull the left scapula posteriorly and down (*arrow D*) toward operator's finger (*B*) using about a pound of force for 2 or 3 seconds. This action is resisted unyieldingly by the operator, whose shoulder is under the patient's axilla (*A*). On the command "Relax" the patient must stop pushing completely, and relax in the balanced position. When relaxation is complete enough, L4 is relocalized one plane of motion at a time; sidebending right (translating the trunk to the left), rotation right, and flexion. After the third isomet-

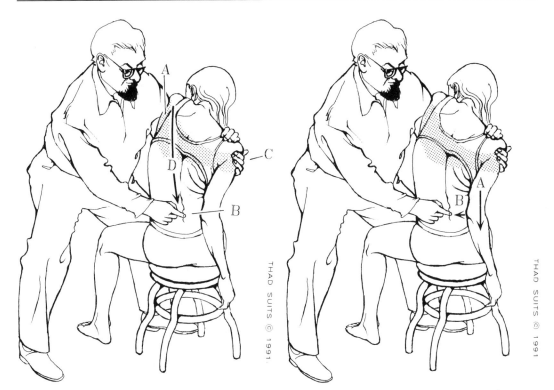

Figure 12.5. Application of ME technique. Example of isometric technique. **Arrow D** through left scapula to L4 at **B**. **A:** Patient's left arm with her hand across chest to top of right shoulder. **C:** Clinician's left hand grasping deltoid region of patient's right arm.

Figure 12.6. Application of ME technique. Example of isotonic technique. **Arrow A:** Patient pushes right hand toward floor forcefully. Left translation occurs at L4 with active right sidebending (see text).

ric contraction of the L4 left extenders and left sidebenders, the patient relaxes and the operator passively relocalizes to the new (usually physiologic by this time) barriers. Then the operator passively guides the left shoulder down between the knees while holding the right shoulder back. When flexion is complete in this rotated position the right shoulder is guided down to a position of symmetrical flexion. (*B*) Index finger monitors L4 localization between the L4 and L5 spinous processes. (*C*) Operator's left hand reaches in front of the patient to hold the far shoulder. (*D*) Direction of patient's isometric force.

While the patient is hyperflexed, the operator checks the transverse processes for symmetry to see if the treatment was successful, and then allows the patient to straighten up.

In Figure 12.6, to treat the same dysfunc-

tion as in Figure 12.5, using isotonic technique, the patient is positioned for localization in the same way as in Figure 12.5. However, the patient is instructed to push his/her right hand toward the floor (*arrow A*) forcefully (20–40 pounds). The operator must be balanced and stable enough to resist (with hand at the right shoulder) a 20–40 lb. force, in order to *prevent the shoulder from descending.* Consequently, a left translation occurs at L4 (*arrow B*), producing active right sidebending as the inhibited left sidebenders permit.

CONCLUSION

Management Strategies

Physician/Patient Paradigms. It is the author's belief that in order to obtain optimum clinical results using manipulative therapy, the clinician's efforts should be guided by a philosophy which accepts the following values as paramount: (1) empowerment of the patient is preferred over treatment of the patient as a passive recipient of therapeutic procedures; (2) understanding of the mechanisms of health is preferred over identification of disease entities; and (3) integrated diagnostic analysis of functional interrelationships within the *whole patient* is preferred to identification of isolated pathological parts (organs or systems) of the patient's body.

One of the important issues in the doctor/patient relationship concerns power and autonomy. Although empowerment of the patient is a basic tenet of the osteopathic philosophy, the subject has been more thoughtfully and thoroughly explored by non-osteopathic practitioners,[11,69,70,71] including the eminent psychologist, Carl Rogers.[72] One powerful psychological effect resulting from the use of ME technique derives from the patient's perception that he is using his own muscles to participate in a collaborative treatment effort, which can be an important step toward increasing autonomy and responsibility for corrective or preventive self-care. It is well known that patient compliance is enhanced when the patient perceives himself to be a participant in the diagnosis and treatment enterprise. Many patients have learned self-treatment home exercises based on ME principles.

This osteopathic bias can be expressed as part of a system of values which regards mobilization of the patient's intrinsic resources to improve health to be more important than too great reliance on the extrinsic resources of the health care system. This is sometimes referred to as the Patient-Centered aspect of the osteopathic philosophy (clearly, a parallel to Carl Rogers' Client Centered psychotherapy). Confidence in the patient's ability to heal him/herself can lead the physician, at the very least, to prudently forego active intervention, when the risk of such intervention is unacceptable: and, at best, to intervene when some manipulable condition is detected, the treatment and correction of which enhances the patient's self healing powers.

Health, Disease, and Holism. In addition to the above mentioned priority, the philosophic orientations toward a *Health versus Disease* and *Integrated Functional Analysis versus Compartmentalization of Pathology* also make sense in the context of the *Patient-Centered* philosophy. The patient is an integrated organism and should be treated as such, not as a collection of organs and other parts which are independent of each other. If one defines health as the ability to respond optimally to stress, it is easier to understand the importance of the perspective of organismic holism, i.e., the view that the parts of the human body are integrated, and, thus, necessarily respond in an interrelated manner to external and internal stressors. The nervous and circulatory systems are important integrators of the body; as the "primary instrument of life," so, too, is the musculoskeletal system. An understanding of these integrating health mechanisms is necessary for the rational practice of medicine.

Indications for Manipulation

One of the most common errors of medical management grows out of an emphasis on symptom control. The thinking which leads to this misguided practice attributes the symptoms of disease to the "disease entity" (whatever that is!). Sir William Osler is often quoted in this regard: "Listen to the patient, Doctor. He is telling you the diagnosis." This aphorism is commonly interpreted as saying that, if one listens to the patient's recital of symptoms long enough, the diagnosis will become apparent, and physical examination will not be necessary. And, of course, once one has "the Diagnosis," the treatment for it can be looked up, if need be. A moment's reflection brings the realization that the symptoms are produced by the host, not the disease. One might even say (granting there may be exceptions) that the worse the patient feels, the better (harder?) his healing mechanisms are working! Osler also said, "Pain is a liar." If one treats the part where the patient experiences the pain, one will be treating the wrong part of the body most of the time. We have previously discussed the concept that in the musculoskeletal system pain almost always develops and persists in the structures which are stressed the most by the *adaptation* to the dysfunction. Thus, if one emphasizes manipulative treatment of the *site* of the patient's pain, one will usually be incorrectly focusing on the adaptation rather than the dysfunction.

The automatic nature of these adaptive mechanisms is exemplified by impairments of the locomotor system. Steindler's[73] "principle of the path of least resistance" describes the way in which the body adapts to functional impairment as the "quickest solution to the problem," usually involving substitutions of movement functions which require normal parts of the body to function in abnormal ways. This discloses a serious flaw in the "wisdom of the body": it has no foresight; its quick solutions, which may have enhanced survival at the moment, at least in prehistoric times, create conditions which are often painful and ultimately maladaptive.

Determination of the method, sequence, frequency, and dosage of manipulative treatment (in fact, *all* treatment) should all be based on a precise analysis of the patient's somatic dysfunctions and the adaptive mechanisms which have ensued. Symptom (pain) or disease directed therapy is hazardous, and, too often, ineffective. The only indication for manipulative treatment is the presence of somatic dysfunction (Neumann[30] p. 4).

In order to impress upon his students the importance of being thorough, the founder of Osteopathy, Andrew Taylor Still, M.D., exhorted them to start at the occiput and go down through the body, making sure each articulation works perfectly.[74] In later times, some of the more structural-mechanical minded pedants have urged manipulators to start at the feet and work upwards, treating as you go. Such a Search and Destroy method would surely result in frequent overtreatment or mistreatment, and certainly waste a lot of the therapist's time in the treatment of adaptations assumed to be dysfunctions. The holistic approach requires that all parts of the whole body system be examined and considered before formulating a comprehensive treatment plan.

The selection of the appropriate manipulative modality should be based on the diagnosis. Within the ME paradigm the selection of techniques derives from a description of a specific joint's ranges of motion in all planes, a distinction between various possible restricting mechanisms, and an estimation of the acuteness or chronicity of the dysfunction.

REFERENCES

1. Chapman F, Chapman AH, Owens C: Chapman's reflexes. Salisbury, NC: Rowan Printing Company, 1932.

2. Magoun HI. Osteopathy in the cranial field. 3rd ed. Meridian, Idaho: The Cranial Academy, 1976.

3. Mitchell FL. The balanced pelvis and its relationship to reflexes. Yearbook of The Academy of Osteopathy, 1948:146–151.

4. Mitchell FL. Structural pelvic function. Yearbook of the Academy of Applied Osteopathy, 1958:71–90.

5. Korr IM. The spinal cord as the organizer of disease processes. Part 2, The peripheral autonomic nervous system. J Am Osteopath Assoc 1979; 79:82–90.

6. Greenman PE. Principles of manual medicine. Baltimore: Williams & Wilkins, 1989.

7. Rumney I. The relevance of somatic dysfunction. J Am Osteopath Assoc 1975; 74:723–725.

8. International Classification of Diseases—Hospital Adaptation (H-ICDA, Ed. 2, 1978). Commission on Professional and Hospital Activities. Ann Arbor, Michigan, 1978.

9. International Classification of Diseases, 9th Ed. Clinical Modification, 3rd ed. U.S. Department of Health and Human Services. March 1989. DHHS Publication No. (PHS) 89-1260, Vol. 1:637.

10. Mitchell FL Jr. Towards a definition of somatic dysfunction. Osteop Ann 1979; 7:12–25.

11. Lewit K. Manipulative therapy in rehabilitation of the locomotor system. London: Butterworths, 1985:17–22.

12. Mitchell FL, ed, Moran PS, Pruzzo NA. An evaluation and treatment manual of osteopathic muscle energy procedures. Valley Park, Missouri: Institute for Continuing Education in Osteopathic Principles, 1979.

13. Bowles CH. Functional orientation for technic (report on a functional approach to specific osteopathic manipulative problems developed in the New England Academy of Applied Osteopathy during 1953–54). Part I, 1955:177; Part II, 1956:107; Part III, 1957:53.

14. Bowles CH. Musculo-skeletal segment as a problem-

solving machine. Yearbook of the Academy of Applied Osteopathy, 1964:175.

15. Hoover HV. Functional technic. Yearbook of the Academy of Applied Osteopathy, 1958:47; reprinted 1969:91.

16. Johnston WL. Segmental behavior during motion. I. A palpatory study of somatic relations. II Somatic dysfunction, the clinical distortion. J Am Osteop Assoc 1972; 72:352–361. III Extending behavioral boundaries. J Am Osteopath Assoc 1973; 72:462–475.

17. Mitchell FL. Clinical significance of cranial suture mobility. In: Retzlaff EW, Mitchell FL, Jr, eds. The cranium and its sutures. New York: Springer-Verlag, 1987:13–26.

18. Jones LH. Strain and counterstrain. Colorado Springs, CO: American Academy of Osteopathy, 1981.

19. Maigne R. Douleurs d'origine vertebrale et traitments par manipulations. Paris: Expansion Scientifique, 1968.

20. Frymann, Viola. Personal communication.

21. Upledger JA. personal communication.

22. Lippincott, HA. The osteopathic techniques of Wm. G. Sutherland, D.O. In: Yearbook of the Academy of Applied Osteopathy, 1949; 49:1–45.

23. Travell JG, Simon DJ. Myofascial pain and dysfunction: the trigger point manual. Baltimore: Williams & Wilkins, 1983.

24. Stoddard A. Manual of osteopathic technique. 2nd ed. London: Hutchinson, 1966.

25. Stoddard A. Manual of osteopathic practice. London: Hutchinson, 1969.

26. Lovett RW. Lateral curvature of the spine and round shoulders. Philadelphia: Blakiston's, 1912.

27. Halladay HV. Applied anatomy of the spine. 2nd ed. Yearbook of the Academy of Applied Osteopathy 1957:119.

28. Fryette HH. Principles of osteopathic technic. Second Printing. Carmel, CA. Academy of Applied Osteopathy, 1966:20–35.

29. Kapandji IA. Physiology of the joints. 2nd ed. Vol. 3. Edinburgh, London and New York: Churchill Livingstone. Longman Group Ltd, 1979:64–83.

30. Neumann HD. Introduction to manual medicine. Berlin, Heidelberg: Springer-Verlag, 1989.

31. Wyke BD. The neurology of low back pain. In: Jayson MIV, The lumbar spine and back pain. London: Pitman Medical, 265, 1980.

32. Basmajian JV. Muscles alive. 4th ed. Baltimore: Williams & Wilkins, 1978:5–17.

33. Burke RE, Edgerton VR. Motor unit properties and selection in movement. In: Wilmore JH ed. Exercise and sport science reviews. New York: Academic Press, 1975:31–81.

34. Janda, V. Muscles, central nervous motor regulation, and back problems. In: Korr IM ed. Neurobiologic

mechanisms in manipulative therapy. New York and London: Plenum Press, 1978:27–41.

35. Janda V. On the concept of postural muscles and posture in man. The Aust J Physiother 1983; 29:83–84.

36. Burke, RE, Levine DN, Zajac FE III, Tsairis P, Engel WK. Mammalian motor units: physiological-histochemical correlation in three types in cat gastrocnemius. Science 1971; 174:709–712.

37. Edgerton VR, Gerchman L, Carrow R. Histochemical changes in rat skeletal muscle after exercise. Exp Neurol 1968;24:110–123.

38. MacConaill MA. The movements of bones and joints. 2. Function of the musculature. J Bone Joint Surg 1949; 31-B:100–104.

39. MacConaill MA, Basmajian JV. Muscles and movements: a basis for human kinesiology. Baltimore: Williams & Wilkins, 1969.

40. Emminger E. Die anatomie und pathologie des blockierten Wirbelgelenks. *Therapie über das Nervensystem*, Vol. 7, Chirotherapie-Manuelle Therapie:117. Gross, D. ed. Stuttgart: Hippokrates, 1967.

41. Mennell J McM. Joint pain. Boston: Little Brown, 1964.

42. Mitchell FL. The training and measurement of sensory literacy in relation to osteopathic structural and palpatory diagnosis. J Am Osteopath Assoc 1976; 75:874–884.

43. Kimberly P. Syllabi for muscle energy tutorials, Michigan State University, College of Osteopathic Medicine, 1982.

44. Kottke FJ, Clayson SJ, Newman IM, Debevec DF, Anger RW, Skowlund HV. Evaluation of mobility of hip and lumbar vertebrae of normal young women. Arch Phys Med 1962; 43:1–8. (Reports changes in pelvisacral angle.)

45. Weisl H. The movements of the sacro-iliac joint. Acta Anat 1955; 23:80–91.

46. Fryette HH. Four innominate lesions—their cause, diagnosis and treatment. J Am Osteop Assoc 1914; 14:105–114. Reprinted In: The Yearbook of the Academy of Applied Osteopathy, 1966:79–88.

47. Mitchell FL, Pruzzo NA. Investigation of voluntary and primary respiratory mechanisms. J Am Osteopath Assoc 1971; 70:1109–1113.

48. Mitchell FL. Voluntary and involuntary respiration and the craniosacral mechanism. In: Tilley M ed. Collected osteopathic papers. New York: Insight Publishing Co., Inc., 1979.

49. Anson BJ, ed. Morris' human anatomy, 12th ed. New York: Blakiston, 1966:151–158.

50. Anson BJ, ed. Atlas of human anatomy. Philadelphia: Saunders, 1950, 342.

51. Brantigan OC. Clinical anatomy. New York, McGraw-Hill Blakiston Division, 1963:294ff.

52. Grant JCB. A method of anatomy, 6th ed. Baltimore: Williams & Wilkins, 1958:335.

53. Grant JCB. Grant's atlas. Baltimore: Williams & Wilkins, 1943:117–118.

54. Hafferl A. Lehrbuch der topographischen Anatomie. 2nd ed. Berlin: Springer-Verlag, 1957.

55. Hollinshead WH. Textbook of anatomy. 2nd ed. Hagerstown, MD: Harper & Row, 1967.

56. Lockhart RD. Anatomy of the human body. Philadelphia: Lippincott, 1959:102.

57. McMinn RMH, Hutchings RT. Color atlas of human anatomy. Chicago: Yearbook Medical Publishers, Inc., 1977.

58. Snell RS. Atlas of clinical anatomy. Boston: Little Brown, 99–103, 1980.

59. Sobotta J, Johannes, McMurrich JP. Atlas and textbook of human anatomy. Philadelphia and London: Saunders, 1914:28.

60. Warwick R, Williams PL. Gray's anatomy. 35th British ed. Philadelphia: WB Saunders, Co., 1973:801–804.

61. Wicke L. Atlas of radiologic anatomy. 4th ed. (Taylor AN, trans and ed). Munich, Baltimore: Urban & Schwarzenberg, 1987.

62. Roy R, Ho KW, Taylor J, Heusner W, Van Huss, W. Observations on muscle fiber splitting produced by weight lifting exercise. Abstract. American Osteopathic Association Research Convention, 1977.

63. Janda V. Personal communication.

64. Gowitzke BA, Milner M. Understanding the scientific bases of human movement. 2nd ed. Baltimore: Williams & Wilkins, 1980.

65. Patterson MM. The reflex connection: history of a middleman. Osteopath Ann 1976; 4:358–367.

66. Retzlaff EW. Personal communication.

67. Korr IM. Personal communication.

68. Spackman R. Two man isometric exercise for the whole man. Dubuque, Iowa: W.C. Brown, 1964.

69. Magraw RM. Ferment in medicine. Philadelphia: WB Saunders, 1966.

70. Meyer A. The commonsense psychiatry of doctor Adolf Meyer. Lief A, ed. New York: McGraw-Hill, 1948.

71. Szasz TS, Hollender M. A contribution to the philosophy of medicine—the basic models of the doctor-patient relationship. Arch Intern Med 1956; 97:585.

72. Rogers CR. Client centered psychotherapy. Boston: Houghton-Mifflin, 1951.

73. Steindler A. Kinesiology of the human body under normal and pathological conditions. Springfield: Charles C. Thomas, 1955.

74. Still AT. Philosophy of osteopathy. Kirksville, MO: A. T. Still, 1899.

13

Strain and Counterstrain

RANDALL S. KUSUNOSE

Observing a skilled strain and counterstrain practitioner you are immediately impressed with how gentle and nontraumatic this technique is for the patient and the operator. How quickly they are able to assess the musculoskeletal system for the areas of dysfunction and the involvement of the patient in assisting to guide the operator to the final treatment position.

This innovative system for the treatment of somatic dysfunction was developed by Lawrence Jones, DO, FAAO. He defines strain and counterstrain as a "passive positional procedure that places the body in a position of greatest comfort, thereby relieving pain by reduction and arrest of inappropriate proprioceptor activity that maintains somatic dysfunction."

From the definition it is clear that the strain and counterstrain concept is not directed toward tissue injury or tissue damage but aberrant neuromuscular reflexes within that tissue. Specifically, the primary proprioceptive nerve endings are singled out as reporting false information to the central nervous system and maintaining somatic dysfunction.[1] The operator will affect this system by passively positioning the patient's dysfunctional segment toward comfort or ease and away from pain, bind, and restricted barriers. The position results in maximal shortening of the involved muscle and its proprioceptors and eventual reduction of neuromuscular firing to tonic levels. Strain and counterstrain is an indirect technique because its action is away from the restricted barrier.

ORIGIN

Jones was motivated to experiment with the concept of positional release in part from his frustration with the rationale of his time for the osteopathic lesion (which has since changed names to somatic dysfunction). He was schooled to believe that somehow joints became locked or subluxed and the only way to treat them was to burst them loose via high velocity thrust techniques. His results were generally good, but occasionally a case would enter his office that resisted all of his manipulative skills, until Jones states, "only stubbornness kept me from admitting I was stumped." He recounts that he was treating just such a case when he discovered positional release.[2,3]

A young man with psoasitis (stooped posture, unable to come completely erect with severe pain across the low lumbar area) had been treated by Jones using high velocity techniques for 6 weeks with no relief of symptoms. He had been treated previously by two chiropractors for 2-½ months with similar results. He complained of pain in bed and an inability to find a comfortable position that he could stay in for any longer than 15 minutes. So, Jones devoted one treatment session to finding a reasonably comfortable position for the patient to sleep in. After 20 minutes of experimentation, a position of amazing comfort was found. Jones relates that: "He was nearly rolled into a ball with the pelvis rotated about 45 degrees and laterally flexed about 30 degrees." This was the first positive response the patient had had after 4 months of treatment, so Jones propped him in the position and went off to treat another patient. When he returned, he helped the patient upright and was astonished to find he could stand completely erect in total comfort. Examination revealed full and near pain-free range of motion. All Jones had done was put the patient in a position of comfort and the results were dramatic after his best efforts had repeatedly failed.

This was the inspiration that started Jones' experimenting with positional release and applying it to all somatic dysfunctions. During this developmental period he observed that the return to neutral done very slowly was important to the outcome of the positional release. If the patient was moved too quickly, especially in the first 15 degrees of motion, the benefit from the positioning was lost. Also, after initially supporting the patient in the position of release for 20 minutes, he was systematically able to reduce the period to 90 seconds. Anything less than 90 seconds and his results were inconsistent; but more than 90 seconds did not appear to increase the benefit to the patient.

The second feature to strain and counterstrain was the discovery of palpable myofascial tender points and their correlation to specific somatic dysfunction. Jones describes tender points as "small zones of tense, tender, edematous muscle and fascial tissue about a centimeter in diameter." These points, found by moderate palpatory pressure, are directly related to somatic dysfunction and with such consistency that they became his diagnostic tool. Tender points are four times more tender than normal tissue. Palpation with less than sufficient pressure to cause pain in normal tissue will elicit a sharp local pain characteristic of a strain and counterstrain tender point. Most of the tender points are found overlying the muscle involved in the dysfunc-

tion. Tender points found in the paravertebral musculature or over spinous processes are especially valuable for diagnosing segmental dysfunction in the vertebral column.

RESEARCH DATA

Prior studies have shown the efficacy of palpation on pressure-sensitive points in accurately diagnosing spinal dysfunction.[4-6] Quantitative studies done by Denslow and associates[7] showed how spinal dysfunction could be objectively confirmed with gauged pressure on the spinous processes and measurement of the motor reflex threshold.

Denslow[7] observed that when he pushed on a dysfunctional vertebral segment on either side of the spinous process or in the paravertebral area he would elicit local pain and a muscular contraction in the erector spinae group. From this clinical observation he designed a study to measure the amount of pressure it would take to elicit an initial muscle response from these points, which was called motor reflex threshold. Pressure was applied to the spinous processes by a self-designed pressure meter, and electromyographic electrodes were placed in the paravertebral musculature. The exact amount of pressure necessary to elicit a muscle response was measured. What he found was that at levels where he had made a palpatory diagnosis of vertebral dysfunction he was consistently able to correlate a lower motor reflex threshold. It took less pressure to elicit pain and a corresponding muscle contraction. Nondysfunctional segments responded with little or no pain and muscle contractions at the highest pressure settings.

Denslow correlated a second characteristic of joint dysfunction with a lower motor reflex threshold, this being differences in tissue texture. At sites of low threshold he describes palpable changes in tissue texture as "doughy and boggy." He used these terms to describe the tense, edematous feel of the tissue. Tissue texture changes and reflex muscle contraction with palpatory pressure were so consistent that he was able to predict low motor threshold levels with 95% accuracy.

Another observation of Denslow's, using electromyograms, was that muscle completely at rest was characterized by an absence of action potentials. At low threshold segments, despite the apparent relaxation of the subject, he found "rest activity," action potentials from the paravertebral musculature even at rest. He states, "It was often necessary to position and reposition the shoulder girdle, upper extremity, head and at times the lower extremities in order to eliminate rest activity."

Denslow concluded that "low threshold segments are apparently hyper-excitable not only to pressure stimuli applied to the corresponding spinous process but also to impulses from proprioceptors associated with positioning."

The phenomenon of the elimination of EMG "rest activity" may be associated with strain and counterstrain. Denslow's study tested the thoracic levels 4, 6, 8, and 10. The strain and counterstrain treatments for posterior thoracic dysfunction at those segments would include passive positioning of the shoulder girdle, upper extremity, head, and lower extremities to find the position of release.

TENDER POINTS

Tender points are not only found over spinous processes or paravertebral musculature. Figure 13.1 shows the magnitude of the number of diagnostic tender points that Jones has mapped out over the entire body. This illustration represents just a small portion of the close to 200 tender points that Jones has correlated with specific dysfunction. Tender points in the posterior torso over spinous processes or paravertebral musculature are closely associated with the area and level of posterior pain complaint. Tender points in the anterior torso and pelvis are also closely associated with an area and level of posterior pain. Patients usually have no awareness of these anterior tender points until they are probed. Many osteopathic clinicians believe

the discovery of anterior tender points, their related dysfunctions, and their correlation to posterior pain to be one of Jones's most significant contributions to the treatment of musculoskeletal dysfunction. Jones feels that 50 percent of the dysfunction that produces the patient's posterior pain is represented on the anterior aspect of the body. Failure to consider these dysfunctions may lead to disappointing results.

An added characteristic of tender points besides their value as a diagnostic tool is their use as a monitoring point. By monitoring the tender point for changes in tissue tension and the patient's feedback of either increasing or decreasing sensitivity, the operator is guided to a position of maximum palpatory relaxation beneath the monitoring finger. Marked and prompt decrease in subjective tenderness ensues. Jones calls this the "mobile point." It is the point of maximum ease or relaxation where movement in any direction will increase tissue tension beneath the monitoring finger. The mobile point signifies the ideal position for release.

Jones[2] explains the use of tender points in this way. "A physician skilled in palpation techniques will perceive tenseness and/or edema as well as tenderness, although the tenderness (often a few times greater than that of normal tissue) is for the beginner the most valuable diagnostic sign. He maintains his palpating finger over the tender point to monitor expected changes in tenderness. With the other hand he positions the patient into a posture of comfort and relaxation. He may proceed successfully just by questioning the patient as he probes intermittently while moving toward the position. If he is correct, the patient can report diminishing tenderness in the tender area. By intermittent deep palpation he monitors the tender point, seeking the ideal position at which there is at least two thirds reduction in tenderness." Finding the position of release in this way, holding this position for 90 seconds and returning to neutral very slowly are the major components of a strain and counterstrain technique.

A common question is the relationship of

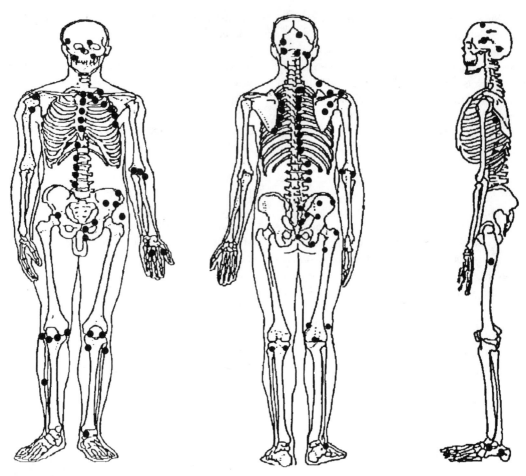

Figure 13.1. Location of tender points. With permission, Jones LH. Strain and counterstrain. Newark, OH: American Academy of Osteopathy, 1981.

strain and counterstrain tender points to Travell's trigger points, Acupuncture points, Chapman reflex points, Shiatsu points, etc. There is, of course, a great deal of overlap in point locations and the palpatory feel of the tissue. However, there are two major differences. First, strain/counterstrain tender points tend to be more segmental in origin. Points along the vertebral column designate segmental dysfunction at the corresponding vertebral level. The other philosophies[8] identify points as related to full body systems and are more holistic in nature. Second, Jones feels strain and counterstrain tender points are a sensory manifestation of a neuromuscular or musculoskeletal dysfunction. The points are used to

make the diagnosis and to monitor the effectiveness of the treatment technique. Treatment is not directed at the tender point but at the dysfunction that produces the tender point. If the treatment is effective the tender point diminishes in tenderness, tissue tension, and edema. In the other philosophies the treatment is directed toward the painful point, by injection, needling, deep pressure, electrical stimulation, and vapocoolants.

RATIONALE

The rationale for strain and counterstrain is based on a neurologic model first proposed by Dr. Irvin Korr in 1975.[6,9] His hypothesis incriminated the muscle spindle or primary proprioceptive nerve endings as the basis for joint dysfunction. His concept is derived from: a) the consensus on the importance of decreased joint mobility or decreased joint range of motion for determining somatic dysfunction, and b) on the muscle's function as a "brake" to retard or resist joint motion. Korr explains, "While usually thinking of muscles as the motors of the body, producing motion by their contraction, it is important to remember that the same contractile forces are also utilized to oppose motion. By the application of controlled counteracting forces, contracting muscle absorbs momentum (for example, of a swinging limb) and regulates, resists, retards and arrests motion." He expanded on his observation of "ease" and "bind," the behavior of a dysfunctional joint to move freely and painlessly in certain planes of motion and the painful resistance to motion in the opposite direction. Korr reasoned that impairment of joint motion in distinct planes was produced by a unilateral active contraction of muscles pulling the joint in a certain direction. Contraction of these muscles around the joint would resist (bind) motion in directions that would tend to lengthen or stretch the muscles and surrender (ease) to motion in directions that would shorten or approximate the muscles.

Korr's premise is that high gamma discharge exaggerates afferent firing from the muscle spindle producing a reflex muscle spasm which fixates the joint in a certain direction and resists any attempts to return to neutral. At this point a review of the structure and function of the muscle spindle[11,12] is in order to establish a common understanding (Fig. 13.2).

MUSCLE SPINDLE

Muscle spindles are highly specialized sensory receptors which are scattered throughout the extrafusal fibers of muscle. Muscle spindle density will vary with function. Phasic muscles have more muscle spindles than postural muscles due to the precision of control required. Each spindle is fluid-filled and contained in a connective tissue sheath about 3–5 mm long, enclosing 5–12 thin specialized muscle fibers known as intrafusal fibers. They lie in parallel to the extrafusal fibers and are attached to them at each end. There are two types of intrafusal fibers: larger fibers with centrally located nuclei aggregated into a bag-like pouch called a nuclear bag fiber, and smaller fibers containing only a single row of nuclei in their central portion called a nuclear chain fiber. These fibers can be thought of as having three regions, a central or equatorial portion where the nuclei are concentrated, and the

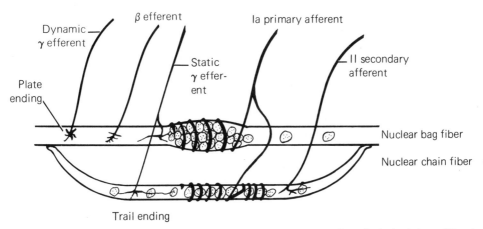

Figure 13.2. Muscle spindle. With permission, Ganong WF. Review of medical physiology. 9th ed. Los Altos, CA: Lange Medical Publications, 1979.

two polar ends which contain the contractile material. In the equatorial portion lie the primary afferent nerve endings also called the annulospiral endings which coil around the nuclear regions. Secondary or flower spray afferent nerve endings terminate on either side of the primary endings closer to the contractile polar ends.

Innervating the intrafusal fibers are gamma motor neurons whose cells originate in the ventral horn, pass through the ventral root, and terminate on the contractile polar ends. In contrast to the alpha motor neurons innervating the extrafusal fibers, these neurons are small and their axons thin.

The muscle spindle is sensitive to length changes. When the extrafusal fibers are stretched the muscle spindle is stretched, causing the annulospiral and flower spray nerve endings to fire. These fibers end monosynaptically directly at the motor neurons of the muscle containing the excited spindles. The excitatory effect produces a reflex contraction of the extrafusal muscle fibers, resisting the stretch. This is the familiar stretch reflex.

The frequency of firing of the annulospiral and flower spray nerve endings is in direct proportion to the change in length. The annulospiral nerve ending has the additional characteristic that its frequency of firing is in proportion to changes in the rate of stretching. Therefore, the annulospiral nerve ending measures length plus velocity of the stretch and the flower spray nerve ending measures only length. Though the effect of these nerve endings is excitatory on the motor neuron of the involved agonist muscle, accessory impulses are transmitted to adjacent interneurons which form an inhibitory pathway to the motor neurons of the antagonist muscle. This is called reciprocal inhibition (see Fig. 13.3).

Gamma efferent stimulation of the intrafusal fibers will also stimulate afferent spindle firing. Impulses transmitted through the gamma efferent neurons will evoke contraction of the polar ends of the intrafusal fibers. Contraction of the polar ends stretches the nuclear portion stimulating the annulospiral and flower spray nerve endings to fire. The response is equal to that produced by stretching the extrafusal fibers. By controlling the contraction of the intrafusal fibers through gamma stimulation the central nervous system

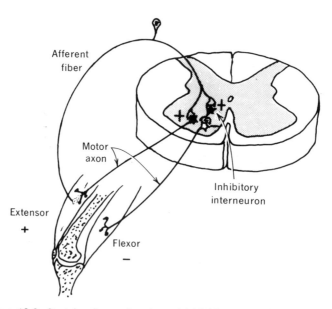

Figure 13.3. Stretch reflex and reciprocal inhibition. Astrand P-O, Rodahl K. Textbook of work physiology. New York: McGraw-Hill, 1970.

is able to set and reset muscle length, muscle tone, and muscle spindles' sensitivity to stretch. This mechanism provides for a state of preparedness for the muscle to respond to slight changes in length. Thus the higher the gamma stimulation the greater the spindle sensitivity to stretch. Stretch of the muscle with high gamma stimulation produces a more intense spindle discharge and therefore a stronger reflex muscle contraction (see Fig. 13.4).

Approximation of the muscle by active contraction or passive shortening will decrease spindle discharge proportionately, and with maximal shortening may even silence it. With high gamma stimulation the muscle must shorten even more to approach the same proportionate reduction in spindle discharge.

MUSCLE SPINDLE AND SOMATIC DYSFUNCTION

Discussion of the role of the muscle spindle in somatic dysfunction would be best initiated with a definition of somatic dysfunction. The current, accepted definition is: impaired or altered function of the related components of the somatic (body framework) system, skeletal, arthroidial, and myofascial structures; and related vascular, lymphatic and neural elements. It is widely accepted that somatic dysfunction involves alterations in systems other than the musculoskeletal. Sympathic involvement in somatic dysfunction is well documented but poorly understood and not within the scope of relevance for this topic. The somatic dysfunctions considered here are primarily produced during mechanical trauma.

The components of somatic dysfunction important to a strain and counterstrain diagnosis would be: first, tissue texture changes described as tense, ropey, and boggy. This is most commonly represented as muscle hypertonicity and tissue edema involving a muscle or muscles investing a particular joint; second, specific tender points which, when palpated, elicit exquisite local pain. Each point indicates a specific somatic dysfunction; and third, impairment in the amplitude and quality of joint

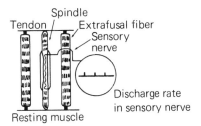

Spindle
Tendon / Extrafusal fiber
Sensory nerve
Discharge rate in sensory nerve
Resting muscle

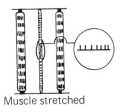

Muscle stretched

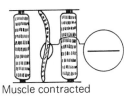

Muscle contracted

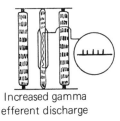

Increased gamma efferent discharge

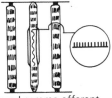

Increased gamma efferent discharge - muscle stretched

Figure 13.4. Effect of various conditions on muscle spindle discharge. Adapted from Ganong WF. Review of medical physiology. 9th ed. Los Altos, CA: Lange Medical Publications, 1979.

range of motion. Jones[2] states, "It is well known that for each painful joint there is a specific direction of position that greatly aggravates the pain and stiffness. Movement of the joint in this direction results in immediate reflex and voluntary muscle resistance, to the point of rigidity. The converse is also true; for each painful joint there is a specific direction of position that greatly relieves pain and muscle tension. Movement of the joint in this direction results in immediate and progressive reflex and voluntary muscle relaxation, to the point of complete relaxation and comfort."

Muscle spindle involvement in somatic dysfunction will be described using an illustration (see Fig. 13.5). This is a sequence of a generic joint. It has a Muscle A and a Muscle B. Below is represented the firing frequency of the annulospiral nerve endings. Plate 1 depicts a joint in neutral. Muscles A and B are in balance and the annulospiral firing frequencies are equal, indicating a tonic rest condition of the muscles. Plate 2 depicts a joint in "strain." Muscle A is severely overstretched and Muscle B is maximally shortened. The annulospiral firing frequency is increased because of the stretch on Muscle A and its spindle. The firing frequency of Muscle B is practically nil. Shortening of the muscle slacks the spindle and reduces afferent firing and the stretch on Muscle A reciprocally inhibits Muscle B. Now, if the body reacts to this strain position in a slow and deliberate manner to return to the neutral position then the

stretched Muscle A is eased back to resting length with no pain and afferent firing returns to tonic levels. What occurred was an overstretching and nothing more. But if the body reacts to this strain position with a quick, sudden, or forceful movement, a panic reaction, to restore the joint to neutral then Muscle B and its spindle are quickly stretched.

Now, since the responsibility of the spindle in Muscle B is to detect the rapid rate of change of the extrafusal fiber lengths and the frequency of firing of the annulospiral nerve ending is in direct proportion to that rate of change, the spindle in Muscle B begins to report a stretch to the CNS even before the muscle reaches its normal resting length. This results in a sharp reflex muscle spasm, not in Muscle A, the overstretched muscle, but in Muscle B, the hypershortened muscle. Plate 3 depicts a joint in dysfunction. Muscle B in spasm fixates the joint in a certain direction and resists any attempts to lengthen and return the joint to neutral. The annulospiral firing frequency of Muscle B is immensely increased, reporting to the CNS a continuing message of strain which maintains the muscle in spasm. Korr[6] explains, "Under the influence of gravitational forces, antagonists and postural reflexes, which would be tending to stretch the muscle back toward resting length,

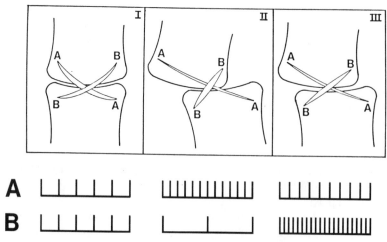

Figure 13.5. Somatic dysfunction at a joint.

the spindle would be continually discharging and through the CNS ordering the muscle to resist. The more the stretch, the much more the resistance."

It comes to mind that if Muscle B is spasmed and its attachments approximated this would shorten and slack the spindle, reduce the afferent discharge to the CNS, and relieve the spasm. Korr postulates that in the position of strain (with Muscle B maximally shortened and its afferent firing practically nil) the CNS, receiving no information from Muscle B, would greatly increase gamma neuron discharge to the intrafusal fibers until the spindle resumes reporting. This is what osteopaths refer to as "high gamma gain." With "high gamma gain" you increase spindle sensitivity to stretch. Now, with a panic reaction stretch to the hypershortened Muscle B the resultant spasm is of such an intensity that the body is unable to reduce it on its own. Korr[6] states, "The higher the gamma activity because of its influence on the excitatory spindle discharge, the more forceful the muscle contraction and the greater its resistance to being lengthened. During high gamma activity the spindle may, in effect, be calling for a contraction when the muscle is already shorter than its resting length."

Therefore, somatic dysfunction occurs not because of strain, but because of the body's reaction to strain. If the reaction is slow and deliberate somatic dysfunction is avoided. If the reaction is panic-like, the velocity of movement sets off the reflex muscle spasm producing dysfunction.

Patient accounts of their mechanism of injury bear this out. The person who is bending forward or squatting and experiences an excessive strain forward will react with a strong backward movement toward neutral. The patient will describe pain not in the strain position but with the return to neutral. The person involved in a minor motor vehicle accident is rear-ended at a speed which would not appear to cause tissue injury, but the person's cervical spine in maximal flexion underwent a quick extension. The complaint of posterior cervical pain is aggravated with extension movement, and muscle guarding would be noted. Flexion movement is pain-free and relaxing. Examination reveals numerous anterior cervical tender points and related anterior cervical joint dysfunction.

PURPOSE OF STRAIN AND COUNTERSTRAIN

What strain and counterstrain attempts to accomplish with its position of comfort is to relax the muscle spasm by reducing aberrant afferent flow from the muscle spindle. This is accomplished by mimicking the original strain position or applying a "counterstrain." By passively mimicking the original strain position the operator moves the joint in a direction of ease and maximally shortens the involved muscle. Holding for 90 seconds allows the spindle to slow down its afferent firing frequency. Returning to neutral in a slow and deliberate manner avoids reexciting the previously spasmed muscle. Korr[6] explains, "The shortened spindle nevertheless continues to fire, despite the slackening of the main muscle, and the CNS is gradually enabled to turn down the gamma discharge, and, in turn, enables the muscle to return to 'easy neutral' at its resting length. In effect, the physician has led the patient through a repetition of the lesioning process with, however, two essential differences: first, it is done in slow motion with gentle muscular forces, and second, there has been no 'surprise' for the CNS; the spindle has continued to report throughout."

CASE STUDY

Most of the knowledge about the nature of somatic dysfunction and what strain and counterstrain accomplishes with its position of comfort is based on patient accounts of their mechanisms of injury, their response to positional treatment, and the observations of skilled practitioners. Neurophysiologic studies in this area are woefully limited. Therefore, the presentation of a case study seems an appropriate way to lend support and give the reader insight into the rationale.

This case, Jones's favorite, involves a middle-aged man who had a habit of falling asleep supine on the sofa. While asleep his right arm would occasionally fall off the edge and hang in marked extension at the elbow. For years, his wife, noticing her husband napping in this position, would slowly and gently replace the arm across his chest without awakening him (a slow return to neutral). And for years the man would awaken from his nap with no complaint of discomfort. One day, while his wife was out, he was awakened abruptly by the ring of a telephone near his head, while his elbow was in marked extension. He was so startled that he violently jerked his right elbow into flexion. He immediately began to feel pain in the right bicep especially with movement into flexion. A diagnosis of bicep strain was made for his condition on the basis of painful elbow flexion, even though palpation revealed no clinical evidence of strained or injured tissue. By the time he saw Jones he had been disabled for 2 years with pain and progressive weakness of the biceps. Examination of the biceps failed to reveal any information as to the nature of the problem. However, palpation of the distal triceps uncovered exquisitely sharp tender points (evidence of triceps dysfunction). The triceps had been maximally shortened then suddenly lengthened with a panic response.

Treatment consisted of positioning the elbow in hyperextension so that the triceps was maximally shortened (mimicking the original strain position), holding the position for 90 seconds while monitoring the tender points, and slowly returning to the neutral position. After three treatments full and pain-free function was restored.

This case demonstrates: first, how important the slow return from a strain position is in avoiding joint dysfunction; second, that the palpable evidence of dysfunction is frequently found on the opposite side of pain in the antagonist of the overstretched muscle; and third, how treatment techniques mimic the original strain position. The apparent weak-ness in the biceps was attributed to disuse and reciprocal inhibition due to the continuous contraction of the triceps.

STRAIN AND COUNTERSTRAIN IN THE MANUAL MEDICINE ARMAMENTARIUM

Strain and counterstrain can be used as a sole treatment modality or as an adjunct to other manual medicine techniques. Its therapeutic uses range from the very acute to the chronic patient.

Its value with the acute patient is unmatched because it is so gentle and nontraumatic. The operator is guided by what feels good to the patient, and often dramatic changes are made in subjective pain, muscle guarding, and edema.

The gentleness of strain and counterstrain makes it safe and effective for treating somatic dysfunction on fragile patients (i.e., elderly, osteoporotic, fractures, pregnancy) and infants.

Strain and counterstrain is valuable with chronic patients for two reasons, first, a scan for tender points provides a quick assessment of the problem areas of the body and allows the operator to delineate the areas of dysfunction contributing to the pain complaint, and second, the treatment will reduce the aberrant flow of afferent impulse in the involved muscles which have maintained the joint in chronic dysfunction.

The approach with strain and counterstrain is to passively put a slight strain into a dysfunctional joint. Patients with severely limited range of motion (adhesive capsulitis, cervical spondylosis) find strain and counterstrain helpful to reduce secondary muscle guarding. Positions of comfort are easily found, but within the available range which will be in lesser degrees of motion than patients with full range of motion. Measurable gains in range and quality of motion can be made.

Pain associated with hypermobility can also be treated. The approach is still to put a strain upon the joint; therefore hypermobile patients are usually treated in greater degrees of motion than patients with normal range.

Strain and counterstrain can make a significant contribution when integrated with other manual medicine techniques. Used in conjunction with articular techniques (i.e., joint mobilization, high velocity manipulation) which restore position and motion, it will normalize the imbalance of muscle tension affecting the joint so that recurrence of dysfunction is decreased.

Strain and counterstrain and muscle energy can be combined with effective results.[9,10] Isometric muscle energy's inhibitory effect on contracted muscle by increasing Golgi tendon organ discharge or through reciprocal inhibition can enhance strain and counterstrain's inhibitory effect on the same muscle. Muscle energy can also be valuable to strengthen the antagonist muscle (weakened by reciprocal inhibition) to bring the joint back to postural balance.

Strain and counterstrain can be used before myofascial release techniques. By clearing corresponding tender points, counterstrain can assist in reducing neurophysiologic barriers, allowing myofascial release to break down biomechanical barriers with greater ease.

CONCLUSION

Strain and counterstrain is an indirect manipulative technique of extreme gentleness for the treatment of somatic dysfunctions. It is based on a neurologic model that proposes, for some, a new concept for the production of somatic dysfunction. The hypothesis is aberrant afferent flow from the muscle spindle produces a reflex muscle spasm that fixates a joint in a certain direction and resists any attempts to return the joint to neutral. Diagnosis is made by the presence of a specific tender point that overlies the muscle. Using the tender point as a monitor the operator is guided into a position of comfort that reduces aberrant afferent flow and returns the muscle to "easy neutral." Holding the position of comfort for 90 seconds and returning to neutral slowly following the positional release

are two very important aspects of this procedure.

Though research data are limited in this area to support the model, the observations of practitioners, recounting the immediate changes in palpable pain, tissue tension, and ease of movement following positional release, point to a neural basis.

Recognition must be given to Lawrence Jones for decades of arduous experimentation on patients and his own body to develop strain and counterstrain. His book, *Strain and Counterstrain*,[2] has mapped out hundreds of the most common tender points and positions for treatment. To the beginner, the treatments appear straightforward and easily mastered, but development of the palpatory skills required to find the optimal position of release takes practice and perseverance. A complete study of the book and the teachings of Lawrence Jones are highly recommended.

REFERENCES

1. Korr IM. Proprioceptors and somatic dysfunction. J Am Osteopath Assoc 1975; 74:638–50.
2. Jones LH. Strain and counterstrain. Newark, OH: American Academy of Osteopathy, 1981.
3. Jones LH. Spontaneous release by positioning. D.O. 1964; 4:109–16.
4. Greenman PE. Principles of manual medicine. Baltimore: Williams & Wilkins, 1989.
5. Korr IM. The segmental nervous system as mediator and organizer of disease processes. The physiological basis of osteopathic medicine. The Postgraduate Institute of Osteopathic Medicine and Surgery, 1970.
6. Korr IM. The neural basis of the osteopathic lesion. The collected papers of Irvin M. Korr. Newark, OH: American Academy of Osteopathy, 1979.
7. Denslow JS, Korr IM, Krems AD. Quantitative studies of chronic facilitation in human motorneuron pools. The collected papers of Irvin M. Korr. Newark, OH: American Academy of Osteopathy, 1979.
8. Travell JG. Simons DJ. Myofascial pain and dysfunction: the trigger point manual. Baltimore: Williams & Wilkins, 1983.
9. Korr IM. The facilitated segment: a factor in injury to the body framework. The collected papers of Irvin M. Korr. Newark, OH: American Academy of Osteopathy, 1979.
10. Chaitow L. Soft-tissue manipulation. Rochester, VT: Healing Arts Press, 1980.
11. Ganong WF. Review of medical physiology. 9th ed. Los Altos, CA: Lange Medical Publications, 1979.
12. O'Connell AL, Gardner EB. Understanding the scientific basis of human movement. Baltimore: Williams & Wilkins, 1972.

14

Functional Technique

WILLIAM L. JOHNSTON

When classified according to the directions of operator forces, manipulative techniques termed functional are generally placed in an *indirect* category. *Direct* techniques will include those procedures in which the operator introduces some physical force in a direct method to encounter and overcome directions of restricted joint motion. Indirect methods will engage opposing directions, away from the restrictive sense of barrier.[1]

There are a number of techniques that apply aspects of an indirect method,[2] including those termed "balance and hold," "exaggerating the lesion position," "strain/counterstrain," and certain techniques termed "combined." What sets functional technique apart from these is essentially the functional orientation in *diagnostic* approach. It is accepted that osteopathic/medical diagnosis initially rules out conditions where manipulation may not be an appropriate consideration in management—and rules in those instances where manipulation may be an appropriate adjunct, and even a primary consideration in the approach to treatment. Then functional diagnosis makes use of palpable signs of disturbed segmental motion function as the basis for development of a manipulative approach in treatment. Other approaches to indirect technique may use a sense of positional or ligamentous rebalancing, tissue approximation, or facet unlocking. Essentially, functional technique uses information/clues from *motion tests* to predict those precise directions

of motion in manipulation which will initiate palpable signs of improving motor function at a lesioned segment.

HISTORICAL PERSPECTIVE

Anyone surveying the early history of manipulation cannot fail to be impressed by how frequently palpable findings in the somatic system have emerged within the anatomic concept of a joint. Whether the palpatory tests probed bony position, deep tissue tensions, or limited mobility, the joint became an acceptable frame of reference: one bone and how it was positioned on the bone below; which direction of joint movement the muscle spasm was constraining; which facet was locked; on which side of the joint the ligaments were weakened. Despite early admonition by McConnell[3] not to regard the bony item, or the muscle, or the ligament as an idol in the conceptual framework for somatic lesioning, the palpable findings at an area of "osteopathic lesion" had emerged early as descriptive of a joint with bony displacement.

This early osteopathic clinical experience, however, had established a focus for clinical attention. Physical mobility was recognized as a vital body function, and appropriate emphasis was given to this important concept by Korr[4] when he described the musculoskeletal (msk) system as the primary machinery of life. Further, recognizing interaction between the msk system and other body systems was essential to completeness in the understanding, within the whole, of other vital body functions. Especially, disturbances in motor function were frequently evident when disturbance was being manifested in another systemic function, for example in the cardiovascular, lymphatic, immunologic, digestive, or respiratory system. When these interactions were observed, the clinical finding of segmental lesioning was a key feature in diagnosis and management. The location of a lesioned segment was a major clinical target for manipulation to make changes in pain, mobility, posture, and spinal reflex activity. Successfully improving limitations of local and regional mobility had a positive impact on the interactions between somatic and visceral systems, sometimes with wide-ranging clinical effects.

During the first half of this century, the continued successful use of indirect manipulative techniques by osteopathic physicians began to stimulate recognition of a need to broaden the narrow conceptual base provided by joint structure and bony position alone.[5-8] During the past 40 years, an orientation to function, i.e. motor function, has made possible a new and valuable direction for descriptive research about palpable findings in the msk examination. Describing palpable findings is not a simple task.

Still, the use of manipulative procedures *without* descriptive attention to the problem being addressed implies duplication of a manual procedure in a routine fashion that is less

sensitive to the condition of the patient. Earlier concepts had allowed for certain general descriptors of palpable findings to emerge as cardinal signs of somatic dysfunction: asymmetry of structural position, tissue texture abnormality, and restricted motion. Such palpable findings, however, are frequent on examination of the msk system. Needed was a framework of tests and criteria for 1) more carefully describing segmental motor function; 2) organizing palpable findings to bring into focus new knowledge about disturbed motor function, and 3) clearly distinguishing location of a primary lesioned segment as a clinical focus for manipulative intervention.

A FUNCTIONAL MODEL FOR A MOBILE SYSTEM

A systems approach defines a group of dynamically-related components, operating in concert, or in related fashion, for the purpose of achieving a specified goal or set of goals. For the human body, a major specified goal of the somatic system is movement. The dynamically-related components are mobile segments. Together, the mobile segments respond to a central command for a whole pattern of body movement to be generated through local spinal control centers.[9,10] Figure 14.1 illustrates a model for movement function.

The concept of a mobile segment includes one bony component, with articular surfaces for movement, and the adnexal tissues that

NEURAL PATTERN GENERATOR:
FOR BODY MOVEMENT

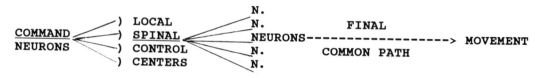

Figure 14.1. A diagrammatic model for movement function.

can 1) stabilize and fix its position, 2) allow movement, and 3) implement movement.[11] Participation of the mobile segment is accomplished along the final common motor path by spinal control of muscle effectors and a monosynaptic feedback system of afferent input from proprioceptor sensors that measure behavior and effect performance, illustrated in Fig. 14.2.

The system responds to commands for movement, whether active or in the form of a passive motion test. Actively, it may be to reach for an object; it may be to step and walk, bend and twist, even breathe and talk. At any particular moment, the command is for a whole movement, not, for example, for thoracic(T)4 to sidebend and rotate in particular directions on T5. What emerges is a series of mobile segments moving in concert, in response to a command for overall movement that is organized in the central nervous system,[10] as illustrated in Fig. 14.3.

To describe palpatory tests for movement function, attention is first of all directed to the axes or coordinates about which movement of an object can be described. Elementary body movements can be reproduced in a series of tests for obtaining clinical informa-

tion, initially about the overall performance in response to a whole movement commanded, but also about the local behavior of a mobile segment during that movement. As tests introduced by the examiner, passive movements offer certain advantages: they minimize active interference by the patient; they permit standardization of a procedure for the examiner; and they contribute to reliability for clinical use, and for research.

A test pattern for passive movements involves six possible directions of elementary movement (Figs. 14.4-**A** and -**B**). There are three degrees of freedom for translational movement (straight-line): up/down along a z coordinate; right/left on a y coordinate; and anterior/posterior along an x axis. In addition, there are three degrees of freedom for primary rotations: axial rotation about the vertical z axis; flexion/extension about y; sidebending or lateral flexion about the x axis. These six directions for passive movement are seen as elementary tools for testing the body's response to movement.

When applied in physical examination, testing the various regions of the body for *regional performance* in response to gross movement demands, the criteria for a palpable

FEEDBACK:
FOR CONTROL

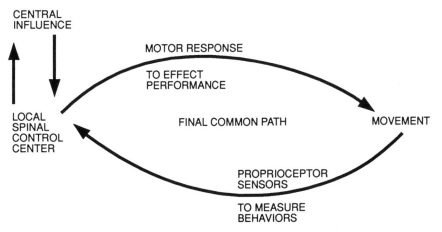

Figure 14.2. Schematic focus on the segmental organization.

THE COMMAND SYSTEM

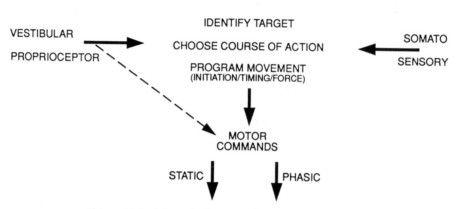

Figure 14.3. Schematic focus on the central organization.

finding of asymmetry are not measurements made visually at the end-point or range—after the response has taken place.[12] Instead, criteria are established for the palpable quality of the motion response *during* the range, and for the quality of the end-point. Regional resistance to an elementary motion test, palpated earlier in one direction than in the opposing direction, is a tentative sign of somatic dysfunction[13] in the body region being tested. Such regional tests screen overall movement function for a first impression of the presence of a clinical disturbance in the mobile system. In this way, physical examination appropriately initiates a sequence of clinical decisions in problem solving for the msk system.[11] The screening tests address the question "is there a problem?" and may begin to narrow attention to a given body region. The region is then scanned with passive gross motion tests, while the examiner monitors from segment to segment, palpating to identify limitation in a segment's motion function. Once located, the segment's dysfunction is characterized by describing its motor asymmetries.

As a movement system, the soma is made up of bony and soft tissues. Bowles[6] initiated a mechanism for bringing together the palpable cues of bony restriction and soft tissue tension. In a very practical way he *united* them

as indicators of movement function as expressed in this principle: the tissues about a moving bony part constantly reflect its behavior as they participate in and comply with the demands for position and movement of the whole system. Tissue findings such as muscle spasm, trigger points, tender points, are not isolates. They can be indicators of dysfunction in a mobile system. To investigate the motor dysfunction clinically, we put the tissue findings back into a moving system by examining how they respond during motion tests. Readers should carefully distinguish tests for motor function from the conceptual framework and procedures of motion tests that isolate and put a muscle on stretch. Also, the conceptual framework is not of a joint and how one bone moves in relation to the bone below. Consider, rather, the concept of mobile segments, spinal, appendicular, and costal, integrated into the process of how one segment moves *in relation to the whole system, when the system moves.*

DIAGNOSIS OF SEGMENTAL DYSFUNCTION

To organize clinical diagnostic tests for *local behavior of a mobile segment* in a mobile system, procedures are developed with a regard for 1) positioning of the patient, 2) where motion

Translations

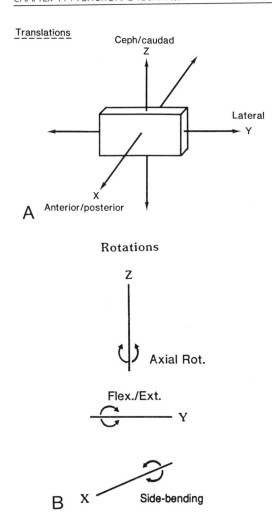

A

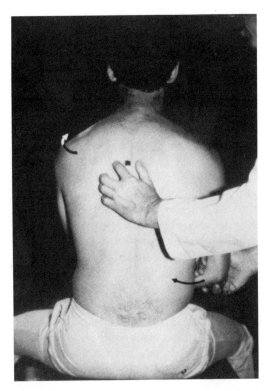

Figure 14.5. Subject is seated; arms are folded. Examiner's left hand contacts the paravertebral tissues bilaterally at T6 (indicated by marker). Left thumb and forefinger monitor response to axial rotation of the shoulders and trunk to the right, introduced by the examiner's right hand at subject's right elbow. (Reproduced with permission, Johnston, WL. Segmental definition: Part 1. A focal point for diagnosis of somatic dysfunction. J Am Osteopath Assoc 1988; 88:99–105).

Figure 14.4. A. coordinate system illustrating straight-line directions of movement, used in description of translatory motion tests. In **B**, the coordinate system illustrates directions of movement about axes, used in description of rotary motion tests. (Reproduced with permission, Johnston, WL. Segmental definition: Part 1. A focal point for diagnosis of somatic dysfunction. J Am Osteopath Assoc 1988; 88:99–105).

is being introduced into the body, and 3) the direction of the motion test. An example is demonstrated in Fig. 14.5, with the patient seated: arms are folded; the examiner is standing posterior; axial rotation right is introduced through the shoulders and trunk by the examiner's right hand at the right elbow; the examiner's left hand monitors response at tissues overlying thoracic T6. The procedural

principles are applicable with the patient supine, prone, or sidelying, with motions introduced through the head and neck, or through the extremities, as appropriate to the segment being examined. Historically, rotations were frequently the extent of the directional nomenclature; motion tests and manipulative procedures instinctively included translations, but the directions and the palpable cues being followed were seldom communicated.

Recognizing the difficulties inherent in developing palpatory skills, it is important to try to clarify the *sensory* aspects of this diagnostic technique for palpating a segment's tissues as they respond to a motion test. Both anatomic and physiologic research supports the fact that *fingerpads* have pressure sensors; physiologists don't describe tension receptors here. In spite of reported clinical findings that may refer to "tone" and "tension," these terms are usually interpretive of a palpated sense of *resistance to pressure*, evoked in a compression test of soft tissues. At a segment to be monitored, finger pad compression is light, yet sufficient to sense the resistance of underlying segmental musculature. During a passive gross motion test, does the tone/tension of the segment's tissues increase—decrease—or stay the same, as reflected to the fingers locally monitoring tissue resistance to the standardized compression?

Figure 14.6 indicates tone on the vertical scale, and range on the horizontal with an example of axial rotation in opposing directions, right and left. Once initial contact is established, finger pads compare responses at the underlying segmental tissues during introduction of opposing directions of a move-

ment test. Comparison of responses to opposing directions provides a basis for reporting symmetry or asymmetry in function of a mobile segment.

What are our expectations for using the term symmetry? Knowledge of anatomy does not lead us to expect the human body to be structurally symmetric. Not even symmetry of motion range would be a reasonable expectation, though Fig. 14.6 does illustrate ranges in rotation right and left that appear symmetric. Some motion ranges are symmetric, but certainly many bony articular surfaces, especially appendicular, are not constructed to allow equal range for sidebending in opposing directions, or for internal/external rotations. So, range to the end-point is not necessarily a reliable indicator for palpating symmetry at a mobile segment.

Instead, symmetry of a segment's mobile function is measured at the *beginning* of motion. Monitoring a mobile unit in a mobile system during initiation of a gross movement

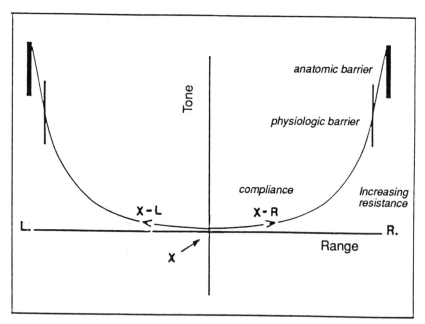

Figure 14.6. Schematic representation for symmetry at a nonlesioned segment. Although represented here for axial rotation only, this illustration is applicable graphically to all six degrees of freedom, and to active respiration. The line X–L through X–R indicates initial motion where symmetry in response to oppos-

ing directions of motion reflects low level of change in palpable resistance to pressure (dynamic neutral). (Reproduced with permission, Johnston, WL. Segmental definition: Part 1. A focal point for diagnosis of somatic dysfunction. J Am Osteopath Assoc 1988; 88:211–217).

in opposing directions reveals an immediate compliance in either direction. There is no *immediate* palpable change in muscular tone, no rise on the tone scale as illustrated in Fig. 14.6, *X* toward *XL*, or *X* toward *XR*.

The standard, therefore, for making decisions on a segment's motor symmetry consists in the palpable sense of initial compliance to opposing directions of a motion test. The compliant phase, illustrated between *XL* and *XR*, represents a dynamic neutral that is energy efficient. The body uses proprioceptive feedback (see Fig. 14.2) as a control mechanism, to keep much of our movement relatively close to a balance-center and energy efficient. Most respiratory movement, for example, would appear to take place within this same dynamic neutral range, without necessarily engaging end of range during either inhalation or exhalation. This suggests how eupneic respiratory activity 24 hours a day may also be relatively energy efficient.

Segmental motion asymmetry is a positive finding, expressed by a detectable difference in palpated resistances when opposing directions of a motion test are compared. Figure 14.7 illustrates at point *x-1*, elevated on the tone scale, an example of the *dys*functional segment, where palpation of tissues reveals increased tension (resistance to pressure), even at rest. When opposing directions are tested, the resistance to pressure at these tissues underlying the palpating hand increases or decreases *immediately*, dependent on the direction of the test. The examiner relates a finding of resistance objectively to the direction of the motion test used to elicit it, rather than conceptually to how one bone fails to move on the bone below, or to how a muscle is being stretched.

At the dysfunctional segment, whether spinal, appendicular, or costal, findings reveal that the segmental motion asymmetry is *complete*, involving all six passive gross motion tests when opposing directions are compared. Asymmetry is even expressed during respira-

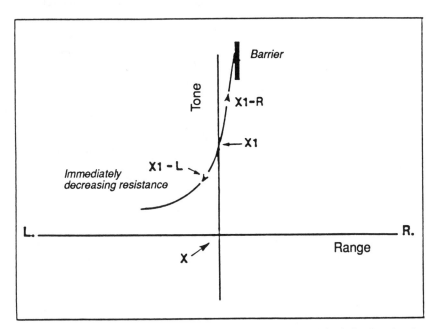

Figure 14.7. Schematic representation for asymmetric behavior at a dysfunctional segment (only axial rotation is indicated). The inclined line X1 through X1–L shows initial early range of motion during which increments of increasing compliance (decreasing resistance) are available during functional manipulation. (Reproduced with permission, Johnston, WL. Segmental definition: Part 1. A focal point for diagnosis of somatic dysfunction. J Am Osteopath Assoc 1988; 88:211–217).

tion, revealing the lesioned segment's total functional asymmetry. Under these circumstances, respiration becomes an extremely effective *active* motion test. As a non-stressful testing procedure, it provides an informative diagnostic cue of motor disturbance, and suggests useful information in developing manipulative technique that has a functional orientation.

Does this segmental dysfunction exist as an isolated finding among normally symmetric adjacent segments? Examination of adjacent segments will reveal that the primary finding is not isolated. The degree of tissue tension at adjacent segmental levels is not as marked, yet still palpably elevated on the tone scale. The same motion tests reveal presence of functional asymmetries, but resistances are in opposing directions of motion to those of the more centrally located primary segmental defect. There is, predictably, a complete opposing asymmetry in the six degrees of freedom, and in active respiration, when testing the adjacent segments above and below a primary segmental dysfunction. The term "mirror image" describes this adaptive behavior at adjacent segments; the phrase "fundamental unit of segmental dysfunction" refers to this three-segment unit in which a central asymmetric function is the primary defect, with secondary mirror image asymmetries at adjacent segments.[8,14]

FUNCTIONAL MANIPULATIVE TECHNIQUE

Up to this point we have considered resistance to a direction of motion test as if "restriction" described the segment's problem, that is, as if there was limited rotation right, but with still normal response to rotation left. True, increasing resistance is a very tangible cue of disturbance, for fingertips monitoring tissue change. As illustrated in Figure 14.7, however, the response to rotation left is not "normal"; there is immediate *decrease* of the existing tension and an increasing compliance when rotation is tested to the left. Importantly, the *palpable sense of decreasing tension* provides the

basis for consideration of an indirect approach in manipulative technique, one that does not encounter the so-called restrictive barrier to overcome it. Rather, it suggests developing manipulative procedures in which specific directions of motion will decrease tissue tension sufficiently to mitigate the asymmetric function.

In functional technique, attention is drawn to a number of features for effective application and development of this manipulative skill. Since response to motion tests in all six degrees of freedom and to respiration are asymmetric at a dysfunctional segment, each aspect of these elementary motions can be used to advantage in functional technique. Each motion test contributes a specific direction of motion (away from resistance) in which there is increasing compliance/decreasing tension/improving function palpable at the fingertips. The increment of change from $X1$ to $X1$-L in Fig. 14.7 is for a short distance only, before compliance begins to level off and approach a normally increasing resistance at the end of range toward the left. To take advantage of this incremental aspect of increasing compliance in the short range, distances in functional technique, therefore, are initial only. More important than extending range is the ability to sum all aspects of the initially increasing compliance by combining the appropriate directions of each rotary and translatory motion. Combining small amounts of each results in an eventual torsion arc or pathway of movement that rapidly and maximally reduces tension at the dysfunctional segment (monitored by palpation as decreasing resistance-to-pressure). A relatively final step in procedure is to direct the patient to slowly inhale or exhale, whichever phase of the respiratory motion contributes increasing compliance (rather than resistance) to the improving function. A successful outcome registers as a palpable *sense of release* of holding forces, allowing a compliant return to midline resting position in directions previously resisted.

Throughout the procedure, the clinician is guided by a continuous signal of increasing ease (decreasing tissue resistance to pressure) at fingertips monitoring the lesioned segment. The final respiratory phase is not a time for holding/waiting, but rather an opportune moment for final skillful use of the directional "tools" to reduce tension and implement adequate tissue release.

The criterion for success in application of a manipulative procedure is similar for all manipulative methods. Retesting of directions of motion previously resisted reveals a return to compliance and symmetry of motion function in each.

Notably, recognizing presence of the mirror-image asymmetries at adjacent segments contributes to reliability for location, and for focussing manipulative attention on the central primary dysfunctional segment. After successful manipulation, tissue tension is reduced throughout the entire three-segment unit; retesting mobility at adjacent segments reveals a similar return to symmetric function. This predictable clinical response to treatment is the basis for considering the mirror-image phenomenon as secondary and adaptive, as clinical evidence of a fundamental somatosomatic reflex response.

THEORETICAL BASIS FOR A FUNCTIONAL STRATEGY

The rationale for clinical response in functional manipulation arises from the palpatory evidence gained at the fingertips during the procedure. As described, functional technique is a type of indirect manipulation in which the clinician guides the manipulative procedure by palpating at the dysfunctional segment for a continuous feedback of information about improving physiologic response to motion. The motor disturbance of the tense dysfunctional segmental tissues is already evident at rest, before motion is introduced. The segment actively resists the particular resting position of the body at the moment of this initial examination. This palpable increased tissue resistance to pressure is also reflected through to the cord segment as increased afferent input, that is, sensory information reflected by the stressed bony position, hypoxic tissue, and asymmetric tone/tension of ligament, muscle, and fascia. When motion is tested, the palpating fingers are monitoring the asymmetric motor function *moment to moment*. They sense the changing resistance to pressure of segmental musculature as it gives clues to the erratic traffic on afferent pathways. The input continually changes depending on the direction of motion; this represents a significant alteration from the homeostatic control of the expected symmetric response to initial motion.

Moment-to-moment control of the segmental behavior being monitored resides especially in the functions of the muscle spindle. Its degree of sensitivity as a kind of servomechanism is controlled centrally through gamma motor efferents, but its sensitive modulation of muscle stretch provides basis for local feedback control (see Fig. 14.2) in a monosynaptic reflex connection with motor effectors, often to the same muscle. In functional technique, improving trends in that motor control function are monitored throughout the procedure as each direction of increasing compliance projects palpable cues of decreasing afferent input. The eventual controlled reduction in afferent proprioceptor bombardment allows normal control mechanisms to effect the return to symmetry in motor response that becomes evident during motion retesting.

In light of the known physiologic mechanisms for motor control, the palpable findings reported here suggest a concept of afferent reduction as an appropriate model for beginning to interpret the clinical results with functional manipulation. Details of a physiologic mechanism for explaining the mirror image asymmetries at adjacent segments need further study. One hypothesis, however, might be drawn regarding volleys of proprioceptor afferents from the central segment acting on segmental interneurons to facilitate synapses in the spinal networks that involve propriospinal neurons for motor control of adjacent segments. Following treatment of the primary functional defect at the central segment, the palpable return to symmetry in these adjacent segments presents clinical evidence for reduced spinal reflex behavior, which appears to have been adaptive. This additionally supports consideration of the concept of afferent reduction as a mechanism in the response to functional technique.

Where segmental dysfunction is present, the volleys of proprioceptor and especially nociceptor afferents during daily movement contribute to facilitation of synaptic transmission at the cord segment. With pathways established and synapses facilitated, the asymmetric motor function becomes self-maintaining. Facilitation of both motor and vasomotor pathways has been postulated for the palpable signs of neuromuscular tension and neurovascular changes in the tissues of these dysfunctional segments. Case studies have documented kinematic and myoelectric changes in regional mobility[15] and thermographic changes in skin temperature[16] following successful manipulative treatment that was functionally oriented.

CLINICAL APPLICATION OF FUNCTIONAL TECHNIQUE

There are no known contraindications for a functional approach where manipulative intervention is clinically indicated. No painful ranges of motion are either tested or used in treatment. The operator's application of physical force is minimal, and no effort is required of the patient, except to control relaxation subjectively and permit the motions initiated and controlled by the clinician. These features present decided advantages, especially when planning management of the acutely ill, in the elderly, and in patients following physical trauma and surgery.

A clinical perspective is offered for the following: 1) the term *somatic dysfunction* is a general descriptor of disturbed motor performance; 2) the term *segmental dysfunction* is a more specific descriptor of problem location and manipulative focus; and 3) there is significant relationship between segmental and somatic dysfunction. Table 14.1 suggests a sequence of events that exist as stages in the natural history of decreasing mobile function. The advanced stage, indicated as item 6, involves disability, ranging from moderate impairment of daily work activities to marked impairment of ability for self care. Reversing the sequence back up the scale, there has been history of some type of gradually accumulating functional impairment, with activity marred by pain and loss of dexterity or strength. Certainly, in time, postural adaptations have occurred to compensate for decreasing mobile function. There is evidence of limited motion range (item 4) in most students examined during stages of higher education. By their early 20s, as "healthy" subjects for research study, these students already reflect physical signs of limitation in some regional ranges of motion. Limited mobility is preceded by beginning regional asymmetries as demonstration of the asymmetric motor function present at primary lesioned segments. The original localization may arise from some initial occasion(s) of physical/motion stress, maybe sudden, maybe gradual, maybe reflex. In almost all humans, dependent on their history, significant segmental dysfunctions are already becoming well established after only 5, 10, 15, 20 years of movement experience; the signs of reduced motor

Table 14.1

From Physical Signs to Presenting Complaints: Factors for Consideration in the Natural History of Decreasing Mobile Function

Decreasing Mobile Function
Natural History:
1. Initial stress point
2. Asymmetric function of a mobile segment
3. Regional motion asymmetry
4. Limited motion range
5. Functional impairment: • Strength   • Postural position   • Dexterity   • Activity limited by pain
6. Disability

performance are evident on a screening physical examination.

Clinical studies[17,18] of kinematic and myoelectric activity in the cervical region support the assumption that this onset of subclinical decreasing mobile function begins early in life. *Asymptomatic* subjects, at the mean age of 25 years, were grouped according to symmetry or asymmetry of cervical region mobility based on their response to a palpatory test comparing passive gross cervical sidebending right with left. During active and passive head rotations, kinematic and myoelectric data identified the presence of 1) significant reductions in *all* rotary motion ranges for the asymmetric subjects, and 2) reduced time and strength of muscle contractions that were also more slowly initiated by the asymmetric subjects. By the time a palpable indication of regional cervical spine asymmetry was present on a screening physical examination, a functional disturbance with significant physiologic correlates was instrumentally measurable.

Descriptively, by reversing the sequence of decreasing mobile function from items 6 to 1 in Table 14.1, we placed clinically relevant pain patterns, muscle spasm, trigger points, tender points, and finally, disability, all as end products. They exist as eventual presenting complaints in the office, having emerged from a gradually developing pattern of somatic dysfunction, with segmental dysfunction as the fundamental unit in the natural history of decreasing mobile function.

As end products, these "isolated" tissue changes (and their pain patterns) are intimately related to key areas of segmental dysfunction. If one is palpated during motion tests as a tissue component of a mobile segment, and the tissue expresses the complete asymmetric response of a motor dysfunction, then that intimate relationship is confirmed. These tissues exist as hypoxic areas of chronicly accumulated irritability and tension, a product of a mobile segment's continual day-to-day asymmetric motor activity. Manipulative attention to restore symmetry to the dysfunctional segmental complex is a major goal of functional technique, and complements other treatment regimens that may be directed toward reducing the clinical pain pattern.

SUMMARY

Attention has been drawn to the primacy of human movement function. On physical examination for the location and extent of somatic dysfunction, a trained professional can recognize initial loss of integrity in this mobile system. Precision in the palpatory diagnosis of primary segmental dysfunction has defined the presence of a somatic component, significant for consideration in wellness, resistance to infectious disease, recovery from systemic illness and from the physical stresses exemplified in pregnancy, surgery, and traumatic injury. Functional manipulation of diagnosed segmental motor asymmetries has broad application in health care; it is a particularly vital factor in conservative patient management.

REFERENCES

1. Hoover HV. Fundamentals of technique. In: Yearbook of the Academy of Applied Osteopathy, 1949. Ann Arbor, MI: Edwards Bros. Inc: 25–41. (Currently: American Academy of Osteopathy, Newark OH).
2. Lippincott HA. Basic principles of osteopathic technique. In: Barnes MW, ed. Yearbook of the Academy of Applied Osteopathy, 1961. Carmel CA: American Academy of Osteopathy: 45–48. (Currently: American Academy of Osteopathy, Newark OH).
3. McConnell CP. Osteopathic art, V. J Am Osteopath Assoc 1935; 34:369–374.
4. Korr IM. The sympathetic nervous system as mediator between the somatic and supportive processes. In: Kugelmass IN, ed. The physiological basis of osteopathic medicine 1970. New York: Postgraduate Institute of Osteopathic Medicine and Surgery, 1970.
5. Hoover HV, Nelson CR. Basic physiologic movements of the spine. In: Page LE, ed. Yearbook of the Academy of Applied Osteopathy, 1950. Ann Arbor MI: Cushing-Malloy Inc, 1950; 63–66. (Currently: American Academy of Osteopathy, Newark OH).
6. Bowles CH. A functional orientation for technic. In: Page LE, ed. Yearbook of the Academy of Applied Osteopathy, 1955. Ann Arbor MI: Cushing-Malloy Inc, 1955; 177–191. (Currently: American Academy of Osteopathy, Newark OH).
7. MacBain RN. The somatic components of disease. J Am Osteopath Assoc 1956; 56:159–165.

8. Johnston WL. Segmental behavior during motion. I. A palpatory study of somatic relations. J Am Osteopath Assoc 1972; 72:352–361.

9. Stein PSG. Motor systems, with specific reference to the control of locomotion. Ann Rev Neurosci 1978; 1:61–81.

10. Ghez C. Introduction to the motor systems. In: Kandel ER, Schwartz JH, eds. Principles of neural science. New York: Elsevier, 1985.

11. Johnston WL. Interexaminer reliability studies. Spanning a gap in medical research. J Am Osteopath Assoc 1982; 81:819–829.

12. Johnston WL. Passive gross motion testing: Part I. Its role in physical examination. J Am Osteopath Assoc 1982; 81:298–303.

13. Project on osteopathic principles education: glossary of osteopathic terminology. J Am Osteopath Assoc 1981; 80:552–567. Reprinted in: Yearbook and Directory of Osteopathic Physicians, 1991. Chicago IL: American Osteopathic Association, 1991: 678–690.

14. Johnston WL, Hill JL. Spinal segmental dysfunction: incidence in cervicothoracic region. J Am Osteopath Assoc 1981; 81:67–76.

15. Johnston WL. Inter-rater reliability in the selection of manipulable patients. In: Buerger AA, Greenman PE, eds. Empirical approaches to the validation of spinal manipulation. Springfield IL: Charles C. Thomas, 1985.

16. Kelso AF, Grant RG, Johnston WL. Use of thermograms to support assessment of somatic dysfunction or effects of osteopathic manipulative treatment. J Am Osteopath Assoc 1982; 82:182–188.

17. Johnston WL, Vorro J, Hubbard RP. Clinical/biomechanic correlates for cervical function: Part I. A kinematic study. J Am Osteopath Assoc 1985; 85:429–437.

18. Vorro J, Johnston WL. Clinical/biomechanic correlates for cervical function: Part II. A myoelectric study. J Am Osteopath Assoc 1987; 87:353–367.

15

Exercise and Training for Spinal Patients

PART A. MOVEMENT AWARENESS AND STABILIZATION TRAINING
PAMELA MAY

PART B. FLEXIBILITY TRAINING
MARY McCLURE

PART C. STRENGTH TRAINING
WRAY PARDY

PART D. AEROBIC EXERCISE
LOIS B. WOLF

Exercises have been widely recommended to help prevent the development of spinal pathology,[1] to decrease pain[2-4] and to increase function.[5] Four types are recognized as necessary to prevent, restore, or maintain a healthy and functional musculoskeletal system: strength training, flexibility training, endurance training, and neuromuscular control training. An exercise program should be individualized to account for specific spinal dysfunction or pathology, level of fitness, age, and personality type. Patient goals should be established, and the exercise program should be designed to assure patient compliance, even after symptoms have resolved. Patient education is essential. Understanding body structure and the nature of biomechanical imbalances and faulty movement patterns will help patients perform their exercises more safely and efficiently. Motivation to continue with an exercise program is enhanced when knowledge is obtained about how motion disorder(s) contribute to symptoms.

PART A.
MOVEMENT AWARENESS AND STABILIZATION TRAINING

Exercise brings to mind varied perceptions. Many people believe exercise is synonymous with exertion, but to a patient with low back pain the probability of pain increases with exercise exertion. To the physical therapist, exercise completes or rounds out the rehabilitation process. In some situations, however, exercise as an essential component of treatment is overlooked. It becomes an afterthought at the end of a treatment session or a routine passed on to many patients despite their having differing dysfunctions. Without proper time, attention, and specificity, the exercise component of a rehabilitation program will be of questionable value. For true benefit, physical therapists must devote time and employ skill in developing exercise specificity for individual patients, who, in turn, must devote time and attention to the exercise movements. A better understanding of exercise is needed by both the physical therapist and the patient for optimal benefit and promotion of self reliance.

Exercise has many aspects and goals. Primarily, it is used: 1) to improve mobility and flexibility, 2) to promote better stability and strength, 3) to increase endurance and control, and 4) to promote aerobic conditioning. The questions and/or confusion surrounding exercise stem from what goals to achieve and how to start: mobility versus stability, flexibility versus strength. The type of motion dysfunction as well as the pain level are essential elements in determining how to initiate an exercise program. These questions will be addressed in this chapter with focus on the musculoskeletal spinal pain patient.

ROLE OF EXERCISE

The importance of exercise in the treatment of the musculoskeletal spinal patient has been widely acknowledged.[1–10] Improving the general fitness of the individual has long been considered a positive adjunct to specific exercise routines in rehabilitation of the lumbar spine patient. Improvement in flexibility, muscle strength, and endurance is thought to facilitate the healing process, decrease mechanical stress, and lessen the chance of reinjury. Many low back pain patients have had a long history of back problems which ultimately leads to decreased activity secondary to pain. Deconditioning occurs with resultant loss of muscle flexibility, joint mobility, muscle strength, and joint stability. Exercise is a key element in the rehabilitation process of patients for optimal response to treatment and reversal of the deconditioning process. The therapist must carefully select the appropriate exercise program for each individual based on the degree of functional impairment and level of pain. In some cases, the patient may be in acute pain and movement aggravates the condition. Awareness of when rest is the most appropriate management strategy is therefore also critical in en-

hancing recovery. In some situations, the best intervention is no intervention.

Neither a stretching or strengthening approach may be appropriate initially if pain is a significant factor. This is also true if one is dealing with a patient having a more involved long-term history where many adaptive changes have been incorporated into the patient's posture and movement patterns. To bring about dynamic changes in the musculoskeletal system, long standing compulsive patterns need to be modified or removed from the nervous system. Imposing traditional exercise movements upon changed or faulty postures and movement patterns will oftentimes only perpetuate the existing condition.[11]

Research has shown that the body begins to compensate to the changes imposed from an injury within 3–5 days post injury.[12] Adaptive changes are the result of the body's attempt to attain pain-free postures and movements. Altered postures and movement patterns observed within 5 days are characteristically similar to those in patients evaluated 1 to 5 years post injury.

According to the above-noted study,[12] the difference between acute and chronic patients was in awareness. The acute patients were aware of postural changes and muscle activity compensations. The chronic patients were unaware of any postural or muscle changes, stating that their muscles were relaxed despite EMG findings to the contrary. Over time chronic pain patients began to accept the postural and muscle compensations as being normal.

The existing faulty postures and movement patterns become habits for the patient.[13] The habitual patterns are imprinted in the nervous system, become familiar, and are repeated over and over.[11] As a result, when the patient reacts to external stimuli of the nervous system, the response is a habitual ready-made pattern. In dealing with chronic spinal pain patients, faulty postures and inefficient movement patterns must be reorganized. Changing habitual, dependent movement patterns and postures is essential for optimizing the rehabilitation program of any pain patient.

Example

Let's start with a commonly seen postural dysfunction such as the forward head posture. Axial extension/retraction is often the instruction to the patients with this posture. Routinely the attempt is to eliminate a faulty posture, yet how often does the patient perform the movement correctly? Sometimes the posterior cervical musculature is too tight and the cervical facet joints too immobile. Alternatively, the forward head is the result of the lack of awareness of how the head, neck, and trunk are typically positioned during the course of a day. Patients with chronic musculoskeletal disorders become unaware of their own muscle tone and activity status and consequently adjust to the abnormal muscle state, accepting it as normal. What needs to be addressed with the forward-head patient and all posturally related conditions is awareness of the body. Home exercise programs are ineffective if patients are posturally and kinesthetically unaware.

Patient Learning

Physical therapists, in reviewing home exercise programs, often judge patient's exercise performance to be either right or wrong rather than assisting the patient in learning movement from within his or her body. Just as the fundamental role of a psychologist is to help the person learn and become aware of emotional states, the essential role of a physical therapist is to help patients learn and become aware of their physical state. Once the patient has become more conscious physically, then appropriate exercise movements can be instructed. The close interrelationship between the emotional being and the physical being is often displayed as physical self awareness improves.[12,14] Patients more conscious physically may perceive themselves on a more positive emotional level. Positive outlooks favorably affect the overall rehabilitation process.

Faulty Posture: Forward Bending

Determining faulty postures and movement patterns may be somewhat subjective. However, there are many guidelines published regarding correct posture[2,14,15] and normal movement patterns.[2,10,15] Most clinicians can identify a forward head posture, an increased or decreased lordosis or rounded shoulders. Identifying variations in forward bending of the lumbar spine is accomplished with active range of motion testing. A patient with low back pain, however, may achieve forward bending of the lumbar spine through hip and pelvic motion in order to avoid movement of the lumbar spine. Avoidance of lumbar forward bending can lead to changes in muscle activity and abnormal recruitment of the hip, pelvic, and lumbar spine muscles.[3] The end result will be establishment of an abnormal movement pattern whereby some muscles and joints are overutilized and others avoided. Other areas of the body may also become involved in order to compensate for the lack of movement in the lumbar spine. Clinically, increased forward bending of the thoracic spine may be observed in the absence of lumbar forward bending.

A traditional exercise approach to improving decreased forward bending in the lumbar spine might be use of the Cat back exercise. In a more acute pain patient, a posterior pelvic tilt might be recommended. Yet, how often does the patient have difficulty performing flexion movements despite the additional use of manual treatment directed at restoring soft tissue and joint mobility? Motion recognition of forward bending may be absent. If the patient's body is saying lumbar forward bending is not an accepted movement pattern, then any attempt to promote forward bending of the lumbar spine on a conscious level is totally foreign. Forward bending has become an untested, unused movement. Learning the movement behavior of forward bending at a subconscious level is then critical. The patient's attention must be drawn to how and which muscles work, what body parts move during certain actions, and what parts do not move.

INCREASING AWARENESS

Helping the patient increase awareness can be accomplished in many ways. Various types of movement therapies can facilitate body awareness, including the Feldenkrais method[11,13,16,17] and the Alexander technique.[18,19] Biofeedback[20] is a more traditional psycho-physical approach which helps identify muscle activity at rest or during functional activity. Regardless of the method, time devoted to the task is critical. The patient must allow sufficient time on a daily basis to become physically aware of abnormal behaviors in order to make fundamental change.

Training cannot be assigned through a set number of repetitions which the patient can perform inattentively while reading a book or watching television. Lack of attention to exercise movements is often evident during review of the patient's exercise program.

Very often the patient is performing the exercise with a faulty movement pattern, thus perpetuating the existing problem. Time devoted, frequency of performance, and attentiveness are critical elements in obtaining favorable outcomes with respect to changing posture and motion behavior. The patient must perform the exercise movements slowly and with attention focused on the movement and not on a book or the television. Attention is defined as a selective narrowing or focusing of consciousness and receptivity.

Although it is important for the patient to give attention (focus) to an exercise, it is even more important for the patient to be aware (show realization or knowledge) of the exercise activity as the movement takes place. Only through awareness and knowledge is learning of motion activity obtained.

Beginning the awareness component of an exercise program involves a number of questions directed to the patient. No right or wrong answer should be supplied by the physical therapist. The questions are designed to assist the patient in focusing on one part of the body as well as to the whole; the feeling experienced as muscles contract and joints move is also emphasized. For example, a patient can be asked to simply look to his or her left (rotation of the head, neck and trunk) and look to the right while in a standing position (Fig. 15A.1 **A** and **B**). The patient is then asked which direction of movement feels freer or feels more restricted. Once identified, the patient can then focus more specifically on where the movement is or is not occurring. For example, does the pelvis move with the head, neck, and trunk? Do the knees bend and straighten with the rotation? Do the feet evert and invert with the rotation? In other words, is the whole body moving or only part of it? The physical therapist should not share observations with the patient, as they may be in total conflict with what the patient is perceiving or is aware of. Directing the questions appropriately helps the patient recognize where motion restrictions exist without the physical therapist telling the patient what is happening.

The essential element in the awareness process is that the patient learns how to use his/her body. Learning is not accomplished if the patient is told what is occurring by the physical therapist instead of feeling and sensing within. Once the patient has attained awareness of the rotation movement, he/she can perform the motion as part of an exercise program until the lesson is learned. The goal in this approach—of learning the movement—is to reorganize the neuromuscular system. With reorganization of the movement, it will hopefully become a new habit—not requiring repetition, but awareness.

Perception and Sensory Engrams

Perception as described by Sage,[21] involves the "essential steps of detection, recognition, and identification of incoming information for an interpretation." Thus, perception requires an interaction between the sensory system and the memory process. Perceptual responses are then translated into commands for movement responses. Sensory-motor performance evaluation requires noncognitive, internal stimulus analysis called interoception. The patient is called upon to focus within the body to assess physical behavior with respect to movement and position. Memory patterns in the sensory and sensory association areas are searched for existing inappropriate pat-

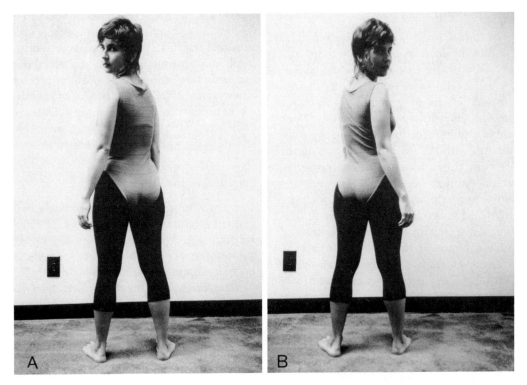

Figure 15A.1A Left rotation: Torso and pelvis appear blocked, right leg not involved with movement.

Figure 15A.1B Right rotation: Note full utilization of body including eversion of left foot and internal rotation of left lower extremity.

terns. The term sensory engram[22] is often used to describe the memory store of different sensory-motor experiences. The CNS translates the engram into action by calling up various motor components needed to reproduce the movement. The motor areas of the cortex are also organized into motor engrams.[22] A motor engram describes a set of prestructured commands when initiated, and results in production of movement sequences.[23] Motor engrams are developed through experience and learning. Movement sequences are differentiated into component parts (movement patterns) which are called upon as movement demands arise.

In the chronic pain patient, the sensory engram utilized for movement may be one that provides a faulty movement pattern, as it may be associated with pain upon lumbar forward bending. However, correction of an un-

desired motor response is relatively easy when existing motor responses are present to compare with.[13,22] The existing motor programs can be called up in a different pattern. Once the patient is provided with the environment and tools for awareness through perception, improving posture and movement patterns can occur.

The goal of promoting patient awareness of physical states is to create efficient postures and movement. In some instances, the process is a total relearning experience for the patient. A developmental perspective of normal motor skill development provides appropriate focus for assessment of posture and movement control. A motor skill development reference also provides guidance for proper questions in sequencing the patient's rehabilitation process. The stages include mobility, stability, controlled mobility, and skill.[24]

Stages of Motor Control

The Initial Stage of Motor Control. This is exhibited by development of functional mobility. During the first few months of life, movements tend to be spontaneous and reflex-based.[13,24] As development progresses, control becomes voluntary, less reflexive. One essential requirement for the voluntary stage of motor control is the ability to initiate the movement through adequate activation of muscles. Another important element is the ability to move through a range with adequate strength. Adequate range of motion and flexibility may be components restored by manual treatment. However, the ability to initiate the desired movement may not be present due to pre-existing abnormal movement patterns in the motor or sensory engram. Awareness of abnormal movement or lack of movement is necessary for restoration of proper motor control for the desired movement. For example, the patient with a forward head posture may initiate cervical forward bending by jutting the jaw forward causing upper cervical backward bending stress. He/she needs to relearn the movement, becoming aware of tucking the chin and rolling the head.

The Second Stage of Motor Control. This stage involves stability. The definition of stability is the ability to maintain a steady position in relation to gravity.[24] The development of stability can be divided into two phases: tonic holding and cocontraction.[25] Tonic holding is the activation of postural muscles in the fully shortened range. Cocontraction refers to simultaneous contraction of the agonist and antagonist muscles to support the body in weight-bearing postures.

The Third Stage of Motor Control Development. The third stage is controlled mobility, the ability to change position and achieve a new position while maintaining postural control. The controlled mobility stage of motor development is achieved through well coordinated patterns of movement and tonal changes.[26]

The Fourth Stage, Skill. The final and highest level of motor control is termed skill.

Skill is a coordinated movement evidenced by discrete motor function superimposed upon proximal stability.[25] Dynamic stability of the trunk and proximal joints is maintained during activities, allowing smooth, controlled movements. The last two stages of mobility are important for accomplishing activities of daily living without experiencing pain and for lessening the likelihood of reinjury.

Facilitating the Learning

The environment for increasing one's body awareness requires few distractions. The tools are time and guidance through appropriate questions and comments. A very basic yet invaluable awareness exercise is breathing.

Breathing. Diaphragmatic breathing has been a mainstay of most home exercise programs, particularly when promoting relaxation. The instructions to the patient often emphasize use of the diaphragm, expansion of the rib cage, and movement of the abdominal wall. This type of instruction assumes that the "how-to directional strategy" is the best method for the learner. The shortcoming, however, is that there is no opportunity for patients to learn what is best for themselves.

In order to improve a breathing pattern, one must first learn the current pattern. There are numerous variables to consider when guiding a patient through a breathing exercise. The patients are asked what they notice about their breathing rate, if their breathing is shallow or deep; if the rib cage (upper or lower) is involved, and, if so, which way the rib cage moves—forward, backward, or laterally, and whether the abdomen moves.

Questions are asked one at a time to facilitate awareness of their breathing pattern. Once a patient has identified their personal breathing pattern, suggestions can be offered to facilitate breathing changes.

Example. With the patient supine, instruct the patient to concentrate and focus on the left side of the body. Ask the patient to feel the rib cage move toward the ceiling, the air expanding the lungs, and the ribs moving out to the side while breathing in. Ask where else movement is felt—the shoulders, collar bone, abdomen, or back? Have the patient move to a right sidelying position with the left arm along the front of the rib cage (Fig. 15A.2). Ask the patient to imagine the left lung as a balloon and feel the entire rib cage move when breathing in an out of the balloon (lung). Feel the air moving into and out of the lungs and mouth. Then, wait a second before breathing in again. Allow the patient to spend several minutes with this exercise. Retest, while backlying. Does your left side feel rested, relaxed, able to breathe more easily? Is there a difference between the left and right sides? If so, balance the sides by repeating the exercise for the right rib cage.

Note that no mention was made of right or wrong movement. There was no instruction to expand the rib cage or abdomen, simply to feel the movement. The amount of movement is also determined by the patient. Large amplitudes of movement are not necessary, especially when learning a new movement pattern. Neuronal stimulus for physical movement is generated prior to actual movement.[27] Thus, the intent to move and/or small movement, are often sufficient for reorganization of a movement pattern. Throughout the entire exercise the patient was allowed to explore and learn a body response to the simple task of breathing. Options for alternate ways to move while breathing are explored.

The Body Responds

Feldenkrais claims that incorrect posture and actions are a direct result of premature or violent demands upon the body.[13] Muscle contractions constantly maintained during all actions, regardless of the movements may express an emotional attitude. The most frequent attitude associated with continuous muscle holding is one of insecurity brought about by feelings of doubt, fear, hesitation, guilt, etc. Physiological stiffening of the body, lowering of the head, sinking of the chest, contracting the abdomen are all protective acts when not performed for purposeful actions. When insecurity is present, patients will fail if instructed in how to do an activity instead of learning from within about the postures they maintain and movements they perform.

With an awareness approach to exercise, pressure to perform an activity in the exact correct way is removed. The body as a whole as well as the specific muscles required can relax and learn. Relaxation is essential in a sensory-motor experience which emphasizes

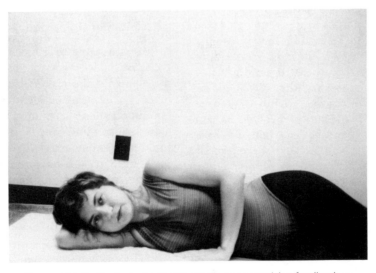

Figure 15A.2. Contact of left arm on rib cage provides feedback as patient focuses on left side while breathing.

self-learning. Without relaxation a patient will continue to impose tension-induced (right versus wrong) movement and postures upon already existing incorrect positions and movements.

The body continues to be in a state of conflict and tension. Manual treatment may have restored the potential joint and soft tissue mobility, but the patient may not take full advantage of the newly available motion if time to learn how to use the new movement activities is not provided. Clinically, one often sees a lumbar spine patient continue to achieve forward bending through anterior tilting of the pelvis and hip flexion despite normal or near normal results from passive motion testing. The ability to employ this new range of motion in the lumbar spine must be relearned by the patient. If the patient is instructed to perform the CAT back exercise; suggestions to focus on each vertebra during the movement can be helpful. Small amplitude, effortless movement of each motion segment can be more beneficial than trying to produce one large amplitude of motion.[17]

Being, Not Doing. Gabrielle Yaron, a Feldenkrais practitioner, indicates that the focus of many therapies is on doing *for* the patient. The patient, however, must learn to do for oneself. Only by handing over the responsibility of movement can true benefit from a home exercise program occur. The greatest contributions made are the guidance and not direction, the enabling and not doing. A patient instructed to do an exercise will, in fact, do exactly that—perform an exercise—but will not internalize the movement or physically experience the activity. An exercise performance that simply involves human doing instead of *human being* is bound to have limited effects, since the essential element for change is communication with the body. "Being" with the body during motion activities is thus essential.

SPINAL STABILIZATION TRAINING

Goals

The purpose of stabilization exercise is to allow a patient to move without pain and with the least amount of protective muscle guarding. The spinal stabilization exercise approach allows the patient to attain dynamic control of movement. The patient learns to eliminate faulty movement patterns leading to repetitive injury. The major goal is to facilitate functional movements necessary for daily activity while protecting the lumbar spine so that the patient can prevent low back injury. The patient must first learn to recognize the functional limits of his/her low back condition and then, with instruction, understand how to stay within the identified limitations.

The functional position will vary amongst patients and be influenced by the type of motion dysfunction as well as by activity. A patient with a spondylolisthesis may only be comfortable in flexion activities of the lumbar spine. For pain avoidance and functional control, the patient may need to keep a posterior pelvic tilt while performing overhead tasks in order to prevent lumbar spine extension. On the other hand, the patient with a lumbar disc derangement may discover positions of lumbar spine extension more comfortable while executing reaching forward and down activities, thus preventing lumbar spine flexion. The point to consider is that no one position or motion activity is best for all patients or every problem.

The Functional Position

As Morgan states, the "functional position is the most stable and asymptomatic position of the spine for the task at hand."[5] Once the functional position is identified the patient can more safely perform activities of daily living. Successful control of back position while performing a variety of activities eventually becomes second nature to the patient. The functional position may become a new posture from which movements are initiated. Movements are therefore performed upon a stable position.

A brief overview of Morgan's approach[5] to functional stabilization follows. Please refer to his works[5] and to Saal et al.[4] for more in-depth descriptions.

Some patients may not be able to actively move their spine to a functional position. "Passive prepositioning" may be necessary when active movement is painful. If a patient is only comfortable with a slightly flexed position of the spine but cannot obtain the position actively, the legs are passively positioned and then supported in 60° of hip flexion. With the hips flexed to 60°, the patient can begin various movements which will recruit the desired muscle activity.

Many people with low back problems need abdominal strengthening exercises.[3,9,28] Traditionally, abdominal strengthening is achieved through concentric abdominal contractions or through lower extremity activities[3] superimposed upon isometric abdominal contractions. However, the acute patient may not tolerate concentric abdominal contractions or lower extremity movements superimposed on isometric abdominal activity. Lower extremity movements also are not feasible when the lower extremities are supported as in passive prepositioning.

Fortunately, upper extremity movements may be tolerated. While in the functional position, the patient can be instructed in various upper extremity movements such as reciprocal overhead flexion or bilateral horizontal abduction. See Fig. 15A.3. Bilateral overhead flexion may initially tend to move the patient's lumbar spine out of functional position. The greater the motion activity, the greater the demand upon the abdominals. The number of repetitions and sets as well as the amount of weight used is determined on an individual basis.

Progression

As the patient progresses, muscle activity is recruited for functional positioning (active prepositioning). The hips may still be flexed to 60°, but abdominal muscle contraction will be necessary to assume the functional position. At this point lower extremity movements can often be utilized as well as upper extremity movements. Lower extremity movements can be as simple as lifting the heels from the ground or partially extending one hip/knee with the foot 6–8 inches from the floor. See Fig. 15A.4A through 15A.4C. Throughout the superimposed movements, the patient must be able to maintain functional position, because inability to do so indicates that the exercise is too advanced. Improper movement patterns could result if the patient substitutes undesired muscle contractions in an attempt to perform the exercise.

Dynamic Spinal Stabilization. This is the next progression in functional stabilization. The patient adopts functional position or range during the superimposed movements. This requires awareness, neuromuscular skill, and continuous adjustments in muscle tension throughout the movements. During hip/knee extension while supine the spine tends to move into extension. As the patient initiates the lower extremity movement of extension, the abdominals and gluteals must be slowly contracted to prevent the tendency for extension movement of the spine.

Transitional Stabilization. The last phase of functional stabilization is transitional stabilization, a type of dynamic stabilization involving a change in the primary muscle stabilizers, agonist, and antagonists. Transitional stabilization exercise is best performed in weight-bearing positions such as kneeling, sitting, or standing. For example, if one lifts an object from the floor to an overhead position, the spine moves from flexion to extension. The patient must learn to stabilize first for the flexion movement then stabilize for an extension movement of the lumbar spine. Stabilization during flexion and extension movements are necessary for performing activities of daily living in a pain-free manner.

The progression of functional stabilization coincides with three stages of motor control. Passive and active prepositioning enables the lumbar spine to achieve stability for motion activity. Controlled mobility therefore can be obtained through dynamic spinal stabilization. Transitional stabilization is an important progression for obtaining and/or improving motor skill.

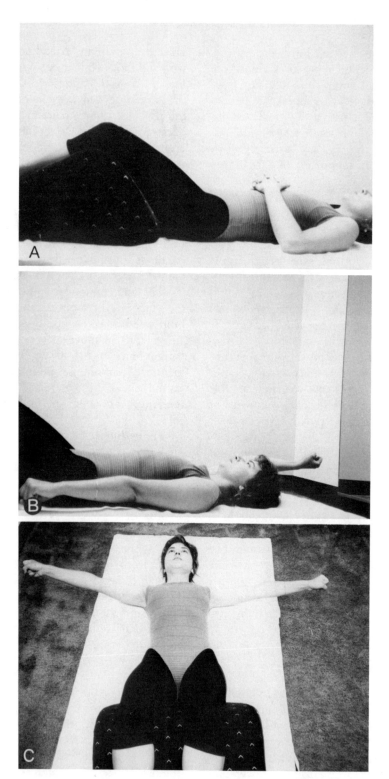

Figure 15A.3A Patient passively supported in functional position.

Figure 15A.3B Reciprocal upper extremity overhead flexion.

Figure 15A.3C Bilateral upper extremity horizontal abduction.

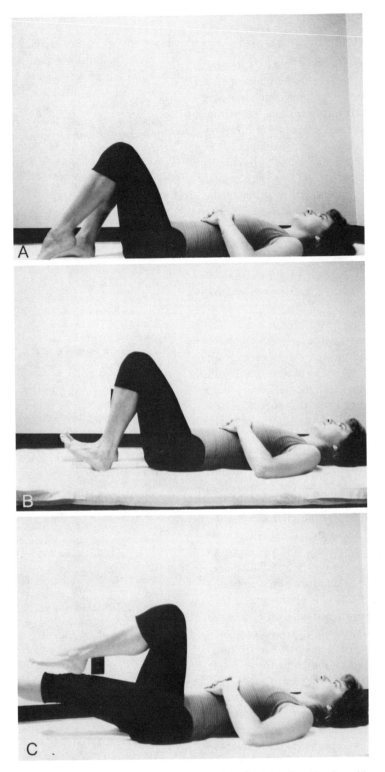

Figure 15A.4A Patient lifts heel while actively maintaining functional position.

Figure 15A.4B Patient can also lift left toes while actively maintaining functional position.

Figure 15A.4C Patient extends right lower extremity with foot 6–8 inches above floor; maintaining functional position during the lower extremity movements.

Individualized Home Program

After achieving transitional stabilization the physical therapist can develop an appropriate home program for the patient which includes ADL exercises and modifications, stretching and strengthening exercises, and cardiovascular training as tolerated. An example of an ADL exercise is rolling from back to side to get out of bed. The patient practices rolling while maintaining functional position of the lumbar spine. The next step is to practice going from sitting to standing while maintaining functional position and moving through functional range. ADL motion activities such as rolling can be complemented by strengthening exercises for the gluteals and quadriceps.

Throughout functional stabilization training, the patient must continue to focus on the motion event. The ability to be kinesthetically aware and the skill to stabilize during dynamic motion activity are fundamental elements of the patient's home program of exercises. Throughout the rehabilitation process the physical therapist and the patient must remember that the entire body is involved with each movement. A section of the body cannot be isolated and treated as an entity in itself as if that part has no effect on other parts. The physical therapist must evaluate and treat the motion disorder as a whole. The patient must constantly assess the entire body for responses and reactions to motion activities. The objective of the awareness and functional approach to exercise rehabilitation is coordinated, well-learned actions performed with an absence of effort and resistance. An improvement in motion control gives patients increased confidence in their body's ability to move safely and without pain.

In our interaction with patients we must not teach the theoretical correct way but instead have patients learn what is correct for them. The result is a person who has sensorimotor awareness as well as the ability to adjust motion activities to the needs of the situation, and ultimately assumes full responsibility for all motion activities. The result is self reliance, fulfilling the major goal of the rehabilitation process.

REFERENCES

1. Jackson C, Brown D. Is there a role for exercise in the treatment of patients with low back pain. Clinical Orthop 1983; 179:39–45.
2. McKenzie RA. The lumbar spine: mechanical diagnosis and therapy. New Zealand: Spinal Publications, 1981.
3. McCune D, Sprague R. Exercise for low back pain. In: Basmajian J, Wolf S, eds. Therapeutic Exercise, 5th ed. Baltimore: Williams & Wilkins, 1990:299–321.
4. Saal J, Saal J. Nonoperative treatment of herniated lumbar intervertebral disc with radiculopathy. Spine 1989; 14:431–437.
5. Morgan D. Concepts in functional training and postural stabilization for the low back injured. Top Acute Care Trauma Rehabil 1988; 2:8–17.
6. Hunter-Griffin L. Orthopedic concerns. In: Shangold M, Mirkin G, eds. Women and exercise physiology and sports medicine. Philadelphia: F.A. Davis Co., 1988; 215–217.
7. Jackson C, Brown M. Analysis of current approaches and a practical guide to prescription of exercise. Clinical Orthop 1983; 179:46–54.
8. Nachemson A. A critical look at conservative treatment for low back pain. In: Jayson M, ed: The lumbar spine and back pain. New York and San Francisco: Grune and Stratton, Inc., 1976.
9. White A, Panjabi M. Clinical biomechanics of the spine. Philadelphia: J.B. Lippincott Co., 1978.
10. Mayer T. Rehabilitation of the patient with spinal pain. In: Mooney V, ed. The orthopedic clinics of North America, evaluation and care of lumbar spine problems. Philadelphia: W.B. Saunders Co., 1983; 623–637.
11. Feldenkrais M. Bodily expressions. Somatics 1988; IV:52–59.
12. Headley B. Postural homeostasis. P.T. Forum 1990; IX:1–4.
13. Feldenkrais M. Potent self. Cambridge: Harper & Row, 1985.
14. Kendall H, Kendall F, Wadsworth G. Muscles testing and function. Baltimore: Williams & Wilkins, 1971.
15. Magee D. Orthopedic physical assessment. Philadelphia: W.B. Saunders Co., 1987; 377–405.
16. Feldenkrais M. The master moves. Cupertino, CA: Meta Publications, 1984.
17. Feldenkrais, M. Awareness through movement. New York: Harper & Row, 1977.
18. Jones F. Body awareness. New York: Schocken Books, 1979.

19. Caplan D. Back trouble. Gainesville, FL: Triad Publishing Co., 1987.
20. Krebo D. Biofeedback in therapeutic exercise. In: Basmajian J, Wolf S, eds. Therapeutic exercise, 5th Ed. Baltimore: Williams & Wilkins, 1990; 109–124.
21. Sage G. Introduction to motor behavior. A neurophysiological approach. Reading, MA: Addison-Wesley, 1977; 215–230.
22. Sullivan S. Strategies to improve motor control. In: Sullivan S, Schmitz T. Physical rehabilitation: assessment and treatment. Philadelphia: F.A. Davis, 1988; 253–280.
23. Schmidt R. Motor control and learning. Champaign, IL: Human Kinetics, 1982.
24. Sullivan S. Motor control assessment. In: Sullivan S, Schmitz T. Physical rehabilitation: assessment and treatment, Philadelphia: F.A. Davis, 1988; 135–158.
25. Stockmeyer S. An interpretation of the approach of Rood to the treatment of neuromuscular dysfunction. Am J Phys Med 1967; 46:900.
26. Bobath B. Adult hemiplegia: evaluation and treatment. London: Wm Heinemann Medical Books, 1978.
27. Lassen N, Inguar D, Skinnj E. Brain function and bloodflow. Sci Am 1978; 238:62–71.
28. Morris J, Lumas B, Bresler B. Role of the trunk in stability of the spine. J Bone Joint Surg 1962; 43A:327.

PART B.
FLEXIBILITY TRAINING

Today's hectic but sedentary work schedules do not allow time for many of us to exercise adequately. Not only does this result in insufficient movement but also frequently restricts the variety of movements that our bodies experience each day. Faulty postural adaptations may develop over the years as a result of the decreased level of activity and abnormal positions and movement patterns. When the body attempts to function outside of the normal postural balance (Fig. 15B.1) length-tension changes can develop in the muscles and connective tissue structures of the body.[6–8] If the length-tension changes are great enough, and if they persist over prolonged periods of time, abnormal shearing, compressive or tension loads to the spinal joints or intervertebral discs may result. Prolonged alterations in the normal biomechanics of the spine may lead to early degenerative changes and pathology in the spinal joints. Thus, spinal stability is contingent upon controlled, balanced muscle and connective tissue behavior. Interruption of the controlled interaction between the trunk and extremity musculature may result in loss of movement control, which could make the intervertebral joints vulnerable to an injury.[8]

RATIONALE FOR STRETCHING

Self-stretching exercises play a critical role in the recovery of patients with spinal dysfunction. They allow patients to increase or maintain gains in range of motion achieved in treatment sessions and help them to assume responsibility for the care of their spine.

The choice of a particular stretching exercise for the spine must be based on a thorough structural and movement analysis of each patient. Exercise prescription will vary from patient to patient. Modification of a standard exercise may be necessary to protect areas of the spine from being over stretched or compressed. Extremity muscle tightness and weakness need to be evaluated to determine their effects on the spine. Treatment of extremity muscle dysfunction is often essential for normal spinal movement.

Patients with the flexion postural dysfunction syndromes described by McKenzie[7] may respond to stretching exercises designed to restore spinal extension. Patients who have excessive amounts of extension at any spinal segment or region need special precaution(s) in extension exercises for other segments and in exercises in other motion planes since restrictions of the spine are not confined to the sagittal plane.

Exercises to promote sidebending and rotation of motion segments also facilitate the force-attenuating properties of the spine. Lateral and rotational deformation of myofascia is equally important in the restoration of spinal range of motion in all planes. Research to substantiate gains in joint and soft tissue extensibility with a particular stretching exercise are inconclusive at this time.

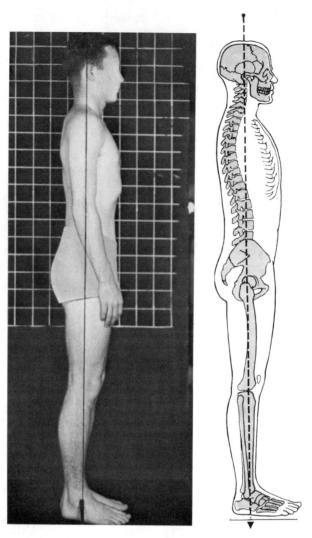

Figure 15B.1 Normal postural balance. With permission from: Kendall FP, McCreary EK. Muscles: testing and function. 3rd ed. Baltimore: Williams & Wilkins, 1983.

Stretching and Myofascial Pain Syndromes

Trigger points in muscles have been recognized for years.[10,11] Trigger points are hypothesized to be the result of vasoconstriction in the muscle. An abnormal, sustained contraction of the muscle secondary to the vasoconstriction causes pain with or without movement. The pain results from the accumulation of metabolites and a decrease in tissue oxidation. Consequently changes occur in the recruitment of motor units and ultimately

may result in altered patterns of muscle contraction.[10,12–15]

Seven myofascial syndromes have been outlined by Kirkaldy-Willis[13] that are associated with low back pain: Multifidus Syndrome, Gluteus Medius Syndrome, Gluteus Maximus Syndrome, Quadratus Lumborum Syndrome, Piriformis Syndrome, Tensor Fasciae Latae Syndrome and Hamstring Syndrome. Each syndrome is characterized by local tenderness in an area that is particular for each muscle and will often have a specific pattern of pain referral.[13] Travell has identi-

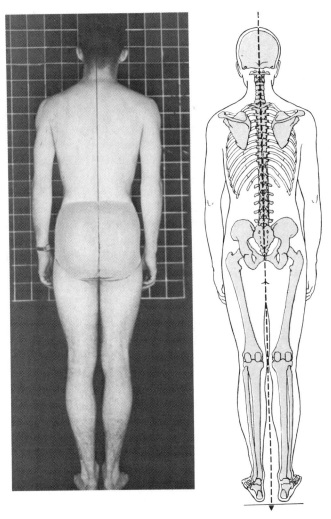

Figure 15B.1 Continued.

fied myofascial trigger point syndromes in almost all of the muscles of the upper quarter.[10]

Treatment through stretching can result
in a reduction or complete relief of symptoms.
If the muscle is stretched correctly, with adequate stabilization of surrounding joint and
myofascial structures, pain symptoms or muscle irritability is less likely. Stretching is usually proceeded by spraying with a coolant
(e.g., Flurimethane or a safer substitute), injection with 0.25% bupivacaine, or by using
post-isometric relaxation techniques.[14,13]
Spray and stretch to lengthen hamstrings,

upper trapezius, masseter, and temporalis
muscles is sometimes successful when other
methods of stretching have proven unsuc-
cessful.

Joint Mechanoreceptor Activation With Stretching

Wyke and Freeman identified four types of
mechanoreceptors present in joints, and three
of these when mechanically stimulated can
inhibit pain. Oscillatory movements at different parts of the available joint range of motion

may activate these mechanoreceptors and reduce pain, improve proprioception and allow increased joint and soft tissue extensibility.[8] This type of stretching is most helpful in highly reactive joints to decrease reflexive muscle guarding and to initiate motion.

Example. A good example of a graded oscillation stretch to reduce pain and initiate and restore motion follows. Patients with acute disc derangement may present with loss of the normal lumbar curve and decreased active and passive lumbar spine extension. Restoration of lumbar extension is believed to shift intradiscal fluid and reduce the bulging anulus.[7] Patients can begin gentle oscillations of their pelvis into anterior rotation while lying prone over a pillow. Lumbar spine extension occurs with anterior rotation of the pelvis. Patients will be able to increase the amplitude of motion as pain is reduced and motion is increased. With increased amplitude of motion the exercise is promoting increased joint range of motion in extension (Fig. 15B.9). The same effects can be achieved with the patients on their hands and knees (Fig. 15B.10). (See p. 375.)

Figures that illustrate exercises mentioned in the text of this Section B follow at the end of Section B, on page 371.

TISSUE MECHANICS

Connective Tissue Response to Stretch

An understanding of normal connective tissue and muscle structure and how these tissues respond to immobilization and stretch is important for safe and effective exercise prescription. Several excellent resources on tissue mechanics are available for additional information.[16–20]

Johns and Wright[21] found that ligamentous joint capsules, tendons, and muscles are responsible for 98% of passive resistance at the normal extremes of joint motion. The composition and spatial arrangement of collagen, elastin, and ground substance will determine how connective tissue responds as a viscoelastic material to changes in tension at various rates.[22,23] Connective tissue elongates proportionately to the magnitude of the locally applied force. This means that a low-force stretching method requires more time to produce the same amount of elongation as a high-force method. However, low-load, long-duration stretching enhances permanent, plastic deformation, so the proportion of tissue lengthening that remains after the tensile stress is removed is greater at lower loads.[24] Permanent elongation of connective tissue may result in some mechanical weakening. Low-force stretching techniques produce less structural weakness than high-load techniques for the same amount of tissue elongation.[25,26]

Williams[19] found that rat soleus muscles immobilized in a shortened position for 10 days in a plaster cast showed a reduction in fiber length and an increase in the proportion of connective tissue. The result was decreased muscle compliance and range of motion. In an attempt to determine the effect of intermittent stretching on these muscle changes, the soleus muscle was passively stretched with a sustained low load force for 15 minutes once each day. Results showed that stretching decreased the accumulation of connective tissue but did not prevent a reduction in muscle fiber length, probably because of the loss of serial sarcomeres.

These results may help explain why patients who present with muscle shortness because of posture or muscle holding habits show a remarkable increase in tissue extensibility during the first few stretching sessions and then seem to plateau. The connective tissue infiltration provides more tissue with viscoelastic properties to undergo plastic deformation. After the connective tissue structures have stretched or realigned, sarcomere addition to muscle fibers is necessary to regain further extensibility. However, intermolecular cross-links in collagen fibers become stiffer and harder to break as they mature,[18] so if shortness has been present for prolonged periods of time even initial gains with stretching may be small.

MUSCLES

Muscles possess both an active contractile component and a passive elastic component. The extensive connective tissue framework of muscle has viscoelastic properties and is thought to provide the major resistance to passive stretch, instead of the myofibrillar elements.[27–29] The passive contractile components in combination with the elastic response of the connective tissue framework are responsible for the muscle's ability to generate tension under load. Refer to Chapters 9, 12, and 13 for further additional related information on muscle histology and physiology.

Type of Stretching Procedure

Several studies have set out to determine whether active, passive, or proprioceptive neuromuscular facilitation (PNF) exercises produce the greatest gains in tissue extensibility. Conclusions varied. Some investigators concluded that PNF was more beneficial than static or ballistic stretching.[31,39] Others found that there was no statistical difference between stretch procedures,[30–34] concluding that passive static stretching was a less complicated and safer method of regaining range of motion.

Caution. *Ballistic stretching* has been recognized as potentially dangerous because of the possibility of exceeding the tissue's physiological range and because it can trigger a protective stretch reflex.[35]

Rationale. The use of static stretching to improve flexibility can be explained physiologically by examining the stretch reflex associated with the muscle spindles and the reflex associated with the Golgi tendon organs. Activation of muscle spindles through stretch stimulates further muscle contraction. The amount and rate of the response are proportionate to the amount of stretching. The Golgi tendon organs have a higher threshold and serve to inhibit contraction throughout the muscle group, protecting the muscle from tearing. Steady stretch affects the two proprioceptive organ systems by depressing the stretch reflex and activating tendon organs, further depressing large muscle tonicity.[36–38]

Proprioceptive neuromuscular facilitation stretching techniques use volitional contractions in an attempt to achieve increased range of motion by minimizing the active component of resistance that is attributed to the spinal reflex pathways.

Developing an Individual Program

At present we do not know the optimal combination of repetitions, duration, and frequency of stretching that will result in maximal flexibility gains. When developing a home program of exercises for a patient, *time* is a critical factor to consider if the patient is expected to be compliant with the exercise program. Patients need to understand the *purpose* of each stretching exercise. *Body awareness* is crucial so the patient can begin to feel specific areas of tightness. *Slow, purposeful movements* coordinated with *gentle diaphragmatic breathing* allow the patients to become aware of subtle muscle holding patterns that need to be changed as they work to increase flexibility. *Concentration* is important for safe and correct stretching to occur.

For most stretching exercises geared to increase length we are recommending five to ten slow stretches to create joint mechanoreceptor stimulation and to warm-up the muscle, followed by a prolonged stretch at the end range of from 30 seconds to 5 minutes, depending upon the muscle that is being stretched. Exercises are to be performed a minimum of one time a day. Stretches that can help to reduce postural stress and pain are instructed to be performed several times a day, as needed. Patients frequently will require passive stretching by the physical therapist before beginning a home program of self-stretching exercises.

Summary. Understanding the mechanical properties of connective tissue and muscle is essential for safe, effective stretching. Low-load, prolonged stretch has been shown to achieve the greatest amount of residual plastic deformation in connective tissue and muscle. Static stretching appears to be the safest, most effective, and least complicated method of gaining increased tissue length for self-stretching programs. Optimal parameters for numbers of repetitions, duration of stretch, and frequency have not been established through clinical trials.

MYOFASCIAL BALANCE

The integrity of the spinal column is dependent upon a balanced muscular system.[4,39] Shortening of the muscles or connective tissue structures that influence spinal function or stability may have an adverse influence on spinal mechanics and result in pathology and pain.[2,40-48] Often clinical practice has shown that the area of pain is not always the site of the primary lesion, and so we must be prepared to evaluate the entire motor system to determine an adequate stretching program.[9,44,49] There is an anatomical and biomechanical relationship between the muscles of the lumbar spine and the pelvis as well as the cervical spine and the shoulders. Muscular and fascial imbalances in one region can set up a chain reaction that may present as dysfunction in any part of the neuromuscular or osteoarticular systems. The imbalances that develop are probably a result of both reflex and mechanical mechanisms.[49]

Stretching Lower Quarter Muscles and Fascial Sheaths

Muscle imbalance is characterized by the development of impaired relationships between muscles prone to tightness and those prone to inhibition and weakness.[9,14,49] The loss of muscle extensibility in trunk, pelvic, lower extremity, and shoulder muscles combined with decreased spinal mobility have been associated with spinal dysfunction and impairment in functional activities.[16,22]

Some muscles of the lower quarter that tend to become shortened and subsequently alter posture and movement of the lumbo-pelvic complex are the iliopsoas, hamstrings, tensor fascia latae, piriformis, erector spinae, and quadratus lumborum.[9] Stretching shortened muscles to restore normal length can help decrease abnormal spinal stress and restore strength. Prior to normalizing muscle balance a thorough evaluation of the musculoskeletal system must be performed so that the factors that are causing or perpetuating the dysfunction can be identified. Length gains made by stretching shortened muscles may be temporary if modifications in posture and movement are not also addressed. Passive stretching of the patient's tight muscles by the therapist may be necessary before the patient is able to make significant gains in a home stretching program.

Iliopsoas. This two-headed muscle functions primarily to flex the hip. However, when the thigh is fixed the iliopsoas can act to flex the lumbar spine.[24,50,51] The vertebral portion of the psoas is believed to play a role in stabilizing the lumbar spine in upright postures,[46] and the iliopsoas muscle to be frequently shortened and hypertrophic in patients with spinal pain.[52] Manifestations of posture and dynamic function can vary depending upon the degree of tightness present and the portion of the muscle that has shortened. Kappler[52] believes that shortening of the vertebral portion of the psoas results in flexion of the upper lumbar spine motion segments with a loss of backward bending, which recruits the erector spinae muscles to contract in an attempt to create backward bending in the lower thoracic/upper lumbar region; instead, the motion occurs in the lumbo-sacral joint. Hypermobility with early degenerative changes in the three-joint complex at L5-S1 may result.[52] Stretching the iliopsoas can help restore upper lumbar mobility and so decrease over-use of the lumbo-sacral segment.

Others believe that bilateral shortness of the iliopsoas muscles may result in hyperextension of the lumbar spine, anterior pelvic tilt, and hip joint flexion.[51] Mechanical imbalances in the spine and pelvis may result from the development of hip flexor tightness. Loss of full passive hip extension may result in increased lumbar extension and more anterior pelvic tilting during the stance phase of gait and during static standing. This change in posture may decrease the mechanical efficiency of gait and may result in abnormal shearing and compressive loading to the lumbar spine. Stress may be imparted to the thoracic spine if the lordosis has extended into the lower thoracic segments.

Once such a pattern is found it becomes necessary to stretch the posterior spinal muscles and fascia as well as the iliopsoas muscles so that a normal pelvic alignment can be obtained before initiating strengthening exercises for trunk and pelvic girdle muscles.[25]

Gluteus Maximus. Electrical activity in the gluteus maximus muscle during active contraction is minimal when the hip is in extreme flexion.[48] The greatest gains in hip extensor strength have been shown to be attained when the hip is exercised in end-range hip extension.[39,45,48] Such a position cannot be achieved in the presence of tight hip flexors. Attempts to strengthen hip extensors might therefore result in over-use of the back extensors perpetuating tightness of the paraspinals.

Hamstrings. Tightness of the hamstring muscles can result in posterior tilting of the pelvis with a resultant decrease of the lumbar curvature.[51] The degree of posterior tilting may be dependent upon the range of hip flexion, which can be limited by tight hamstring muscles when the knees are extended.[47,53] Tight hamstrings can influence spinal loading in sitting as well as standing. With increased angles of backward tilting of the pelvis the posterior ligament tension and posterior muscle activity increase. Spinal compression loads may also increase. Restoring hamstring extensibility affects hip flexion range of motion. If hamstring length is normal[54] and full range of anterior pelvic rotation can occur the spinal posture will be minimally affected by knee extension during sitting.[47] Restoration of hamstring length may play a role in decreasing spinal stress when driving a car since driving requires a position of hip flexion and knee extension. If hip flexion is limited by hamstring tightness, placing the knee in extension can tilt the pelvis posteriorly, increasing spinal flexion and can theoretically increase compressive loading to the lumbar spine.

Quadratus Lumborum. This muscle serves to laterally flex the lumbar spine and provide lateral trunk stability along with the external oblique. Tightness limits lumbar sidebending to the contralateral side and may cause a compensatory thoraco-lumbar segmental motion increase as well as adversely affect pelvic mechanics. Stretching techniques that use gravity assistance are helpful in stretching the quadratus lumborum (see Fig. 15B.20).

Fascial Sheaths. Since the attachment of many muscles is from the deep surface of fascia, and since each muscle is invested by a fascial sheath, the fascia and muscles are treated together. Certain fascial specializations have been labeled "postural fascia" because they have thickened to provide additional tissue strength for spinal support as well as to perform motion that is initiated by muscular activity. Some of the important fascial sheaths that can become shortened along with postural muscles are the *lumbo-dorsal fascia,* the *iliotibial band of the fascia lata,* the *gluteal fascia* and the *cervical fascia.*[41] During weight bearing the tensor fasciae latae flexes, medially rotates, and abducts the hip.[51] It attaches to the iliac crest and to the tibia via the iliotibial band. The fascial investment of the tensor is continuous with the gluteus maximus muscle, and this common fascia blends in with the sacrotuberous ligament and attaches to the sacrum, coccyx, and iliac crest.[43] Loss of normal extensibility in the tensor fasciae latae can result in tension transmission to the pelvis and knee because of the fascial continuity. The extensive fascial sheaths with their multiple insertion sites may help explain why it is difficult to find only one self-stretching exercise that effectively increases tensor fasciae latae length.

Stretching Upper Quarter Muscles and Fascial Sheaths

Any alteration of the function of the lumbar spine, pelvis, and lower extremities will probably lead to the development of upper quarter dysfunction, especially of the head and neck.[9,44,49] Changes in head posture can lead to a series of neck and shoulder myofascial changes. Forward head posture occurs when the head and neck are displaced anterior to the body's line of gravity.[51] The occiput backward bends on the atlas creating shortening of the posterior suboccipital muscles and leading to a functional loss of mid-cervical motion as these segments become protracted.[55] The C7-T1 motion segment develops an increased anteroposterior angle as flexion is increased in the upper and mid-thoracic motion segments.

Increased flexion of the lower cervical and upper thoracic motion segments may result in increased tension in the cervical fascia and the posterior cervical extensors as they attempt to stabilize. Progressive alterations in the upper cervical and mid-cervical range of motion can result as length changes occur in the upper trapezius, levator scapulae, sternocleidomastoid, and pectoral muscles. The shoulder becomes protracted and elevated and the scapulae laterally rotate and abduct. As a result the plane of the glenoid fossa becomes more vertical and increased activity of the upper trapezius and levator scapulae muscles becomes necessary to maintain the head of the humerus in the glenoid fossa both during elevation of the arm and when the arm is hanging by the side of the body.[49] A vicious cycle can ensue that will not be broken until postural balance is restored to the neck-shoulder myofascial complex.

Myofascial asymmetries and tightness that result from a forward head posture may lead to joint imbalances at the sternocostal, costovertebral, and costotransverse joints. The combination of myofascial and joint restrictions could limit the participation of thoracic motion segments in trunk mobility and might predispose transitional areas of the spine such as the cervico-thoracic, thoraco-lumbar and lumbo-sacral regions to increased stress. Stretching exercises for rib cage expansion and thoracic spine mobility frequently are more beneficial if respiratory assist is incorporated into the stretching routine to assist with relaxation.

Flexion Versus Extension

Mobility of the spine contributes to general spinal health and mechanical efficiency. There are few controlled studies designed to determine the effectiveness of flexion versus extension exercises for regaining overall spinal mobility, reducing pain, and improving functional performance. Available studies are contradictory and inconclusive.[56–60] No parameters have been established to determine how much flexion and extension is necessary to provide good health and mechanical efficiency.[61]

Prospective studies have shown that lumbar spine flexion[54,62,63] and extension range of motion are poor predictors of spinal pain. Clinically, symptomatic relief of low back pain has been reported in patients who have undergone spinal flexibility training.[64,65] However, there is not a scientific foundation to support the premise that greater lumbar spine flexibility is associated with a decrease in the risk of developing back problems.[62]

Perhaps the results from the studies would be different if active spinal flexion and extension were examined more completely. There are three aspects of motion that should be addressed: range of motion, direction of motion and control of motion.[66] In addition, regional participation of all spinal segments should be evaluated.

If all these parameters were addressed for both flexion and extension, a pattern of range of motion limitations might be discovered that could help predict an individual's likelihood of developing low back pain at a future time. For example, two individuals might have equal ranges of lumbar spine flexion and extension, as measured by a tape measure or other spinal measuring device. However, while subject A has normal recruitment of thoracic spine and lumbar spine motion segments, subject B has moderate to severe restriction in motion from T3/4 through T9/10 and increased motion from T10/11 through

L5/S1. Subject B may be more predisposed to developing low back pain because of the abnormal mechanical stresses being impacted to the lumbar spine with all functional activities requiring trunk motion.[39] Gross range of motion measurements of the spine alone will not provide this information.

Several investigators attempted to determine which type of exercises were most effective for reducing pain and restoring mobility in patients identified with idiopathic low back pain.[56-60] As mentioned earlier, the results were contradictory and inconclusive. The patients were not chosen to participate in the study on the basis of a particular spinal posture. Nor was identification of restrictions in joint and soft tissue mobility made. All individuals were randomly assigned to treatment groups irregardless of spinal mechanics. Future studies should identify a particular postural dysfunction and assign these individuals to a randomly chosen exercise regime for more controlled and clinically applicable results. Exercise strategies must be based on an individual's biomechanical evaluation and determined motion needs. In addition, the execution of the exercises may have to be altered from patient to patient depending upon the degree of tightness present, the pathological condition of the spine, and the structure of the entire vertebral column, not just the area of dysfunction.

McKenzie reported positive results from a retrospective survey study of 318 patients treated for recurrent low back pain over a 10-year period of time. A home program of extension exercises and postural advice was given.[67] The gains in range of motion, functional status, and pain relief occurred in a high percentage of patients. They may have been due in part to the fact that evaluation disclosed a high percentage of patients who had a decreased lumbar lordosis when sitting due to a slump posture as well as an increase in pain.

Passive extension exercises help increase extensibility in shortened periarticular tissues and promote facet joint backward bending. McKenzie's extension program is designed to increase spinal motion in a direction that was found restricted during initial evaluation. Perhaps restoration of backward bending was partly responsible for reduction of pain. In healthy males during periods of decreased activity, Smith and Mill[68] found that extension-in-lying exercises performed for 2 minutes a day over 4 weeks helped decrease the likelihood of losing passive extension range of motion in the lumbar spine. They were compared to a control group not performing extension-in-lying exercises. In the literature, no studies were found that could document a significant increase in shortened posterior spinal myofascial extensibility with flexion exercises.[58]

Spinal Protection During Passive Stretching

Stretching exercises for the spine should be done in the safest and most effective way. One study[59] by Gracovetsky et al. found that controlling the amount of lordosis in the spine is an important factor in maintaining the distribution of movement between muscles and ligaments. That factor therefore influences the amount of compressive loading on the spine. Pelvic tilting exercises allow patients to adjust the amount of lordosis to the level of comfort, which can be utilized to keep lumbar spine forces minimal and evenly distributed. This study[59] reinforced previous findings[69] that a flexed intervertebral joint offers more resistance to compression. However, previous intervertebral disc studies by Nachemson[70] indicate that compression loading to the spine is increased in recumbent postures when active trunk or hip flexion or hip extension are initiated. Saul and Saul[71] have used the Gracovetsky idea[59] successfully in designing the flexibility portion of their rehabilitation program for patients with disc dysfunction. In order to decrease spinal stress the neutral pelvic position should be assumed and maintained while stretching extremity and most spinal myofascia. When exercises are designed to increase rotation and sidebending of different vertebral segments the neutral pelvic position is maintained to assure that the desired mobility is not compensated for by an increased lordosis in the lumbar spine. For example, when stretching the rectus femoris or the iliopsoas muscle the pelvis should remain in neutral so that the lumbar spine does not hyper-extend and substitute for the shortened hip flexors.

Care must be taken to assure that hypermobile joints and overstretched myofascia are not injured during active and passive stretching procedures. The patient must understand which part of the spine or extremity requires motion and in which area(s) stretching is contraindicated. For example, in performing McKenzie's extension-in-lying exercise, modifications can be made so that motion can be generated in different areas of the thoracic or lumbar spine. If the patient has increased mobility at L4-5 and L5-S1 but is restricted from T2-T12 in backward bending, the instructed exercises should minimize backward bending at the lower lumbar spine and increase motion through the thoracic segments. Modification can be achieved by altering hand position and increasing patient awareness of where and when the stretch has created motion in segments that move excessively (Fig. 15B.12).

Patients with restrictions in mid and upper thoracic rotation and tight anterior shoulder muscles can benefit from rotation stretching exercises. However, care must be taken to assure that motion is confined to the thoracic spine by having the patients bend their knees towards their chest to protect and minimize motion in the lumbar spine as they create a rotation stretch through the thoracic spine (Fig. 15B.5).

Studies have shown that intradiscal pressure is increased in sitting and forward bending from erect standing.[39,72] Patients who have probable disc disease should minimize time spent in flexed weight-bearing postures as much as possible. Hamstring extensibility exercises can be safely and effectively performed in two positions that will not create spinal flexion (Fig. 15B.21 and Figure 15B.22).

SUMMARY OF PART 15B

Muscle and connective tissue tightness can result in abnormal spinal stress distribution and in changes of spinal stability as well as alterations in movement patterns. Restoration of muscle and connective tissue extensibility can enable a person to begin functioning with a balanced myofascial system and thus help reduce abnormal spinal stress and reduce pain. Knowledge of individual muscle function in an abnormal as well as a normal state is necessary to determine which muscles are contributing to a patient's biomechanical imbalance so that appropriate stretching programs can be determined. Since myofascial dysfunction is closely associated with joint dysfunction, restoration of extensibility to myofascial structures will result in an improvement in joint mobility and so reduce the incidence of tissue irritation.[40,44,49]

Flexibility training has been recognized as an important first step in the reconditioning program of patients with spinal pain. Restoring muscle balance prepares the motor system for strengthening, endurance, and neuromotor reprogramming exercises.

RECOMMENDED EXERCISES ILLUSTRATED

The exercises in the series of figures (Figs. 15B.2–15B.34) have been chosen because of their clinical effectiveness. The exercises will be described for the different regions of the spine, for the upper extremities and lower extremities. Many of the stretching exercises can be enhanced by incorporating relaxation and movement awareness principles.

REFERENCES

1. Cady LD, Bischoff DP, O'Connell ER, Thomas PC, Allen JK. Strength and fitness and subsequent back injuries in firefighters. J Occup Med 1979; 21:269.
2. Williams P. Low back and neck pain: causes and conservative treatment. 3rd ed. Springfield: Charles C Thomas, 1974.
3. McKenzie R. The lumbar spine. 1st ed. Upper Hutt, NZ: Wright and Carmen Ltd., 1981.

4. Maitland GD. Mobilization of the spine. 3rd ed. New York: Churchill Livingstone, 1979.

5. Jull GA, Janda V. Muscles and motor control in low back pain: assessment and management. In: Twomey LT, Taylor JR, eds. Physical therapy of the low back. New York: Churchill Livingstone, 1987.

6. Kendall HO, Kendall FB, Boynten D. Posture and pain. Huntington, NY: Robert E. Kriegler, 1977.

7. Janda V. Muscles, central nervous motor regulation and back problems: 28–41. In: Korr IM, ed. The neurobiologic mechanisms in manipulative therapy. New York: Plenum, 1978.

8. Sahrmann S. A program for correction of muscular imbalance and mechanical imbalance. Clinical management in P.T. 1983; 3:21–28.

9. Farfan HF. Biomechanics of the lumbar spine. In: Kirkaldy-Willis WH, ed. Managing low back pain. 2nd ed. New York: Churchill Livingstone, 1988.

10. Travell JC, Simons DG. Myofascial pain and dysfunction—the trigger point manual. Baltimore: Williams & Wilkins, 1983.

11. Rosomoff HC. Comprehensive pain center approach to the treatment of low back pain. Low back pain. Report of the workshop NIDRR. Carron H, Wilson AB, eds. Grant # G00B300043. 1987; 77–85.

12. Kirkaldy-Willis WH. The pathology and pathogenesis of low back pain. In: Kirkaldy-Willis WH, ed. Managing low back pain, 2nd ed. New York: Churchill Livingstone, 1988.

13. Kirkaldy-Willis WH. The site and nature of the lesion. In: Kirkaldy-Willis WH, ed. Managing low back pain. 2nd ed. New York: Churchill Livingstone, 1988.

14. Lewitt K. Manipulative therapy in rehabilitation of the motor system. Boston: Butterworths, 1985; 256–257.

15. Wyke B. In: Jayson M, ed. The lumbar spine and back pain, 1st ed. New York: Grune and Stratton, Inc. 1976; 189–256.

16. Woo SL-Y, Buckwalter GE. Injury and repair of the musculoskeletal soft tissues. Park Ridge, IL: American Academy of Orthopedic Surgeons, 1987.

17. Gossman MR, Salumann SA, Rose ST. Review of length associated changes in muscle. Experimental evidence and clinical implications. Phys Ther 1986; 62:1799–1807.

18. Engles M. Tissue response. In: Donatelli LR, Wooden MJ, eds. Physical therapy. New York: Churchill Livingstone, 1989; 3–29.

19. Williams PE. Effect of intermittent stretch on immobilized muscle. Ann Rheum Dis 1988; 47:1014–1016.

20. John RJ, Wright U. Relative importance of various tissues in joint stiffness. J Appl Physiol 1962; 17:824–828.

21. Williams PE, Cantanere T, Lucey EG, Goedspinh G. The importance of stretch and contractile activity in prevention of connective tissue accumulation in muscle. J Anat 1988; 158:109–114.

22. Abrahams M. Mechanical behavior of tendon in vitro. A preliminary report. Med Biol Eng 1967(Sep); 5:433–443.

23. Stramberg D, Wiederhielm CA. Viscoelastic description of a collagenous tissue in simple elongation. J Appl Physiol 26:857–862.

24. Laban MM. Collagen tissue: implication of its response to stress in vitro. Arch Phys Med Rehabil 1962; 9:461–466.

25. Warren CG, Lehman JF, Koblanski JN. Elongation of rat tail tendon: effect of load and temperature. Arch Phys Med Rehabil 1971; 52:465–474.

26. Warren CG, Lehman JF, Koblanski JN. Heat and stretch procedures: an evaluation using rat tail tendon. Arch Phys Med Rehabil 1976; 57:122–126.

27. Casella C. Tensile force in total striated muscle, isolated fiber and sarcolemma. Acta Physiol Scand 1950; 21:380–401.

28. Stolov W, Weilepp TG, Riddell WM. Passive length-tension relationship and hydroxyproline content of chronically denervated skeletal muscle. Arch Phys Med Rehabil 1970; 51:517–525.

29. Stolov W, Weilipp TG. Passive length-tension relationship of intact muscle, epimysium, and tendon in normal and denervated gastrocnemius of rat. Arch Phys Med Rehabil 1966; 47:612–620.

30. Sady SP, Wortman M, Blanke MA. Flexibility training: ballistic, static or proprioceptive neuromuscular facilitation. Arch Phys Med Rehabil 1982; 63:261–263.

31. Tanigawa MC. Comparison of the hold-relax procedure and passive mobilization on increasing muscle length. Phys Ther 1972; 52:725–735.

32. Mediros J, Smide GL, Burmeister LF, Soderberg GL. The influence of isometric exercise and passive stretch on hip joint motion. Phys Ther 1977; 57:518–523.

33. Osternig LR, Robertson R, Travel R, Hainsen P. Muscle activation during proprioceptive neuromuscular facilitation (PNF) stretching techniques. Am J Phys Med 1987; 66:298–307.

34. Condon SM, Hutton RS. Soleus muscle electromyographic activity and ankle dorsiflexion range of motion during four stretching procedures. Phys Ther 1987; 67:24–30.

35. Schultz P. Flexibility: day of the static strength. Am J Sports Med 1979; 7:109–117.

36. deVries HA. Quantitative electromyographic investigation of the spasm theory of pain. Am J Phys Med 1966; 45:119–134.

37. deVries HA. Electromyographic observations of the effect of static stretching upon muscular distress. Residents Quarterly 1961; 32:468–479.

38. deVries HA. Evaluation of static stretching proce-

dures for improvement of flexibility. Residents Quarterly 1962; 33:222–229.

39. Nachemson A. Physiotherapy for low back pain patients. Scand J Rehabil Med 1969; 1:85–90.

40. Cathie AG. Considerations of fascia and its relation to disease of the musculoskeletal system: American Academy of Osteopathy—Year Book 1974; 85–88.

41. Cathie AG. The fascia of the body in relation to function and manipulative therapy. Unpublished.

42. Snyder G. Fasciae-applied anatomy and physiology. Academy of Applied Osteopathy Yearbook 1956; 65–75.

43. Becker FR. The meaning of fascia and fascial continuity. An Osteopathic Annals, New York: Insight Publishing Co. Inc., 1975.

44. Gustavson R. Training therapy: prophylaxis and rehabilitation. New York: Thieme Inc., 1985.

45. Farfan HF. The biomechanical advantage of lordosis and hip extension of upright activity. Man as compared with other anthropoids. Spine 1978; 3:336–340.

46. Nachemson A. The possible importance of the psoas muscle for stabilization of the lumbar spine. Acta Orthop Scand 1968; 39:47–57.

47. Stokes IA, Abery JM. Influence of the hamstring muscles on the lumbar spine curvature in sitting. Spine 1980; 5:225–528.

48. Fischer FJ, Houtz ST. Evaluation of the function of the gluteus maximus muscle. Am J Phys Med 1968; 17:182–191.

49. Janda V. Muscles and cervicogenic pain syndromes. In: Grant R, ed. Physical therapy of the cervical and thoracic spine. New York: Churchill Livingstone, 1988.

50. Bogduk N, Twomey L. Clinical anatomy of the lumbar spine. New York: Churchill Livingstone, 1987.

51. Kendall HO, Kendall FP, Wadsworth GE. Muscles, testing and function, 2nd ed. Baltimore: Williams & Wilkins, 1971.

52. Kappler RE. Lumbosacral instability and iliopsoas dysfunction. New York: Insight Publishing Co., Inc., 1981.

53. Troup JDC, Hood CA, Chapman AE. Measurement of the sagittal mobility of the lumbar spine and hips. Am J Phys Med 1968; 9:308–321.

54. Biering-Sorensen F. Physical measurements as risk indicators for low back trouble over a one year period. Spine 1983; 9:106–119.

55. Ayub E, Glasheen-Wray M, Kraus S. A case study of the effects of the rest position of the mandible. J Orthop Sports Phys Ther 1984; 5:179–183.

56. Davies JE, Gibson T, Tester L. The value of exercises in the treatment of low back pain. Rheum Rehabil 1979; 18:243–247.

57. Zylbergold RS, Piper MC: Lumbar disc disease: comparative analysis of physical therapy treatments. Arch Phys Med Rehabil 1981; 62:176–179.

58. Pante JD, Jensen GJ, Kent BE. A preliminary report on the use of the McKenzie Protocol versus Williams Protocol in the treatment of low back pain. J Orthop Sports Phys Ther 1984; 6:130–139.

59. Gracovetsky S, Kary M, Pitcher I, Levy B, Said RB. The importance of pelvic tilt in reducing compressive stress in the spine during flexion-extension exercises. Spine 1989; 14:412–416.

60. Kendall PH, Jenkins JM. Exercises for backache: a doubleblind controlled trial. Physiotherapy 1968; 54:154–157.

61. Jackson CP, Brown MD. Analysis of current approaches and a practical guide to prescription exercises. Clin Orthop 1983; 179:46–54.

62. Battie M, Bijos S, Fisher L, et al. The role of spinal flexibility in back pain complaints within industry. A prospective study. Spine 1990; 15:768–773.

63. Troup JDG, Foreman JK, Baxter CE, Brown D. The perception of back pain and the role of psychophysical tests of lifting capacity. Spine 1987; 12:645–657.

64. Mayer TG, Gatchel RJ, Kishino R, et al. Objective assessment of spine function following industrial injury. Spine 1985; 10:482.

65. Mellin G: Physical therapy for chronic low back pain: correlation between spinal mobility and treatment outcome. Scand J Rehabil Med 1985; 17:163–166.

66. Nyberg R. Spinal manipulation and the role of the physical therapist. In: Basmajian J, ed. Manipulation, massage and traction. Baltimore: Williams & Wilkins, 1983.

67. McKenzie RA: Prophylaxis in recurrent low back pain. New Zealand Med J 1979; 89:22–23.

68. Smith RL, Mell DB: Effects of prone spinal extension exercise on passive lumbar extension range of motion. Phys Ther 1987; 67:1517–1521.

69. Adams MA, Hutton WC. Prolapsed intervertebral disc: a hyperflexion injury. Spine 1982; 7:184–191.

70. Nachemson AL The lumbar spine, an orthopedic challenge. Spine 1976; 1:59.

71. Saal JA, Saal JS. Nonoperative treatment of herniated lumbar intervertebral disc with radiculopathy. An outcome study. Spine 1989; 14:431–437.

72. Nachemson AL. The load on lumbar discs in different positions of the body. Clin Orthop 1966; 45:107.

RECOMMENDED STRETCHING EXERCISES

Illustrations 15B.2–15B.34 by Mike Jackson, Riverdale, GA.

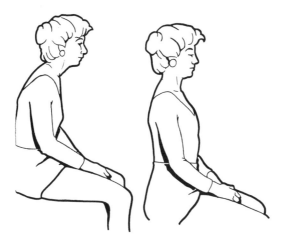

Figure 15B.2 Correcting a forward head posture/nodding

Purpose: 1) To decrease stress to your neck and low back
            2) Improve your spinal alignment and posture
            3) Improve ability to breathe through your diaphragm
            4) Increase mobility in upper cervical spine

Description: Correct trunk position by imagining a string pulling from your chest up and forward, at a 45 degree angle. Tuck your chin straight back, keeping eyes horizontal. Nod your head gently, feeling the stretch at the base of your skull.

Comments: Think tall and wide. Relax into the position with breathing.

         Reps: Sets: Time:

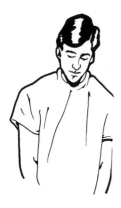

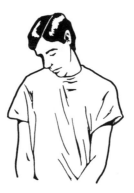

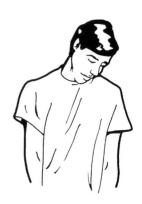

Figure 15B.3 Pit look.

Purpose: 1) To decrease neck and shoulder tension.
             2) To increase neck rotation

Description: Sitting or standing with a straight back and arms resting in lap. Drop head and neck slowly. Move in a forward direction, bringing chin as close to chest as possible. Repeat to the left and right, as if looking at the arm pit.

Comments: Slow, gentle, gravity assist movement. Breathe out at end of motion.

        Reps: Sets: Time:

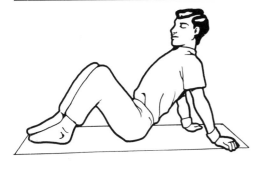

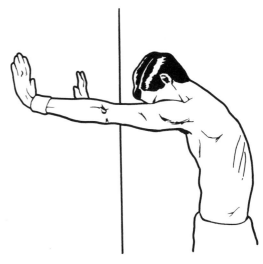

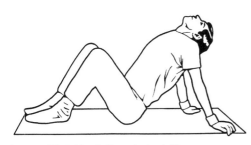

Figure 15B.4 Head tilt and chest lift.

Purpose: To increase neck and mid back mobility and improve posture.

Description: Sitting with knees bent and resting on hands, elbows straight. Your therapist will tell you which head position to use. Lift chest up towards ceiling at 45° angle.

Comments: Breathe in and out to increase the movement.

    Reps: Sets: Time:

Figure 15B.6 Back hunch.

Purpose: To increase movement in mid back, upper arms and neck.

Description: Stand 2–3 feet from a wall. Place hands on wall at shoulder height with elbows straight. Bend elbows and lean towards the wall. Push back from the wall until elbows are straight. Tuck chin to chest as far as you can. Then arch your mid-back.

Comments: Breathe in and out at end position and repeat. Do not raise your shoulders towards ears during the movement.

    Reps: Sets: Time:

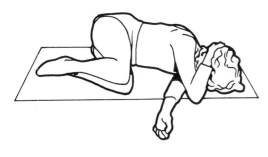

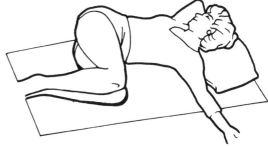

Figure 15B.5 Upper and mid back rotation stretch.

Purpose: 1) Increase mobility in upper and mid back
         2) Promote movement in chest and arm muscles

Description: Assume a sidelying position and bend knees as close to your chest as possible, to isolate motion to your mid and upper back. Place the hand of your upper arm behind your head. Rotate your arm and head back until you feel a comfortable stretch through your midback and chest. Stay in this position through one deep breath, feeling an increase in the movement as you exhale.

Comments: Reps: Sets: Time:

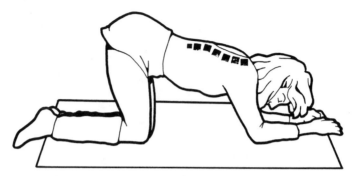

Figure 15B.7 Thoracic spine extension on all fours.

Purpose: To increase backward bending in upper back.

Description: Kneel while propping yourself on your forearms. Keep low
              back flat. Drop midback towards the floor. Return to start-
              ing position.

Comments: Use exhalation to assist with the movement.

      Reps: Sets: Time:

Figure 15B.8 Back straightener.

Purpose: To increase mid back movement and improve posture.

Description: Kneeling with forearms supported on a table and head resting
              on forearms. Let upper and midback sag down towards floor and
              then lift up.

Comments: Breathe out at end of each sag to increase the movement. Keep
              low back flat.

      Reps: Sets: Time:

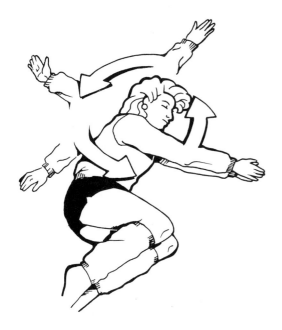

Figure 15B.9 Circumduction.

Purpose: 1) To promote relaxation and stretching of the neck and shoulder area
2) To stretch the mid and lower back muscles and joints

Description: Lie on your side, arms straight out in front of body. Slide the top hand forward, feeling a comfortable stretch. With hand in this position, slowly move top arm in a circle around your body. The head and trunk will rotate as your arm moves behind you.

Comments: Move slowly. Keep top arm relaxed. No discomfort should be felt.

      Reps: Sets: Time:

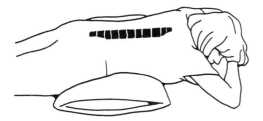

Figure 15B.10 Prone anterior pelvic tilt.

Purpose: 1) To increase mobility in the lower lumbar spine.
2) To coordinate lumbo pelvic motion.

Description: Lie on your stomach, with a pillow under your stomach. Tilt your pelvis forwards (towards the floor) and relax. Hip bones should stay in contact with the pillow as your low back arches.

Comments: Keep the amplitude of the motion within comfort. Tilt during the exhalation phase of your breathing.

      Reps: Sets: Time:

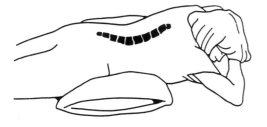

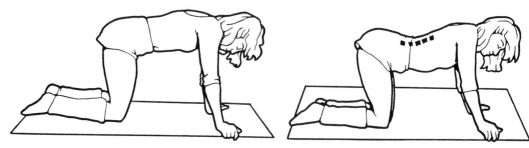

Figure 15B.11 Forward pelvic tilt on all fours.

Purpose: To increase low back backward bending

Description: Get on hands and knees with weight evenly distributed on all four limbs.
             Keep elbows straight.
             Tilt your pelvis toward the floor while sticking buttocks out, allowing your low back to sag.
             Resume the neutral position.

Comments: Use exhalation to assist with the motion.

             Reps: Sets: Time:

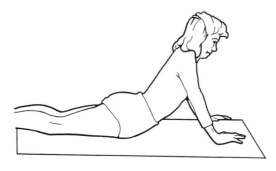

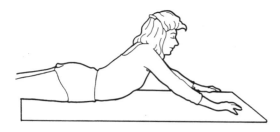

Figure 15B.12 Prone press up.

Purpose: 1) Increase backward bending in low back
          2) Reduce disc pressure

Description: Lie on stomach. Keep back and bottom muscles relaxed. Place hands at the position instructed by your therapist. Slowly push your trunk up with your arms. Stay in this position through one deep breath, feeling your back sag more as you exhale. Return to starting position.

Comments: 1) Concentrate on feeling the motion occurring in your upper and midback first and then moving into your low back. Be sure the involved area of your back is also moving.
           2) Hips should remain in contact with the floor as you push up.

             Reps.   Sets: Time:

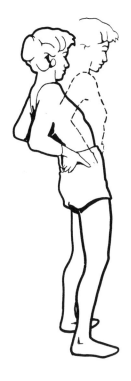

Figure 15B.13 Extension in standing.

Purpose: 1) Increase backward bending in the low back
2) Decrease disc pressure

Description: Stand with feet shoulder width apart. Place your hands in the small of your back to provide support. Shift your weight over your feet, letting your shoulders go back and your hips forward.

Comments: Keep the exercise passive. Don't force the backward motion by contracting your muscles.

Reps: Sets: Time:

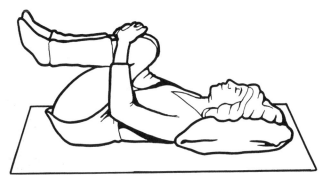

Figure 15B.14 Double knee to chest.

Purpose: 1) To increase abdominal strength.

Description: Do a pelvic tilt. Maintain the pelvic tilt as you slowly raise both knees to your chest. The abdominal muscles will be working to keep your low back flat.

Comments:

Reps: Sets: Time:

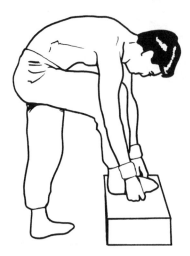

Figure 15B.15 Foot touch.

Purpose: To increase spinal flexion movement and hamstring length.

Description: Standing with one foot on stool or step. Slowly curl forward with arms in front so as to reach for foot on stool or step.

Comments: Slow, gentle, gravity assist motion.

    Reps: Sets: Time:

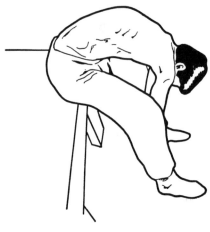

Figure 15B.16 Back curl.

Purpose: 1) To increase spinal flexion movement

Description: Sitting, legs apart and arms between legs, slowly bend head, neck and back forward with arms in front so as to reach for the floor.

Comments: Slow, gentle, gravity assist motion. Attempt to recruit movement at each vertebra in the spine. Exhale slowly at end of movement.

    Reps: Sets: Time:

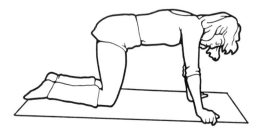

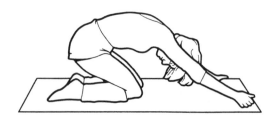

Figure 15B.17 Sphinx.

Purpose: To improve neck, trunk, and shoulder mobility

Description: From a hands and knee position with back straight, tuck chin down toward chest and slowly shift your weight back to your heels. Allow your back to round out. Return to starting position.

Comments: You will feel a comfortable stretch from your pelvis to your neck and through the shoulders. EXHALE as you sit back on your feet.

    Reps: Sets: Time:

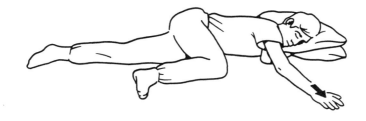

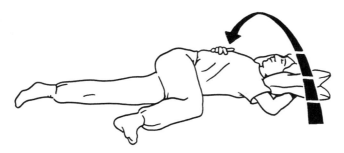

Figure 15B.18 Trunk rotation.

Purpose: 1) To increase spinal rotation range of motion.
             2) To stretch the muscles on the side of the hip.

Description: Lie on side with bottom leg straight and top leg flexed. The amount of top leg flexion determines where the spinal rotation occurs (for ex. when the leg flexes further the spinal rotation is felt higher up in the back). Slide upper arm forward along floor and then back across body while the head, shoulder and upper body also rotate back. Pause 1 or 2 full breaths in the rotated position to facilitate additional relaxation and further movement.

Comments: On the last repetition, hold rotated position for 30 to 60 seconds. Be sure to breath slowly to enhance muscle relaxation.

Reps: Sets: Time:

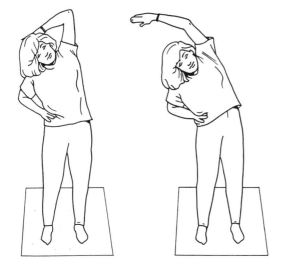

Figure 15B.19 Trunk side bending in stretching.

Purpose: 1) To increase extensibility in lateral trunk muscles.
             2) To help restore lumbo pelvic motion.

Description: Stand erect with feet shoulder width apart. Place your right hand on your hip and your left hand on the top of your head. Slowly side bend to the right while shifting your weight to the left. Feel for a stretch along your left side. Stay in this position through 1 deep breath and return to starting position. To stretch your right side reverse hand positions and directions.

Comments: Allow the opposite hip to move slightly sideways as you complete the side bending motion. Do not strain while you side bend.

Reps: Sets: Time:

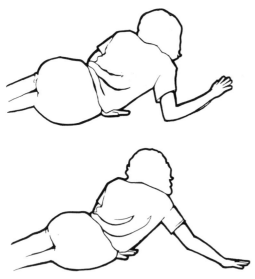

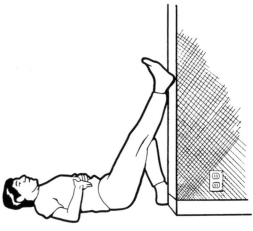

Figure 15B.21 Hamstring Stretch.

Purpose: To increase hamstring length

Description: Lie on your back with the leg to be
                      stretched propped on a door frame so
                      that you feel a comfortable stretch from
                      the buttock to the back of the knee. The
                      other leg may be bent or straight.

Comments: Use exhalation to assist with the stretch.
                      As you gain flexibility, place your heel
                      higher on the door frame. To vary the
                      stretch, rotate your foot inward and out-
                      ward as you hold the stretch.

                            Reps: Sets: Time:

Figure 15B.20 Quadratus lumborum stretch.

Purpose: 1) To lengthen the lateral trunk muscles.

Description: Lie on your right side with your knees
                      comfortably bent. Prop on your forearm,
                      elbow bent. Allow your trunk to "sag"
                      toward the floor. You should feel a com-
                      fortable stretch along the right side of
                      your trunk.

Comments: Remember to breathe, using exhalation
                      to assist with relaxation and stretch.

                            Reps: Sets: Time:

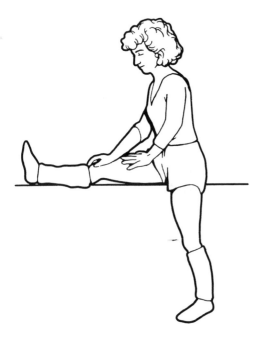

Figure 15B.22 Standing Hamstring Stretch.

Purpose: To increase hamstring length

Description: Place your heel on an object (stair,
                      chair) keeping your back and knee
                      straight, toes toward the ceiling, so that
                      you feel a comfortable stretch from the
                      buttock to the back of the knee. Repeat
                      with the opposite leg.

Comments: As your muscles lengthen, over time,
                      place the heel on a higher object. Use
                      exhalation to assist with the stretch.

                            Reps: Sets: Time:

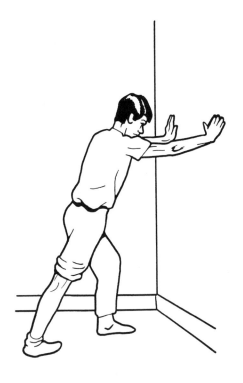

Figure 15B.23 Heel cord stretch.

Purpose: Lengthen calf muscles

Description: Stand with one leg in front of the other
                  and toes straight ahead. Shift weight
                  onto front leg by flexing knee while
                  keeping the back knee straight and the
                  heel of your back foot in contact with
                  the ground.

Comments: Keep back foot pointed straight ahead
                  or slightly turned so you feel the weight
                  on the outside of the foot. Repeat the
                  procedure with your knee slightly bent
                  to lengthen the calf muscle in the lower
                  part of your calf.

                  Reps: Sets: Time:

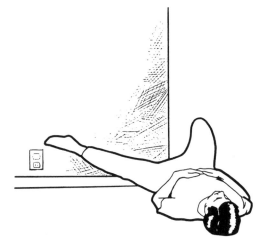

Figure 15B.24 Inner thigh stretch.

Purpose: To lengthen inner thigh muscles

Description: Lie on your back at a door jam. Bend
                  the hip and knee of the leg facing the
                  free corner and place the opposite heel
                  on the wall, keeping your knee straight.
                  Allow the straightened leg to slide
                  down the wall until you feel a stretch in
                  your inner thigh and groin.

Comments: As you stretch out you should be able
                  to move your bottom closer to the wall.

                  Reps: Sets: Time:

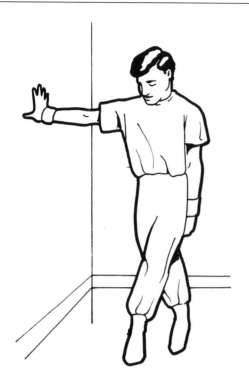

Figure 15B.25 Tensor stretch.

Purpose: To stretch muscles on outside of thigh

Description: Cross leg nearest the wall behind other
                leg. Lean hips in towards the wall until
                a stretch is felt on the outside of the hip
                and thigh.

Comments:

                Reps: Sets: Time:

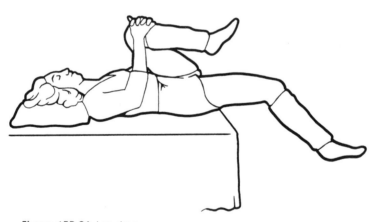

Figure 15B.26 Leg drop.

Purpose: 1) Lengthen muscles in front of hip and thigh
          2) Correct pelvic imbalance

Description: Lie on your back with your hips at the edge of a table.
              Hold _____ knee to your chest.
              Drop _____ leg gently towards the floor.
              Keep your low back flat.
              Hold position for _____.

Comments:

                Reps: Sets: Time:

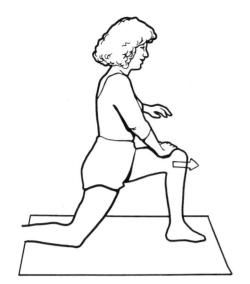

Figure 15B.27 Lunge.

Purpose: To stretch the muscles in the front of the hip and groin.

Description: Kneel on one knee. Shift weight forward onto front foot making sure back remains straight.

Comments: A stretch should be felt in front of the hip and thigh of the back leg.

Reps: Sets: Time:

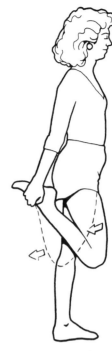

Figure 15B.28 Standing quadriceps stretch.

Purpose: Stretch muscles in the front of the thigh

Description: Stand beside a table or chair and hold on with one hand for balance. Bend the opposite knee and hold the ankle with your free hand. Pull ankle up towards your bottom until you feel a stretch in the front of your thigh.

Comments: Keep your pelvis level and your back flat.

Reps: Sets: Time:

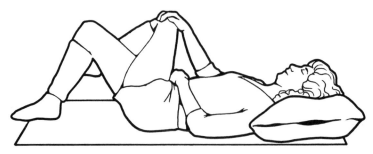

Figure 15B.29 Buttock stretch.

Purpose: To promote motion of the buttock muscles in order to increase hip mobility.

Description: Cross your LEFT leg over your RIGHT leg grasping left knee with your RIGHT hand. Move your LEFT
              knee towards the right shoulder with your RIGHT arm. Repeat to the opposite direction for the
              opposite leg.

Comments: The leg that is not being stretched may be straight rather than bent. You will feel a comfortable
              stretch deep in the buttock. Take up the slack as the muscles relax during EXHALATION. Be sure
              to keep your trunk on the floor.

              Reps: Sets: Time:

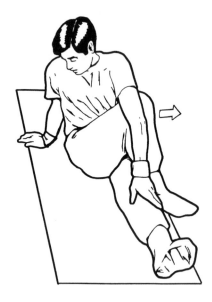

Figure 15B.30 Trunk twist.

Purpose: To relax and stretch the muscles on the
              outside of the hip and thigh.

Description: To exercise the RIGHT side:
              Sit on the floor with your RIGHT leg
              crossed over the LEFT leg. Place LEFT
              elbow on the outside of the RIGHT knee.
              While looking toward your RIGHT hand,
              slowly move your bent leg with your arm
              to the LEFT until you feel a mild stretch
              along buttock, hip, and outside of the
              RIGHT thigh. Repeat with the opposite
              leg.

Comments: EXHALE as you stretch and take up the
              slack as the muscles relax.

              Reps: Sets: Time:

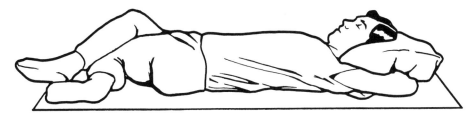

Figure 15B.31 Knee drop.

Purpose: 1) To relax and stretch muscles along the outside of the hip and lower back
          2) To increase lower back rotation

Description: To exercise the LEFT side:
          Lie on your back with your RIGHT knee crossed over the LEFT. Keeping your shoulder blades on
          the floor, slowly drop your legs to the RIGHT until you feel a mild stretch along the LEFT side of
          the lower back and hip. Hold. Return to the starting position. Repeat to the opposite side with
          the LEFT knee over the RIGHT.

Comments: EXHALE to assist with the stretch.

          Reps: Sets: Time:

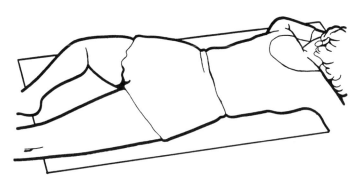

Figure 15B.32 Frog leg exercise.

Purpose: 1) To lengthen the muscles in the inside and front of the thigh and hip.
          2) To improve low back sidebending

Description: Lie on your stomach. Place the bottom of one foot flat against the inside of the calf of the opposite
          leg. Slide knee up and out to the side. Return to starting position.

Comments: Reps: Sets: Time:

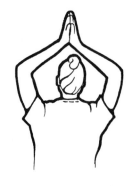

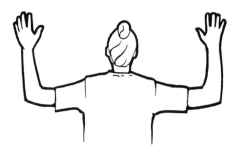

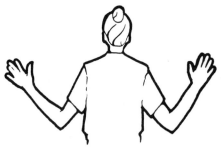

Figure 15B.33 Pull downs.

Purpose: 1) Lengthen muscles in the front of the chest.
          2) Improve control of the shoulder blade stabilizers.
          3) Improve posture.

Description: Start with arms overhead, palms together keep a 90 degree angle between arm and elbow. Bring arms down and back as if trying to place your elbows into your back pockets.

       Reps: Sets: Time:

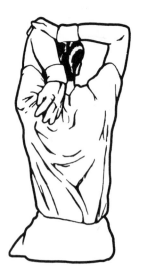

Figure 15B.34 Arm stretch.

Purpose: To stretch the back of the arm.

Description: Sitting or standing with back straight. One hand reaches behind same shoulder and the other is placed on the elbow. Push elbow back slowly and gently.

Comments: Breathe into the stretch. Do not let low back arch.

       Reps: Sets: Time:

PART C.
STRENGTH TRAINING

ROLE OF STRENGTH TRAINING

The rehabilitation process post injury and post healing includes re-establishment of: a) normal joint motion and soft issue extensibility, b) normal strength and control, and c) cardiovascular fitness. This section will address the role of strengthening in the management of the spinal pain patient.

Exercise instruction has been an integral part of rehabilitation of the spinal pain patient, and its importance in the management of patients with spinal motion dysfunction is well documented.[1-5] However, few controlled experimental studies have been published that substantiate the efficacy of strengthening exercises prescribed historically for the spinal pain patient.[6,7] In a study by Mayer et al.,[8] objective functional capacity techniques were employed to evaluate the effectiveness of a functional restoration program in which 66 patients with chronic pain were treated and the results were compared to 38 controls who had not undergone the treatment. Follow-up evaluations were performed at 3 and 6 months post initial evaluation and a telephone survey at 1 year post. Approximately 80% of the patients had improved functional capacity measurements at the follow-up visits. The treatment group had twice the rate of return to work as compared to the comparison group. Additional studies that document treatment outcomes for various spinal rehabilitation programs are necessary.[9]

Studies comparing subjects with low back pain to normal subjects reveal differences in trunk strength between the two groups.[9-11] A study of 286 chronic low back pain patients were compared to normals when isokinetic flexion and extension were evaluated. Torque values were lower in both flexion and extension, with extension loss being greater than flexion loss. Mayer[10] concluded that strength deficits are a major factor in the deconditioning syndrome. Trunk strength was reduced in subjects with low pack pain or sciatica when compared to healthy controls.[12] Comparison of abdominal and back strength between normals and patients who had undergone discectomy revealed a 30% reduction in isokinetic and isometric trunk extensor and isokinetic flexor torque when tested at 4–6 weeks postoperatively and 11–23 months postoperatively.[9] Although few studies have evaluated the results of a spinal strengthening program, evidence is available to support the difference in strength between patients and healthy controls, and thus a need to instruct in an appropriate strengthening program exists.

Strength is defined as the ability of a muscle to produce force.[13,14] Muscular strength is increased most effectively through voluntary maximal contractions.[15] A strengthening program operates on three principles: overload, gradual progression of exercise, and specificity.[14,16,17] In order for the muscle to gain strength it must be overloaded. In other words, the muscle must be worked at a near maximal to maximal resistance.[13,15,17] The mechanism can be challenged by increasing the range of motion, resistance, repetitions or sets, rate of work or exertion, duration of work, or activity.[14] Gradual progression of the exercise routine allows for comfortable and safe strength gains.[16]

The therapist must take into account the current level of fitness of the patient, the injured tissue, the stage of healing, and the goals of the strengthening program. Strengthening considerations for the athlete who presents with a lumbosacral strain will be different from the program established for the deconditioned individual presenting with a lumbar disc bulge.

Specificity

Specificity of exercise initially involves performance of exercise to accomplish short term goals, for example, partial sit-up instruction to increase oblique abdominal strength in the first 30° of trunk flexion. Specificity also includes instruction in strengthening tasks designed to mimic the activity that the patient will be required to perform in daily life.[17–19] Before the spinal pain patient returns to lifting tasks, for instance, simulation and practice of the task should occur under the supervision of the therapist.

TYPES OF STRENGTH TRAINING

The classical types of strength training include isometric, isotonic, and isokinetic. Isodynamic and isoinertial will also be discussed.

Isometric

An isometric contraction occurs against an immovable object, and the muscle maintains a constant length.[15,20] Because there is little or no joint movement during isometric strengthening, this static strengthening may be appropriate when pain or the injury limits the joint range of motion. Isometric-type strengthening lends itself well to the initial stage of strengthening post injury.[13,15–17,20,21] However, caution is suggested in the use of isometrics in individuals with acute or settled disc involvement because of the concurrent rise in intradiscal pressure[4,22] or in individuals exhibiting joint hypermobility, particularly in the cervical region. Olaf Evenjth[23] suggests that isometric contraction in the cervical region promotes further increases in motion at the excessively mobile segments. Isometric exercise, in the presence of lumbar or thoracic hypermobilities has not been shown to increase ligamentous irritability.

When using isometrics, remember that strength gains are specific to the joint angle at which the exercise is being performed.[13,15–17,20,21] *Advantages* to isometric training include: prevention of muscle atrophy, stimulation of mechanoreceptors, increased circulation to the muscle, thereby facilitating healing and edema control, reduced potential for joint or ligamentous irritability (except in the cervical spine), promotion of strength, and few equipment requirements. *Disadvantages* include: promotion of strength only at specific joint angles, increased lumbar intradiscal pressure,[4,22] inability to produce concentric or eccentric contractions, and the potential for

increased blood pressure when contractions are held for more than 6 seconds or when rest periods are shorter than 20 seconds.[13,16,21]

"BRIME" (Brief Repetitive Isometric Maximal Exercise). This protocol requires a 6-second maximum isometric followed by a 20-second rest, 20 times per day.[16] Another suggests several sets of 3–6 second maximal contractions at least three times per week.[15] 75% to 100% contractions held for 2–8 seconds, for 6–8 repetitions, with 2–3 minutes between contractions has also been suggested.[17]

Isotonic

Isotonic is classically defined as meaning "constant tension," but use of free weights or weight training equipment does not result in constant tension exerted by a muscle.[15] Isotonic has also been referred to as meaning "fixed resistance" and was first introduced by DeLorme through progressive resistive exercise (PRE) prescription.[14,16] Isotonic exercise can be achieved with free weights (barbells, cuff weights, water jugs, etc.) or with variable resistance equipment as seen in hydraulic systems (*Hydra-Gym*—Hydra Fitness, Belton, Texas) and machine weights (Nautilus; Deland Florida; Eagle—Cybex, Ronkonkoma, NY; Universal—Cedar Rapids, Iowa). Many forms of proprioceptive neuromuscular facilitation (PNF), the subject of Chapter 11, involve isotonic exercise.[17]

Isotonic exercise can be further divided into *concentric* or a shortening muscle contraction, and *eccentric* or a lengthening muscle contraction.[15–17,20] Eccentric isotonics generate more tension than concentric isotonics or isometrics.[21] There exists controversy over whether the strength gains are greater with eccentric strengthening or concentric strengthening[15], but an individual requires less effort to accomplish an eccentric contraction.[15,21] Eccentric work may be given before initiating concentric strengthening because it is easier to perform.[21] Eccentric work is necessary prior to the completion of the rehabilitation process to accommodate for ADL activity. Descending stairs, lowering to sit from stand, and bending forward are a few examples of activities requiring a lengthening contraction. In the spinal pain patient, 'step-ups' (Fig. 15C.1) are recommended for progression of quadriceps and gluteal eccentric and concentric control.

Advantages of isotonic strengthening include: strength gains through the entire range of motion, ability to produce concentric and eccentric loading, and improved muscular endurance.[16,21] A *disadvantage* of eccentric exercise is residual soreness.[15,16,21] With isotonic strengthening the muscle is loaded most at the weakest point in the range, and the amount of weight lifted is limited by the amount that can be held at that point in the range. The muscle is never working at its maximum potential except at the weakest point in the range. Variable resistance machines, Nautilus for example, accommodate to that point in the range through a cam mechanism to avoid maximally loading the muscle at the weakest position in the range of motion. Traumatic synovitis may occur secondary to excessive joint loading. Patient safety is a factor because isotonics do not accommodate to pain or fatigue.[21]

Protocols. Isotonic strengthening protocol varies somewhat from author to author, but the general consensus advocates working out 3 days per week,[15–17] performing 3–4 sets of 10–12 repetitions,[14,16] with 5–10 minutes between sets.[17] Performance at 50% max, 75% max, and 100% is suggested by Delorme and others.[14,16] A final suggestion to maximize eccentric benefits includes lifting to a count of 3, holding for 2 seconds, and lowering for a count of 4.[14] Some of the recommendations in this section of the chapter will be based on isotonic protocol. However, modification for each patient relative to previous level of fitness, fatigue, gradual progression, etc. needs to be considered.

Inertial Exercise. Developed by bioengineer William McLeod and Steve Davison, Ph.D., this is similar to isotonic exercise in that it allows for concentric and eccentric muscle contraction. However, one author reports that it develops coordination, not strength.[24] Inertial exercise provides a means of improving control over a given mass. Inertial exercise involves acceleration and deceleration of a mass through reciprocally pulling a line along a horizontal track (Fig. 15C.2). The *Impulse Inertial Exercise System* (IMPULSE—E.M.A., P.O. Box 2312, Newnan, GA 30264) allows for 2 variables of control, resistance and frequency.[24] Functional activities can be developed through the use of the IMPULSE.[24,25] The IMPULSE appears to be most beneficial at the end stages of rehabilitation to maximize control over a golf swing, tennis stroke, casting maneuver, or PNF pattern in order to accomplish painfree controlled movements (Figs. 15C.3–15C.6).

Suggested protocol involves movement of 17½ pounds through a 24-inch path (12 inches on either side of midline) accomplishing 30 repetitions in approximately one minute. Once the task is accomplished, the weight of the mass is gradually reduced allowing for

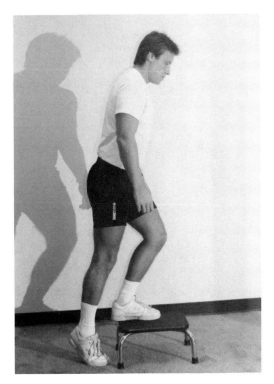

Figure 15C.1. Step-ups.

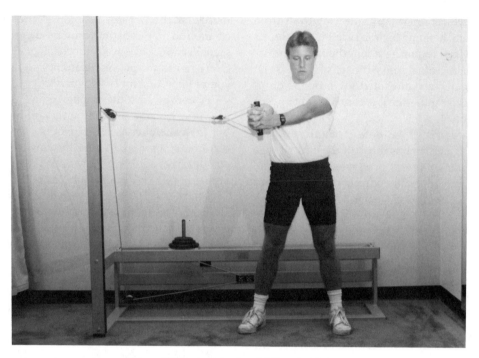

Figure 15C.2. Impulse Inertial Exercise System.

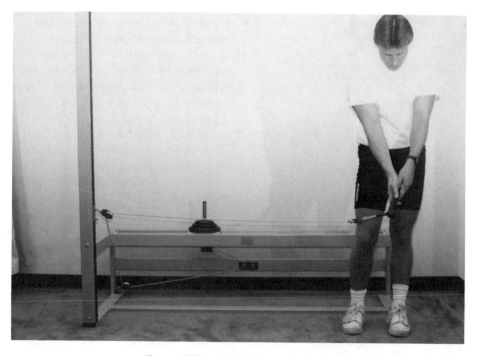

Figure 15C.3. IMPULSE for golf swing.

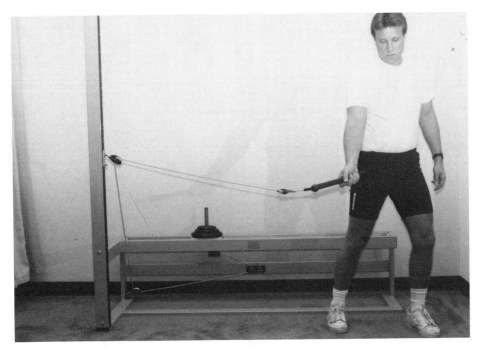

Figure 15C.4. Tennis stroke, etc.

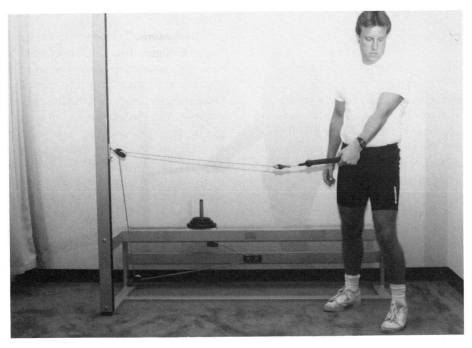

Figure 15C.5. Tennis stroke, etc.

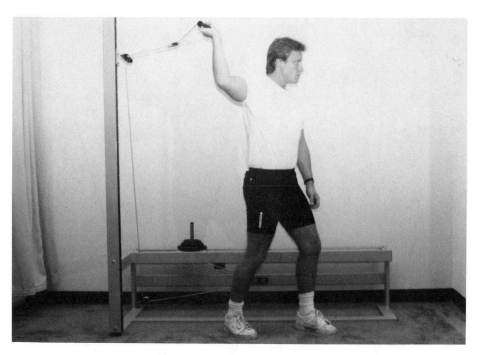

Figure 15C.6. Tennis stroke, etc.

greater control of acceleration and deceleration.[25]

Isokinetic

Isokinetic strengthening was introduced in the 60s.[26] Exercise is performed at a fixed speed and resistance is variable, accommodating to the patient through the range of motion.[21] *Advantages* include: maximal dynamic loading of the muscle through the range (unlike isotonic), patient safety because the resistance matches patient output, specificity of exercise through velocity training, accommodation to fatigue and pain, decreased joint compressive forces at high speeds, overflow of strength gains at faster speeds to slower speeds, and minimal post-exercise soreness (except in units with eccentric capabilities).[15,21] *Disadvantages* include: equipment expense, time, and space. In addition, trunk movement is not isokinetic because the trunk accelerates and decelerates throughout the path of motion; therefore, the existing

isokinetic dynamometers may not be ideal for task simulation and assessment of trunk performance.[26,28]

"Isodynamic." This term was coined by Isotechnologies Inc. (Hillsborough, NC) to describe a computer-controlled triaxial spinal dynamometer that provides constant resistance independently in 3 cardinal planes. Isodynamic refers to a combination of initial isometric type exercise that the subject must overcome while moving against a constant resistance. The *Isostation B200* (Isotechnologies Inc.) measures torque, angular position and velocity of the trunk in 3 planes simultaneously (Fig. 15C.7). The speed, and therefore the acceleration and deceleration, is under control of the subject allowing for realistic reproduction and assessment of trunk movement. Information is recorded from 3 axes simultaneously as described in Chapter 7.[26,27] *Disadvantages* of both the B200 and isokinetic trunk devices include expense of equipment, time and space for set up, and inability of each device to allow lower extrem-

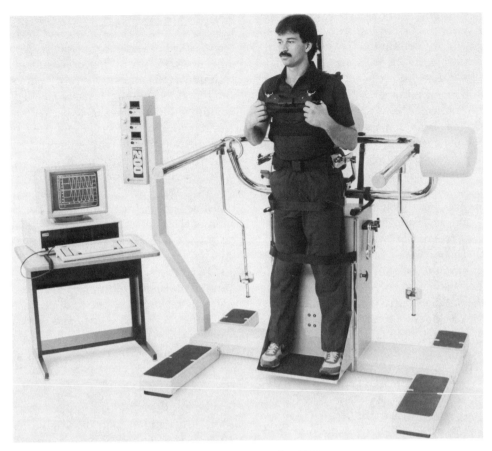

Figure 15C.7. Isostation B200.

ity involvement to totally simulate an actual lifting task.

Advantages of Spinal Dynamometers. These include the ability to collect and store objective measures relating to trunk performance, establishment of normative data, ability to measure and monitor progress, and the ability to assist in establishment of rehabilitation goals. Computer software packages and protocols vary among clinicians. One protocol is typical to the isotonic protocol with the exception that the individual is not exercised at 100% maximum output dynamically. Dynamic strengthening is performed at 25%, 50%, and 75% of the maximal isometric value achieved. Retesting takes place every 4–6 weeks.

PRACTICAL APPLICATIONS AND RATIONALE

The methods and specific exercises in the foregoing review of current strengthening approaches sets the stage for a discussion of their applications to spinal regions. First, the concept of muscle imbalance is presented. Exercise prescription relates, in part, to the presence of typical patterns of muscle imbalance seen in the cervicothoracic and lumbopelvic regions.

Deconditioning and Muscle Imbalance

Rest and reduction of activity is the initial treatment most commonly prescribed by physicians for low back pain.[29] Joint immobility,

muscle atrophy, weakness, fatigue, and reduced cardiovascular fitness are often the consequences of prolonged musculoskeletal
disuse following bedrest or immobilization.[18,19,30] The "disuse syndrome"[30] or "deconditioning syndrome"[18,19] describe the effects of disuse on the musculoskeletal system.
Muscle imbalance and altered muscle activity
are components of the deconditioning syndrome[18,19] and are seen following spinal injury.[31,32] Sahrmann defines muscle imbalance
as "faulty static and/or dynamic properties of
muscle that alter the equipoise between antagonists and synergists and thus disrupts alignment and the quality with which a segment
rotates about its axis."[33] Postural dysfunction
may result in muscle imbalance secondary to
adaptive tissue shortness and accompanying
weakness. According to Janda,[32–34] muscle imbalance describes the situation in which some
muscles become tight and others weak in response to postural demands, pain, or pathology. He compares the presence of a typical
muscle pattern to that of capsular patterns
seen in synovial joints as described by Cyriax.
Generally, the muscles that become tight are
postural in nature. Those that become weak
are antagonistic to the tightened mus-
cles.[31,32,34] Gustavsen[35] reports that extensors
generally become tight and flexors weak.

Altered recruitment patterns and muscle
weakness in the presence of muscle imbalance
have been described by several authors.[5,31–38]
Faulty movement patterns reduce the efficiency and effectiveness of limb or spinal motion[33] and can perpetuate abnormal stresses
on the neuromuscular system spine leading to
further impairment.[31–34]

Stages. Strengthening of weakened muscles is accomplished through several stages.
Initially, the exercise given must achieve activation of the correct muscle. Exercise that
is performed vigorously or against excessive
resistance may result in an incorrect compensatory motion performed by substituting musculature. An example is noted when asking a
patient to perform a sit-up. An uncontrolled
sit-up against gravity may result in contraction of the iliopsoas rather than the expected

abdominals. Initially the emphasis must be
placed on the quality and control of the movement, avoiding fatigue and faulty patterns.
The use of PNF or functional integration
techniques starting in a gravity-eliminated
and supportive position is recommended. Operating within a comfortable partial (or protected) range of motion is suggested before
movement in the full range of motion. As the
patient is able to perform the pattern correctly, exercise positions can be progressively
less supportive and against greater gravitational demands. Progression of an exercise to
additional repetitions or sets is dependent also
on patient fatigue, activation of the correct
muscles, and change in symptoms.

Once correct movement patterns have
been established, additional strengthening
concerns relate to specificity of exercise and
return to previous activities and work environments. Job simulation and trunk performance testing/strengthening is suggested
here.

Regional Options

The following paragraphs will discuss
strengthening options from a regional perspective mentioning typical patterns of muscle
imbalance secondary to postural stresses, frequent patterns of injury and considerations,
brief evaluation methods, and strengthening
suggestions. In an effort to combine all regions, lifting considerations will also be discussed.

Cervical, Upper through Midthoracic
and Shoulder Girdle Regions

These regions are functionally inter-related.
Clinically, injury to one area often affects
the functional abilities of the other areas.
Janda[32–34] describes a muscle imbalance pattern seen typically in the head-shoulder region. The "proximal or shoulder crossed syndrome" describes a situation in which an
imbalance exists between the tight an shortened levator scapulae, upper trapezius, and
pectoralis group and weak lower stabilizers
of the scapula and deep neck flexors

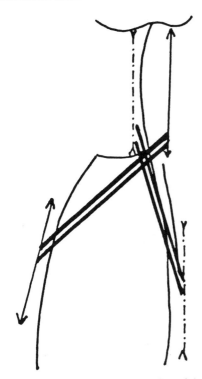

Figure 15C.8. Schematic representation of the proximal crossed syndrome. The thick lines connect shortened and weakened muscles. The short, tight muscles are the levator scapulae, upper trapezius, and pectorals; the weak muscles are the deep neck flexors and lower stabilizers of the scapula. With permission from: Janda V. Muscles and cervicogenic pain syndromes. In: Grant R, ed. Physical therapy of the cervical and thoracic spine. New York: Churchill Livingstone 1988; 153–166.

(Fig. 15C.8).[32,34] A moderate forward head, scapular elevation, winging and abduction, rounded shoulders and increased kyphosis of the upper thoracic segments are seen.[32,36] This patient presents with restricted occipito-atlantoid forward bending and moderately shortened sub-occipital muscles. Excessive mobility and ligamentous irritation at the low mid-cervical or cervicothoracic junction may be seen. Shortened sternocleidomastoid (SCM), scalene and pectoral muscles are often present. Increased upper trapezius tone and tightness is common. Scapular protraction and reduced upper-mid thoracic soft-tissue and joint mobility is noted. Movement patterns of the shoulder are often affected, leading to potential overuse and strain.[36] Clinically, overuse of the upper trapezius during upper extremity elevation and reduced strength/control of the rotator cuff muscles is frequently observed.

Evaluation of strength and proper muscle recruitment has been recommended by Janda for evaluation of the cervico-thoracic region.[31,32] Three movements are tested: flexion of the head on the neck in supine, prone push-up, and shoulder abduction.

Tests and Progression of Exercises

In the first test, in the presence of weak pre-vertebral cervical flexors, an overactive SCM will produce forward jutting of the jaw. Figure 15C.9 demonstrates normal head-on-neck flexion and Fig. 15C.10 depicts SCM overuse.

Gradual strengthening of the neck flexors will be required to restore normal function.[32,38] Gradual strengthening of the cervical flexors can begin provided a position of comfort can be found as well as a position that allows the pre-vertebral flexors to contract without overuse of the SCM. A gravity-eliminated or gravity-assist position such as sitting or sidelying works well initially. Progression through a partial controllable range with emphasis on cardinal plane flexion and diagonal flexion is suggested. Repetition is determined by fatigue; as the individual fatigues, increased firing of the SCM will be noted. Eventually, the patient can be progressed to a supine position and will be able to move through the full range of motion (Figs. 15C.11, 15C.12).

Progressive strengthening of the cervical flexors is consistent with the PNF approach and can be found in Chapter 11. Rocabado discusses the presence of weak posterior sub-occipital muscles in the presence of suprahyoid tightness, and suggests gradual short-arc strengthening of the cervical extensors to accomplish axial extension.[39] Assumption of an all fours or prone prop position with the head and neck held in neutral with gradual increase in "hold" time to 2 minutes is beneficial at the end stage of rehabilitation

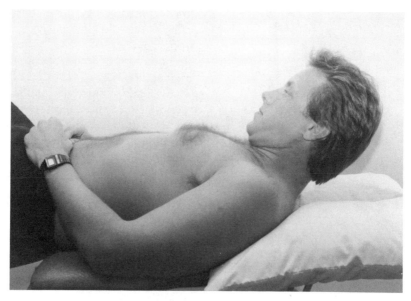

Figure 15C.9. Normal head-on-neck flexion.

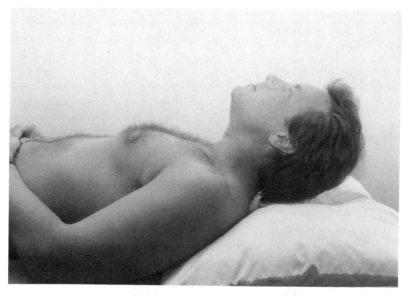

Figure 15C.10. Sternocleidomastoid overuse.

(Chapter 11). Caution is advised against the use of other types of isometric exercise in the cervicothoracic region as isometric loading potentially increased ligamentous stress and irritability at a hypermobile segment.[23] Awareness of correct movement planning and execution is important when performing cer-

vical flexor diagonal strengthening in the individual with ligamentous laxity at the cervicothoracic junction as "fulcrumming" and additional irritation can occur. The same caution must be exercised in individuals with known disc involvement or radiculopathy.

Scapula and Shoulder Girdle. Informa-

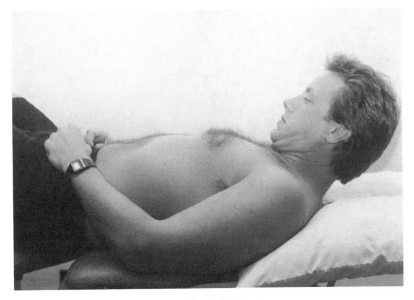

Figure 15C.11. Full flexion.

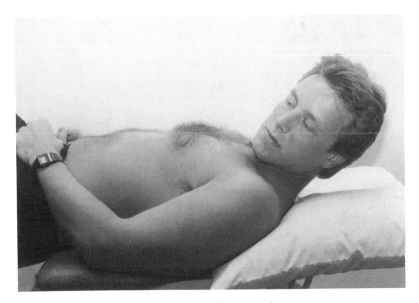

Figure 15C.12. Flexion-rotation.

tion about the stabilization capacity of the scapula is gained from the prone push up (Fig. 15C.13). Winging of the scapula can be seen at the completion of the up phase or initial phase of lowering on the side of impairment (Fig. 15C.14). Strengthening of the serratus anterior, rhomboids, lower trapezius and la-

tissimus dorsi is suggested to regain control of the involved scapula.[31,36,38]

Scapular stabilization ability and shoulder girdle function can also be assessed through elevation of shoulder abduction and repetitive scapular elevation and lowering. Janda[32] discusses a "firing pattern" seen with shoulder

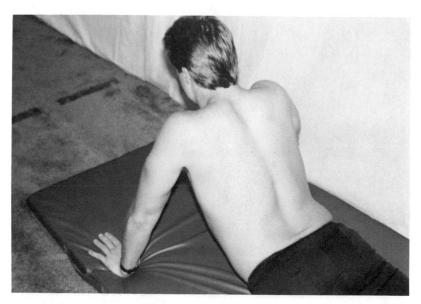

Figure 15C.13. Prone push-up.

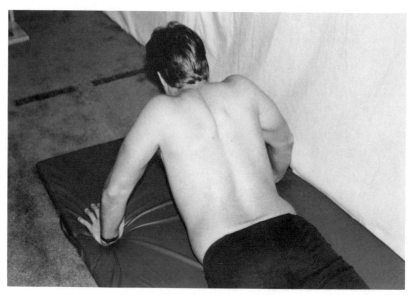

Figure 15C.14. Scapular winging.

abduction. During the initial 5° of scapular abduction, scapular fixation secondary to the contraction of the middle and lower trapezius muscles should be noted followed by contraction of the supraspinatus and deltoid, followed by contraction of the upper trapezius and levator scapula. EMG studies do not seem to agree on a consistent firing pattern for shoulder abduction.[40,41] Clinically, muscle imbalance in this region can be seen with performance of shoulder abduction; watching for initial stabilization of the scapula against the thoracic cage followed by smooth scapular rotation, slight protraction, and elevation of the humerus. One is reminded to pay attention to the normal scapulohumeral rhythm. Increased upper trapezius activity and irregular scapular motion is seen with imbalance. Finally, through observation of shoulder elevation and lowering, eccentric and concentric control of the scapular elevators can be monitored (Fig. 15C.15). With imbalance, a jerky motion, overuse of the trapezius, and scapular winging will be seen particularly during lowering of the scapula suggesting weakness of the scapular stabilizers.

Regaining scapulothoracic and glenohumeral control and strength is accomplished first through a functional or awareness through movement approach as mentioned previously. PNF works well at the initial stages as well (See Chapter 11). Once control has been gained and upper trapezius overuse reduced, additional strengthening can be accomplished in several ways. Isokinetics can be used quite effectively at this stage progressing from a neutral shoulder position through

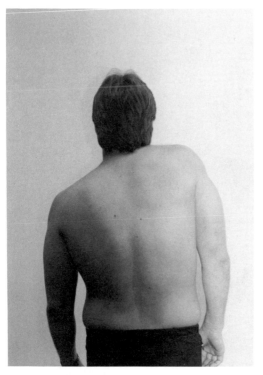

Figure 15C.15. Scapular elevation.

more functional diagonal patterns. The reader is referred to *Clinics In Physical Therapy, Volume 11, Physical Therapy of the Shoulder*, Robert Donatelli, M.A., P.T. (ed) for an isokinetic protocol. If utilizing only isokinetics, do not overlook the need for eccentric work as well.

Isotonic strengthening can be used at this stage. The use of progressive resistance of *Theraband* can accomplish both a concentric and eccentric work-out. Starting from the neutral shoulder position to accomplish internal and external rotation followed by a gradual progression into PNF extension patterns works very well for strengthening of the rhomboids, middle and lower trapezius, rotator cuff and latissimus dorsi muscles (Figs. 15C.16–15C.19). Overhead Theraband can also be used for latissimus and rhomboid strengthening (Fig. 15C.20). Free weights can also be used for parascapular strengthening (Fig. 15C.21). Seated push-ups are also recommended for latissimus dorsi and scapular depressor strengthening (Fig. 15C.22). Care must be taken to observe for upper trapezius overuse, poor postural alignment, and substitution patterns that would undermine strengthening efforts. Progression into a program of 3–4 sets of 10–12 repetitions with emphasis on both concentric and eccentric control (allowing the lengthening contraction to be longer than the shortening contraction), 3 times per week is recommended.

Before completion of the rehabilitation program, inertial work is also suggested. Inertial work can be accomplished using the *Impulse* at the completion of the strengthening phase for parascapular and rotator cuff muscles (Figs. 15C.23–15C.25). The Impulse has been effective for retraining of a golf stroke (Fig. 15C.3), tennis swing (Figs. 15C.4, 15C.5), or casting maneuver (Fig. 15C.6), for examples. The inertial exerciser assists in specificity of training as mentioned previously. Finally, before discharge, additional specificity occurs through having the individual "practice" activities that he plans to resume under PT supervision to address body mechanic, stress reduction, etc.

Strengthening goals for the cervico-

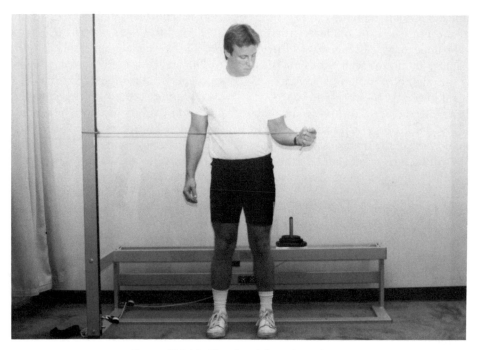

Figure 15C.16. Theraband (lateral rotation).

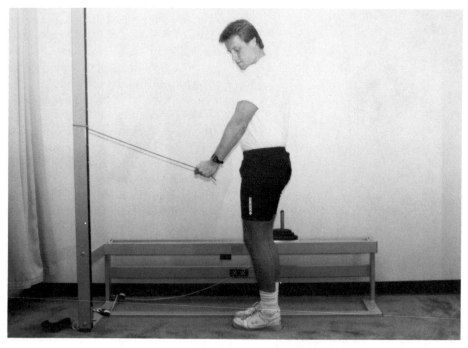

Figure 15C.17. Theraband (extension).

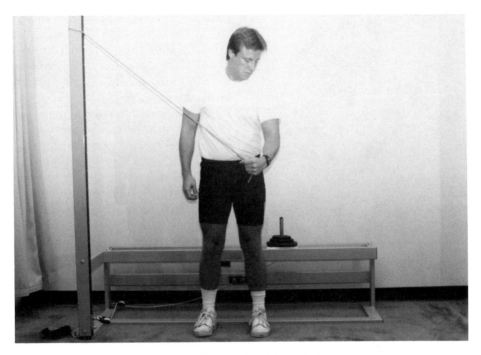

Figure 15C.18. Theraband (combination).

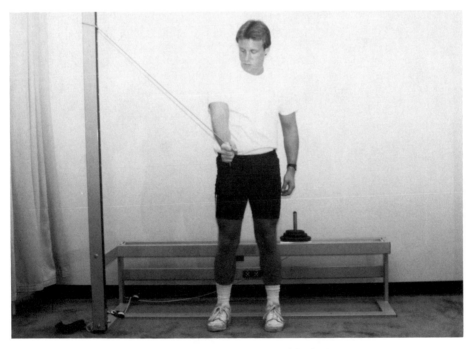

Figure 15C.19. Theraband (adduction).

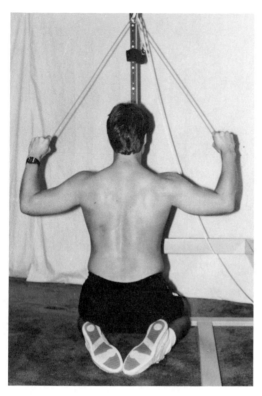

Figure 15C.20. Latissimus and rhomboid strengthening.

thoracic region are generally the same regardless of the dysfunction. The individual who presents with the "proximal crossed syndrome" will share similar strengthening objectives to the individual with post whiplash ligamentous sprain. Tissue healing, functional soft tissue extensibility and joint range of motion, and painfree performance of the requested exercise are necessary prerequisites to performance of a strengthening task. Avoidance of isometrics in the cervical spine has been discussed.[23] Caution is required when an individual with discal involvement, central spinal stenosis, or foraminal encroachment is progressed through a strengthening program.

Low Thoracic, Lumbopelvic, and Lower Extremity Regions

These can be combined when addressing injury or postural dysfunction of the lumbopelvic region. Awareness of typical muscle imbalance patterns, muscular components of spinal stability, and lifting mechanisms are helpful in the understanding of strengthening needs in the lumbopelvic region.

Most common clinical presentations seen in the spinal pain patient include: postural

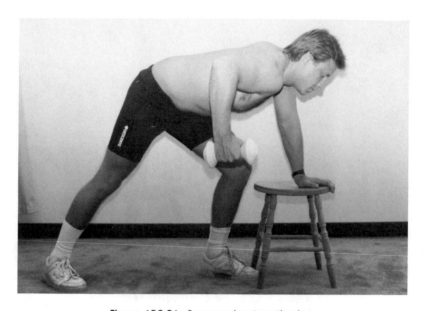

Figure 15C.21. Parascapular strengthening.

dysfunction with accentuated or reduced spinal curves, dysfunction related to reduced spinal mobility, dysfunction related to excessive spinal mobility, combination of 3 and 4, and varying degrees of disc involvement. As seen in the cervical region, strengthening needs are often the same regardless of the presenting diagnosis. However, certain precautions and contraindications do exist and will be presented.

The "pelvic crossed syndrome" is a typical pattern seen in the lumbopelvic region characterized by tightness and shortening of the hip flexors and lumbar errector spinae with weakness of the gluteal and abdominal muscles (Fig. 15C.26). The imbalance encourages a forward pelvic tilt, increased lumbar lordosis, and slight hip flexion. Often the hamstrings are tight in this syndrome. Weakness of the gluteus medius and accompanying tightness of the quadratus lumborum and tensor fasciae latae can also be found.[31] This imbalance displaces the pressure distribution posteriorly on the discs, facet joints, and ligaments of the lumbar spine.[33,36] The potential

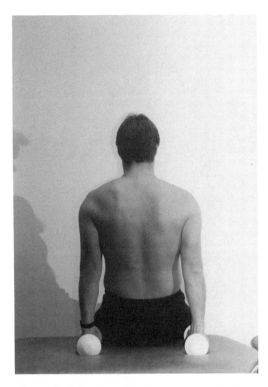

Figure 15C.22. Scapular depressor strengthening.

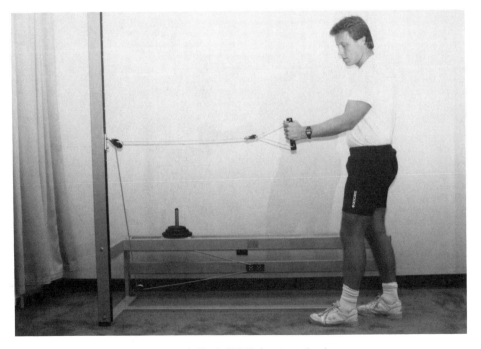

Figure 15C.23. IMPULSE for strengthening.

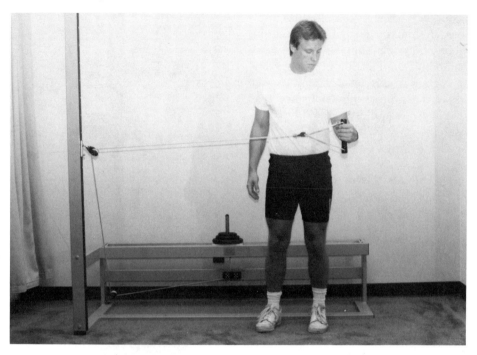

Figure 15C.24. IMPULSE for rotator cuff muscles, etc.

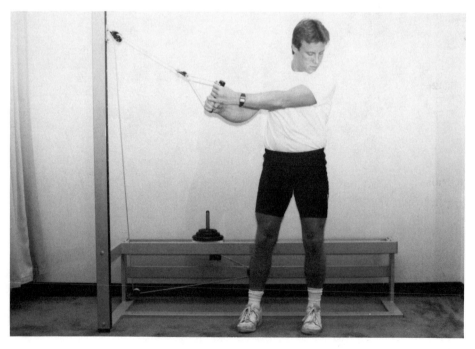

Figure 15C.25. IMPULSE, bilateral effects.

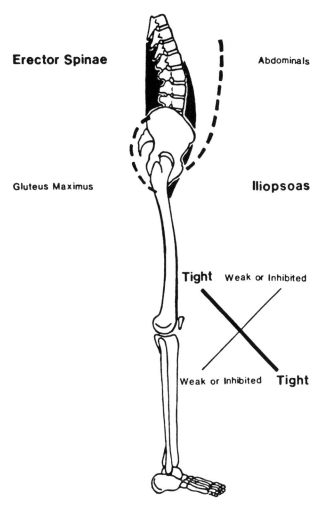

Erector Spinae

Abdominals

Gluteus Maximus

Iliopsoas

Tight Weak or Inhibited

Weak or Inhibited **Tight**

Figure 15C.26. Pelvic crossed syndrome. With permission from: Jull GA, Janda V. Muscles and motor control in low-back pain: assessment and management, In: Twomey LT, Taylor JR, eds., Physical therapy of the low back. New York: Churchill Livingstone, 1987; 253–278.

for degeneration of the lumbar segments is suggested.[36]

Janda also discusses a "layer" syndrome characterized by a combination of the "proximal or shoulder crossed" and the "pelvic crossed" syndrome creating a generalized muscular imbalance evidenced by layers of weakened or shortened musculature. Observing from posteriorly, the layers include tight hamstrings, weak gluteals, weak lumbar erector spinae, tight erector spinae in the thoracolumbar junction, weakness of the mid thoracic musculature, and shortened upper trapezius muscles (Fig 15C.27).[31,32,36]

Sahrmann recognizes trunk imbalance patterns related, in part, to faulty postures. Some of these include increased lordosis or swaybacked postures with excessive pressure posteriorly or the "flatback" posture with decreased hip extensor extensibility.[33]

In the lumbo-pelvic region, hip extension, hip abduction, and the trunk curl up can be used to assess motor control in the presence of faulty posture. Improper firing of the lumbopelvic musculature places undue stress on the lumbar spine. Psoas and abdominal imbalance also affects the stability of the trunk, particularly the lumbar region.[23,33,34,42]

Muscle Hypotrophy   Muscle Hypertrophy

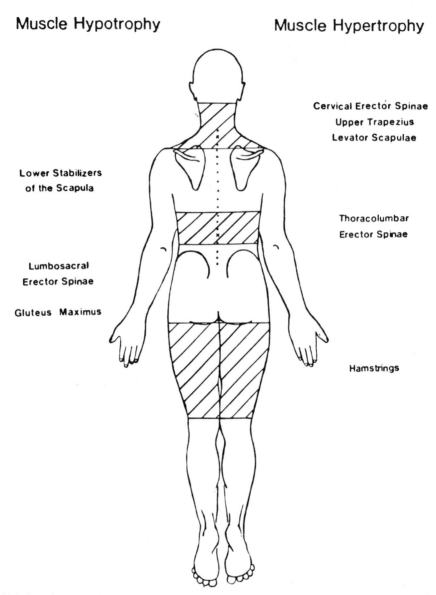

Cervical Erector Spinae
Upper Trapezius
Levator Scapulae

Lower Stabilizers
of the Scapula

Thoracolumbar
Erector Spinae

Lumbosacral
Erector Spinae

Gluteus Maximus

Hamstrings

Figure 15C.27. Layer syndrome. With permission from: Jull GA, Janda V. Muscles and motor control in low-back pain: assessment and management. In: Twomey LT, Taylor JR, eds., Physical therapy of the low back. New York: Churchill Livingstone, 1987; 253–278.

To assess muscle recruitment during hip extension the patient is asked to lift the extended leg into extension from the prone position (Fig. 15C.28). The hamstrings and gluteus maximus act as prime movers and the errector spinae stabilize the pelvis. Janda[37,38] reported that the normal response is contraction of the ipsi gluteus maximus followed by the contralateral errector spinae, followed by the ipsilateral errector spinae. However, Pierce and Lee[43] evaluated 20 healthy subjects and concluded that there existed a variability in the firing order of the errector spinae, gluteus maximus, and biceps femoris. Increased errector spinae activity may be seen in the presence of gluteus maximus weakness.[31,37] In

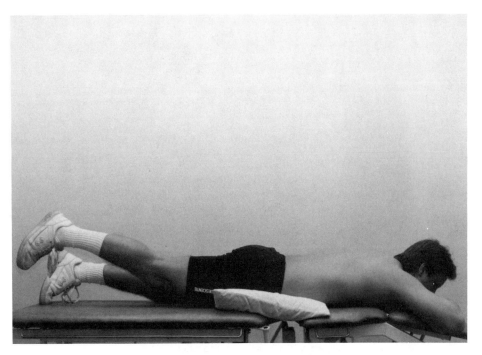

Figure 15C.28. Assessing extension.

this scenario, the lift is accomplished through a forward pelvic tilt and hyperextension of the lumbar spine resulting in posterior compression and anterior shear in the lumbar region. Initial attention must be focused on re-establishment of gluteal firing with hip extension. Again the use of functional integration (as noted previously) or PNF works well initially. Working in prone and requesting a minimal amount of hip extension, an unweighting of the limb with contact on the weak gluteus maximus, is beneficial in the initial stages of muscle re-education. Strengthening of the gluteus maximus is important, in part, because of its role in lifting.

Abduction of the hip is tested in sidelying with the bottom leg flexed and top leg in neutral hip extension. The subject is asked to minimally abduct the top leg (Fig. 15C.29). Firing of the gluteus medius and minimus should occur first. Next, contraction of the tensor fascia lata should be noted. Finally, contraction of the quadratus lumborum should occur.[38] The first sign of weakness may be seen when the hip externally rotates and

the tensor fascia lata initiates the motion. With excessive lateral rotation, the subject will attempt to use the iliopsoas to replace the glutei (Fig. 15C.30). Improper control/recruitment can place undue stress on the lumbosacral region.[31] Again initial re-education can be accomplished through the use of functional integration or PNF or through minimal accomplishment of a side leg-raise with or without manual contact. Isotonic prescription suggests progression to 3 sets of 10–12 repetitions, 3 times per week. Progressive ankle weights or Theraband in supine, sidelying, or standing are useful. Finally, the IMPULSE can be used at the end stages of abductor strengthening (Fig. 15C.31).

Abdominal Muscles

The attainment of strong abdominals has long been advised for protection of the lumbar spine and for assistance during lifting tasks.[44–46] Janda[31] evaluates the relationship between the abdominals and the iliopsoas through performance of a hooklying sit-up. If the

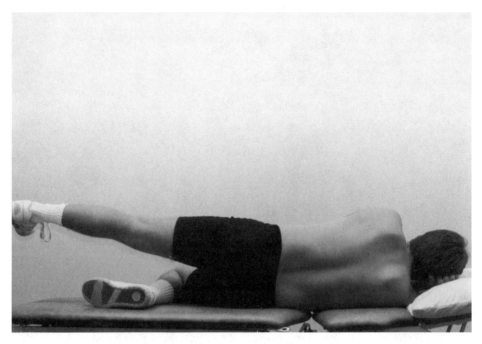

Figure 15C.29. Minimal abduction of hip.

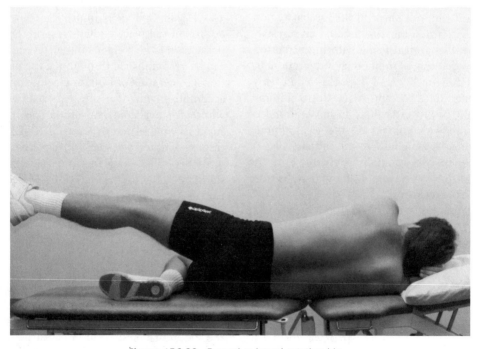

Figure 15C.30. Excessive lateral rotation hip.

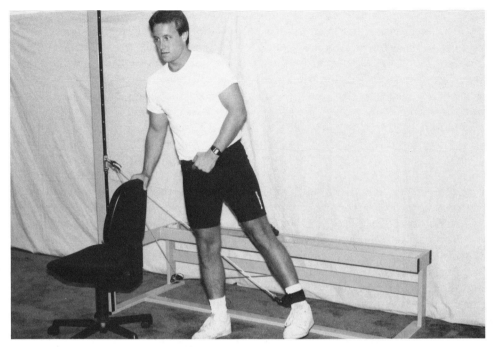

Figure 15C.31. Abdominal strengthening with IMPULSE.

iliopsoas is strong, there will be little to no trunk flexion observed. If the abdominals are strong, trunk flexion will be noted. Kendall and Kendall[42] utilize the leg lowering test to assess for abdominal and psoas control. The controversies surrounding strength testing of the abdominals will not be presented.

"The integrity of the spinal mechanism depends on controlled interaction between the musculature," says Farfan.[47] Stability of the spine is gained from the extrinsic support provided by the trunk musculature and ligamentous system.[4,44,47–51] Trunk muscles maintain the pelvis and axial skeleton in correct position. Isometric contraction of the trunk musculature allows proximal stability and distal (extremity) mobility.[33] Lateral stability of the spine is, in part, dependent on the activity of the quadratus lumborum, latissimus dorsi, vertebral portion of the psoas, and the obliques.[40,44,47] Vertical stability of the spine is assisted by contraction of the psoas.[4,47–49] Intra-abdominal and intra-thoracic pressure also contributes to the vertical stability of the spine.[52–54]

Torque forces which are particularly harmful to the intervertebral disc and joints[4,47,54] are counteracted by the oblique abdominal musculature,[4,44,47] the errector spinae, multifidi, and rotatores.[4,55] The gluteus medius and tensor fasciae latae also aid in torque control as reported by Carlsöö through EMG study.[4]

Shear forces are particularly hazardous to the facet joints.[47] Clinically, increased anterior shear is seen in an individual with an increased lordosis. The posterior components of the motion segments are under greater shear stress when the lordosis increases. The abdominal musculature assists in reducing shear forces in the lumbar spine[44,52,53] by raising intrathoracic and intraabdominal pressure.[52,53] A controversy exists, however, between authors who feel the abdominal musculature, particularly the obliques and transversus abdominis, assist in raising the intra-abdominal pressure[52,56] and those who feel a rise in intra-abdominal pressure is independent of abdominal strength.[57]

The role of musculature, intra-abdominal

pressure, the thoracolumbar fascia, and the posterior ligamentous system in lifting have been studied by many researchers and remains controversial.[44,47–53,56–62] In recent years, computerized testing devices for trunk performance have added an objective dimension to the assessment of the trunk muscles involved in lifting.[8,10,18,63–70]

Lifting

Most researchers agree that the squat lift is superior to the stoop lift with respect to minimizing stress on the low back.[62] However, controversy persists regarding the mechanisms activated in lifting, the position of the lumbar spine during the initial portion of the lift, and the resultant stress on the low back. One group advocates lifting in the lordotic position[59,60,71] and the other advocates lifting in a pelvic tilt position.[4,44,47–53,56–62]

The advocates of the squat lift with the spine in a lordotic posture recommend this posture because the flexion moment of the trunk is reduced and the erector spine activity is the greatest when compared to lifts accomplished from a kyphotic starting position. They assume that disc compression forces are minimal and % strain on the lumbodorsal fascia is 0.[59,60] They ignore the effect of this lift on anterior shear. Also, the point has been made that when lifting an object from the floor, maintaining a lordotic posture is simply not possible.[62]

The second proposed lifting mechanism relates to the role of the thoracolumbar fascia and hip extensors in assisting the initial portion of the lift. The advocates of this mechanism argue that the errector spinae muscles are not capable of resisting the flexion moments encountered in heavy lifts,[4,44,45,47–52,54] and they propose two theories. The first relates to the balloon effect created by intra-abnormal pressure[52,53,55–57] and the second describes the function of the "posterior ligamentous system."[4,44,45,47–54,54,61]

The role of intra-abdominal pressure and its assist in a lift remains controversial as does the role of the abdominal musculature in creating of increased pressure.[52,53,55–57] The supposition is that during lifting the abdominal muscles contract and raise intra-abdominal pressure, creating a balloon with the superior portion being the diaphragm. The balloon supports the thorax and assists the back muscles is raising the trunk.

The second theory contends that a lift can be accomplished through the contraction of the hip extensors (gluteus maximus and hamstrings) and transmission of that force through the lumbar and thoracic spine to the upper extremities.[22] The muscles of the lumbar spine are assisted by the "posterior ligamentous system" consisting of the facet capsules, posterior ligaments, and posterior layer of the thoraco-lumbar fascia.[4,22,44,45,47–52,54,61] The thoracolumbar fascia envelopes the intrinsic muscles of the spine creating a fascial tunnel.[44,45,47,50,51,54] The fascial tunnel assists in increasing tension and the ability of the errector spinae muscles to extend and has been called the "hydraulic amplifier mechanism." The effectiveness of the mechanism is dependent upon contraction of latissimus dorsi, transversus abdominis, and internal obliques.[22,61,62]

In order for the posterior ligamentous system to be effective, the lumbar spine must remain flexed. This flexion is believed to be maintained by the weight being raised and contraction of the abdominal muscles. As the spine approaches the upright posture, the flexion moment is reduced and the errector spinae muscles can complete the lift.[37] An in-depth account of the role of the thoraco-lumbar fascia in lifting can be found by reading papers by Farfan, Gracovetsky, Bogduk, and others.[4,44,45,47–52,54] Despite controversies surrounding the lifting question, the musculature typically involved in a lift include the errector spinae, gluteus maximus, hamstrings, oblique abdominals, transversus abdominis, and latissimus dorsi. Strengthening of these muscles is therefore indicated in individuals who will be required to lift even small loads.

The role of the upper extremity musculature and quadriceps femoris need to be considered when discussing lifting. Strengthening of the latissimus dorsi and scapular stabilizers for proximal stability (see previously) as well as the distal musculature must not be overlooked. Evaluation of the extremities can be completed through isokinetic evaluation and rehabilitation and will not be included in this chapter. Quadriceps strengthening will be included later.

Given the role of the abdominals in stability of the spine and in lifting, strengthening exercises should be focused on activation of the internal and external obliques and transversus abdominis. In an EMG study by Partridge,[73] rotation of the thorax on the pelvis, posterior pelvic tilting in standing and hook-lying, and bent knee hip rolling were found to generate the greatest amount of activity in the internal obliques.[40,72,73] External oblique activity was found to be the greatest with hook-lying sit-ups with trunk rotation.[40,74] Halpern and Bleck[75] evaluated 5 sit-up variations monitoring the rectus abdominis and obliques with surface electrodes. They found the shoulder lift hook-lying sit up, flexing the trunk only to allow for scapular clearance, elicited the greatest activity in all three muscles. Greater abdominal activity was measured through EMG when the hook-lying sit-up was performed with the feet unsupported compared to supported.[76] The abdominal muscles are needed during the first ⅓ of the full hook-lying sit-up.[46,74] The external oblique, rectus abdominis, and rectus femoris muscles were studied using surface electrodes while performing eight sit-up variations. The external obliques and rectus abdominis were most active during the concentric and eccentric phases of the head lift/lower and shoulder lift/lower phases. The hook lying unsupported fast and slow variety elicited the most abdominal activity and least rectus femoris activity.[76] Bilateral leg raising activated all the abdominal musculature minimally[40,73] but when weighed against the significant increase in intradiscal pressure (120kgf)[4,77] is not recommended. Sit-ups with or without the hips generate 175-180kgf on the lumbar discs.[4,77] Halpern and Bleck[75] suggested that the partial or shoulder lift sit up reduces loads on the lumbar disc because of the minimal amount of lumbar flexion required, but disc loads occurring during a shoulder lift sit-up could not be found in the literature. However, the loads are probably only slightly less than when performing a full sit-up.

Strategies in Lift Training

Once re-establishment of pelvic control is gained through functional techniques (see previously) further progression of abdominal strengthening can occur. In the presence of cervical involvement, partial sit-ups are avoided until adequate cervical flexor strength has been gained. A progression from isometric holding patterns with support from a chair in the 90/90 position to hook-lying unilateral straight leg lowering (Fig. 15C.32) can be accomplished. Next, isometric holding patterns from several angles in the hip flexion range can be instructed (Figs. 15C.33, 15C.34). Hip rolling is also effective for abdominal and transversospinalis strengthening (Fig. 15C.35). An advanced exercise for the abdominals demands control of the abdominals with the legs at a 90/90 starting position moving into unilateral hip and knee extension (Fig. 15C.36).

With sufficient cervical strength, recommendations for additional abdominal strengthening are in agreement with the literature. Variations of the partial sit-up in the hook-lying, feet unsupported position are instructed. Patients are instructed to curl the chin to the chest curling only far enough to clear the scapulae from the floor (Figs. 15C.37, 15C.38).

Because of the significant loads placed on the lumbar discs during sit-up activities[4,77] caution is advised with the discal patient. If the symptoms have resolved and the patient can perform active forward bending repeatedly and repeated flexion in lying without increased symptoms, gradual abdominal work can usually begin. Continued monitoring of symptoms and signs and re-establishment of the neutral lordosis is imperative following abdominal work. With all strengthening rou-

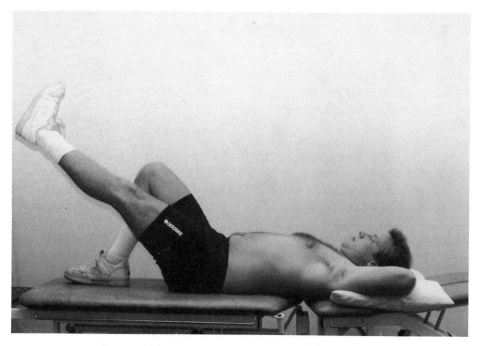

Figure 15C.32. Posterior pelvic tilt and straight leg raise.

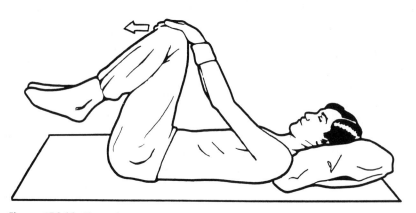

Figure 15C.33. Knee stopper.

Purpose: To strengthen the abdominal muscles.

Description: Lying. Raise knees and put hands on thighs. Push knees into hands for 5 seconds and then lower feet.

Comments:

Reps: Sets: Time:

tines, care must be taken to avoid substitution patterns and fatigue. Isometric prescription suggests 5 repetitions of each exercise, held for 5 seconds, at 75–100% of maximal effort with 30 seconds of rest between each contrac-tion. Once isotonic work begins, 10–12 rep-etitions for 2–3 sets, three times per week is suggested. Inertial exercise can be used for trunk strengthening at the completion of the rehabilitation process. Truncal rotation as

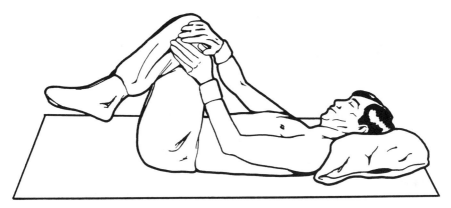

Figure 15C.34. Side knee stopper.

Purpose: To strengthen oblique abdominals.

Description: Lying. Raise knees and place both hands on side of 1 knee. Push knees into
hands for 5 seconds and then lower feet to floor. Repeat to opposite side.

Comments:

        Reps: Sets: Time:

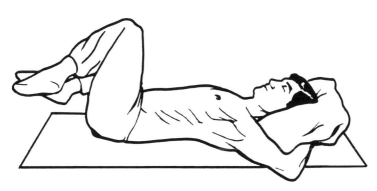

Figure 15C.35. Rotary trunk stretch/strengthener.

Purpose: 1) To stretch the lower back and trunk muscles
        2) To strengthen the lower abdominal muscles
        3) To strengthen the short rotators of the spine

Description: Lie on your back with your hips bent to 90 degrees or more until back is flat. Keeping your knees
together and shoulders on the floor, slowly drop your knees to the RIGHT until you feel the LEFT
shoulder start to raise up. Return to the starting position. Repeat to the opposite direction.

Comments: Only move as is comfortable without straining your low back or abdominal muscles. Breathe
comfortably through the exercise.

        Reps: Sets: Time:

well as chop-lift patterns can be accomplished with the Impulse (Figs. 15C.39, 15C.40).

Lower Limb Factors. Gluteus maximus and hamstring strengthening exercises have also been studied with EMG by Fischer and Houtz,[40] who monitored the gluteus max-imus, erector spinae, hamstrings, and quadriceps musculature during various exercises and activities. Gluteus maximus 'muscle setting' elicited a large degree of activity regardless of the position. Maximus activity was also greatest at the end range of hip extension with the hamstrings being more active from a hip flexed through a hip extended position. Hyperextension of the hip combined with external rotation exhibited the strongest contraction of the maximus.[40,78] The application of Janda's pelvic crossed syndrome to a spinal pain patient reveals that individuals often present with tight hip flexors thus reducing hip extension and exhibit gluteal weakness. Once hip flexor extensibility has been restored, gluteus maximus strengthening can occur. Those who cannot extend the hips beyond neutral need to be concentrating on gluteal setting exercises for the maximus and hamstrings until hip extension can be accomplished.

Isokinetic dynamometers can be used for lower extremity strengthening. Step-ups are suggested for concentric and eccentric work for the gluteals and quadriceps primarily, although they are well suited for total lower extremity strengthening (Figs. 15C.41, 15C.42, 15C.43). On a standard step stool, the patient performs 2–3 sets, 10–12 repetitions each, of step-ups in 3 positions. Raising the body is accomplished in 2–3 seconds and lowering in 3–6 seconds. Gluteal strengthening can also be accomplished from the all-fours position (Figure. 15C.44). Although the literature[40,78] suggests hip hyperextension for maximal gluteus maximus strength gains, hyperextension is avoided because of the accompanying increase in lumbar lordosis and movement out of a functional pelvic position (see previously). *Theraband* also can be used for hip extensor strengthening in the standing position. The straight leg is extended from 45 degrees of hip flexion to neutral hip extension. Isotonic protocol is recommended. The *Impulse* can also be used for hip extensor training (Fig. 15C.45).

Intrinsic Spinal Muscles in Lifting

Paraspinal strength differences between normal individuals and those with low back pain have been studied.[8–12,63,66] The role of the erector spinae and transversospinalis or intrinsic back musculature has also been discussed with regards to lifting. Strengthening of intrinsic muscles is important in the reha-

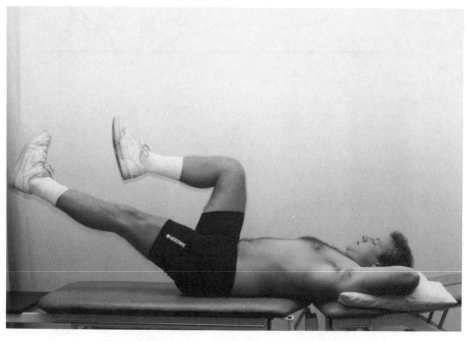

Figure 15C.36. Advanced abdominal strengthening.

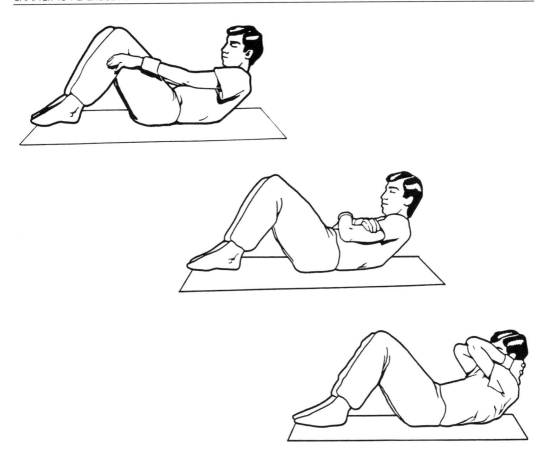

Figure 15C.37. Abdominal curl

Purpose: To strengthen the abdominal muscles

Description: Lie on your back with hips and knees bent and feet flat on the floor. Place hands: 1. on your thighs, 2. across your chest or 3. behind your head as instructed by your therapist. Flatten your back into the floor, bend your chin toward your chest, and slowly curl your trunk forward until your shoulder blades clear the floor. Slowly "unroll" back to the starting position.

Comments: EXHALE as you curl up.

    Reps: Sets: Time:

bilitation of the spinal patient. The erector spinae group spans many segments in the spine in its course from the aponeurotic attachment to the sacrum, ilium, and spinous processes to the head and therefore is capable of creating mass trunk backward bending, eccentric forward bending, eccentric and concentric sidebending, and truncal rotation.[40,79] The transversospinalis group spans only 4–6 segments at its longest point to 1–2 segments at its shortest and will provide proximal control and stability.[80] Initial strengthening may place emphasis on the transversospinalis group through PNF or isometric approaches followed by a gradual progression of midrange work to promote proximal control/stability. Nicolaison and Jorgenson found that the isometric endurance of trunk flexors and extensors was shorter in a group of patients who could not work because of back pain.[11] Use of the *Isostation B200* is the isometric mode is one suggestion for initial strengthening of the intrinsic musculature. Use of heavy resistance theraband can also be used to begin

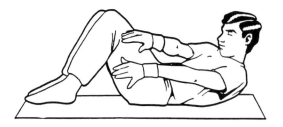

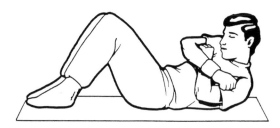

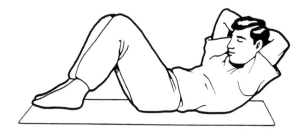

Figure 15C.38. Abdominal laterals.

Purpose: To strengthen the lateral abdominal muscles

Description: Lie on your back with your hips and knees bent and feet flat on the floor. Place hands: 1. on your thighs, 2. across your chest or 3. behind your head as instructed by your therapist. Flatten your back, bend your chin toward your chest, and slowly curl toward the outside of the RIGHT knee until the shoulder blades clear the floor. Return to the starting position. Repeat to the opposite side.

Comments: EXHALE as you curl up.

        Reps: Sets: Time:

mid-range trunk rotation, lateral bending, or diagonal patterns. Inertial exercise is also beneficial when promoting mid-range rotation for proximal control/stability (Fig. 15C.39).

Erector Spinae Strengthening. Various methods have been suggested.[3,5,33,35,36,38,72,83] Jackson recommends prone extension from 45° of trunk flexion to neutral from the prone position to maximize the extensor moment.[72] Eccentric work is also recommended because of the eccentric role of the errector spinae in forward bending.[40,83] Kahanovitz et al.[83] dem-

onstrated errector spinae isokinetic strength gains from a program of prone trunk extension, prone leg lifts, and arm and leg lifts from an 'all fours' position over 20 treatment sessions, 5 days per week for 4 weeks. Sinaki[3] demonstrated increased erector spinae strength following 3 months of prone extension from neutral and leg lifts from an 'all-fours' position as measured isometrically by a strain-gauge. Subjects performed 15 repetitions four days per week for 3 months. When strengthening the paraspinals, attention to ec-

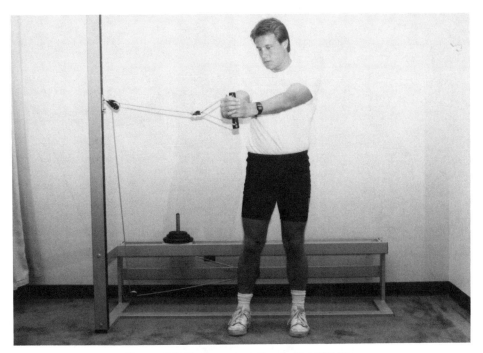

Figure 15C.39. Truncal rotation (with IMPULSE).

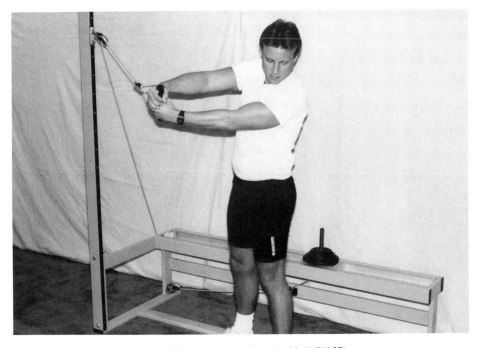

Figure 15C.40. Truncal chops (with IMPULSE).

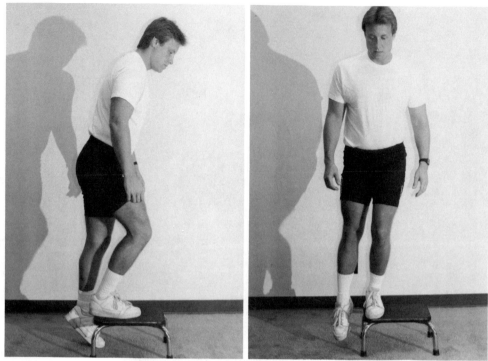

Figure 15C.41   **Figure 15C.42**

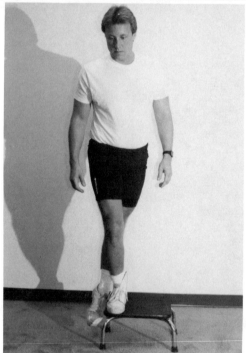

Figure 15C.43

Figure 15C.41 to Figure 15C.43. Various one-step step-ups.

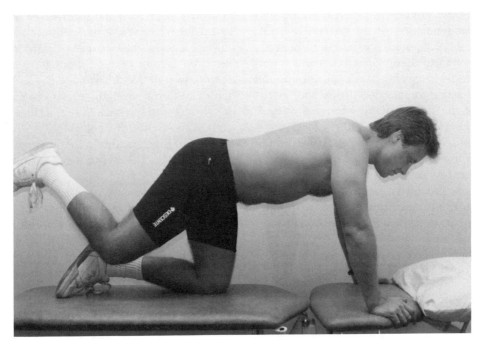

Figure 15C.44. Hip extension strengthening.

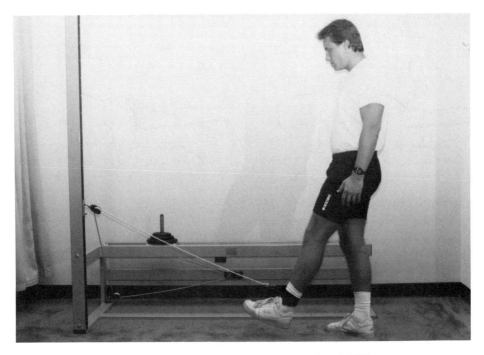

Figure 15C.45. Hip extensor training (with IMPULSE).

centric and concentric strengthening and eventual simulation of on the job or ADL activities is suggested. Awareness of the stress placed on the posterior spinal elements as well as potential narrowing of the spinal canal and intervertebral foramen occurring with extension of the spine beyond neutral is critical. "Bird Dog" (Fig. 15C.46) allows for paraspinal strengthening and maintenance of the neutral lordosis.

Recent advances in spinal testing equipment have provided a mechanism for intrinsic strengthening. Additionally, data regarding extensor to flexor ratios, torque production, range of motion, and velocity measurements according to the type of contraction (isometric, isotonic, isodynamic, isokinetic) can be collected. Beimborn and Morrissey[81] present an exhaustive review of the literature addressing trunk performance studies. Extensor force has been found to exceed flexor force in isometric, isotonic, and isokinetic modes.[81] Extensor to flexor strength ratios were reduced in subjects with low back pain or sciatica when compared to healthy controls.[8,10,12,81] Peak torque extensor to flexor ratios range from 1.0–2.0 with 1.3 being most commonly cited.[81]

Normative data are essential for the clinician when evaluating test results and establishing rehabilitation goals. Use of spinal dynamometers in conjunction with a rehabilitation program is valuable.[8,18,19,82] Levene et al.[69] used an isodynamic device that allows

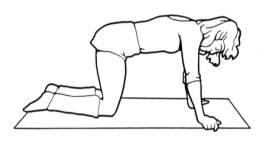
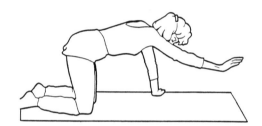
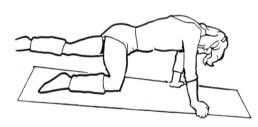
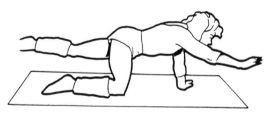

Figure 15C.46. Bird dog.

Purpose: Increase strength and control of trunk muscles

Description: Start on hands and knees, weight equally distributed.
      a) Lift your right arm out in front of your body.
      b) Lift your left leg straight out behind your body until your leg is level with your trunk.
      c) Repeat with opposite arm and leg.
      d) Lift right arm and left leg at the same time.
      e) Lift left arm and right leg at the same time.

Comments:

      Reps: Sets: Time:

data collection of three planes of motion simultaneously. They identified coupling patterns of motion between the primary axis of motion and the secondary and tertiary axes as well as trends in torque production for static and dynamic tests, velocity, and strength ratios for men and women. Smidt et al.[82] studied the effects of high intensity exercise using the *KIN/COM trunk testing unit* (Chattex Corporation, Chattanooga, TN) over a 6-week training period followed by reassessment 6 weeks following completion of the study. One group received eccentric training, the second group received concentric training and the third served as a control. Subjects exercised, in the sagittal plane, three times per week for 6 weeks performing three sets of ten repetitions per session. Results indicated that trunk strength gains were highest within the same mode of exercise used in training. Training transfer did occur but to a lesser degree. Trunk extensors showed the greatest strength gains in the eccentric mode. Strength and endurance measurements were retained, for the most part, 6 weeks following completion of the program.

Studies establishing protocols and investigating the efficacy of treatment programs with trunk performance devices are limited but soon may be forthcoming. Given normal database information, expected ratios, peak torque to bodyweight information, etc., use of computerized spinal dynamometers can be beneficial starting from the subacute to settled stages of dysfunction progressing to return to work. Several of the units can simulate lifting patterns and out of cardinal plane activities. Unfortunately, as mentioned previously, strengthening protocols for back conditions have not yet been firmly established and continued research is necessary.

Testing. Once pelvic control has been mastered, testing and rehabilitation utilizing the *Isostation B200* has served as a beneficial adjunct to the rehabilitation process. B200 testing focuses on torque production, velocity, range of motion, and power in 3 planes simultaneously.[28] Contraindications to testing

include: healing vertebral fracture or osteoporosis, presence of a lateral shift, sciatica, neurological changes, and failure of the pre-test.

The pre-test consists of a resistance free range of motion test. and isometric testing in the standing position. Flexion/extension, lateral flexion, and rotation are tested (Figs. 15C.47, 15C.48, 15C.49). Recreation or an increase in symptoms constitutes failure of the pre-test.

Testing includes evaluation of range of motion and isometric torque in all planes (6 directions). Dynamic testing is performed with the resistance set at 50° maximum torque production for each plane and is evaluated in six directions as well. Upon completion of the test, a program is established and the patient progresses to performance of a routine consisting of three sets of 12 repetitions in each direction, three times per week. *Re-testing* takes place every 4–6 weeks. Progress and

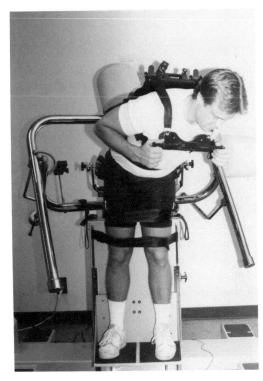

Figure 15C.47. Isostation B200—flexion-extension.

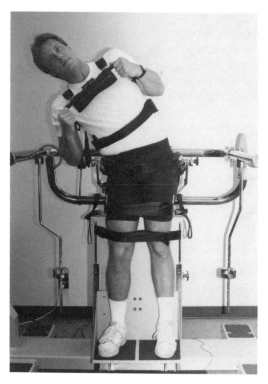

Figure 15C.48. Lateral flexion.

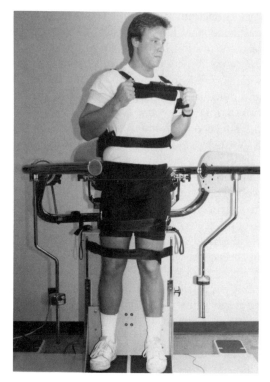

Figure 15C.49. Rotation.

return to work status can be determined through comparison to normal values or through the use of commercial software packages now available.

Pelvic Girdle

The mechanical dysfunctions of the pelvic girdle generally can be classified into categories of hypomobility of hypermobility related to trauma, postural strains, inflammatory disorders, infection, metabolic disorders, or miscellaneous causes. Clinically, the presentation is often one of ipsilateral hypomobility and contralateral hypermobility particularly when the dysfunction is secondary to trauma. Alterations in muscle function also accompanies or may be responsible for pelvic girdle disorders.[84] Evaluation, passive mobilization/muscle energy techniques to correct a hypomobility, or external stabilization to reduce hypermobility precedes strengthening and is not included in this chapter. The reader is

referred to *The Pelvic Girdle* by Diane Lee for further information.[84]

The rehabilitation of the pelvic girdle is not complete without attention to the musculature responsible for the control of the articulations. In keeping with Janda's philosophy, the musculature in the lumbopelvic region that tend to tighten include: the erector spinae, quadratus lumborum, hamstrings, rectus femoris, iliopsoas, tensor fasciae latae, adductors, and piriformis muscles.[31,34,36,84] Stretching techniques have been addressed earlier in the chapter. The muscles that tend to weaken include the abdominals, gluteal muscles, and quadriceps.[31,34,36,84] Lack of progression through a strengthening program for these muscles, addressing both concentric and eccentric control, may account for an increased frequency of re-injury often seen in patients with sacro-iliac (SI) dysfunction. Functional technique (previously addressed) or PNF work (Chapter 11) is well suited for the SI region. Additional exercises that can be easily given as part of the program for the lumbo-pelvic region have been discussed.

In summary, this section of this chapter has presented a means of evaluating for muscle imbalance, improper recruitment patterns, and weakness. Rationale for targeting certain key muscles has also been presented. Recommendations for strengthening exercises and protocols have been given.

REFERENCES

1. Grieve GP. Common vertebral joint problems. Edinburgh: Churchill Livingstone, 1981; 451–455.
2. Caillet R. Low back pain syndrome. 2nd ed. Philadelphia: FA Davis, 1976; 59–77.
3. Sinaki M, Grubbs NC. Back strengthening exercises: quantificative evaluation of their efficacy for women aged 40 to 65 years. Arch Phys Med Rehabil 1989; 70:16–20.
4. Panjabi AW, White MM. Clinical biomechanics of the spine. Philadelphia: J.B. Lippincott Company, 1978.
5. McQuarrie A. Physical therapy. In: Kirkaldy-Willis WH ed. Managing low back pain. New York: Churchill Livingstone, 1988; 345–354.
6. Davis JE, Gibson T, Tester L: The value of exercises in the treatment of low back pain. Rheum Rehabil 8: 1979; 243–247.
7. Jackson CP, Brown MD: Is there a role for exercise in the treatment of patients with low back pain? Clin Orthop 1983; 179:39–45.
8. Mayer TG, Gatchel RJ, Kishino N, Keeley J, Capra P, Mayer H, Barnett J, Mooney V. Objective assessment of spine function following industrial injury: a prospective study with comparison group and one-year follow-up. Spine 1985; 10:482–493.
9. Kahanovitz N, Viola K, Gallagher M: Long-term strength assessment of postoperative diskectomy patients. Spine 1989; 14:402–403.
10. Mayer TG, Smith SS, Keeley J, Mooney V. Quantification of lumbar function part 2: sagittal plane trunk strength in chronic low-back pain patients. Spine 1985; 10:765–772.
11. Nicolaisen T, Jorgensen K. Trunk strength, back muscle endurance and low back trouble. Scand J Rehabil Med 1985; 121–127.
12. Triano JJ, Schultz AB. Correlation of objective measure of trunk motion and muscle function with low-back disability ratings. Spine 1987; 12:561–565.
13. Kraemer WJ, Daniels WL. Physiologic effects of training. In: Bernhardt DB, ed. Sports physical therapy. New York: Churchill Livingstone, 1986; 29–53.
14. Roy S, Irvin R. Sports medicine: prevention evaluation management and rehabilitation. Englewood Cliffs: Prentice-Hall, Inc, 1983.
15. Fleck SJ, Schutt RC. Types of strength training. Orthop Clin North Am 1983; 6:449–458.
16. Davis JM. Rehabilitation of sports injuries: a practical approach. In: Bernhardt DB, ed. Sports physical therapy. New York: Churchill Livingstone, 1986; 155–171.
17. Falkel JE. Methods of training. In: Bernhardt DB, ed. Sports physical therapy. New York: Churchill Livingstone, 1986; 65–79.
18. Mayer TG. Assessment of lumbar function. Clin Orthop 1987; 221:99–109.
19. Mayer TG, Gatchel RJ. Functional restoration for spinal disorders: The sports medicine approach. New York: Lea and Febiger, 1988.
20. Atha J. Strengthening muscle. Exerc Sport Sci Rev 1981; 9:2–73.
21. Davies GJ. A compendium of isokinetics in clinical usage. LaCrosse: S and S Publishers, 1984; 2–17.
22. Bogduk N, Twomey LT. Clinical anatomy of the lumbar spine. Melbourne: Churchill Livingstone, 1987; 88–92.
23. Evenjth O. Class Notes Graduate Program, Institute of Graduate Health Sciences. Atlanta, 1980.
24. Thein LA. Impulse inertial exercise systems protocol. University of Wisconsin, Madison. May 8, 1990.
25. Engineering Marketing Associates P.O. Box 2312, Newnan, GA, 30264, operational literature. January 1985.
26. Rothstein JM, Lamb RL, Mayhew TP. Clinical uses of isokinetic measurements: critical issues. Phys Ther 1987; 67:1840–1844.
27. Isotechnologies, Inc., Operational literature. Hillsborough, NC, 1984.
28. Parniapour, M, Nordin M, Sheikhzadeh A. The relationship of torque, velocity, and power with constant resistive load during sagittal trunk movement. Spine 1990; 15:639–643.
29. Waddell G. A new clinical model for the treatment of low-back pain. Spine 1987; 12:632–644.
30. Bortz W. The disuse syndrome. West J Med 1984; 141:691–694.
31. Jull GA, Janda V. Muscles and motor control in low-back pain: assessment and management. In: Twomey LT, Taylor JR, eds. Physical therapy of the low back. New York: Churchill Livingstone, 1987; 253–278.
32. Janda V. Muscles and cervicogenic pain syndromes. In: Grant R, (ed). Physical therapy of the cervical and thoracic spine. New York: Churchill Livingstone, 1988; 153–166.
33. Sahrmann SA. Diagnosis and treatment of muscle imbalance associated & musculoskeletal pain. Washington University School of Medicine, St. Louis, October 1987.
34. Janda V. Muscles, central nervous motor regulation, and back problems. In: Korr IM ed. The neurobiologic mechanisms in manipulative therapy. New York: Plenum Press, 1978; 27–42.

35. Gustavsen R. Training therapy: prophylaxis and re-habilitation. New York: Thieme Inc, 1985.

36. Janda V, Schmid HJA. Muscles as a pathogenic factor in back pain. International Federation of Orthopaedic Manipulative Therapists, 4th Conference, New Zealand, 1980; 1–24.

37. Lewit K. Manipulation therapy in rehabilitation of the motor system. Boston: Butterworth, 1985.

38. Buswell JS. Normal muscle dysfunction-teaching notes.

39. Rocabado M. Head, neck and dentistry I. Course Notes Physiotherapy Dept, Aukland Technical Institute, Australia, 1983.

40. Basmajian JV, DeLuca CJ. Muscles alive. 5th ed. Baltimore: Williams & Wilkins, 1985.

41. Bagg SD, Forrest WJ. Electromyographic study of the scapular rotators during arm abduction in the scapular plane. Am J Phys Med 1986; 65:111–124.

42. Kendall HO, Kendall FP, Wadsworth GE. Muscles testing and function. Baltimore: Williams & Wilkins, 1971.

43. Pierce MN, Lee WA. Muscle firing order during active prone hip extension. J Orthop Sports Phys Ther 1990; 12:2–9.

44. Farfan HF. Muscular mechanism of the lumbar spine and the position of power and efficiency. Orthop Clin North Am 1975; 6:135–144.

45. Gracovetsky S, Farfan H, Helleur C. The abdominal mechanism. Spine 1985; 10:317–324.

46. Liemohn W, Snodgrass LB, Sharpe GL. Unresolved controversies in back management—a review. J Orthop Sports Phys Ther 1988; 9:239–244.

47. Farfan HF. Biomechanics of the lumbar spine. In: Kirkaldy-Willis WH ed. Managing low back pain. New York: Churchill Livingstone, 1988; 15–27.

48. Nachemson A. The possible importance of the psoas muscle for stabilization of the lumbar spine. Acta Orthop Scand 1968; 39:47–57.

49. Nachemson A. Electromyographic studies on the vertebral portion of the psoas muscle. Acta Orthop Scand 1966; 37:177–190.

50. Macintosh JE, Bogduk, N. The anatomy and function of the lumbar back muscles. In: Twomey LT, Taylor JR eds. Physical therapy of the low back. New York: Churchill Livingstone, 1987; 103–134.

51. Macintosh JE, Bogduk N, Gracovetsky S. The biomechanics of the thoracolumbar fascia. Clinical Biomechan 1987; 2:78–83.

52. Twomey LT, Taylor JR. Lumbar posture, movement, and mechanics. In: Twomey LT, Taylor JR eds. Physical therapy of the low back. New York: Churchill Livingstone, 1987; 51–84.

53. Bartelink DL. The role of abdominal pressure on the lumbar intervertebral disks. J Bone Joint Surg [Br] 1957; 39:718–725.

54. Gracovetsky S, Farfan HF. The optimum spine. Spine 1986; 11:543–571.

55. Morris JM, Benner G, Lucas DB. An electromyographic study of intrinsic muscles of the back in man. J Anat 1962; 96:509–520.

56. Ortengren R, Anderson GBJ: Electromyographic studies of trunk muscles, with special reference to the functional anatomy of the lumbar spine. Spine 1977 2:44–52.

57. Hemborg B, Moritz U. Intra-abdominal pressure and trunk muscle activity during lifting. Scand J Rehabil Med 1985; 17:5–13.

58. McGill SM, Norman RW. Partitioning of the L4-L5 dynamic moment into disc, ligamentous and muscular components during lifting. Spine 1986; 11:666–678.

59. Hart DL, Stobbe TJ, Jaraiedi M. Effects of lumbar posture on lifting. Spine 1987; 12:138–145.

60. Delitto RS, Rose SJ, Apts DW. Electromyographic analysis of two techniques for squat lifting. Phys Ther 1987; 76:1329–1334.

61. Gracovetsky S, Farfan HF, Lamy C. The mechanism of the lumbar spine. Spine 1981; 6:249–262.

62. Sullivan MS. Back support mechanisms during manual lifting. Phys Ther 1989; 69:52–59.

63. Thorstensson A, Arvidson A. Trunk muscle strength and low back pain. Scand J Rehab Med 1982; 14:69–75.

64. Smith SS, Mayer TG, Gatchel RJ, Becker TJ. Quantification of lumbar function part 1: isometric and multi speed isokinetic trunk strength measures in sagittal and axial planes in normal subjects. Spine 1985; 10:757–764.

65. Mayer TG, Barnes D, Kishino ND, Nichols G, Gatchel RJ, Mayer H, Mooney V. Progressive isoinertial lifting evaluation: a standardized protocol and normative database. Spine 1988; 13:993–997.

66. McNeill T, Warwick D, Anderson G, Schultz A. Trunk strengths in attempted flexion, extension and lateral bending in healthy subject and patients with low back disorders. Spine 1980; 5:529–538.

67. Batt'ie MC, Bigos SJ, Fisher LD, Hansson TH, Jones ME, Wortley MD. Isometric lifting strength as a predictor of industrial back pain reports. Spine 1989; 14:851–856.

68. Nordin M, Kahanovitz N, Verderame R, Parniapour M, Yabuts, Viola K, Greenidge N, Mulvihill M. Normal trunk muscle strength and endurance in women and the effect of exercises and electrical stimulation, part 1: Normal endurance and trunk muscle strength in 101 women. Spine 1987; 12:105–111.

69. Levene JA, Seeds RH, Goldberg HM, Frazier M, Fuhrman GA. Trends in isodynamic and isometric trunk testing on the Isostation B200. J Spin Dis 1989; 2:20–35.

70. Lagrana NA, Lee CK. Isokinetic evaluation of trunk muscles. Spine 1984; 9:171–175.

71. Troup JD: Dynamic factors in the analysis of stoop and crouch lifting methods: a methodological approach to the development of safe material handling standards. Clin North Am 1977; 8:201–209.

72. Jackson C, Brown MD. Analysis of current approaches and a practical guide to prescription of exercise. Clin Orthop 1984; 179:46–54.

73. Partridge M. Participation of the abdominal muscles in various movements of the trunk in man: an EMG study. Phys Ther Rev 1959; 39:791–800.

74. Flint MM. Abdominal muscle involvement during the performance of various forms of sit-up exercises. Am J Phys Med 1965; 44:224–234.

75. Halpern AA, Bleck EE. Sit-up exercises: an electromyographic study. Clin Orthop 1979; 145:172–178.

76. Godfrey KE, Kindig LE, Windell EJ. Electromyographic study of duration of muscle activity in sit-up variations. Arch Phys Med Rehabil 1977; 58:132–135.

77. Nachemson A, Morris JM. In vivo measurements of intradiscal pressure. J Bone Joint Surg 1964; 46:1077–1092.

78. Fischer FJ, Houtz SJ: Evaluation of the function of the gluteus maximus muscle, an electromyographic study. Am J Phys Med 1968; 47:182–191.

79. Hollingshead WH, Rosse C. Textbook of anatomy. 4th ed. Philadelphia: Harper and Row, 1985.

80. Donisch EW, Basmajian JV. Electromyography of deep muscles of the back in man. Am J Anat 1972; 133:25–36.

81. Beimborn DS, Morrissey MC. A review of the literature related to trunk muscle performance. Spine 1988; 13:655–660.

82. Smidt GL, Blanpied PR, White RW. Exploration of mechanical and electromyographic responses of trunk muscles to high-intensity resistive exercise. Spine 1989; 14:815–830.

83. Kahanovitz N, Nordin M, Verderame R, Yabut S, Parniapour M, Viola K, Mulvihill M. Normal trunk muscle strength and endurance in women and the effect of exercises and electrical stimulation, part 2: comparative analysis of electrical stimulation and exercises to increase trunk muscle strength and endurance. Spine 1987; 12:112–118.

84. Lee D. The pelvic girdle. New York: Churchill Livingstone, 1989.

PART D.
AEROBIC EXERCISE

FITNESS AND BACK PAIN

General fitness programs are often suggested as an additional exercise component in the rehabilitation of patients with back pain.[1-7] While fitness implies movement, Webster defines fitness as being "physically and mentally sound."[8] In this regard, aerobic exercise of sufficient intensity and duration produces an increase in beta-endorphins in the blood plasma and spinal fluid which may, in part, play a role in reducing pain as well as producing a state of well-being.[1,9,10] In addition, a retrospective study[11] looking at life conditions in persons with and without low back pain reported that back-healthy persons viewed their need for medical care less than the individuals with low back pain.

A prospective longitudinal study investigated changes in health behavior in sedentary men between 49–59 years after exercising 1 hour, three times a week for 18 months. Significant differences between the experimental and control groups were reported with respect to work performance, attitude toward work, a positive feeling about their health, and increased ability to handle stress and tension.[12] Therefore, a person's attitude toward health may be a significant factor for occurrence of low back pain. The relationship between aerobic training and the release of neurotransmitters, which may modify behavior via regulatory mechanisms of the neural-endocrine systems, is a possible explanation for health attitude changes.

Fitness can also be measured by physiological parameters such as muscle endurance and strength, aerobic and anaerobic power, and cardiorespiratory function. Numerous investigations regarding the physical effects of regular exercise have been performed and are outlined in Table 15D.1.

Rationale

Exercise for back pain patients has been an integral part of the rehabilitation process, but the efficacy and rationale for such programs are lacking.[5] A further complication in understanding the benefits of prescribing exercises for the treatment of patients with back pain is that often the cause and pathophysiology underlying most back problems cannot be determined.[12,13] Although, some patients will be diagnosed with a herniated nucleus pulposus, radiculopathy or unstable spondylolisthesis to explain their systems, the majority of patients will be labeled with a multitude of

Table 15D.1
Effects of Habitual Physical Exercise (Modified after Åstrand P-O. Exercise physiology and its role in disease prevention and in rehabilitation. Arch Phys Med Rehabil 1987; 68:305–309)

- Increase in maximal oxygen uptake and cardiac output-stroke volume
- Reduced heart rate at given oxygen uptake
- Reduced blood pressure
- Reduced heart rate × blood pressure product
- Improved efficiency of heart muscle
- Improved myocardial vascularization?
- Favorable trend in incidences of cardiac morbidity and mortality
- Increased capillary density in skeletal muscle
- Increased activity of "aerobic" enzymes in skeletal muscles
- Reduced lactate production at given percentage of maximal oxygen uptake
- Enhanced ability to utilize free fatty acid as substrate during exercise-glycogen saving
- Improved endurance during exercise
- Increased metabolism—advantageous from a nutritional viewpoint
- Counteracts obesity
- Increase in the HDL/LDL ratio
- Improved structure and function of ligaments, tendons, and joints
- Increased muscular strength
- Reduced perceived exertion at given work rate
- Increased release of endorphins
- Enhanced fiber sprouting?
- Enhanced tolerance to hot environment—increased rate of sweating
- Reduced platelet aggregation?
- Counteracts osteoporosis
- Can normalize glucose tolerance

nondescript diagnoses. A few examples are lumbar strain, mechanical back pain, back spasm, and nonspecific low back pain.

Schmidt has reported that chronic low back pain patients have a decreased aerobic capacity when compared to individuals without low back pain.[14] Cady and fellow investigators conducted a prospective study on 1652 firefighters to evaluate five strength and fit-ness parameters and subsequent back injuries for the years 1971 to 1974. The results of the study indicated that individuals with higher fitness levels had fewer subsequent back injuries.[7]

Bowne and his co-workers classified 669 sedentary office workers into five fitness categories based on their performance on a submaximal treadmill test which measured maximal oxygen uptake.

Disability and medical costs, heart rate, percent body fat, serum cholesterol, serum triglycerides, body weight, and blood pressure were measured over a 5-year time span. The participants in the study were instructed to exercise for a minimum of 20 minutes at their target heart rate, which was 70%–80% of their predicted maximum for their age. The results of the study demonstrated a 45.7% reduction in major medical costs in the post entry year with a reduction of 20.1% in the number of disability days. The most significant changes in cardiorespiratory fitness were resting heart rate and percent body fat.[15]

Because the etiology of back pain is unknown for the majority of cases, the mechanism which links aerobic fitness to a reduction in pain and disability is speculative. However, Mayer has identified factors associated with a "deconditioning syndrome" in back pain patients. Many of these factors contribute to the deconditioned patient and are improved with aerobic exercise.[2]

PHYSICAL EFFECTS OF INACTIVITY

Deconditioning

Lumbar motion, trunk strength, cardiovascular fitness and lifting capacity comparing chronic low back pain patients and age, gender, body matched control groups, indicate significant group differences.[2] Mayer has labeled this phenomenon as the deconditioning syndrome. The deconditioning syndrome is described as a progressive process with an onset difficult to determine. Internal factors such as poor blood supply and external factors like cigarette smoking may delay healing and contribute to deconditioned effects. The deconditioned effects include joint hypomobility, muscle atrophy, loss of endurance, tightening of connective tissue, inhibition of neural outflow, and eventual loss of cardiovascular fitness. Further symptoms, such as chemical muscle guarding may appear as a result of sustained muscle activity which results in decreased blood flow and accumulation of lactic acid in the muscle. Gradually, the duration of inactivity increases due to "new injuries" and perpetuates the disuse phenomenon.[2]

As noted earlier, several physiologic parameters are negatively affected as a result of inactivity. But the most deleterious effects are seen in the cardiovascular and musculoskeletal systems.[16] Many investigations have been performed using the bedrest model to study the consequences of inactivity on the heart, muscle, and connective tissue.[9,16–24]

Demineralization of Vertebrae

The biological adaptation of the skeletal system to immobilization is demineralization through the excretion of calcium which results in bone atrophy.[16,19,20,24–26] This phenomenon is also seen with inactivity, weightlessness, and bedrest.[16]

Krolner and Toft[24] investigated the consequences of short-term bedrest (mean 27 days) on the bone mineral content (BMC) of the second, third, and fourth lumbar vertebrae. Fifteen subjects hospitalized for protrusions of the lumbar discs were monitored by dual-photon absorptiometry when admitted, at the end of the bedrest period and after 15 weeks of re-ambulation. The BMC of the lumbar vertebrae decreased 0.9% per week during the bedrest period. A partial recovery in the BMC was reported after the 15-week ambulation phase, but it was only 0.54%, .51 units lower than at admission. Hansson[25] has reported similar findings with a reduction in bone mass of 2% per week in the fourth lumbar vertebra in patients immobilized after scoliosis surgery.

In addition, the amount of bone loss may be specific to the immobilized area. Patients with paralyzed upper and lower extremities demonstrated a more rapid decrease in BMC in the lower extremities.[26]

Collagen Loss

Animal experimentation on ligament and tendons following inactivity have demonstrated structural and biomechanical changes.[9,21] The number and size of collagen fiber bundles decrease with immobilization. Alterations in the collagen crosslinks include significant increases in the number of reducible intermolecular crosslinks.[21] As a result of the anatomical changes due to inactivity, the strength of the connective tissues decreases. The forces generated by the ligaments and tendons also diminish.[9,21]

Muscle Atrophy

Human muscle tissue is negatively affected with inactivity and will decrease in mass to half normal size within 1–2 months after immobilization.[17] The antigravity muscles of the lower extremity appear to be most affected, as evidenced by a decrease in limb circumference, urinary excretion of muscle breakdown products, and diminished strength.[17] A decrease in oxidative potential of the immobilized skeletal muscle and a reduction in capillary density are also associated with inactivity.[9,21] Type II fiber atrophy has been seen during aging and with disuse.[23] Larsson[23] investigated males between the ages of 22–65 to determine if progressive disuse may be a dominant factor in the decline in muscle strength in old age. The subjects were placed on an exercise program for 15 weeks with morphological and strength measurements taken before and after the training session. Needle biopsies were taken from the left vastus lateralis muscle. Results from this study demonstrated that muscle fiber atrophy was reduced after the training period, thereby suggesting fiber atrophy may relate to progressive disuse.

General Physiologic Changes

General deconditioning from prolonged bedrest results in decreased maximal oxygen uptake (VO$_2$ max) and physical work capacity.[18] Specific changes in cardiac function as a result of inactivity are elevated heart rate and a reduced stroke volume, thereby diminishing the efficiency of the myocardium.[18] Additional effects of deconditioning are loss of orthostatic tolerance and changes in fluid and electrolyte balance.[16] Vascular fluid volume is diminished after bedrest and may alter cardiovascular hemodynamics, resulting in a decreased VO$_2$ max.[18]

Specific Vertebral Muscle Effects

The adaptive response of skeletal muscle has been noted previously, but an additional consequence of inactivity is that atrophied muscle is incapable of adequately supporting the axial skeletal structure. Sandler[17] believes atrophied supportive spinal musculature may lead to the development of low back pain. Devries has demonstrated a method for evaluating muscle fatigue based on electromyographic (EMG) fatigue curves.[27] Increased electrical activity in the muscle tissue occurs over time when the muscle works against a consistent force isometrically or isotonically. A primary factor in the elevated myoelectrical activity associated with muscle fatigue is a combination of recruitment and increased neuromuscular stimulation.

These neural adjustments appear to be required to compensate for the decreased tension development in the muscle fiber.[27] Devries[28] hypothesized that since postural muscles contain tonic-type motor units, the EMG fatigue curves should be flat in order for the muscles to maintain erect posture over a long period of time. Eight of twelve subjects participating in this study had chronic low back pain. Participants were asked to stand for 22 minutes while the electrical activity from the back extensors was monitored with surface electrodes. EMG fatigue curves for the back extensors were flat for nine subjects who did not experience low back pain. However, 3 subjects developed low back pain during prolonged standing with an associated rise in electrical activity.

Those limited results must be interpreted with caution due to the fact that the standing position was not controlled for extraneous movements. It has been demonstrated that movement of the pelvis, head, and arms affect the electrical activity of the longissimus portion of the erector spinae during quiet standing.[29]

Despite the difficulty with monitoring electricity activity in a prolonged standing position, decreased muscle endurance (resistance to fatigue) indeed may be a factor in the etiology and perpetuation of low back pain. Decreased blood flow to skeletal muscle as a result of inactivity causes marked changes in the EMG fatigue curve. The same effects have been demonstrated with arterial occlusion to skeletal muscle.[27]

PHYSICAL EFFECTS OF AEROBIC EXERCISE

Numerous investigations have been performed which demonstrate the positive physiologic responses to exercise and the adaptive nature of the biological tissue.[1,7,9,14–26,30,31] For example, VO$_2$ max is elevated with aerobic exercise concomitantly with an increase in capillary density to the skeletal muscle.[9,21] Due to the changes in capillary density to the muscle tissue, mitochondrial volume, oxidative enzymes, and muscle fiber size are increased in both fast and slow twitch fibers.[9,21,23]

The capillary proliferation, which is one of the vascular responses to physical training, may permit for a longer time period in which an exchange of substrates, metabolites, and gases between the blood and tissue can occur which may facilitate tissue repair after injury.[9]

Bone

Bone is a dynamic biological tissue which is affected by mechanical loading and hormonal control. Gravitational forces and muscle contraction are necessary to maintain the bone mineral content (BMC). Each skeletal segment may require a certain threshold for mechanical stimuli to cause tissue adaptation.[19] Thus, a certain amount of mechanical loading could produce a decrease in bone mass in the femur but hypertrophy in the radius.[19,30] Studies comparing bone densities in active populations and sedentary individuals reveal increased bone mass in the active populations.[19] The BMC of tennis players and swimmers were compared with a control group, and there was a 22% superior difference in BMC in the tennis players.[31] In fact, the BMC of the lumbar vertebrae in tennis players was significantly greater than the control group. No significant differences were noted in the BMC of the lumbar vertebrae between the swimmers and the control group.[31] Therefore aerobic activity, which incorporates a weight-bearing component, is preferred when attempting to maintain or increase bone density.[19,32]

Nachemson's[33] review of experimental data suggests motion may be more beneficial than rest in healing the soft tissues and joints.[33,34] Studies investigating tensile loading conditions of connective tissue demonstrate that overloading the ligaments and tendons result in the tissues becoming stronger before yielding to an increase in deformation.[21] Increased strength of the transitional zones, the junction between the ligaments and bones, will occur with endurance training.[21] Tipton and his colleagues[21] summarized the results of animal studies which investigated the anatomical and biochemical changes in connective tissue as a result of exercise. Studies reviewed demonstrated increased collagen concentration in the ligaments and tendons in mice after exercise.

These findings need confirmation in other tissues with other animals. Anatomical and biochemical changes in connective tissue with training will require specific exercise programs and experimental designs to demonstrate dramatic results. But the clinical implications from the animal studies indicate that exercise will increase the forces transmitted to the ligaments and tendons which may also increase the functional capacity of these structures.[21]

PSYCHOSOCIAL EFFECTS OF INACTIVITY AND EXERCISE

Pain is a subjective experience which usually involves a combination of physiological, psychological, and social factors. Patients with back pain may express feelings of anxiety, lack of energy, inability to sleep, withdrawal, increased stress, and depression.[16] The intensity of these psychobehavioral responses may vary depending on the duration of the symptoms. While controversy exists regarding the effects of exercise on the psychological problems associated with painful conditions, the strongest evidence suggests a positive effect.[12,35-39]

Psychochemistry

Knowledge regarding the biochemistry of brain function and the role of the central nervous system in hormonal regulation has enhanced the understanding of the physiological functioning of beta-endorphins and monoamines. Many studies which have investigated the relationship between the release of endorphins with physical exertion have concurred that physical activity results in elevated levels of endorphins.[10,36,37,40-42] Plasma levels of catecholamines and adrenocorticotropin (ACTH) are also increased with aerobic exercise.[10,37,41] These chemical substances are associated with analgesia and the body's ability to respond to stress.[10,41]

In addition, the monoamines, dopamine, serotonin, and norepinephrine, have also reported to be involved with sleep behavior and depression.[10,35] Neurons which secrete monoamines are located in the brain stem and reticular formation. Aminergic synaptic transmission also occurs from neurons which project into the hypothalamus, limbic system, and basal ganglia. Emotional and motivational states, and motor behavior are affected respectively by aminergic transmission.[10] Although the exact physiological significance of these substances in relation to exercise have not been clearly elucidated, changes in health behavior occur with physical training.[12]

Dearman and her colleagues[10] studied the quantitative differences in plasma levels of endorphins, cortisol, and catecholamines in nine athletes running 26.2, 6, and 2 miles. The VO_2 for each subject was determined on treadmill testing. A significant increase in all the measured substances was seen for the post-exercise levels despite the duration of exercise. The percentage increase in endorphins was large between 2.0 and 6.0 miles but decreased between 6.0 and 26.2 miles. Large increases in endorphins were demonstrated after developing maximal intensity levels within 8–15 minutes on the treadmill test. Fraoli et al.[41] reported similar findings. Therefore, large increases in endorphins can result with short-duration, high-intensity exercise.

Quantitative studies measuring levels of endorphins do not address mood changes which occur after exercise. Markoff and his associates[36] studied mood changes in ten runners by administering the Profiles on Mood States (POMS) before and after the subjects ran a mean distance of 10.9 miles. Naloxone, an opiate antagonist, was injected subcutaneously immediately after the post-run POMS and the POMS was administered again after 20 minutes. The naloxone failed to reverse the mood changes noted after running and suggests that the mood change is not endorphin-mediated. Despite deficiencies in the research design of this study, significant reductions were noted in the anger-hostility and depression-dejection mood scales after running.

Ramsford[37] summarized several studies on the anti-depressant effect of exercise. Some of the positive psychological effects associated with exercise were improvements in emotional stability, interpersonal functioning, social and emotional adjustment, self conceptualization, and positive personality traits. Physical fitness apparently reduces depression through enhanced aminergic transmission. Several investigators suggest depression may be affected by altered synaptic transmission because reduced levels of the urinary metabolites of serotonin, dopamine, and norepinephrine are found in depressed patients. Also, antidepressant medication tends to en-

hance aminergic transmission.[37] Since studies have demonstrated increased levels of monoamines in plasma after exercise, physical activity appears to be a viable option in managing depression.[10]

Finally, dynamic exercises, such as walking and jogging or static activities like lifting or holding heavy objects affect slow wave sleep (SWS).[38,39] SWS appears to be associated with a restorative function for the body.[39] These studies demonstrated that the amount of SWS increased after exercise and that physically fit subjects have significantly longer durations of SWS than unfit individuals.[38,39]

AEROBIC EXERCISE: RECOMMENDATIONS FOR THE BACK PATIENT

Suggestions for aerobic exercise should delineate frequency, intensity, duration, type of activity, initial level of fitness, and progression of physical activity. A thorough medical examination should be performed before initiating a program.[43]

ACSM Recommendations

The American College of Sports Medicine has outlined recommendations for developing and maintaining fitness in healthy adults.[44] Some of the recommendations are listed below:

- The *type* of activity should require exercises such as walking and running which use large muscle groups over a prolonged period.
- The *intensity* of the exercise session should be 65–95% of age-predicted maximum heart rate or 50–85% of VO_2 (functional capacity).
- The *duration* of the aerobic activity should be 15–60 minutes of discontinuous or continuous activity.
- The *frequency* of a conditioning program should be 3–5 times per week.
- The *conditioning effects* begin to take place between 6–8 weeks after the program is initiated, and, in most cases, the work load can increase during each session; therefore the rate of progression is based upon adjusting

the duration and intensity or a combination of both.

Preliminary Test

Before initiating a fitness program, a functional test to determine the extent of deconditioning should be given. Patients whose heart rates take more than 5 minutes to return to their resting values after jogging or climbing stairs for 2 minutes are considered to be in poor cardiovascular condition. These patients may require further testing.[1]

Program Design

Modifications of the general guidelines will occur when recommending an aerobic program for the back patient. The mode of activity must be scrutinized for potential positional elements which could aggravate a back problem. Duration and intensity of exercise may require adjustments based on the stage of condition and tissue reactivity. Designing an exercise program for any patient involves clinical decision making and judgment based on experience.

The general guidelines listed in Table 15D.2 are based on biomechanical considerations of the patient and the aerobic activity, but any exercise or treatment involves careful analysis of the patient's signs and symptoms. For example, a patient with a discogenic problem who presents with positive neurological signs which are worsening would not be instructed to increase walking distance or cadence.

As mentioned earlier in the chapter, most back patients, regardless of the diagnosis, are deconditioned and could benefit from aerobic exercise. Therefore, once the patient with discal signs and symptoms stabilizes, a walking program would be recommended. The stabilizing signs would be negative neurological signs, increased spinal mobility, a decrease in leg pain, and centralization of the pain. A walking program for this individual may be simply to encourage a five-minute walk daily at a comfortable pace and ignoring heart rate, time, and mileage. Progression with the ac-

tivity will be based on the response to minimal activity. As duration and intensity of walking are increased, the therapist evaluates patient response to exercise. Table 15D.3 is a guideline for progressing a walking program. Mileage may vary from 9–26 miles a week upon completing the advanced walking routine. Walking velocities may vary from 2–4 mph at the beginning of the program to 4–6 mph with the advanced routine.[45] Patients with limited lumbar spine extension, sacroiliac joint dysfunction, or limited hip range of motion may need slower velocities and a longer duration of exercise.

As walking velocities increase, stride length may increase which will result in increased lumbar and hip extension, and anterior ilial rotation during the toe-off position of the stance phase of gait. Moderate levels of exercise, perhaps 30–40% maximum heart rate, over a lifetime may be more advantageous than intense aerobic workouts followed by months of inactivity. The duration of walking is more important than the intensity for the reduction of body fat.[46] Patients can self-monitor their exercise progression by measuring heart rate, time to complete activity, and mileage using a pedometer and recording the data on a form. See Fig. 15D.1. Joint reaction forces are reduced with walking when compared to fast walking or jogging. Rydell[47] measured joint reaction forces at the hip from unilateral stance to running and found the force to be 1.3–5 times body weight respectively. Also, if walking speed was increased to 1.4 m/sec, the joint reaction force increased to 3.3 times body weight. Therefore, viscoelastic inserts,[48] proper running shoes[49] and appropriate running surfaces[50] are recommended to attenuate the forces to the low back.

Walking Posture. This is a fundamental component to enhancing the aerobic workout and should be reviewed with the patient before the workout. The patient is instructed to walk with the eyes focused forward, head level, shoulders back, and to breath deeply. The buttocks and stomach are tucked in. The upper extremities are held close to the trunk

Table 15D.2
Recommendations for Aerobic Exercise for Patients with Spinal or Pelvic Pain

Syndromes	Signs	Aerobic Exercise	Justification
Disc protrusion	Increased pain with sitting Decreased lumbar lordosis Slump sitting Lateral shift Restricted lumbar mobility	Walking (level surface) Swimming (Freestyle backstroke) Bicycle (as condition stabilizes)	Promote lumbar extension Decrease compressive load Decrease forward lean load
Disc-herniation	Previously had "protrusion" signs Prolonged standing may be worse Sitting may be less painful Extension may increase pain	Walking—3 times a day (10 min per session) Bicycle	Promote activity to increase circulation—to heal tissue Decrease compressive load
Stenosis (spinal canal intervertebral foramen)	Flexion relieves pain Extension increases pain Long history of back pain Lumbar and leg pain after exercise in standing	Bicycle Swimming (side stroke)	Avoid extension
Spondylolisthesis	Stress fracture pars interarticularis congenital defect Athletics involving forceful extension (gymnastics) Ligamentous ache (require change of posture hyperlordotic, hypermobility of motion segment)	Rowing machine Bicycle	Promote forward bending

Condition	Signs/Symptoms	Activities	Goals
Sacroiliac joint (hyper or hypomobile)	Symptoms usually unilateral Increase pain on affected side with walking or stairclimbing sitting history of falling on ischial tuberosity pain with rolling over bed	Swimming (freestyle) with buoy between legs	Avoid stressing sacroiliac joint
Postural syndrome	Poor Postural habits Increase or decrease lumbar lordosis Foward head and shoulders Sedentary lifestyle Decreased strength trunk musculature May have few symptoms but neck and back pain may develop	Depends on structure/Mobility i.e., decrease lumbar lordosis Forward head/shoulders Swimming (freestyle) Walking i.e., increase lumbar lordosis Rowing Bicycle	Promote activities which attempt to counter poor posture
Instability	Excessive range of motion with hypomobility neighboring segments Longstanding poor postural habits overuse of manipulation Hyperlordosis	Walk 3 times per day 10 min per session Bicycle	Promote increasing muscular efficiency without over-stressing hypermobile segment
Fibromyalgia	Muscle fatigue multiple areas of tenderness Sleep disturbances Anxiety/Depression	Walking Bicycle Swimming	Increase circulation to muscles Increase endurance Antidepressant Improve sleep

Table 15D.3
Sample Walking Program for Deconditioned Patients with Back Pain

Week	Time	Heart Rate (% Maximum Heart Rate)
Week 1	5–10 minutes daily	Heart rate below target zone
Week 2	5–10 minutes daily	60–65%
Week 3	5–10 minutes/2 times per day	60–65%
Week 4	5–10 minutes/3 times per day	60–65%
Week 5	15 minutes/5 times a week	60–65%
Week 6	18 minutes/5 times a week	60–65%
Week 7	20 minutes/5 times a week	60–65%
Week 8	30 minutes/3 times a week	60–65%
Week 9	35 minutes/3 times a week	60–65%
Week 10	40 minutes/3 times a week	60–65%
Week 11	45 minutes/3 times a week	60–65%

Advance walking program follow routine for additional 15–18 weeks walking 45 min, 3 times per week, 70–75% maximum heart rate.

and should swing freely with hands unclenched. In addition, the patient is advised to walk on level terrain since walking uphill causes forward bending of the spine and downhill walking promotes lumbar extension, which could aggravate an existing back problem.[45]

Weights. Hand-held weights or weighted belts have become part of the walking routine for some individuals desiring to increase strength or the intensity of the workout. Studies have failed to show an increase in maximal oxygen uptake or heart rate during walking with hand-held weights of 2.27 kg while maintaining a normal arm swing. Also, vigorous arm swings with weights may alter the mechanics of walking.[51] Patients with degenerative disc or joint disease are not encouraged to use weights, due to the potential for increased compressive loading to the spine.

Jogging. Frequently, back patients have reported jogging prior to the onset of spinal pain and identify returning to jogging as one of their goals of treatment. Initially, jogging is not a recommended activity for patients with acute and subacute spinal pain, but once the acute episode of spinal pain has subsided and mobility of the spine has increased, the patient may start a walking program. As muscle and cardiorespiratory endurance increase,

the patient may progress to the walk/jog program outlined in Table 15D.4.

An important element in management of spinal conditions is patient education. The patient should be informed about the effects of running activities on the lumbar disc and facet joints. A recent study measured a significant decrease in vertebral column height after one hour of running compared to 7.5 hours of static activity. Vertebral column height decreased as a result of fluid loss from the disc due to the compressive loading. The disc is less able to attenuate shock and distribute loads due to the decrease disc height.[52]

The patient at least 25 pounds above ideal body weight should be advised to walk or bicycle. The additional weight plus increased joint reaction forces encountered with running would potentially exacerbate or produce pain in the joints of the lower extremities and/or spine. Recommendations regarding stage of condition, running surfaces, and shoes will be similar to walking.

A level running surface is also advised for jogging to encourage an upright posture and avoid increased intersegmental forces from the forward lean in uphill running.[53,54]

Swimming. Often swimming is recommended to back patients without regard to type of stroke, level of skill, and mobility re-

Endurance Program Data Base
Physical Therapy

Client Name: _____   Age: _____

Endurance Program: Stationary Bicycle _____   Walking _____   Running _____   Swimming _____   Rowing _____

Resting Pulse: _____   Target Pulse: _____

Precautions: _____

_____

Method: _____

_____

Date	Laps Completed or Time Required to Perform Activity	Distance	Resting Pulse	Post-Ex. Pulse	Comments	Examiner (Initials)

Figure 15D.1. Sample of data base record for individual patients.

Table 15D.4
A Starter Program for Joggers

Once you can comfortably walk two miles in 30 minutes, you are ready to start jogging. How fast you can increase your mileage for jogging depends on your level of fitness. A safe method is to increase your mileage by 10 per cent every week. Gradually progress to a 30-minute jog three or four times a week.

Step	Exercise Time (minutes)		Repetitions (times repeated)		Workout Time (minutes)
	Jog	Walk	Jog	Walk	Total
1	1	1	12	12	24
2	2	1	8	8	24
3	3	1	6	6	24
4	4	1	5	5	25
5	5	1	4	4	24
6	7	1	3	2	23
7	10	1	2	2	22
8	12	1	2	1	25
9	15	1	2	1	31
10	20	—	1	—	20
11	25	—	1	—	25
12	30	—	1	—	30

strictions which could aggravate the lumbar spine and sacroiliac joint. Freestyle, backstroke, and butterfly gain forward propulsion through the water primarily with the upper extremities. Rotation of the trunk in freestyle and backstroke is necessary to allow the shoulders to function in a neutral position. The lower extremities are secondary to the upper extremities, except in breaststroke, for forward propulsion in the water, and function primarily to balance the rotation of the trunk.[55]

The butterfly is contraindicated for lumbosacral dysfunction due to increased stress placed at the lumbosacral junction for forward movement by utilizing a bilateral flutter kick and lumbosacral flexion and extension to propel the body forward.

Freestyle is ideally performed by allowing the head to roll to the side to inhale which promotes trunk rotation instead of lifting the head out of the water. Eighty percent of the propulsive force for freestyle comes from the upper extremities.[55] During the recovery phase of the stroke (when the arm is out of the water), the elbow is higher than the hand, the head is rolling to the side, and the trunk rotates to the same side as the head. If a

patient presents with hypomobility in the thoracic segments, especially extension and rotation, the possibility exists for increased stress to the lower lumbar spine and shoulder. This observation emphasizes the importance of a complete structural and mobility assessment for the back pain patient. Patients with sacroiliac dysfunction may experience discomfort with freestyle due to the mechanics of the flutter kick. Normal range of motion for the knee in freestyle, backstroke, and butterfly is from full extension to 90° flexion. A biomechanically incorrect flutter kick may include less flexion and result in increased stress at the sacroiliac joint and the lower lumbar spine.

Sidestroke is not performed at the competitive level, but is useful for patients beginning a swimming program. The aerobic benefits of sidestroke are dubious, but the important factor is to motivate the patient to become involved in an enjoyable activity. A scissor kick provides for propulsion and the upper extremities glide on the surface after a downward stroke is performed with the top extremity. The mechanics of the stroke include minimal rotation of the trunk with forward bending of the lumbar spine. Sidestroke may be utilized as an exercise for relaxation or as a rest interval between other strokes.

Breaststroke is associated most with the complaints of back pain in swimming. Early elbow flexion and increased arm abduction during the pull-through phase propels the torso above the water and aggravates a lordotic posture.[56] Therefore, the breast stroke is not a recommended activity for the hyperlordotic spine, lumbar facet irritation, or individuals with spondylolisthesis.

Swim Fins have been recommended by manufacturers to increase caloric expenditure and fitness levels. Scientific studies have failed to show changes in the metabolic rate with swim fins.[57] Swim fins do make the lower extremity muscles work harder, but also increase the lever arm of the leg. The increased lever arm length could potentially stress the lumbosacral junction or sacroiliac joint.

Bicycling. Rehabilitation programs for orthopedic patients frequently include stationary bicycle ergometry. The rationale for incorporating stationary biking is to improve cardiovascular fitness, muscle strength, and endurance. However, bicycle ergometry may be uncomfortable for patients with lumbar facet restrictions and discogenic problems due to the forward inclination of the trunk.

The recommended position for bicycling is a standard pedal shaft (7 inches length), aligning the metatarsal heads directly over the axis of the pedal, toe clips to maintain the foot position, and adjusting the seat height so the knee is flexed to 15° when the pedal is in the down position. The handlebars are adjusted so the trunk is flexed to 20°.[58] Modifications for the back patient may emphasize an upright posture during bicycling until forward bending loads supported through the upper extremities are tolerated. The patient is instructed to gradually progress to 30 min. of bicycling with a cadence of at least 80 revolutions per minute despite the resistance.

Electromyographic activity of the rectus abdominis and erector spinae muscles during bicycling is minimal with the leg muscles demonstrating increased activity.[59] Therefore, bicycling benefits the cardiorespiratory system and increases lower extremity strength but appears to have little effect on the trunk musculature.

Rowing. Although this should be an excellent aerobic activity, a back patient may need to defer to another activity because of the difficulty in assuming the exercise position on the machine. Also, the mechanics of rowing are usually performed with a rounded back which places increased forward bending loads on the lumbar spine. Once the patient has been instructed on how to get up and down safely from the floor and can perform the movement without pain, rowing may be an appropriate selection.

The patient is instructed to place both feet in the stirrups, slide the buttocks close to the feet, and grip the handle with palms down. The back should be kept erect while the patient pushes away from the stirrups followed by pulling with the upper extremities, keeping the elbows raised. The handle is brought toward the chest with the rib cage elevated and shoulders back. As the patient slides back to the start position, emphasis should be placed on keeping the arms straight, knees flexed, and back in an upright posture. Patients with sacroiliac dysfunction may experience difficulty with rowing due to the hyperflexed position of the hips and posterior rotation of the pelvis. Rowing would not be appropriate for the severely deconditioned patient due to the difficulty in maintaining the correct posture throughout the exercise.

Electromyographic analysis of the rectus abdominis and erector spinae during rowing demonstrated peak activity when the subject was farthest away from the feet.[60] The rowing machine maximally works the upper and lower body musculature, and patients may develop muscle strength and endurance as well as increasing aerobic capacity.

Stair Climbing and Bench Aerobics. These have gained recent popularity. One of the main difficulties with the stair climber is the forward bent posture assumed during the activity. Patients should be encouraged to use the arm support and maintain an erect posture.

Bench aerobics is similar to the stair climber but without upper extremity support. The activity has been introduced into aerobic classes as a safe, low-impact exercise, but as the exercise participant begins to fatigue, the potential for increased loading to the knee and faulty posture increases. Participants may step on and off a bench ranging from 4 to 12 inches. The higher the step, the greater the risk for muscle fatigue, increased loading of patellofemoral joint, and forward bending stress to the lumbar spine.[61]

Intensity of Activities

The intensity of exercise can be based upon heart rate, related perceived exertion, or METS. The intensity of exercise is usually determined as a percentage of functional capacity and to achieve conditioning should not exceed 85% or be lower than 50% of functional capacity.[62] A nonlaboratory method for determining an age-adjusted target heart rate is calculated by subtracting the age of the individual from 220 and multiplying this value by a certain training percentage. For example, a 36 year old patient would have a maximum heart rate of 184. The target heart rate would be 184 times .70 = 129. This method underestimates the target heart rate for a given MET by 15%, so the target heart rate is adjusted by adding 15% to the calculated target heart rate.[63] Because of physiological or pathophysiological limitations, the exercise intensity may be lowered, but generally 60–70% of functional capacity is customary for average conditioning intensity.[62]

Duration of Program

A general consensus for prescribing duration of a conditioning program is 15–60 minutes, exclusive of the warm up and cool down periods of the training program.[43,44,63] Generally, most conditioning phases last between 20–30 minutes. Significant cardiovascular improvements have been noted with high intensity, short duration exercise sessions, but low intensity, long duration conditioning programs are recommended for sedentary and symptomatic individuals.[43,44,53] Milesis and coworkers[64] compared different durations of running performed 3 times per week at 85–90% maximal heart rate with a control group. This study concluded that a 15-minute program at moderate to high intensity performed 3 times a week produced an increase in cardiorespiratory fitness compared with the control group. Debusk[64] reported that three 10-minute bouts of exercise per day may be just as beneficial as 30 minutes performed at one time.

The frequency of exercise may vary from several sessions daily to 5–6 times per week.[1,9,43] Exercising 6–7 times per week enhances aerobic fitness and allows for the exercise to become a part of the patient's daily routine.[1]

Summation

One of the primary goals in developing an aerobic program for the back pain patient is to encourage movement and responsibility for managing the condition. Quite often, back pain patients have reduced activity levels and may initially require encouragement to perform minimal daily exercises. Even minimal, regular physical activity may reverse the deconditioning effects brought about by back pain and decrease the depression and anxiety associated with pain.[18]

REFERENCES

1. Nutter P. Aerobic exercise in the treatment and prevention of low back pain. Occup Med 1988; 3:137–145.
2. Mayer TG, Gatchel RJ. Functional restoration for spinal disorders: The sports medicine approach. Philadelphia: Lea & Febiger, 1988.
3. Bower DW. The role of exercises in the management of low back pain. In: Grieve GP: Modern manual therapy of the vertebral column. Edinburgh; New York: Churchill Livingstone, 1986.
4. Jackson CP, Brown, MD. Analysis of current approaches and a practical guide to prescription of exercise. Clin Orthop 1983; 179:46–54.
5. Jackson CP, Brown MD. Is there a role for exercise in the treatment of patients with low back pain? Clin Orthop 1983; 179:39–46.

6. Bowne DW, Russell ML, Morgan JL, et al. Reduced disability and healthcare in an individual fitness program. J Occup Med 1984; 26:809–816.

7. Cady LD, Bischoff DP. Strength and fitness and subsequent back injuries in firefighters. J Occup Med 1979; 21:269–272.

8. Merriam-Webster Dictionary, HB Woolf ed. New York: Simon & Schuster, 1974.

9. Astrand PO. Exercise physiology and its role in disease prevention and in rehabilitation. Arch Phys Med Rehabil 1987; 68:305–309.

10. Dearman MS, Francis KT. Plasma levels of catecholamines, cortisol, and beta-endorphins in male athletes after running 26.2, 6, and 2 miles. J Sports Med Phys Fitness 1983; 23:30–38.

11. Saraste H, Hultman G. Life conditions of persons with and without low back pain. Scand J Rehabil Med 1987; 19:109–113.

12. Heinzelmann F, Bagley RW. Response to physical activity programs and their effects on health behavior. Public Health Rep 1970; 85:905–911.

13. White AA, Gordon SL. Synopsis: Workshop on idiopathic low back pain. Spine 1982; 7:141–149.

14. Schmidt A. Cognitive factors on performance level of chronic low back pain patients. J Psychosom Res 1985; 29:183–189.

15. Cady LD, Thomas PC, Karwasky RJ. Program for increasing health and physical fitness of firefighters. J Occup Med 1985; 27:110–114.

16. Sandler H, Vernikos J. Conclusion. In: Sandler H, Vernikos J, eds. Inactivity: physiological effects. Orlando: Academic Press, 1986.

17. Sandler H. Effects of inactivity on muscle. In: Sandler H, Vernikos J, eds. Inactivity: Physiological effects. Orlando: Academic Press, 1986.

18. Convertino VA. Exercise responses after inactivity. In: Sandler H, Vernikos J, eds. Inactivity: Physiological effects. Orlando: Academic Press, 1986.

19. Smith EL, Raab DM. Osteoporosis and physical activity. In: Astrand PO, Grimby G, eds. Physical activity in health and disease. Acta Med Scand Symposium Series, No. 2, Stockholm: Almqvist & Wiskell International, 1986.

20. Sinaki M. Exercise and osteoporosis. Arch Phys Med Rehabil 1989; 70:220–229.

21. Tipton CM, Vailas AC, Mathes RD. Experimental studies on the influences of physical activity on ligaments, tendons and joints: A brief review. In: Astrand PO, Grimby G, eds. Physical activity in health and disease. Acta Med Scand Symposium Series. No 2, Stockholm: Almqvist & Wiskell International, 1986.

22. Heinriksson J, Reitmann JS. Time course changes in human skeletal muscle succinate dehydrogenase and cytochrome oxidase activities and maximal oxygen uptake with physical activity and inactivity. Acta Physiol Scand 1977; 99:91–97.

23. Larsson L: Physical training effects on muscle mor-

phology in sedentary males at different ages. Med Sci Sports Exerc 1982; 14:203–206.

24. Krolner B, Toft B. Vertebral bone loss: an unneeded side effect of therapeutic bedrest. Clin Sci 1983; 64:537–540.

25. Hansson TH, Roos BO, Nachemson A: Development of osteopenia in the fourth lumbar vertebrae during prolonged bedrest after operation for scoliosis. Acta Orthop Scand 1975; 46:612–630, 1975.

26. Whedon GO. Disuse osteoporosis physiological aspects. Calcif Tissue Int 1984; 36:146–150.

27. Devries H. Method of evaluation of muscle fatigue and endurance from electromyographic fatigue curves. Am J Phys Med 1968; 47:175–181.

28. Devries H. EMG fatigue curves in postural muscles. A possible etiology for idiopathic low back pain. Am J Phys Med 1968; 47:175–181.

29. Wolf SL, Wolf LB, Segal RL. The relationship of extraneous movements to lumbar paraspinal muscle activity: Implications for EMG biofeedback training applications to low back pain patients. Biofeedback Self Regul 1989; 14:63–74.

30. Lanyon EE. Functional strain as a determinant for bone remodeling. Calcif Tissue Int 1984; 36:56–61.

31. Jacobsen P, Beaver W, et al. Bone density in women, college athletes, and older athletic women. J Orthop Res 1984; 2:328–332.

32. Siscovick DS, Laporte RE, Newman JM. The disease-specific benefits and risks of physical activity and exercise. Public Health Rep 1985; 100:180–188.

33. Nachemson A. Work for all. Clin Orthop 1983; 179:77–85.

34. Deyo R, Diehl AK, Rosenthal M. How many days of bedrest for acute low back pain? N Engl J Med 1986; 315:1064–1070.

35. Taylor CB, Salles JF, Needle R. The relation of physical activity and exercise in mental health. Public Health Rep 1985; 100:195–202.

36. Markoff RA, Ryan P, Young T. Endorphins and mood changes in long distance running. Med Sci Sports Exerc 1982; 14:11–15.

37. Ransford CP. A role for the amines in the anti-depressant effect of exercise: A review. Med Sci Sports Exerc 1982; 14:1–10.

38. Browman CP. Sleep following sustained exercise. Psychophysiology 1980; 17:577–580.

39. Griffin SG, Trinder J. Physical fitness, exercise, and human sleep. Psychophysiology 1978; 15:447–450.

40. Colt EW, Wardlaw SL, et al. The effect of running on plasma B-endorphins. Life Sci 1981; 28:1637–1640.

41. Fraoli F, Moretti C, Paolucci D, et al. Physical exercise stimulates marked concomitant release B-endorphin and adrenocorticotropic hormone (ACTH) in peripheral blood in man. Experientia 1980; 36:987–989.

42. Carr DB, Bullen BA, Skrinar GS, et al. Physical conditioning facilitates the exercise induced secre-

tion of beta-endorphin and beta-lipoprotein in women. N Engl J Med 1981; 305:560–563.

43. Heath GH. Exercise programming for the older adult. In: Blair SN, Painter P, eds. Resource manual for guidelines for exercise testing and prescription. Philadelphia: Lea and Febiger, 1988.

44. American College of Sports Medicine Position Statement on: The recommended quantity and quality of exercise for developing and maintaining fitness. Med Sci Sports 1978; 10:7–9.

45. Yanker GD. A complete book of exercise walking. Chicago: Contemporary Books, Inc., 1983.

46. Burton K, Yanker G. Walking medicine: lifetime guide to preventative and therapeutic exercise walking programs. New York: McGraw-Hill, 1990.

47. Rydell N. Biomechanics of the hip joint. Clin Orthop 1973; 92:6–15.

48. Voloshin A. An in vivo study of low back pain and shock absorption in the human locomotor system. J Biomechan 1982; 15:21–27.

49. Cook SD, Brinker MR, Poche M. Running shoes: Their relationship to running injuries. Sport Med 1990; 10:1–8.

50. Chadbourne RD. A hard look at running surfaces. Phys Sport Med 1990; 18:103–109.

51. Owens SG, Al-Ahmed A, Moffatt RJ. Physiological effects of walking and running with hand-held weights. J Sport Med Phys Fitness 1989; 29:384–387.

52. White TL, Malone TR: Effects of running on intervertebral disc height. J Orthop Sports Phys Ther 1990; 12:139–146.

53. Bach DK, Green DS, Jenson GM, Savinor E. A comparison of muscular tightness in runners and nonrunners and the relation of muscular tightness to low back pain in runners. J Orthop Sports Phys Ther 1985; 6:315–323.

54. Cappozzo A. Force actions in the human trunk during running. J Sports Med 1986; 5:14–22.

55. Richardson AR. The biomechanics of swimming: The shoulder and knee. Clin Sports Med 1986; 5:103–113.

56. Fowler PJ: Swimming injuries of the knee, foot and ankle, elbow and back. Clin Sports Med 1986; 5:139–148.

57. Gall SL. Swim fins—adding splash to the laps. Phys Sport Med 1990; 18:91–96.

58. Goodwin C, Cornwall MW. Effect of an adjustable pedal shaft on ROM and phasic muscle activity of the knee during bicycling. J Orthop Sports Phys Ther 1989; 11:259–262.

59. Despires M. An electromyographic study of competitive road cycling conditions simulated on a treadmill. Biomechanics IV. Baltimore: University Park Press, 1974; 349–355.

60. Rodriguez BS, Rodriguez RP, Cook SD, Sandborn PM. Electromyographic analysis of rowing stroke biomechanics. J Sport Med Phys Fitness 1990; 30:103–108.

61. Haraste A. Bench aerobics: A step in the right direction? Phys Sport Med 1990; 18:25–26.

62. Kavanagh I. General deconditioning. In: Basmajian JV, Kirby RL, eds. Medical rehabilitation. Baltimore: Williams & Wilkins, 1984.

63. Milesis CA, Pollock ML, Bah MD. Effects of different durations of physical training on cardiorespiratory function, body composition, and serum lipids. Res Q 1976; 47:716–725.

64. Debusk RF, Stenestrand U, Sheehan M, Haskell WL: Training effects of long versus short bouts of exercise in healthy subjects. Am J Cardiol 1990; 65:1010–1013.

16

Ergonomic Considerations

DANIEL ORTIZ and RUSSELL SMITH

Ergonomics is the multidisciplinary science concerned with adapting the workplace to meet the physical and mental capabilities of the worker. The word is derived from the Greek "ergon" meaning "work" and "nomos" meaning "laws of." Concepts in ergonomics are developed from research in work physiology, anthropometry, medicine, psychology, and engineering. The goal is to maximize compatibility between the individual and the task and environment, to promote human performance and health.[1-3]

Problems associated with productivity, quality control, and worker health arise when workers are exposed to jobs that exceed their mental or strength capabilities.[4] For example, poorly designed seated and standing workstations and jobs that force individuals to assume stressful work postures and/or handle excessive loads are connected to musculoskeletal aches and pains and possibly disease and injury.[2] Indeed, the back is often the target of poor work design and lay-out.[1,3] While the back is the primary focus of this chapter, a significant class of disorders known as cumulative trauma disorders affecting the upper extremities also are associated with poor work design and organization.[2,5,6] We have observed that application of ergonomic concepts in industry has grown substantially in the last 5 years. Industry's growing sensitivity is partly due to the rule enforcement activity of the Department of Labor's Occupational Safety and Health Administration and their development of an ergonomic guideline,[6] excessive workers compensation losses, and increased union activity with respect to ergonomics.

Central to the manual therapist's practice is the skillful manipulation of forces applied to the patient. Clinically, these forces may result from manual techniques, therapeutic exercises, and/or forces from a chosen posture (e.g., standing or sitting). Also essential to the manual therapist is the emphasis placed on function during evaluation and treatment. The field of ergonomics shares similar emphases, studying the relationship between an individual and the work and environment. Although not exhaustive, the ergonomic concepts presented in this chapter may provide another perspective for the therapist in the patient assessment process. In particular, it pertains to the limitations of the recovering worker and the various requirements of the task that may be assigned.

THE NATURE OF WORK

Depending on the task, industrial work is done seated, standing, and rarely, both seated and standing. Seated work is generally recommended for jobs that require precise movements of the hands over an entire shift. Standing is recommended for jobs that require a wide range of motion and considerable forces to accomplish the task.[7] Fine assembly tasks and driving are generally done seated, while many heavy manual material-handling jobs are done standing.

Whether sedentary or standing the dimensions of the workplace with respect to the worker can cause the individual to assume stressful, inefficient postures and motions to accomplish the task. Examples include trunk flexion, frequent or sustained reaches with arms fully extended, and work that requires shoulder abduction for long durations.[8,9] Awkward and/or sustained postures, including prolonged standing or sitting, can create static loads on the muscles of the body and spine, possibly impairing worker comfort and performance.[1,3,5,10]

The potential postural incompatibilities posed by sitting and standing are further compounded by the load handling requirements of some tasks. Jobs that require the handling of heavy loads are prevalent in many industries and are associated with back injuries.[11,12] Because of their potential impact on the back, materials handling and sitting and standing will be treated separately.

STATIC VERSUS DYNAMIC WORK

Many jobs contain both static and dynamic elements.[1] In dynamic work, muscle fibers rhythmically contract and relax (i.e., muscle length changes) in response to nerve stimulation. This cyclic change in muscle length facilitates blood circulation. Muscles involved in static exertions, however, are contracted for long periods. Postures that are sustained for extended periods, therefore, involve static exertions and promote muscle fatigue from the resultant blood vessel compression by the contracted muscle group. This compression results in a restriction of blood flow through the affected muscle group and causes: *a*) the heart to work harder; *b*) a build-up of metabolites, especially lactic acid, carbon dioxide, and potassium; and *c*) energy source depletion.[1,13]

Although the exact mechanism of muscle fatigue has not been elucidated, the accumulation of metabolites, energy source depletion, and the CNS recruitment of motor units are

thought by some researchers to be associated with a reduction in muscular performance.[1,5,13] Indicators of muscle fatigue—localized pain and discomfort, loss of work tolerance, and EMG changes—are widely studied.[1,8]

Static loading of the muscles can affect work tolerance and the worker's ability to maintain the muscle exertion.[8] At 60% of the muscle's maximum voluntary contraction there is almost total occlusion of blood flow through the muscle. The length of time the exertion can be maintained at this level is less than 60 seconds. However, if the exertion can be held to under 15–20 percent of MVC, blood flow is normal and it can be maintained for relatively long periods.[1,5] Some researchers suggest that only static exertions less than 5–8% of MVC can be maintained indefinitely.[14]

Under similar conditions, a static effort compared to a dynamic effort leads to a higher energy consumption and elevated heart rate. Subsequently, rest periods of 20–50 times the contraction period may be necessary.[1,5] As many jobs have both static and dynamic components, they should be carefully evaluated to determine if the static components can be reduced or eliminated through job reorganization or redesign.[9]

To help reduce static loading of the back and upper extremity muscles the work should be located so the worker can maintain the elbows down close to the body with a 90° forearm flexor angle.[1,2] Consequently, working height is a concern.[1,15] Suggestions for work height differ from below elbow level (5–10 cm) for most work activities to above elbow level (5 cm) for visually demanding work. To avoid the potentially harmful effects of maintaining prolonged positioning in stressful postures, an adjustable workbench would be ideal to determine the most appropriate height for the specific individual during a specific function. Additionally, work activities should also be located so that forward reaches in the sagittal plane are kept within 14–16 inches (length of small lower arm) of the worker.[2]

STANDING AND SEATED WORK

Standing and sitting postures have been associated with reports of pain to the lumbar region among workers.[3,16] To avoid prolonged posture and alter the stresses to the individual, a workplace which combines sitting and standing has been recommended.[1,15] The use of a saddle-chair has been proposed as a possible mechanism to support a standing posture, especially with reduced leg space.[15] The support-standing posture offers the worker the advantages of sitting as compared to standing (i.e., improved worker precision with decreased total energy consumption) with a more neutral posturing of the spine.[1,15] The practice of frequent postural changes during standing, whether by the use of support-standing devices, weight shifting and/or foot rests or rails, is to be encouraged in environments requiring prolonged standing. The use of compressible mats or surfaces has also been proposed to help evenly distribute load on the feet, decrease ground reactive forces, and promote comfort.[10]

Seated Work

Although standing is a posture commonly seen in work environments, probably sitting is a posture more characteristic of our times.[17] Consideration of the forces during sitting and the response of the human body to the various sitting postures is important in planning a total treatment approach. The human body's response to forces during sitting have been considered a cause of low back pain.[18–20]

Stability. The base of support during sitting (with the addition of the buttocks and posterior thigh) is greater than in standing, thus allowing greater stability with a resultant decrease in total energy demand.[1] A portion of the improved stability is diminished with the loss of the passive locking mechanism at the hips, present during standing. The loss of this locking mechanism during sitting decreases the stability of the trunk over the hips, necessitating support from muscle activity and/or external support including chair features and/or ergonomic aids.[1,15,21]

Movements. Observations of seated individuals have revealed movement patterns during sitting.[22,23] One movement pattern described includes small oscillatory movements of the trunk over the ischial tuberosities. This dynamic behavior of the body during sitting may be an effort to avoid sustained postures. Avoiding sustained postures may result in a decrease in static forces preventing or slowing the fatigue of the muscles attempting to stabilize.[1]

Spinal Posture and Line of Gravity. Another factor affecting the level of muscle activity is the posture of the spine and of the extremities adopted by the seated individual.[1,24] Proposed unsupported sitting postures, based on the location of the center of gravity and percent of body weight transmitted to the feet are the anterior, the middle, and the posterior sitting postures.[25] The anterior sitting posture shifts the center of gravity anterior to the ischial tuberosities with greater than 25% body weight transmitted to the feet. The anterior shift of the center of gravity relates to either an anterior pelvic tilt (with the spine flexed, extended, or in neutral) or a neutral pelvis with flexion of the spine. The middle sitting posture presents with the center of gravity above the ischial tuberosities, and approximately 25% body weight is transmitted to the feet. The middle sitting posture can be maintained in a more upright (erect), slightly flexed, or straight posturing of the spine.

During posterior sitting, the center of gravity is typically posterior to the ischial tuberosities. The body weight transmitted to the feet is relatively decreased as compared to the previous postures (less than 25%). A posterior tilt of the pelvis with thoracic and lumbar kyphosis is present with the posterior posture.

Muscular Responses. The difference in the line of gravity between the three sitting postures results in different forces applied to the spine which influence the responses of the individual to sitting (e.g., muscle activity). During an anterior sitting posture, increased EMG activity of the erector spinae generally and of the hip extensors has been noted.[26,27] If the anterior displacement of the center of gravity occurs primarily due to trunk flexion (rather than hip flexion), the EMG activity of the lumbar erector spinae muscle will decrease with increased hip extensor activity.[27] The middle sitting posture, especially erect, reportedly necessitates increased activity of the erector spinae secondary to the inherent instability of balancing over the ischial tuberosities.[21] Posterior sitting posture will result in decreased activity of erector spinae with increased EMG activity of the iliopsoas,[28] and cervical extensors.[29] EMG activity of the posterior cervical muscles increases with increased flexion of the thoracic and lumbar spine.[29]

Disc Pressures. These vary according to the sitting posture.[24,26] Lumbar disc pressure at the L3/4 segment was found to be lowest in the erect sitting posture (approximately three times greater than in standing). Posterior sitting increased disc pressure (approximately two times) relative to the middle posture. Anterior sitting with increased thoracic and lumbar flexion gave the greatest level of disc pressure (approximately three times the pressure during the middle sitting posture).

External Supports. As might be expected, a chair back, lumbar support, or arm support have been demonstrated to influence the mechanics of the sitting posture. Disc pressures decrease with the use of a lumbar support or a backrest.[30] A slightly (approximately 10°) inclined backrest will decrease lumbar disc pressures and will decrease EMG activity of erector spinae in the thoracic, lumbar, and cervical spine.[29,30] Ergonomic aids have, also, been demonstrated to decrease EMG activity. For example, elbow supports during sitting reduce the activity of posterior cervical and thoracic muscles.[29]

Personal and Environmental Influences. Other factors influencing the forces brought to bear on the seated individual (and subsequent response by the individual to the forces) relate to the individual,[31] the environment, and the task.[32] Of interest to the manual therapist may be the influence of individual pa-

tient variances in functional abilities on the posture attained during sitting. An example is the correlation identified in female subjects between range of hip mobility (both hip extension and flexion with knee extended) and position of lumbar spine in sitting.[7] A decreased hip mobility correlated positively to decreased lumbar lordosis in sitting postures.[31] This finding highlights the importance of not losing sight of the individual's specific limitations during observation and/or training of sitting posture.

Workstation. Workplace design and the surrounding environment influence the posture and other responses of the seated individual. Workplace design includes chair features[24,33,34] and desk features.[15,34] Environmental factors are the lighting and visual demands of the task.[35] Recommended "ideal" chair and desk features vary from author to author,[1,15,18,31,34] and "ideal" remains an idea and not a fact for everyone. The normal variation of structure and function in the general population may partially account for the conflicting recommendations. Although the actual features may differ among authors, concepts are consistent between them. They can be applied to the worker by featuring adjustability of the furniture and congruency between the furnishings (i.e., between chair and desk) and with the task and/or individual.[1]

Chair Design and Choice

During the process of determining which chair or desk feature is desired, it is important to establish their specific purposes. Also to be evaluated is the ability of the individual to attain and maintain the facilitated postures without discomfort. The uniqueness, functionally and structurally, each individual brings to the seated posture needs to be appreciated by the clinician.[36] Limited mobility, as well as instability, will influence the effects of the various features prescribed. As discussed, hip mobility has been related to the amount of lordosis achieved during sitting.[31] Also, restriction in flexion of the lower lumbar segments may significantly affect the amount of kyphosis achieved during sitting, due to the chief role of the lower lumbar segments during sitting in lumbar kyphosis.[24] Inability or difficulty in adequately stabilizing the spine in a particular posture may result in an avoidance of the desired posturing. Facilitating a posture that a person desires to avoid may produce greater stress as the individual works at resisting the imposed stresses.

Features of Chairs

The general purpose of a chair or desk is to provide "optimal stability with minimal restraint."[21] The clinician will creatively balance the need for mobility with the need for stability, attempting to minimize static contractions of postural muscles and allowing for dynamic activity. One chair feature demonstrating the balance between mobility and stability to be considered is the seat.[1,37,38] Proper seat height will distribute the weight between the ischial tuberosities and posterior thighs. A low seat height will localize the weightbearing posteriorly on the ischial tuberosities.[21] A seat too high could produce pressure on the thighs restricting blood flow and promoting user discomfort.[2] A footrest or support may be needed with chairs that lack an adequate range of adjustability. The seat edge should not contact the popliteal fossa, because it will compromise the ability of the individual to alter leg position.[18] A rounded seat edge will facilitate mobility of the leg.[18] The favored seat contour is a flat surface with a slight depression for the buttocks to help resist sliding out of the chair.[21] A more concave contour will increase weightbearing through the greater trochanter, resulting in internal rotation of the femur and potentially restricting movement of the legs.[39] The correct angle of the seat is debated in the literature with support for backward sloping seats, forward sloping seats, and flat seats.[24,34,40]

The Kneeling Chair (e.g. Balans Chair). This has received much attention and presents with a forward sloping seat. Again, disagreement is found in the literature regarding the effects and indications of the kneeling chair.[23,41–43] Proponents suggest the seat facilitates an erect posturing of the spine with increased ease of function anteriorly.[21,43] Other studies suggest no longterm improvement in posturing and increased EMG activity of the erector spinae.[41,42,44] The opponents also argue that the chair inhibits mobility of the seated individual. The kneeling chair may be indicated for short timeperiod activities performed anteriorly, but not indicated during longer activities.

The seat-to-backrest angle is another chair feature of interest.[24,29,45] The consensus appears to support a seat-to-backrest angle of 95–105° with resultant decreased EMG of the erector spinae (lumbar, thoracic, and cervical) and decreased disc pressure.[1,19,24]

Features of Desks and Tables

Desk/worksurface features considered to influence postural stresses include height, slope, and distance from the seated individual. Table height is related to seat height.[1] Grandjean[1] has demonstrated the ideal desk height for office workers to be 27–30 cm above the seat, regardless of the individual's body type. Chair and desk should be adjusted to allow the individual to work with elbows down by the side, flexed at approximately 90° with the hand functioning on the desk.[1] Slanted desk surfaces (10°–20°) have been related to more erect posturing of the spine, decreased fatigue, decreased complaints of pain, and decreased EMG activity when compared to flat desk surfaces.[15,46]

MANUAL MATERIALS HANDLING

Static loads on the muscles of the body can have a negative effect on worker comfort and health. As pointed out in the foregoing sections the target of postural stress due to static exertions is often the structures of the back. This is particularly true with jobs that involve load handling and transfer. The manual handling or transfer of material, either finished goods, raw materials, or materials in process, is an activity prevalent in industry.[47] These activities can create large loads on the spine and back muscles and expose workers to potential injury.

Injuries related to materials handling represent roughly 25% of annual worker compensation claims. Over 79% of these injuries affect the lower back, with most involving the erector spinae, discs, and/or facet-joints.[47,48] Overexertion is said to be the primary cause of these injuries.[47] Moreover, approximately two-thirds of all overexertion claims involve lifting loads, and about 20% involve pushing or pulling loads.[5] Heavy industry (e.g., construction and mining) has the highest incidence of back injuries, but other industries report problems as well.[49] Occupations at risk include miscellaneous laborers, garbage collectors, warehouse workers, mechanics, and nursing aides.[11]

Lifting Guide

The high prevalence of back pain and injuries among the working population establishes the need for developing lifting limits. Incorporating information from analytical approaches in epidemiology, biomechanics, psychophysics, and physiology, the National Institute for Occupational Safety and Health (NIOSH) developed a lifting guide[12] for assessing employee risk for back injury. The general concepts of this guide are discussed below.

From the standpoint of epidemiology, the following task characteristics are considered to be job risk factors associated with back injury:[12]

a) *object weight:* the heavier the load the greater the risk;

b) *the location of the load center of gravity* from the worker: the greater the distance from the body the greater the risk;

c) *lifting frequency and duration:* the higher the lift frequency the greater the risk;

d) *the location of the load* at the start of the lift/lower: lift from floor is the most hazardous.

Twisting, severe trunk flexion, and jerking motions can substantially increase the stresses on the low back and are, therefore, considered to be risk factors as well.[12,49]

Biomechanical Models. These are used to assess the forces and torques acting on the different parts of the body. Predicting the compressive force acting on the L5/S1 disc is of great interest because the stresses at this point can be high, exposing individuals to possible injury.[50] Based on cadaver and epidemiologic studies NIOSH concluded that compressive forces in excess of 650 kilograms create a serious back injury risk to most workers. Compressive forces greater than 350 kilograms may be associated with a sudden increase in the incidence of low back pain. Consequently, the 350 kg value is suggested as an upper limit for lifting by NIOSH.

Static biomechanical models that assess the forces due to gravity on the L5/S1 disc are commercially available. Dynamic biomechanical models take into consideration the torques and forces due to acceleration. One study[51] showed that depending on lifting method (leg lift, back lift, trunk kinetic lift, and load kinetic lift), dynamic compressive force due to inertia on the lumbosacral spine could be 33–60% greater than the predicted static compression. Consequently, the dynamic aspect of manual lifting is an important factor in the risk assessment process.

Maximum Acceptable Weights. The application of psychophysics to predicting the acceptability of material handling jobs has been explored by a number of researchers.[50] One researcher[48] asked subjects to perform lifting, lowering, carrying, pushing, and pulling tasks under different controlled conditions (e.g., frequency, height at start of activity, distance travelled, object width). Subjects were also asked to adjust the weight of the load to the maximum level acceptable to them under the defined conditions. From this experimentation, maximum acceptable weights (MAWs) or forces that are acceptable to 10, 25, 50, 75, and 90% of the industrial population were derived by gender for the different material handling categories. Apparently, employees working at jobs that are acceptable to less than 75% of the working population are three times more likely to develop an overexertion strain or sprain. Consequently, the

MAW for 75% of the working population should be used as the lower limit of acceptability.

Action Limit and Maximum Permissible Limit. From the foregoing information, NIOSH derived an equation for calculating an Action Limit (AL) and a Maximum Permissible Limit (MPL) for lifting. It is outside the scope of this chapter to discuss the details of this equation. However, NIOSH provides an in-depth explanation of the derivation of the equation and provides examples of its application for interested parties.[12] The Action Limit for lifting is the product of four factors and a constant (90 pounds):

$$AL = 90(HF)(VF)(DF)(FF)$$

HF is the horizontal factor that takes into consideration the distance of the load from the worker's body. VF is the vertical factor that takes into consideration the location of the object at the start of the lift. DF is the distance factor that takes into consideration the distance the load is lifted. Finally, the lifting frequency is represented by FF the frequency factor. The maximum value each factor can be is one. Consequently, under optimal conditions the maximum Action Limit is 90 pounds. As conditions become less than optimal the AL decreases. The MPL is simply three times the AL:

$$MPL = (3)(AL)$$

The actual loads handled under the given lifting conditions can be compared to the calculated AL and MPL for those same conditions. Jobs at the AL would be acceptable to 75% of women and 99% of men producing a compressive force of 350 kg on the L5/S1 disc. Conversely, only 25% of the men and less than 1% of the women would have the muscle strength to do lifting tasks at or above the MPL and compressive forces would equal or exceed 650 kg on the L5/S1 disc. Jobs below the AL create a small risk of injury to most healthy workers. Jobs between the AL and MPL create a moderate to severe risk of injury with jobs at or above the MPL classified as "high hazard" from the standpoint of back injury.

Significantly, this guide assumes ideal lifting conditions (e.g., smooth, sagittal plane lift and comfortable ambient temperature), that often do not exist in the workplace. Consequently, the limits that are developed probably underestimate employee risk of back injury. At the time of this writing the *NIOSH Work Practices Guide for Manual Lifting* was being revised to take factors concerning coupling devices and twisting into consideration.

Control Strategies

Engineering (e.g., job and tool redesign) and administrative (e.g., training) controls should be implemented to reduce the exposure to overexertion injuries. Both types of controls are necessary when a job exceeds the AL. Administrative controls include medical screening, pre-employment strength testing, and employee methods training. The long held, yet waning, notion that the straight back bent knee method is by itself an effective intervention strategy is unsubstantiated. One published study shows that a "free style" method is energetically more efficient, requires less time, and is preferred by employees over the straight back bent knee method.[52] The importance of sound biomechanics and physical fitness should be the emphasis of any training program. Employees should be made aware of the high risk motions and postures (e.g., bending, twisting, and accelerating the object), possibly increasing the probability of risk factor avoidance.

In industries or jobs that are not amenable to engineering changes (e.g., certain construction, fire-fighting, and some warehouse operations) pre-employment strength testing is often given as a possible intervention. The concept is based on matching the worker to the job. One method involves comparing a worker's isometric strength capability to the strength requirement of the job in question. The risk of back injury has been demonstrated to be about three times greater at jobs that equal or exceed a worker's isometric strength capability.[53]

Any strength testing procedure must be carefully designed for the job or jobs of interest. The Equal Employment Opportunity Commission requires that any test used as a screening tool exactly simulate the strength requirements of the job in question (i.e., test validity is required). Selection criteria used in any testing regimen cannot discriminate against the prospective worker population. Moreover, the Americans with Disabilities Act of 1990, that requires the employer to make reasonable accommodation for the disabled worker, may further limit the possible use of this method in industry.

Jobs at the MPL are considered to be high risk, and only through engineering controls can they be made acceptable to most employees. A few examples of engineering controls are given as follows:

1. Hydraulic lift (e.g., scissors lift) to maintain the object height at the level of work and eliminate the lift/lower component
2. Self-leveling dispensers to eliminate the lift/lower component
3. Unit load concept (e.g., the use of pallets) so that a forklift can be used instead of manual labor during truck loading operations
4. Automation

The efficacy of back schools, back belts, medical screening, and employee training in preventing or reducing the incidence of musculoskeletal injuries is apparently low or as of yet unproven.[54] Strength and fitness training does show promise, however. An effective approach to controlling back injuries will be the use of both engineering and administrative controls. Through sound job design alone the incidence of back injury might be reduced by as much as 33%.[54] Considering the magnitude of the problem, this figure is impressive.

CONCLUSIONS

The basic ergonomic principles concerning standing, sitting, and manual materials handling have been discussed. Understanding of the mechanics of the standing and sitting postures and the effects on the postures of alterations in workstation design or individual worker characteristics is clinically beneficial in evaluating a patient or client as he/she interacts with his/her work environment. Comprehension of the various forces generated during manual material handling is critical for a total management approach to patients who encounter such tasks as a regular part of their work. Integration of sound biomechanical principles and anatomical considerations to the work environment will greatly assist the manual therapist in functionally preparing the patient for his/her work environment and vice versa.

REFERENCES

1. Grandjean E. Fitting the task to the man. 4th ed. London: Taylor and Francis, 1988.
2. Tichauer ER. The biomechanical basis of ergonomics: anatomy applied to the design of work situations. New York: Wiley-Interscience Publication, John Wiley & Sons, 1978.
3. van Wely P. Design and disease. Appl Ergonomics 1970; 1:262–269.
4. Pulat BM. Introduction. In: Industrial ergonomics: a practitioner's guide, Alexander DC, Pulat BM, eds. Norcross GA: Industrial Engineering and Management Press, Institute of Industrial Engineers, 1985; 1–7.
5. Chaffin DB and Andersson G. Occupational biomechanics. New York: John Wiley & Sons, 1984.
6. U.S. Department of Labor, Occupational Safety and Health Administration. 1990. Ergonomics program management guidelines for meatpacking plants. OSHA 3123.
7. Eastman Kodak Company, The human factors section. Ergonomic design for people at work; Vol. 1. Belmont, CA: Lifetime Learning Publications, 1983.
8. Chaffin, DB. Localized muscle fatigue: definition and measurement. J Occup Med 1973; 15:346–354.
9. Greenberg L, Chaffin DB. Workers and their tools: a guide to the ergonomic design of hand tools and small presses. Midland, MI: Pendell Publishing Co., 1976.
10. Konz S. Work design. Columbus: Grid Publishing, Inc., 1979.
11. Bureau of National Affairs, Inc. Back injuries: costs, causes, cases and prevention. A BNA Special Report. Washington, DC: BNA; 1988.
12. National Institute for Occupational Safety and Health. A work practices guide for manual lifting. U.S. Government Printing Office, Washington, DC, 1981.
13. Kroemer KHE, Kroemer HJ, Kroemer-Elbert KE. Engineer physiology: bases of human factors/ergonomics. 2nd ed. New York: Van Nostrand Reinhold, 1990.

14. Corlett EN. Analysis and evaluation of working posture. In: Ergonomics of workstation design. Kvalseth, TO, ed. Boston: Butterworth, 1983.

15. Bendix T, Krohn L, Jessen F, Aaras A. Trunk posture and trapezius muscle load while working in standing, supported-standing and sitting positions. Spine 1985; 1:433–439.

16. Kelly MJ, Ortiz DJ, Folds DJ, Courtney TK. Human factors in advanced apparel manufacturing. In: Human aspects of advanced manufacturing and hybrid automation. Karwowski W, Rahimi M, eds. Amsterdam: Elsevier, 1990.

17. Grandjean E, Hunting W. Ergonomics of posture-review of various problems of standing and sitting posture. Appl Ergonomics 1977; 8:135–140.

18. Keegan JJ. Alterations of the lumbar curve related to posture and seating. J Bone Joint Surg 1953; 35A:589–603.

19. Kottke FJ. Evaluation and treatment of low back pain due to mechanical causes. Arch Phys Med Rehabil 1961; 42:426–440.

20. McKenzie RA. The lumbar spine. New Zealand: Spinal Publications, 1981.

21. Zacharkow D. Posture: Sitting, standing, chair design and exercise. Illinois: Charles C Thomas, 1988.

22. Branton P. Behavior, body mechanics and discomfort. In: Grandjean E, ed. Proceedings of the symposium on sitting posture. London: Taylor and Francis; 1969; 202–213.

23. Dillon J. The role of ergonomics in the development of performance tests for furniture. Appl Ergonomics 1981; 12:169–175.

24. Andersson GB, Murphy RW, Ortengren R, Nachemson AL. The influence of back rest inclination and lumbar support on lumbar lordosis. Spine 1979; 4:52–58.

25. Schoberth H. Cited by: Zacharkow, D. Posture: sitting, standing, chair design and exercise. Illinois: Charles C Thomas, 1988; 54–57.

26. Andersson GB, Jonsson B, Ortengren R. Myoelectric activity in individual lumbar erector spinae muscles in sitting. A study with surface and wire electrodes. Scand J Rehabil Med 1974; 3(suppl):19–108.

27. Carlsöö S. How man moves. London: Heinemann; 1972.

28. Keagy RD, Brumlik J, Bergan JJ. Direct EMG of the psoas major muscle in man. J Bone Joint Surg 1966; 48A:1377–1382.

29. Schuldt K, Ekholm J, Harms-Ringdahl K, Nemeth G, Arborelius UP. Effects of changes in sitting work posture on static neck and shoulder muscle activity. Ergonomics 1986; 29:1525–1537.

30. Andersson GB, Ortengren R, Nachemson A, Elfstrom G, Broman H. The sitting posture: an electromyographic and discometric study. Orthop Clin North Am 1975; 6:105–120.

31. Bridger RS, Wilkinson D, Van Houweninge T. Hip

32. Hsiao H, Keyserling WM. A three-dimensional ultrasonic system for posture measurement. Ergonomics 1990; 33:1089–1114.

33. Corlett EN. Aspects of the evaluation of industrial sitting. Ergonomics 1989; 32:256–269.

34. Mandal AC. The correct height of school furniture. Hum Factors 1982; 24:257–269.

35. Smith M. Health issues in VDT work. In: Visual display terminals. Useability, issues, and health concerns. Bennett S, Case D, Sandelin J, Smith M, eds. Englewood Cliffs, NJ: Prentice-Hall, 1984.

36. Vollowitz E. Furniture prescription for the conservative management of low-back pain. In: Topics in acute care and trauma rehabilitation, Edgelow P, Farrell J, eds. 1989; 2:18–37.

37. Tijerina L. Optimizing the VDT workstation. Ohio: CLC, 1983.

38. Tijerina L. Video display terminal workstation ergonomics. Ohio: OCLC, 1984.

39. Diffrient N. The Diffrient difference. Leading Edge 1984; 5:41–59.

40. Corlett EN, Eklund JA. How does a backrest work? Appl Ergonomics 1984; 15:111–114.

41. Lander L, Korbon GA, DeGood DE and Rowlingson JC. The Balans chair and its semi-kneeling position: An ergonomic comparison with the conventional sitting positions. Spine 1987; 12:269–271.

42. Lueder RK. Seat comfort: A review of the construct in the office environment. Hum Factors 1983; 25:701–711.

43. Soderberg G, Blanco MK, Cosentino TL, Kurdelmeier K. Analysis of posterior trunk musculature during flat and anteriorly inclined sitting. Hum Factors 1986; 28:483–491.

44. Frey JK, Tecklin JS. Comparison of lumbar curves when sitting on the Westnote Balans Multi-Chair, sitting on a conventional chair, and standing. Phys Ther 1986; 66:1365–1369.

45. Boudrifa H, Davies BT. The effect of back rest inclination, lumbar support and thoracic support on erector spine muscles when lifting. Eur J Appl Physiol 1985; 54:538–545.

46. Eastman MC, Kamon E. Posture and subjective evaluation at flat and slanted desks. Hum Factors 1976; 18:15–26.

47. Garg A. Lifting and back injuries: A review of the causes of this industrial health problem, and the major methods used to combat it. Plant Engin. December 22, 1983; 67–71.

48. Snook SH. The design of manual handling tasks. Ergonomics 1978; 21:963–985.

49. Tak-sun Y, Roht LH, Wise RA, Kilian DJ, and Weir FW. Low back pain in industry: an old problem revisited. J Occup Med 1984; 26:517–524.

50. Herrin GD, Jaraiedi M, Anderson C. Prediction of

joint mobility and spinal angles in standing and in different sitting postures. Hum Factors 1989; 31:229–241.

overexertion injuries using biomechanical and psychophysical models. Am Ind Hyg J 1986; 46:322–
330.

51. Leskinen TPJ. Comparison of static and dynamic
biomechanical models. Ergonomics 1985; 28:285–
291.

52. Garg A and Saxena U. Physiological stresses in warehouse operations with special reference to lifting

technique and gender: a case study. Am Ind Hyg
Assoc J 1985; 46:53–59.

53. Chaffin DB, Herrin GD, Keyserling WM. Pre-
employment strength testing: An updated position.
J Occup Med 1978; 20:403–408.

54. Snook SH. Comparison of different approaches for
the prevention of low back pain. Appl Ind Hyg J
1988; 3:73–78.

17

Rationale for the Use of Spinal Manipulation

RICH NYBERG and JOHN V. BASMAJIAN

Spinal manipulation as a viable treatment strategy for patients with low back conditions has gained noticeable acceptance among medical practitioners in recent times.[1] Once considered unorthodox practice, spinal manipulation is now a common practice in many health disciplines. Manual clinicians use theoretical and clinical rationale to justify the use of spinal manipulative therapy since scientific validation is still a subject in need of further investigation. The following section discusses three possible mechanisms by which spinal manipulation may work.

MECHANICAL INFLUENCES ON TISSUES

Connective Tissue Immobilization

The effects of immobilization of joints have been extensively studied by many investigators. Joint restriction is the result of a loss of extensibility in the periarticular soft-tissue structures about the joint, i.e., capsules, ligaments, connective tissue, and myofascia. The periarticular biochemical changes of soft tissue resulting from enforced immobilization, immobilization after injury, or perhaps lack of use involve the loss of glycoaminoglycan (GAG) molecules. A parallel loss of water content occurs in response to the decrease in GAGs. Authorities contend that the water between collagen fibrils serves as a diffusion me-

dium for cellular transport and as a lubricating mechanism to allow for greater extensibility. A loss of fluid volume between collagen fibers along with the stationary attitude of the fibers allows the fibers to approximate, thereby increasing the potential for abnormal crosslink formation.[2] One histologic study demonstrates an increased number of adhesions between collagen fibers after 9 weeks of immobilization.[3] Motion may also be inhibited by an abnormal waveform disposition and arrangement of new collagen fibrils which resists tensile force. In summary, joint stiffness is the result of: *a*) a loss of the normal lubricating mechanism between collagen fibers due to decreased numbers of GAGs; *b*) the approximation and stationary attitude of collagen fibers which leads to an increased number of adhesions; and *c*) the smaller crimp angles found in the collagen fibrils.[4]

Motion-Induced Changes in Connective Tissue Extensibility

Restoration of extensibility to the joint capsule and ligaments as well as the myofascial tissues about the joint is a significant part of spinal manipulation theory for practitioners who favor passive motion through the use of manipulation. Movement may, in fact, inhibit a contracture process by stimulating GAG synthesis, thereby restoring lubricating efficiency and normal three-dimensional spatial patterns in the matrix. Apparently, a critical fluid barrier must be maintained between collagen fibers to allow realignment in the direction of imposed stress or movement. Movement activity assists in regular synthesis, deposition, and spacing of newly synthesized collagen fibrils, thereby inhibiting abnormal cross-link formation. Stress or motion responsiveness of collagen is important in preventing random haystack patterns in deposition and stationary fiber-to-fiber attitudes.[2] Spinal movement therapies may therefore restore, maintain, or promote tissue extensibility, thus facilitating range of motion.

Rupture of the abnormal cross-links which form between fibers[3] is another possible way in which spinal manipulation may work. Intra- and extra-articular joint adhesions may be broken as a result of a specific manipulative force. Spinal manipulators speculate that thrust manipulation is effective in rupturing joint adhesions because of the high velocity used in the technique. The possibility of normal capsular tissue being overstretched or torn by thrust manipulative technique must be considered. Therefore, repetitive use of thrust technique on a patient at the same segmental level is not advisable. The potential end result of repetitive thrust manipulation is joint instability which ultimately may lead to early degenerative joint changes, such as articular cartilage wear, capsular thickening, and bony hypertrophy. On the other hand, the benefit of thrust technique in creating joint release and freedom of motion cannot be ignored.

Muscle-Tendon Immobilization

Muscles immobilized passively in a shortened position for at least 5 days reduce the number of sarcomeres in series to adjust to the functional length of the muscle. Active muscle contraction in a shortened muscle results in rapid sarcomere loss within 12 hours.[6–8] Decreasing sarcomere numbers in series enables a shortened muscle to maintain maximal overlap of myosin cross bridges and actin fila-

ments. Extensibility as well as tension development of muscles immobilized in a shortened position is significantly decreased within a 4–6 week period. Length tension curves are very short, active tension is reduced, and passive tension curves are steeper in immobilized, shortened muscles than in normal muscles or muscles immobilized in a lengthened position.[8] Active tension development as measured by average contraction time (time from onset of tension to maximum tension during a muscle twitch) is slower due to a loss in weight and contractile protein within fibers of immobilized muscle.[9]

Immobilized Tendons Becoming Irregular in Size and Shape

Incised canine flexor tendons immobilized up to 42 days demonstrate fibrous adhesions which obliterate the space between the tendon and tendon sheath. A disorganized pattern of collagen and reticular fibers is found between cells. Various stages of collagen degradation and resorption are also present.[10] Vascular examination of the incised, immobilized tendons shows a reduction in peritendinous vessel density and a coiling, transverse, vessel orientation as opposed to the straight, longitudinal vessels in normal tendon.[11]

Motion-Induced Changes in Muscle-Tendon Extensibility

Hypoextensibility of muscle associated with a decrease in sarcomere number can be reversed by movement activity. The soleus muscles of guinea pigs immobilized in shortened positions for 12 hours recovered almost full extensibility within 36–48 hours after immobilization.[6] Remobilization of immobilized muscle also restores weight, increases contractile protein and oxidative capacity within fibers, and improves active tension development. Passive stretch adaptation of innervated skeletal muscle also results in subsequent hypertrophy.[12]

The effects of early intermittent passive mobilization on healing canine flexor tendons is positive with respect to tendon excursion.

Tendon gliding function as measured by angular rotation, and linear extension in early passive mobilization groups is similar to uninjured, contralateral control tendons within 12 weeks post injury. In contrast, immobilized tendons and delayed mobilization tendon groups had angular rotation values of 19% and 60%, respectively, when compared to intact controls after 12 weeks. Gliding function of the delayed mobilization group, however, was the same as the controls after 12 weeks, but only 58% of control values in the immobilized group.[13] The histologic characteristics of mobilized tendon which appear to relate to improvement in tendon excursion include: *a*) vascular remodeling in a longitudinal orientation (parallel to the tendon fibers), *b*) reduced adhesion formation, *c*) extensive proliferation of fibroblasts, and *d*) parallel orientation of fibroblasts and collagen. Reinstatement of tendon motion function in the early mobilized groups possibly relates to the induction of a cellular response from the epitenon which inhibits inflammatory cell ingrowth to the repair site.[10,11] The investigators emphasize that the amount of stress applied to the tendon repair site is critical. Careful, controlled motion stress is essential in preventing repair site rupture. The use of manipulation to injured tendon, therefore, must consider the extent of repair to determine the type and amount of loading utilized in treatment.

Motion-Induced Changes in Connective Tissue and Muscle-Tendon Strength

Endurance exercise trained dogs developed larger diameter collagen fiber bundles, higher collagen content, and greater weights in the ligaments of the exercised limbs than the ligaments in non-endurance trained dogs.[14] Separation force per body weight for the ligament-bone complex is also greater in exercised trained animals than in non-exercised or immobilized groups.[14,15] Likewise, the strength of healing canine flexor tendons as measured by ultimate load value is significantly greater 12 weeks post injury in early,

mobilized groups when compared to delayed mobilized or immobilized groups.[13] Motion-activated connective tissue or muscle-tendon, particularly if normal length-tension relations are maintained, are probably less susceptible to injury since higher or longer duration loads are necessary for disruption.[8,16]

Immobilization of Articular Cartilage

The intra-articular effect of prolonged immobilization of joints has been studied extensively in rats, rabbits, and monkeys.[17-19] Regardless of the method of immobilization (plaster casts, internal fixation, compression clamps) the histologic changes are quite similar.[20] A consistent finding in immobilized joints is the progressive proliferation of fibrofatty connective tissue into the joint cavity. With prolonged immobilization the separation between fibrofatty tissue and hyaline cartilage becomes less distinct as mature fibrous connective tissue is deposited, ultimately obliterating the joint space. Contact of articular surfaces through compression causes pressure necrosis with liquefaction of articular cartilage, fibrillation, and articular erosion[17] as well as the formation of intra-cartilaginous cysts.[19] In addition, mesenchymal tissue produced from underlying bone marrow spaces damages and eventually replaces the deep layers of the articular cartilage. The zone of calcified cartilage thickens[18] with prolonged periods of joint immobilization which may lead to a total replacement of articular cartilage with intra-articular fibrous or bony ankylosis.[20] One noteworthy and clinically relevant finding is that significant degenerative change is possible in immobilized joints not subjected to abnormal pressure by forced positions or weight bearing, but instead by normal, intermittent muscle contractions.[19]

Pressure necrosis of articular cartilage probably results from the restriction of synovial fluid from reaching the contact surfaces as well as the impedance of nutritive fluid diffusion within the intercellular areas of the cartilage.[17] Consequently, chrondrocyte cells die and the intercellular substances become disorganized. Degeneration of joints from immobilization and/or persistent pressure is a clearly recognized factor in limiting mobility. The degree of stiffness appears to be proportional to the severity of articular degeneration, particularly with respect to fibrofatty and adhesion presence.[20]

Motion-Induced Changes in Articular Cartilage

Early motion activity and weight bearing have been found to enhance the repair of full-thickness cartilage defects.[21] Active motion without normal joint loading from weight bearing, however, may not maintain normal articular cartilage.[22] Use of continuous passive motion to joints with full thickness articular cartilage defects accelerates repair and produces tissue that resembles normal hyaline cartilage morphologically and histologically.[23] The healing of articular cartilage is not only more rapid, but more complete with continuous passive motion as compared to immobilization or intermittent active motion treatment.

The absence of intra-articular adhesions in joints receiving continuous passive motion relates to the restoration of normal range of motion. In contrast, immobilized joints were found to have intra-articular adhesions in 50% of the adult rabbit knees studied and limitation in range of motion by 50%.[23] The clinical relevance of continuous passive motion treatment to manipulative therapists facilitating articular cartilage healing and joint range of motion is evident, since manipulation is a form of passive movement. Caution should be exercised in selecting the type of motion stress to augment repair of articular cartilage, since studies substantiate that vigorous activity or early weight bearing can be detrimental.[24,25]

RESTORATION OF VERTEBRAL POSITION

Correcting abnormal position of vertebrae is a proposed mechanism of spinal manipulation. To accept that spinal manipulation repositions vertebrae requires an underlying assumption that vertebrae displace. Vertebral subluxations and dislocations from traumatic injury brought about by fracture and/or ligament rupture result in a biomechanically unstable segment. If potential cord damage exists, reduction by skeletal traction and adequate stabilization is recommended. Manual manipulative treatment is contraindicated.

Vertebral displacements or facet joint incongruities of less magnitude may benefit from manipulative therapy. The only problem is in detection. How does one correct vertebral or facet alignment when evaluative measures are unable to identify a positional problem?[26] The concept of chiropractic subluxation is, therefore, difficult to accept. The lack of a precise, quantitative definition and the failure to scientifically substantiate a vertebral subluxation disorder anatomically or biomechanically relegates the existence of such a problem to belief or theory.

One study, however, does reveal positional adjustment from a manipulative procedure. Using 20 patients who fulfilled criteria for sacroiliac joint dysfunction, investigators measured innominate tilt before and after unilateral posterior rotation manipulation.[27] Data analysis revealed a statistically significant change in innominate tilt on the same side manipulated as well as an equal and opposite tilt on the contralateral non-manipulated side. The manipulative procedure, therefore, had a bilateral effect on innominate position despite only one side being manipulated. Although this pelvic study supports the influence of manipulation on positional relations, no experimental study confirms individual segmental realignment following manipulation.

Rotary spinal manipulation, however, was shown to correct trunk lists in 8 out of 10 lateral shift patients with back and leg pain within 2 days. The remaining 2 had improved position, but not totally. In contrast, the 4 trunk list patients not receiving manipulation continued to have lists during the 8-week study or until surgery.[28]

REDUCTION OF A
DISC HERNIATION

Spinal manipulation for patients with known disc herniations remains a subject of considerable controversy. In a clinical study on 27 patients with known myelographic defects consistent with a disc protrusion, nine obtained sciatic pain relief within 24 hours after manipulation under anesthesia. Myelographic re-examination, however, failed to demonstrate any change in the defects.[28] Interestingly, the authors did not question the relevance of the assumed underlying pathology (disc protrusion) as determined by myelogram. The question clearly in need of explanation is: What is the mechanism of pain relief after rotary manipulation of the spine if the disc is not affected? Perhaps other pain-sensitive structures within the spine need additional consideration when analyzing the etiology of low back and sciatic pain.

In the same study a total of 39 patients with consistent clinical findings suggestive of a disc protrusion received rotary spinal manipulation under anesthesia. Twenty out of 39 had complete relief or only occasional symptoms with no activity restrictions in a 3-year follow-up study. The study findings support Mensor's 50% good to excellent results on 205 patients following rotary spinal manipulation under anesthesia.[29] The authors[28] conclude that manipulation has a definite role in the conservative management of disc patients, especially if the myelogram is negative.

In a preliminary communication, Matthews and Yates reported a reduction in the size of small disc protrusions on two patients with positive epidurograms after rotary thrust manipulation.[30] Two control subjects with similar epidurographic findings did not demonstrate any diminution in the size of the concavity produced by small disc deformities after similar non-thrust maneuvers. Reduction of a disc protrusion by rotary manipulation is thought to occur in response to the imparted torsion stress. Torsion stress imparted by a rotation manipulation increases the tension in intact posterior longitudinal ligament and annulus fibrosus fibers. The supposed centripetal force created within the disc applies pressure to the intra-discal contents, facilitating reduction of bulging disc material. Although the proposed mechanism of disc reduction has supporters,[31] the specific, actual mechanisms for therapeutic change following spinal manipulation is unknown. Also a reminder to the manual practitioner is the fact that the magnitude of therapeutic force necessary to affect a positive result is largely undetermined. Consequently, care should be exercised in delivery of spinal manipulation force so as to not exceed the physiologic limits of the affected tissue, particularly, when annular or ligament mechanical failure tolerances are low.

Hydrodynamic Effects

Disturbance in hydrodynamic balance within the disc after derangement is a proposed mechanism for rationalizing extension movement manipulation and/or exercise. Disruption in continuity or weakening of the posterior annulus presumably allows fluid transport into the affected area. As fluid volume and resultant hydrostatic pressure increases in the posterior compartment the disc deforms, producing a radial bulge.

Proponents of the extension concept in treating posterior disc derangements utilize posterior-anterior directed manipulation pressures and/or extension exercises to compress the posterior aspect of the disc. The repeated or sustained loads are intended to transport intradiscal fluids out of the posterior disc area. Posterior annular fibers are thereby relieved of increased fluid pressure and, thus, allowed to approximate and heal. The beneficial effects achieved by extension programs for certain back-troubled patients is recognized by many clinicians; however, exact mechanisms for the therapeutic change need validation.

In a preliminary report extension exercises

as recommended by McKenzie were performed by 16 patients with CAT scan results suggestive of disc protrusion.[32] Nineteen disc-confirmed CAT scan patients serving as controls received non-steroidal anti-inflammatory drugs, bed rest, and a "trivial" exercise. By comparing a 3-month post-treatment CAT scan to the pre-treatment CAT scan, investigators found no significant differences in the disc bulge of either group. To evaluate the position and configuration of the nucleus pulposus NMR studies were performed on 3 patients placed in an extended spinal posture for a prolonged time period (exact time length not provided in report). The extended position did not appear to alter the shape or position of the nucleus when examined by NMR study.

Despite preliminary findings which contradict the supposed hydrodynamic concept of the extension program, clinical observations seem to support the theory. Many clinicians relate patient reports of difficulty in returning to erect posture after repetitive or sustained flexion activities to an increase in posterior fluid volume within the disc. The accumulation of fluid posteriorly apparently blocks or resists easy return to the upright position by preventing posterior vertebral margin approximation. Obtaining a vertical trunk position is eventually attained by a series of graduated extension movements which theoretically shift the fluid content anteriorly, allowing restoration of the normal lumbar curve. Successful return to the erect position is eventually achieved by backward-bending despite experimental evidence of posterior disc bulging during extension movement.[33] Apparently the disc bulge produced by extension or return from flexion is a limiting, but not preventive, factor in many instances for individuals trying to regain vertical position after flexion.

While some biomechanical authorities report that nuclear position is essentially unaffected by flexion-extension movements,[34,35] others show evidence of possible nuclear deformation or displacement during movement.[35,36] Most likely, the ability of a nucleus

to change shape or displace during a motion event is dependent on many factors such as: range obtained, number of movements, length of time in the movement position, magnitude and velocity of the load, as well as the biochemical and biomechanical integrity of the annular fibers. Additional investigation of the physical properties of the intervertebral disc will need to account for loading variables and the condition of the disc itself.

Advocates of an extension approach contend that a disc is more stable when the lumbar spine assumes a normal anterior curve. Support for this argument is provided by stress analysis studies on the disc. By loading vertebra-disc-vertebra specimens from the thoracic and lumbar spines with tension and compression forces, Markolf found discs to be less stiff in tension than under compression.[38] Although normal tensile forces are attenuated well by the alternating direction of the layers of annular fibers, the disc has no apparent mechanism for resisting the shear stress created by tension. As a result, disc failure is more likely with tensile loading than compression loading.[26] Promotion of extension range of motion to achieve a normal lumbar anterior curve may increase compression stress, but reduces tensile loading to the disrupted or weakened posterior annulus. The potential for further internal disruption is theoretically decreased, since the posterior annulus is capable of resisting compression better than tension. Furthermore, the maintenance of an anterior lumbar curve also apposes facet joints which in turn helps the disc to resist torque[39] and anterior shear loading.[40]

FACET JOINT EFFECTS

Spinal rotatory manipulation is presumed to create separation between processes in lumbar facet joints. Despite many claims by manual therapists that facet joints can be gapped or opened by manipulation, few studies substantiate the allegation.[41,42] However, the mechanism of a crack or pop produced in a joint by manipulation has been verified by Unsworth, Dawson, and Wright.[43] With 10–16 kg loads the metacarpophalangeal joints of 5 subjects were separated on the average of 0.5 mm. The separation of the joint was associated with a cracking noise. The authors suggest that cavitation takes place in the synovial fluid between the cartilagenous surfaces of the joint when tension force is applied. As a result of cavity formation in the joint, fluid flows into the low pressure area. As fluid flows into the low pressure region the vapor collapses, energy is released, and a noise is heard. Therefore, the collapse not the formation, of a vapor bubble causes the crack.

Unsworth, Dawson, and Wright also found non-cracking joints to have rest positions 25% greater than cracking joints. Close approximated joint surfaces apparently provide the right conditions for cavitation. Cracking during a lumbar spinal manipulation therefore may relate to the separation of facet joint surfaces that have come together and opposed movement. Forceful manipulation to a non-cracking joint is ill advised due to the probability of the articular surfaces being already separated.

Gapping of facet joints by slowly applied rotation forces is not a consistent phenomenon. In one study on 12 fresh spines separation of facet joint surfaces was observed in only a minority of mobile segments.[42] The authors support the contention of intra- and extracapsular fat pad adaptive movement in manipulated facet joints, but maintain that in normal spinal segments the articular facet processes do not separate significantly. Manipulation that displaces fat pad synovial tissue of facet joints, however, may decrease pain, since the pads are innervated by nociceptive nerve endings.

Meniscus Entrapment

The meniscus entrapment theory in the synovial facet joints and subsequent rationale for the use of manipulation is based on the compression of articular processes.[44] As the articular processes appose the firm connective tissue apex of the meniscus, meniscoid is believed to be caught and imprints a recess in the cartilagenous surface. Entrapment of the meniscus itself is not painful. The pain results from the tension on the joint capsule from the imprisoned meniscus. Movement activity that challenges the affected joint further strains the capsule accentuating the pain. Reflex muscle guarding develops to protect the joint from additional aggravation. Manipulation is performed to distract the articular surfaces, release the meniscus and relieve the capsule of tension stress.

Although the meniscoid entrapment concept is subscribed to by a number of investigators[44-46] some limitations to the theory exist. Bogduk points out that connective tissue rims are too short to be trapped and the adipose tissue pads too soft to create a recess. According to Bogduk, imprisonment of a meniscus in not likely to create tension in the capsule because the meniscus contains only loose connective tissue and probably would divide rather than transmit tension.[47] Therefore, the histologic features of the meniscoid are perhaps inconsistent with the imprisonment hypothesis.

The scientific basis for the dramatic pain relief sometimes obtained by spinal manipulation warrants further examination into the mechanisms of injury. Other causes of acute locked back conditions aside from facet meniscoid entrapment may involve sudden or creeping facet subluxation resulting in capsular tension or compression between joint surfaces, fracture of a vertebral end plate from compression overload during an uncoordinated weight lift, peripheral-outer annular tears due to forced axial rotation resulting in loose disc fragments or distortion of the disc into pain sensitive tissues.[48] The use and type of manipulative procedure for acute back conditions require consideration of all possible causes of the condition.

NEUROPHYSIOLOGIC EFFECTS

Pain

Aside from mechanical effects, spinal manipulation or motion therapy is believed to produce changes in neurophysiologic activity in tissues. Improvement in spinal mobility following manipulation may not relate to the biomechanical effects on tissue, but to a reduction in pain. The work of Wyke and Freeman helps substantiate a scientific basis for pain relief after spinal manipulation. Through experimental study, Wyke and Freeman, determined the existence of four types of synovial joint receptors.[49] Types I, II, and III are classified as mechanoreceptors which function to convert mechanical stimuli into electrical energy. Mechanoreceptors offer positional and kinesthetic information from the respective joint structure to the central nervous system. Type IV receptors are nociceptors and are responsible for signaling pain.

According to the Gate Control theory proposed by Melzak and Wall[50] in 1965, mediation of incoming stimuli through afferent nerve fibers from the various body tissues, somatic and visceral, occurs in the cells of the substantia gelatinosa in laminas two and three of the spinal cord. Mechanoreceptor discharge has an inhibitory effect on the presynaptic cells of the substantia gelatinosa which, in turn, depresses nociceptive activity. Wyke states that the perception of pain from an irritated spinal structure is inversely related to the amount of mechanoreceptor activity from the embryologically associated spinal tissues.[51] Mechanical force generated from spinal manipulation is transmitted to the affected spinal segment and may activate mechanoreceptor endings. In essence, mechanoreceptor discharge would assist in closing the gate to pain. Manual practitioners recognize pain determination as a central summation phenomenon and a function of postsynaptic neuronal regulation as well as presynaptic influence.[50]

Experimental Evidence of Pain Relief

Numerous clinical studies have evaluated the effects of manipulation on spinal pain, yet little emphasis has been placed on the investigation of measured pain tolerance changes induced by manipulation. Glover, after finding areas of increased sensitivity adjacent to assumed dysfunctional spinal segments used a rotational manipulation to the lesioned level.[52] After manipulation, Glover reported an 89% success rate in diminishing the hyperaesthesia, although no quantification of pain threshold or tolerance was attempted.

In a subsequent study,[53] baseline paraspinal pain threshold levels were assessed on 50 asymptomatic subjects by measuring the electrical current strength of a pain stimulus in milliamperes. At least one paraspinal area of increased pain sensitivity was detected in 94% of the asymptomatic subjects. The existence of hyperaesthesia regions in a majority of asymptomatic individuals supports the contention of sub-clinical facilitation of cutaneous sensory reflex pathways. Manipulation applied to the presumed, associated spinal segment resulted in a statistically significant elevation in pain tolerance (140%) when compared to a non-manipulated control group. Sensory activation of cutaneous, myofascial, and articular receptors by manipulation is proposed to lower cutaneous pain reflexes by modulation of nociceptive afferent activity.

Clinical Evidence of Pain Relief

The high incidence of spontaneous recovery from low back pain requires examiners of manipulation to ensure proper controls during investigations. Any improvement in subjective pain report from manipulative therapy must be analyzed with respect to a control group. Clinical research evaluating the effectiveness of spinal manipulation for pain relief is complicated by the variability and subjectivity in pain measurement, use of random selection method, difficulty in identifying specific criteria for patient selection, precise determination of the treatment intervention, use of multiple procedures, patient-therapist interaction, as well as the natural recovery process.

The majority of clinical studies on spinal manipulation which use proper controls show manipulated groups to have shorter duration of symptoms, but no significant longterm benefits. In one study, 152 patients with recent, acute low back pain were selected at random and divided into two treatment groups.[54] One group received unspecified manipulative treatment and the other group bedrest and analgesics. Fifty percent of the manipulated patients were symptom-free in 1 week versus 27% in the bedrest, analgesic group.

Evans, in a controlled crossover investigation, evaluated the effects of rotary manipulation along with rescue analgesia for 3 weeks and then analgesics for 3 weeks in one group of low back pain patients.[55] The second group of patients had the treatment phases reversed during the two 3-week periods. Using a 0–3 daily pain score which correlated (r = .92) to the number of codeine capsules consumed per weeks, the authors concluded that pain relief is obtained more quickly with manipulation and rescue analgesics than with analgesics alone.

Short-term benefits of spinal manipulation on patients diagnosed to have intervertebral disc syndromes were evidenced in Chrisman's study.[28] Fifty-one percent of the manipulated group reported a significant improvement in sciatic symptoms within 24 hours, while 16 out of 22 patients in the non-manipulated groups required disc surgery within 8 weeks. The immediate subjective effects of manipulation on pain was frequently described to be dramatic.

A randomized clinical trial of rotational manipulation administered to 95 patients with low back pain also supports the contention of immediate, short-term benefit from manipulation.[56] The randomly assigned groups were comparable in pretreatment measures. An experimental group receiving rotational manipulations was compared to a control groups obtaining lumbosacral soft tissue massage. The immediate effects of manipulation after the first treatment with respect to the amount of pain relief is significantly greater (p < .05) than the degree of relief produced by soft tissue massage. After 3 weeks both groups demonstrated improvement in symptoms, and no significant difference in pain levels was detected.

Likewise, spinal manipulation was found to offer significantly more pain relief than a detuned short-wave diathermy placebo treatment within the first 15 minutes of the first session.[57] At 3 and 7 days after treatment, however, both groups were markedly improved with no difference in regard to pain relief. Although immediate pain reduction was greater in manipulated patients, an immediate improvement was also noted in the placebo group. Authors ascribe the immediate change in pain status to the following factors common to both groups: interest and treatment rendered within a research unit, discussion of test results, reassurance of no signs of spinal tumor, disc prolapse or other disease, localized treatment to the area of pain, and the encouragement that the pain will soon improve. Clinical practitioners must realize the entire spectrum of interventions accounting for changes in patient condition. The therapeutic value of any of the above factors cannot be underestimated.

In another clinical investigation 48 patients with low back pain, but no neurologic signs, were assigned randomly to two treatments: lumbar mobilization and manipulation patients were compared to patients having a regimen of microwave diathermy, isometric abdominal exercises, and ergonomic advice.[58] The mobilized-manipulated group required 3.5 ± 1.6 treatments to become symptom-free, while the diathermy, exercised, ergonomic groups needed 5.8 ± 2.3 treatments to reach symptom-free status. Pain responses in both groups after 3 weeks, however, were almost identical, indicating no potential longterm benefit in the manipulated patients.

In summary, most studies demonstrate spinal manipulation to have positive short-term effects on low back pain, yet no significant impact on longterm results when compared to other treatment interventions. In one such study, manipulation was shown to be marginally better than "definitive physiotherapy," corset use, or analgesics after 3 weeks of treatment.[59] Some patients, although not definitively identified with respect to evaluative findings, responded quickly to manipulation. A follow-up questionnaire at 3 and 6 months, however, did not reveal any significant differences among groups in pain status.

Other studies[60,61] also indicate no long-term advantage in using spinal manipulation treatment for nonspecific low back pain conditions. The probability of hastening back recovery with manipulation is mentioned as a potential benefit. The apparent value of accelerating recovery from a back problem is not to be underestimated, particularly with respect to time off from work, income loss, and hardship to both the injured and uninjured fellow workers. On the other hand, a clear recognition of the role of spinal manipulation in the context of an entire management plan is needed to address the issues of reoccurrence and prevention. The clinical impression of most manipulative practitioners reinforces the importance of patient education and self-responsibility in longterm effective management of back conditions. The main influence or determining factor in successful management of a back problem may, in fact, relate to the actions of the individual.

Myofascial Tone

In accordance with the facilitated segment concept, a joint lesion may cause the segmentally-related musculature to become hyper-responsive. According to one hypothesis, the fusimotor neuron (Gamma) discharge to the affected intrafusal muscle fibers is being sustained at high frequencies. Consequently, the intrafusal fibers are kept in a chronic shortened state, and the muscle spindle becomes hypersensitive to incoming stimuli. The spindles reflexly control the tensional state of the extrafusal muscle fibers. Local muscle spasm is sometimes palpated in the area of dysfunction, and reflex muscle contractions are occasionally elicited after pressure. The joint surfaces become tightly apposed, and an increased resistance to motion, usually in one direction, results.[62]

During spinal manipulation, the affected joint is moved, and muscles about the joint are stretched. A barrage of afferent impulses is generated from the mechanical force of the manipulation which may order the central nervous system to reduce the fusimotor neuron discharge. Stretching of the muscle by spinal manipulation may also transmit tension to the tendon. The golgi tendon organs may then inhibit fusimotor neuron discharge and serve to relax both intrafusal and extrafusal fibers.[62] Another possible mechanism by which spinal manipulation may normalize myofascial tone is reflex inhibition from Type III mechanoreceptors in the joint capsule.[63] Apparently, the Type III mechanoreceptors have a reflex inhibitory effect on the associated musculature about the joint. Although the spinal reflex inhibitory theory is not supported by the work of Wyke, many clinicians sense palpable change in local paraspinal muscle tone after spinal manipulation as well as in hamstring tension.

Support for the contention that spinal manipulation affects myofascial tension status is provided in a study by Fisk.[64] By incorporating a tension gauge into a pulley system, the limit of tolerable comfort was measured in the hamstrings of patients with unilateral low back pain before and after spinal manipulation. Although exact measures were not provided in the article, statistical analysis showed a significant difference in hamstring tension for a given arc of elevation in patients receiving rotary spinal manipulation on the affected side when compared to a manipulated, asymptomatic control group. Fisk suggests that manipulation causes a reflex reduction in gamma motor nerve discharge to the muscle spindles through stimulation of Type III mechanoreceptors in facet joint capsules.

Further evidence of changes in hamstring tension is provided in a study on 51 patients with myelographic confirmed disc protrusions.[65] Half were provided a conventional treatment approach using short-wave diathermy, isometric pelvic tilt hold exercises, and lifting and postural education strategies while the other half received oscillatory rotation manipulative therapy as well as posture and lifting advice. Spinal range of motion assessments using a spondylometer and straight leg raise measurements using a hydrogoniometer were taken before and after the 6-week treatment period. Straight leg raising increased from a mean of 31° to 35° in the conventional treatment group, whereas the manipulated patients had pre-treatment straight leg raise means of 29° and post treatment means of 68°. Greater increases in spinal flexion-extension, side bending, and rotation were also reported for the manipulated patients than for the conventional treatment group.

Proprioception

An additional consideration is the possibility of spinal manipulation affecting proprioceptive function. Capsular or ligamentous injury from overstretch, repeated trauma, disuse, and accelerated aging changes results in a loss and deactivation of mechanoreceptors. The proprioceptive role of the affected segment is adversely affected as a result.[66] Spinal manipulation may help activate inactive receptors and thus improve postural and kinesthetic awareness. Reviving inactive mechanoreceptors and restoring proprioceptive control reduces the chance of reinjury and, hence, is an important consideration in preventive care. No studies relating spinal manipulation to proprioceptive function were disclosed.

Nerve Tension

Force generated during extremity, trunk, and head/neck movements causes repeated "piston like" movements of the neuromeningeal complex in and proximal to the intervertebral foramen.[67] The position of the nerve structures within and medial to the foramen changes in response to the tension force induced by the spinal cord during trunk movements and/or the traction effect from peripheral nerves during limb movements. Research evidence demonstrates a medial and superior drawing tension of nerve roots/sleeves within the foramen during spinal flexion and a posterior-inferior movement and relaxation of nerve roots-sleeves during spinal extension.[68] Likewise, the spinal cord-dura lengthen and the nerve roots tense on the convex side of

the curve during bending activity while the concave side is folded and relaxed.[69] Axial rotation causes posterior roots on the same side to relax while anterior roots are stretched. A persistent vertebral rotation position is theorized to move a nerve root around the contralateral pedicle by 0.5 to 1.0 cm.[70] In regard to lower extremity movement effects on nerve root tension, straight leg raising, adduction, and internal rotation increase tension whereas hip extension, abduction, and external rotation decrease tension.[69]

Biomechanical knowledge of the central and peripheral nervous systems allows for some interesting speculation as to the neurologic effects of manipulative or motion-based therapies. For example, if manipulation or motion treatment is not capable of reducing or positionally altering a disc protrusion, perhaps a positive result from movement therapy is related to decreasing tension or changing position of affected nerve structures. A reduction in nerve or dural tension brought about by spinal and/or limb movements may not only help to offer pain relief, but could conceivably allow associated, protective, hyperactive muscles to turn down a ready alert-on guard status.

Theoretically an irritable left-sided S1 nerve root under tension from a 2.0 mm posterior-lateral disc protrusion may find relief from one or a combination of spinal or limb movements. In this scenario, spinal extension and/or right-side bending as well as left hip extension, abduction, and/or external rotation are all movements that have the potential to reduce nerve root-sleeve tension or actually move the affected S1 root away from the offending disc material. The results of one study support the implication that spinal extension movement can relieve nerve root tension and decrease the compressive forces produced on a nerve root negotiating a protruded disc.[71] Other studies of this nature would be of interest to the manipulative therapist.

Many questions come to mind when considering changes in nerve tension or movement brought about by movement activity as a possible mechanism of pain relief. Are the types of movements necessary to achieve nerve tension or position change predictable? What range of motion needs to be obtained? Is the velocity of the movement important? If successful in pain relief, will the patient still be vulnerable when moving in non-corrective directions?

CRANIOSACRAL THERAPY

Craniosacral therapy advocates propose another neurophysiologic effect by which manipulation may work. In craniosacral therapy, specifically directed gentle pressures are applied to the cranium or sacrum to redirect cerebral and spinal blood flow as well as cerebrospinal fluid fluctuation. Congestion or retardation of venous drainage or cerebrospinal fluid within the cranium and the spinal column is hypothesized to be the cause of local biochemical changes which lead to tissue irritability.[72] Redistribution of venous blood or cerebrospinal fluid would then prevent stasis and help to lubricate inflamed, irritable nerves or membranes. By enhancing fluid flow the hypersensitive tissues would be soothed and bathed, thus decreasing pain.

Redirection of blood or cerebrospinal fluid by manual pressures to the cranium or sacrum has yet to be experimentally verified. Opponents are therefore quite skeptical. Advocates are equally convinced of the therapeutic value in treating pain patients. Some support for craniosacral theory was demonstrated in May's study.[73] Mays found that injection of autogenous cerebrospinal fluid into the lumbar subarachnoid space in select post-laminectomy chronic pain patients gave significant pain relief within 10–15 minutes and lasted about 15 minutes. The composition and hydrodynamic action of cerebrospinal fluid is believed to impart a significant influence upon the electrical activity of the nervous system.

Another theory advanced by craniosacral practitioners relates to the releasing of membranous tension. When contacts are made or pressures delivered, cerebrospinal fluids may distribute to intracranial or spinal membranes which have abnormal tension.[74] Cerebro-

spinal fluid pressure changes have been calculated to vary from 5–15 mm, depending on pulse and respiratory activity.[75] Fluid alterations induced by manual contacts are believed to subject the taut membranes to hydrodynamic pressures sufficient to normalize membrane tension in the involved region(s).

The effects of craniosacral therapy may also be explained on the basis of autonomic nerve regulation. One study appears to offer support for an autonomic regulatory action.[76] In this study parasympathetic tone was assessed by quantifying the amplitude of respiratory sinus arrhythmia from the heart rate pattern and by measuring heart rate in two groups of healthy subjects. One group of 20 subjects was treated with a pelvic lift manipulation, while another group of 10 subjects received moderate bilateral pressure to the anterior deltoid muscle. The pelvic lift manipulation involved posterior-directed sacral pressure and moderate epigastrium pressure on subjects in supine position (a similar procedure called lumbosacral decompression is described in craniosacral texts). The pelvic lift was found to significantly increase parasympathetic nerve activity as measured by cardiac vagal tone for the duration of the treatment when compared to the control group. Parasympathetic enhancement through manipulative therapy may be responsible for improving breathing patterns, reducing muscle tension and stimulating circulation.

PSYCHOLOGIC EFFECTS

Treatment strategy is determined by the objective physical findings and by the subjective report of pain described by the patient. The patient's pain behavior and description sometimes suggest a strong emotional factor in the problem. Recognition that emotional and stress-related factors contributed to pain perception and that pain is a poorly measured clinical phenomenon is imperative for successful management. Effectiveness of a manipulation approach therefore must be based on two components—objective clinical changes such as range of motion and the patient's report of pain.

The tactile nature of spinal manipulative therapy is acknowledged to have a powerful psychological effect. Manual clinicians attempt to provide a rational explanation for the effectiveness of spinal manipulation by mechanical and neurophysiologic mechanisms, but often they do not appreciate fully the degree to which the laying on of hands contributes to pain relief. While manipulators prefer to believe that spinal manipulation is effective at least partially on a biomechanical basis, they must accept the powerful role of tactile healing.

Further reinforcement of the psychologic effect of spinal manipulation is exhibited through the interest and concern of the evaluator during the examination. After having been thoroughly assessed, patients are often impressed by the expertise of the manual practitioner. Psychologically, they experience a sense of satisfaction because the condition has been closely examined. Advising patients about the nature of the condition as well as informing them about what they don't have alleviates unnecessary anxiety and fear. Communication, compassion, and support are important elements in successful management of back pain patients. The thoughtful manual therapist remembers that non-physical interactions play as much of a part in neuro-sensory-motor modulation as the physical treatment. Often as a result, a patient's pain may decrease after the evaluation alone.

The psychologic impact of spinal manipulation on low back pain has been investigated. In one study the success of manipulation was evaluated by patient's pain report and MMPI given immediately and 5 days after the treatment.[77] Scores on hysteria, hypochondriasis, and functional low back pain measured by the MMPI did not correlate with patient's immediate pain relief. However, 5 days post manipulation the absence of pain relief significantly correlated with the MMPI results. Presumably, spinal manipulation alone can be responsible for immediate pain relief. Prevention of reoccurrence, however, appears to require attention to predisposing psychologic factors.

During some manipulations, an audible sound occurs. The pop, snap, or clunk may signify to the patient that a correction has been made. Patients frequently associate the sound with a repositioning or movement of a vertebra. The type of sound is often predictive of the event that occurred and therefore has meaning to the therapist as well. However, psychologic dependence on sounds produced by manipulation is not desirable. Association of joint noise with correction of the problem may place the clinician in a situation where the patient desires repetitive manipulation, a treatment strategy most would not recommend.

WHAT TYPE OF BACK PROBLEM RESPONDS BEST TO MANIPULATIVE THERAPY?

In reviewing the literature on spinal manipulation treatment for back pain a fairly uniform consensus is revealed with respect to the best back to manipulate. In most clinical studies, the manipulation performed was a thrust or high velocity type. Therefore, the following five criteria relate to the use of one form of manipulative therapy:

1. Short pain duration (preferably presenting with 2–4 weeks of pain)[78,79]
2. Sudden onset of back or leg pain[80]
3. Spinal motion restrictions[81] suggestive of a mechanical back condition
4. Negative myelogram[28]
5. No neurologic deficits[82]

Contraindications

Adverse reactions from lumbar manipulations are possible under the following conditions: large disc herniation with positive neurologic signs (SLR < 20°), spinal osteoporosis, recent vertebral fracture, bowel or bladder incontinence, spinal tumor, unstable spinal segments, and pregnancy. The use of high-velocity manipulation is a contraindication for the above conditions. Relative contraindications, however, exist for using other types of manipulation on the same conditions.

Necessity of Patient Exercise

The value of therapeutic exercise performance in managing low back pain is fairly well established. Research validation on the effectiveness of regular exercise activity in management of back pain allows the clinician to properly focus attention on patient education and responsibility. Successful longterm outcomes are a function of back care education and patient commitment to posture-control strategies, proper body mechanics, and a steady exercise routine.

A study on low back patients placed on exercise regimes clearly demonstrates significant improvements in self-rated pain scales, reductions in the frequency of pain, and greater levels of physical activity than patients not exercising.[83] Another study on 142 patients with subclassified mechanical low back pain found education in back care and exercise to be the most effective forms of treatment in regard to pain relief and activity level when compared to spinal manipulation, back supports, and analgesic medicine.[84]

The preventive effects of an exercise program have also been analyzed. Exercise groups have been found to have a 50% reduction in the number of episodes of back pain and the number of sick-leave days attributable to back pain during a 1½-year treatment period when compared to the year and half prior to the intervention.[85] In contrast, absenteeism attributed to back pain increased in a non-exercised control group.

Clinical evidence also shows nonoperative treatment of herniated lumbar disc patients through aggressive exercise training and back school to produce successful functional outcomes with respect to activity level, pain level, work status, and further medical care.[86] A 90% good to excellent outcome and a 92% return to work rate demonstrates that patients with herniated lumbar discs and radiculopathy can be treated successfully with patient education and exercise programs. The authors

conclude that the presence of disc herniation or weakness in the lower extremity is not sufficient evidence that surgery is mandatory.

CONCLUSION

In summary, the use of manipulation alone in the treatment of back pain is useful in early management stages. Benefits of manipulation in longterm management of back conditions are speculative at this time. The issue, however, seems to be more of an academic or research dilemma than a clinical debate. In the clinical setting the practice of manipulation for a low back patient is within context of an entire management program which includes patient education strategies. Performance of manipulation alone for a low back condition is analogous to a surgeon conducting surgery in the absence of anaesthesia, sterile operating-room conditions, a recovery room, or post-surgical protocols.

Spinal surgery and manipulation are simply preliminary interventions to permit the body to repair and recover. The patient is the true healer and rehabilitator, while the clinician is merely a facilitator to the process. When assisting in the recovery process we need to remain humble to the miracles of the restorative body, since patient experiences remind us that the best intervention is often nothing more than support and encouragement.

REFERENCES

1. Rosenthal E. Hands-on back therapy is winning respectability. The New York Times, July 3, A1 and B6, 1991.
2. Woo S L-Y, Matthews JW, Akeson WH, Amiel D, Convery FR. Connective tissue response to immobility. Correlative study of biomechanical and biochemical measurements of normal and immobilized rabbit knees. Arthritis Rheum 1975; 18:257–264.
3. Akeson WH, Amiel D, Mechanic GL, Woo S L-Y, Harwood FL, Hamer ML. Collagen cross-linking alterations in joint contractures: changes in the reducible cross-links in periarticular connective tissue collagen after nine weeks of immobilization. Connect Tissue Res 1977; 5:15–19.
4. Betsch DF, Baer E. Structure and mechanical properties of rat tail tendon. Third International Con-

gress of Biorheology Symposium on Soft Tissues Around A Diarthrodial Joint. Biorheology 1980; 17:83–94.

5. Akeson WH, Amiel D, Woo S L-Y. Immobility effects of synovial joints: the pathomechanics of joint contracture. Biorheology 1980; 17:95–110.

6. Tabary JC, Tardieu C, Tardieu G, Tabary C. Experimental rapid sarcomere loss with concomitant hypoextensibility. Muscle Nerve 1981; 4:198–203.

7. Tabary JC, Tabary C, Tardieu C, Tardieu G, Goldspink G. Psychological and structural changes in the cat's soleus muscle due to immobilization at different lengths by plaster casts. J Physiol 1972; 224:231–244.

8. Williams PE, Goldspink G. Changes in sarcomere length and physiological properties in immobilized muscle. J Anat 1978; 127:459–468.

9. Cooper RR. Alterations during immobilization and regeneration of skeletal muscle in cats. J Bone and Joint Surg 1972; 54-A(5):919–953.

10. Gelberman RH, Vande Berg JS, Lundborg GN, Akerson WH. Flexor tendon healing and restoration of the gliding surface. J Bone and Joint Surg 1983; 65-A(1):70–80.

11. Gelberman RH, Menon J, Gonsalves M, Akeson WH. The effects of mobilization on the vascularization of healing flexor tendons in dogs. Clin Orthop 1980; 153:283–289.

12. Faulkner JA. Structural and functional adaptations of skeletal muscle. In: Rousses C, Macklem PT, eds. The thorax. New York: Marcel Dekker, 1985; 1329–1351.

13. Gelberman RH, Woo S L-Y, Lothringer K, Akeson WH, Amiel D. Effects of early intermittent passive mobilization on healing canine flexor tendons. J Hand Surg 1982; 7:170–175.

14. Tipton CM, James SL, Mergner W, et al. Influence of exercise on strength of medial collateral knee ligaments of dogs. Am J Physiol 1970; 218:894–902.

15. Vailas AC, Tipton CM, Matthes RD, Gart M. Physical activity and its influence on the repair process of medial collateral ligaments. Connect Tissue Res 1981; 9:25–31.

16. Woo S L-Y, Gomez MA, Amiel D, et al. The effects of exercise on the biomechanical and biochemical properties of swine digital flexor tendons. J Biomech Eng 1981; 103:51–61.

17. Salter RB, Field P. The effects of continuous compression on living articular cartilage. J Bone Joint Surg 1960; 42-A(1):31–49.

18. Trias A. Effect of persistent pressure on the articular cartilage. J Bone Joint Surg 1961; 43-B(2):376–386.

19. Thaxter TH, Mann RA, Anderson CE. Degeneration of immobilized knee joints in rats. J Bone Joint Surg 1965; 47-A(3):567–585.

20. Enneking WF, Horowitz M. The intra-articular effects of immobilization on the human knee. J Bone Joint Surg 1972; 54-A:937–985.

21. DePalma AF, McKeever CD, Subin DK. Process of repair of articular cartilage demonstrated by histology and autoradiography with tritiated thymidine. Clin Orthop 1966; 48:229–242.

22. Palmoski MJ, Colyer RA, Brandt KD. Joint motion in the absence of normal loading does not maintain normal articular cartilage. Arthritis Rheum 1980; 23:325–334.

23. Salter RB, Simmonds DF, Malcolm BW, Rumble EJ, Macmichael D, Clements ND. The biological effect of continuous passive motion on the healing of full-thickness defects in articular cartilage. J Bone Joint Surg 1980; 62-A(8):1232–1251.

24. Michelsson JE, Riska EB. The effect of temporary exercising of a joint during an immobilization period. Clin Orthop 1979; 144:321–325.

25. Evans EB, Eggers GW, Butler M, Blumel T. Experimental immobilization and remobilization of rat knee joints. J Bone Joint Surg 1960; 42-A:737–758.

26. White AA, Panjabi MM. Clinical biomechanics of the spine. Second Edition. J. B. Lippincott, Philadelphia, 1990.

27. Cibulka MT, Delitto A, Kolderhoff RM. Changes in innominate tilt after manipulation of the sacroiliac joint in patients with low back pain. Phys Ther 1988; 68:1359–1363.

28. Chrisman OD, Mittnacht A, Snook G. A study of the results following rotary manipulation in the lumbar intervertebral-disc syndrome. J Bone Joint Surg 1964; 46-A(3):517–524.

29. Mensor MC. Non-operative treatment, including manipulation, for lumbar intervertebral disc syndrome. J Bone Joint Surg 1955; 37-A(5):925–936.

30. Matthews JA, Yates DA. Reduction of lumbar disc prolapse by manipulation. Br Med J 1969; 20:696–697.

31. Cyriax J. Textbook of orthopaedic medicine, Vol. I, 6th ed. London: Bailliere Tindall, 1975.

32. Korenko PM, Boumphrey FR, Bell GR, Modic MT, McKenzie RL. Extension exercises in the treatment of acute disk prolapse: a prospective study. Presented at the annual International Society for the Study of the Lumbar Spine Conference, April, 1985.

33. Reuber M, Schultz A, Denis F, Spencer D. Bulging of lumbar intervertebral disks. J Biomech Eng 1982; 104:187.

34. Roaf R. A study of the mechanics of spinal injuries. J Bone Joint Surg 1960; 42-B(4):810–823.

35. Brown T, Hanson R, Yorra A. Some mechanical tests on the lumbo-sacral spine with particular reference to the intervertebral discs. J Bone Joint Surg 1957; 39-A:1135–1164.

36. Shah JS, Hampson WG, Jayson MI. The distribution of surface strain in the cadaveric lumbar spine. J Bone Joint Surg 1978; 60-B(2):246–251.

37. Krag MH, Seroussi RE, Wilder DG, Pope MG. Internal displacement distribution from in vitro loading of human thoracic and lumbar spinal motion

segments, experimental results and theoretical pre-dictions. Spine 1987; 12:1001–1007.

38. Markolf KL. Stiffness and dampening characteristics of the thoraco-lumbar spine. Proceedings of work-shop on bioengineering approaches to the problems of the spine. NIH, Sept., 1970.

39. Adams MA, Hutton WC. The relevance of torsion to the mechanical derangement of the lumbar spine. Spine 1981; 6:241–248.

40. Cyron BW, Hutton WC. Articular tropism and the stability of the lumbar spine. Spine 1980; 5:168–177.

41. Kirkaldy-Willis WH. Managing low back pain. New York: Churchill Livingstone, 1983; 25–29.

42. McFadden KD, Taylor JR. Axial rotation in the lumbar spine and gaping of the zygapophyseal joints. Spine 1990; 15:295–299.

43. Unsworth A, Dowson D, Wright V. Cracking joints. A bioengineering study of cavitation in the metacarpophalangeal joint. Ann Rheum Dis 1971; 30:348–358.

44. Kos J, Wolf J. Les menisques intervertebraux et leur role possible dans les blocages vertebraux. Ann Med Phys 1972; 15:203–218.

45. Lewit K. Manipulative therapy in rehabilitation of the motor system. London: Butterworths, 1985; 17–22.

46. Kraft GL, Levinthal DH. Facet synovial impinge-ment. A new concept in the etiology of lumbar ver-tebral derangement. Surg Gynecol Obstet 1951; 93:439–443.

47. Bogduk N, Engel R. The menisci of the lumbar zygapophyseal joints. A review of their anatomy and clinical significance. Spine 1984; 9(5):454–460.

48. Farfan HF. The scientific basis of manipulative pro-cedures. Clin Rheum Dis 1980; 6(1):159–177.

49. Wyke B. The neurology of joints. Ann Roy Coll Surg Engl 1967; 41:25.

50. Melzack R, Wall PD. Pain mechanisms: a new the-ory. Science 1965; 150:971–979.

51. Wyke B. Neurological aspects of low back pain. In: Jayson M ed. The lumbar spine and back pain. New York: Grune and Stratton, Inc. 1976; 189–256.

52. Glover JR. Back pain and hyperaesthesia. Lancet May 1960; 1165–1169.

53. Terrett AC, Vernon H. Manipulation and pain tol-erance. A controlled study on the effect of spinal manipulation on paraspinal cutaneous pain tolerance levels. Am J Phys Med 1984; 63:217–225.

54. Coyer AB, Curwen IH. Low back pain treated by manipulation. A controlled series. Br Med J March 1955; 705–707.

55. Evans DP, Burke MS, Lloyd KN, Roberts EE, Rob-erts GM. Lumbar spinal manipulation on trial. Part 1—Clinical Assessment. Rheum Rehabil 1978; 17:46–53.

56. Hoehler FK, Tobis JS, Buerger AA. Spinal manip-ulation for low back pain. JAMA 1981; 245:1835–1838.

57. Glover, Morris JG, Khosla T. Back Pain: A random-ized clinical trial of rotational manipulation of the trunk. Br J Ind Med 1974; 31:59–64.

58. Farrell JP, Twomey LT. Acute low back pain. Com-parison of two conservative treatment approaches. Med J Aust Feb. 1982; 1:160–164.

59. Doran DM, Newell DJ. Manipulation in treatment of low back pain: a multicentre study. Br Med J 1975; 2:161–164.

60. Zybergold RS, Piper MC. Lumbar disc disease: com-parative analysis of physical therapy treatments. Arch Phys Med Rehabil 1981; 62:172–199.

61. Jayson MI, Sims-Williams H, Young S, Baddeley H, Collins E. Mobilization and manipulation for low back pain. Spine 1981; 6:409–416.

62. Korr IM. Proprioceptors and the behavior of lesioned segments. In: Osteopathic medicine-clinical review series, Stark EI, ed. Acton, MA: Publishing Sciences Group, 1975; 183–200.

63. Paris SV. Mobilization of the spine. Phys Ther 1979; 59:988–995.

64. Fisk JW. A controlled trial of manipulation in a selected group of patients with low back pain favour-ing one side. New Zealand Med J Oct. 1979; 288–291.

65. Nwuga VC. Relative therapeutic efficacy of vertebral manipulation and conventional treatment in back pain management. Am J Phys Med 1982; 61:273–278.

66. Wyke. Conference on the aging brain, cervical ar-ticular contributions to posture and gait: their rela-tion to senile disequilibrium. Age Aging 1979; 8:251.

67. Sunderland S. Meningeal-neural relations in the in-tervertebral foramen. J Neursurg 1974; 40:756–762.

68. Reid JD. Effects of flexion-extension movements of the head and spine upon the spinal cord and nerve roots. J Neurol Neurosurg Psychiatry 1960; 23:214–220.

69. Brieg A. Biomechanics of the central nervous system. Some basic normal and pathological phenomena. Stockholm: Almquist and Wiksell, 1960.

70. Farfan H. Mechanical disorders of the low back. Philadelphia: Lea and Febiger, 1975.

71. Schnebel BE, Watkins RG, Dillin W. The role of spinal flexion and extension in changing nerve root compression in disc herniations. Spine 1989; 14:835–837.

72. Magoun HI. Osteopathy in the cranial field. Kirks-ville: The Journal Printing Co., 1976.

73. Mays KS, et al. Relief of postlaminectomy syndrome in selected patients by injection of the autogenous cerebrospinal fluid. Spine 1981; 6:274–278.

74. Upledger JE, Vredevoogd JD. Craniosacral therapy. Chicago: Eastland Press, 1983.

75. Bowsher D. Cerebrospinal fluid dynamics in health and disease. Springfield: C.C. Thomas, 1960.

76. Cottingham JT, Porges SW, Lyon T. Effects of soft

tissue mobilization (Rolfing Pelvic Lift) on parasympathetic tone in two age groups. Phys Ther 1988; 68:352–356.

77. Tobis JS, Hoehler FK. Musculoskeletal manipulation in the treatment of low back pain. Bull N Y Acad Med 1983; 59:660–668.

78. Hadler NM, Curtis P, Gillings DB, Stinnett S. A benefit of spinal manipulation as adjunctive therapy for acute low-back pain: a stratified controlled trial. Spine 1987; 12:703–706.

79. MacDonald RS, Bell CM. An open controlled assessment of osteopathic manipulation in nonspecific low-back pain. Spine 1990; 15:364–370.

80. Riches EW. End results of manipulation of the back. Lancet May, 1930; 957–960.

81. Sims-Williams H, Jayson MI, Young SM, Baddeley H, Collins E. Controlled trial of mobilization and manipulation for low back pain: hospital patients. Br Med J 1979; 2:1418–1320.

82. Haldeman S. Spinal manipulative therapy. A status report. Clin Orthop 1983; 179:62–70.

83. Deyo RA, Walsh NE, Martin DC, Schoenfeld LS, Ramamurthy S. A controlled trial of transcutaneous electrical nerve stimulation (TENS) and exercise for chronic low back pain. N Engl J Med 1990; 322:1627–1634.

84. Sikorski JM. A rationalized approach to physiotherapy for low back pain. Spine 1985; 10:571–579.

85. Kellett KM, Kellett DA, Nordholm LA. Effects of an exercise program on sick leave due to back pain. Phys Ther 1991; 71:283–293.

86. Saal JA, Saal JS. Nonoperative treatment of herniated lumbar intervertebral disc with radiculopathy. An outcome study. Spine 1989; 14:431–437.

Index